Surgical Critical Care and Emergency Surgery

Surgical Critical Care and Emergency Surgery

Clinical Questions and Answers

EDITED BY

Forrest O. Moore, MD, FACS
Assistant Professor of Clinical Surgery
Department of Surgery
Division of Trauma & Surgical Critical Care
LSU Health Sciences Center, Shreveport, LA

Peter M. Rhee, MD, MPH, FACS, FCCM, DMCC
Professor of Surgery and Molecular Cell Biology
Vice Chair of Surgery
Director of Trauma, Critical Care and Emergency Surgery
University of Arizona Health Sciences Center, Tucson, AZ

Samuel A. Tisherman, MD, FACS, FCCM, FCCP
Professor, Departments of Critical Care Medicine and Surgery
University of Pittsburgh Medical Center, Pittsburgh, PA

Gerard J. Fulda, MD, FACS, FCCM, FCCP
Associate Professor, Department of Surgery
Jefferson Medical College Philadelphia, PA
Director, Surgical Critical Care and Surgical Research
Christiana Care Health Systems, Newark, DE

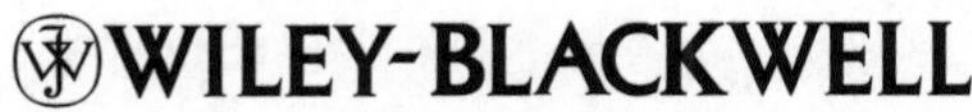

A John Wiley & Sons, Ltd., Publication

This edition first published 2012 © 2012 by John Wiley and Sons, Ltd.

Registered office: John Wiley & Sons, Ltd, The Atrium, Southern Gate, Chichester, West Sussex, PO19 8SQ, UK

Editorial offices: 9600 Garsington Road, Oxford, OX4 2DQ, UK
The Atrium, Southern Gate, Chichester, West Sussex, PO19 8SQ, UK
111 River Street, Hoboken, NJ 07030-5774, USA

For details of our global editorial offices, for customer services and for information about how to apply for permission to reuse the copyright material in this book please see our website at www.wiley.com/wiley-blackwell

Library of Congress Cataloging-in-Publication Data

Surgical critical care and emergency surgery : clinical questions and answers / edited by Forrest O. Moore ... [et al.].

p. ; cm.
Includes bibliographical references and index.
ISBN 978-0-470-65461-3 (pbk.)
I. Moore, Forrest O.
[DNLM: 1. Critical Care–methods. 2. Surgical Procedures, Operative–methods. 3. Critical Illness–therapy. 4. Emergencies. 5. Emergency Treatment–methods. 6. Wounds and Injuries–surgery. WO 700]

617′026–dc23

2011044211

A catalogue record for this book is available from the British Library.

Wiley also publishes its books in a variety of electronic formats. Some content that appears in print may not be available in electronic books.

Set in 9/11.5pt Times by Aptara Inc., New Delhi, India
Printed and bound in Malaysia by Vivar Printing Sdn Bhd

1 2012

Contents

Contributors

Editors

Forrest O. Moore, MD, FACS
Assistant Professor of Clinical Surgery
Department of Surgery
Division of Trauma & Surgical Critical Care
LSU Health Sciences Center
Shreveport, LA

Peter M. Rhee, MD, MPH, FACS, FCCM, DMCC
Professor of Surgery and Molecular Cell Biology
Vice Chair of Surgery
Director of Trauma, Critical Care and Emergency Surgery
University of Arizona Health Sciences Center
Tucson, AZ

Samuel A. Tisherman, MD, FACS, FCCM, FCCP
Professor
Departments of Critical Care Medicine and Surgery
University of Pittsburgh Medical Center
Pittsburgh, PA

Gerard J. Fulda, MD, FACS, FCCM, FCCP
Associate Professor, Department of Surgery
Jefferson Medical College
Philadelphia, PA
Director, Surgical Critical Care and Surgical Research
Christiana Care Health Systems
Newark, DE

Contributors

Jared L. Antevil, MD
Cardiothoracic Surgeon
Naval Medical Center Portsmouth
Portsmouth, VA

Vishal Bansal, MD
Assistant Professor of Surgery
University of California San Diego School of Medicine
Department of Surgery
UCSD Medical Center
San Diego, CA

Stephen L. Barnes, MD, FACS
Associate Professor and Chief, Division of Acute Care Surgery
Program Director, Surgical Critical Care Fellowship
Frank L Mitchell Jr MD Trauma Center
University of Missouri Department of Surgery
Columbia, MO

Stacy A. Brethauer, MD
Assistant Professor of Surgery
Cleveland Clinic Lerner College of Medicine
Staff Surgeon, Bariatric and Metabolic Institute
Cleveland Clinic
Cleveland, OH

Carlos V.R. Brown, MD, FACS
Associate Professor of Surgery
University of Texas Southwestern – Austin
Trauma Medical Director
University Medical Center Brackenridge
Austin, Texas

Mark Cipolle, MD, PhD, FACS, FCCM
Medical Director, Trauma Program
Christiana Health Care System
Newark, DE

Jeffrey P. Coughenour, MD
Medical Director, Trauma and Surgical ICU
Assistant Professor of Surgery
Division of Acute Care Surgery
University of Missouri School of Medicine
Columbia, MO

Brett D. Crist, MD, FACS
Assistant Professor of Orthopedic Surgery
Co-director, Orthopedic Trauma Service
Co-director, Orthopedic Trauma Fellowship
Department of Orthopedic Surgery
University of Missouri
Columbia, MO

Gregory J. Della Rocca, MD, PhD, FACS
Assistant Professor of Orthopedic Surgery
Co-director, Orthopedic Trauma Service
Department of Orthopedic Surgery
University of Missouri
Columbia, MO

Heather Dolman, MD, FACS
Assistant Professor of Surgery
Wayne State University
Detroit Receiving Hospital
Detroit, MI

Jay J. Doucet, MD, MSc, FRCSC, FACS
Associate Professor of Clinical Surgery
University of California San Diego School of Medicine
Department of Surgery
UCSD Medical Center
San Diego, CA

Therese M. Duane, MD, FACS
Associate Professor of Surgery
Division of Trauma, Critical Care, Emergency General Surgery
Director of Infection Control STICU
Chair Infection Control
VCU Health System
Richmond, VA

Lt Col Joseph J. DuBose, MD, FACS, USAF MC
Assistant Professor of Surgery
University of Maryland Medical System
R Adams Cowley Shock Trauma Center
Director of Physician Education
Air Force/C-STARS
Baltimore, MD

Juan C. Duchesne, MD, FACS, FCCP
Associate Professor of Surgery
Director, Tulane Surgical Intensive Care Unit
Division of Trauma and Critical Care Surgery
Tulane and LSU Departments of Surgery and Anesthesiology
New Orleans, LA

Marquinn D. Duke, MD
Chief Resident, General Surgery
Tulane Department of Surgery
New Orleans, LA

Meghan Edwards, MD
Surgical Critical Care Fellow
Cedars-Sinai Medical Center
Los Angeles, CA

Hoylan Fernandez, MD, MPH
Chief Resident, General Surgery
St. Joseph's Hospital and Medical Center
Phoenix, AZ

Raquel M. Forsythe, MD, FACS
Assistant Professor of Surgery and Critical Care Medicine
Director of Education, Trauma Services
University of Pittsburgh Medical Center
Pittsburgh, PA

Adam D. Fox, DPM, DO
Assistant Professor of Surgery
Division of Trauma Surgery and Critical Care
Department of Surgery
UMDNJ
Newark, NJ

Randall S. Friese MD, MSc, FACS, FCCM
Associate Professor of Surgery
Division of Trauma, Critical Care and Emergency Surgery
Department of Surgery
University of Arizona Health Science Center
Tucson, AZ

Frederick Giberson, MD, FACS
Clinical Assistant Professor of Surgery
Jefferson Medical College
Program Director, General Surgery Residency Program
Christiana Care Health System
Newark, DE

Timothy Harrison, MS, DO
Trauma, Surgical Critical Care and General Surgery
Crozer Chester Medical Center
Upland, PA
Formerly Trauma and Surgical Critical Care Fellow
Department of Surgery
Christiana Care Healthcare System
Newark, DE

Daniel N. Holena, MD
Assistant Professor
Division of Traumatology, Surgical Critical Care and Emergency Surgery
Department of Surgery
Hospital of the University of Pennsylvania
Philadelphia, PA

Charles Kung Chao Hu, MD, MBA, FACS, FCCP
Associate Medical Director, Trauma Services
Director, Surgical Critical Care
Scottsdale Healthcare Osborn Medical Center
Scottsdale, AZ

Kenji Inaba, MD, FRCSC, FACS
Assistant Professor of Surgery
Medical Director, Surgical ICU
Division of Trauma and Critical Care
University of Southern California
LAC+USC Medical Center
Los Angeles, CA

Marcin A. Jankowski, DO
Assistant Director of Trauma and Surgical Critical Care
General Surgery
Crozer Chester Medical Center
Uplan, PA
Formerly Trauma and Surgical Critical Care Fellow
Department of Surgery
Christiana Care Health System
Newark, DE

Bellal Joseph, MD
Assistant Professor
Division of Trauma, Critical Care and Emergency Surgery
Department of Surgery
University of Arizona Health Science Center
Tucson, AZ

Lewis J. Kaplan, MD, FACS, FCCM, FCCP
Associate Professor of Surgery
Section of Trauma, Surgical Critical Care and Surgical Emergencies
Yale University School of Medicine
New Haven, CT

Leslie Kobayashi, MD
Assistant Professor of Surgery
Division of Trauma, Critical Care and Burns
UCSD Medical Center
San Diego, CA

Narong Kulvatunyou, MD, FACS
Assistant Professor
Division of Trauma, Critical Care and Emergency Surgery
Department of Surgery
University of Arizona Health Science Center
Tucson, AZ

Rifat Latifi, MD, FACS
Professor of Surgery
Division of Trauma, Critical Care and Emergency Surgery
University of Arizona Health Science Center
Tucson, AZ
Director, Trauma Services, Hamad Medical Corporation
Doha, Qatar

Felix Lui, MD, FACS
Assistant Professor of Surgery
Section of Trauma, Surgical Critical Care and Surgical Emergencies
Yale University School of Medicine
New Haven, CT

Michael C. Madigan, MD
Chief Resident, Department of Surgery
University of Pittsburgh Medical Center
Pittsburgh, PA

Gary T. Marshall, MD, FACS
Assistant Professor of Surgery and Critical Care Medicine
University of Pittsburgh Medical Center
Pittsburgh, PA

Adrian A Maung, MD, FACS
Assistant Professor of Surgery
Section of Trauma, Surgical Critical Care and Surgical Emergencies
Yale University School of Medicine
New Haven, CT 06520

Patrick McGann, MD
Trauma and Surgical Critical Care
Grant Medical Center
Columbus, OH

Christopher S. Nelson, MD
Surgical Critical Care Fellow
Department of Surgery
Division of Acute Care Surgery
University of Missouri Health Care
Columbia, MO

Scott H. Norwood, MD, FACS
Clinical Professor of Surgery
University of South Florida School of Medicine
Tampa, Florida
Director of Trauma Services
Regional Medical Center Bayonet Point
Hudson, Florida

Andre Nguyen, MD
Assistant Professor
Division of Trauma and Surgical Critical Care
Department of Surgery
Loma Linda University School of Medicine
Loma Linda, CA

Terence O'Keeffe, MB ChB, MSPH, FACS
Associate Medical Director, Surgical ICU
Associate Program Director, Critical Care Fellowship
Assistant Professor of Surgery
Division of Trauma, Critical Care and Emergency Surgery
Department of Surgery
University of Arizona Health Science Center
Tucson, AZ

Scott R. Petersen, MD, FACS
Trauma Medical Director
General Surgery Residency Program Director
St. Joseph's Hospital and Medical Center
Phoenix, AZ

Herb A. Phelan, MD, FACS
Associate Professor
University of Texas Southwestern Medical Center
Department of Surgery
Division of Burns/Trauma/Critical Care
Dallas, TX

Harrison T. Pitcher, MD
Assistant Professor of Surgery
Division of Acute Care Surgery
Jefferson Medical College
Philadelphia, PA
Formerly Trauma and Surgical Critical Care Fellow
Christiana Care Healthcare System
Newark, DE

Ali Salim, MD, FACS
Associate Professor of Surgery
Program Director, General Surgery Residency
Cedars-Sinai Medical Center
Los Angeles, CA

Anthony Sciscione, MD
Director of Maternal Fetal Medicine and Ob/Gyn residency program
Department of Obstetrics and Gynecology
Christiana Care Health System
Professor, Department of Obstetrics and Gynecology
Drexel University School of Medicine
Philadelphia, PA

Stacy Shackelford, MD, FACS
Colonel, USAF
Trauma and Surgical Critical Care Fellow
University of Southern California
LAC+USC Medical Center
Los Angeles, CA

Michelle Strong, MD, PhD
Trauma/Critical Care Surgeon
Trauma Trust
Tacoma Trauma Center
Tacoma, WA

Andrew Tang, MD
Assistant Professor
Division of Trauma, Critical Care and Emergency Surgery
Department of Surgery
University of Arizona Health Science Center
Tucson, AZ

Nicholas Thiessen, MD
Chief Resident, General Surgery
St. Joseph's Hospital and Medical Center
Phoenix, AZ

Julie L. Wynne, MD, MPH, FACS
Assistant Professor of Surgery
Division of Trauma, Critical Care and Emergency Surgery
Department of Surgery
University of Arizona Health Science Center
Tucson, AZ

Andrew Young, MD
Resident, General Surgery
VCU Department of Surgery
Richmond, VA

Preface

This project was born out of the needs of those taking the surgical critical care examination administered by the American Board of Surgery. We realized that, although there are many good critical care review texts, none was focused exclusively on the unique problems posed by and care required for the surgical patient. In the popular question-and-answer format, this review book serves as an excellent resource when caring for the surgical patient with an acute process, whether the patient requires critical care or surgical intervention. In addition, the evolving specialties of acute-care surgery and emergency general surgery, and the role of caring for patients with other surgical emergencies/trauma, are inseparable from surgical critical care. The same surgical specialists care for acute care/emergency surgery patients. Thus, it makes sense to incorporate these fields into one review book.

Medical students, residents, fellows, and practicing surgeons, will find this text useful, as will nonsurgical specialties who care for the critically ill and injured surgical patient. While it is primarily a method of study for those planning to take the critical care boards, many prefer the question-and-answer format as a method of learning. This text is divided into two main sections: surgical critical care and emergency surgery. Each question is accompanied by a vignette and associated references used to support the answer. Some of the references cited were recent and some of the questions reflective of changing practice, but the main goal overall was to provide current standard of care answers to each question. We gathered experts in the field of surgical critical care and emergency general surgery who worked diligently to put this book together and we are indebted to them for their time and effort. The senior editor and mentors were paired with those who recently had taken the exam to ensure that the format and focus were relevant.

In summary, this review book has all the necessary elements to aid in reviewing for the exam and to learn how to care for the critically ill patient with a surgical problem.

Forrest O. Moore, MD, FACS
Peter M. Rhee, MD, FACS
Samuel A. Tisherman, MD, FACS
Gerard J. Fulda, MD, FACS

PART ONE
Surgical Critical Care

Chapter 1 Respiratory and Cardiovascular Physiology

Marcin A. Jankowski, DO and Frederick Giberson, MD, FACS

1. *All of the following are mechanisms by which vasodilators improve cardiac function in acute congestive heart failure except:*

A. Increase stroke volume

B. Decrease ventricular filling pressure

C. Increase ventricular preload

D. Decrease end-diastolic volume

E. Decrease afterload

Most patients with acute heart failure present with increased left-ventricular filling pressure, high systemic vascular resistance, high or normal blood pressure and low cardiac output. These physiologic changes increase myocardial oxygen demand and decrease the pressure gradient for myocardial perfusion resulting in ischemia. Therapy with vasodilators in the acute setting can often improve hemodynamics and symptoms.

Nitroglycerine is a powerful venodilator with mild vasodilitory effects. It relieves pulmonary congestion through direct venodilation, reducing left and right ventricular filling pressures, systemic vascular resistance, wall stress, and myocardial oxygen consumption. Cardiac output usually increases due to decreased LV wall stress, decreased afterload, and improvement in myocardial ischemia. The development of tolerance within 16 to 24 hours of starting the infusion is a potential drawback of nitroglycerine.

Nitroprusside is an equal arteriolar and venous tone reducer, lowering both systemic and vascular resistance and left and right filling pressures. Its effects on reducing afterload increase stroke volume in heart failure. Potential complications of nitroprusside include cyanide toxicity and the risk of "coronary steal syndrome."

In patients with acute heart failure, therapeutic reduction of left-ventricular filling pressure with any of the above agents correlates with improved outcome.

Increased ventricular preload would increase the filling pressure, causing further increases in wall stress and myocardial oxygen consumption, leading to ischemia.

Answer: C

Hollenberg, MS (2007) Vasodilators in acute heart failure. *Heart Failure Review* **12**, 143–7.

Marino P (2007) *The ICU Book*, 3rd edn, Lippincott Williams & Wilkins, Philadelphia, PA, Chapter 14.

Nohria A, Lewis E, Stevenson, LW (2002) Medical management of advanced heart failure. *Journal of the American Medical Association* **287** (5), 628–40.

2. *Which is the most important factor in determining the rate of peripheral blood flow?*

A. Laminar flow

B. Length

C. Viscosity

D. Radius

E. Pressure gradient

The forces that determine peripheral blood flow are derived from observations on ideal hydraulic circuits that are rigid and the flow is steady and laminar. This is quite different from the human circulatory system which is compressible and flow is pulsatile and turbulent. The Hagen-Poiseuille equation states that flow is determined by the

Surgical Critical Care and Emergency Surgery: Clinical Questions and Answers, First Edition. Edited by Forrest O. Moore, Peter M. Rhee, Samuel A. Tisherman and Gerard J. Fulda.

fourth power of the inner radius of the tube ($Q = \Delta p \pi r^4/8\mu L$), where P is pressure, μ is viscosity, L is length, and r is radius. This means that a twofold increase in the radius will result in a sixteenfold increase in flow. As the equation states, the remaining components of resistance, such as pressure difference along the length of the tube and fluid viscosity, are inversely related and exert a much smaller influence on flow. Although this equation may not accurately describe the flow state in our circulatory system, it has useful applications in describing flow through catheters, flow characteristics of different resuscitative fluids and the hemodynamic effects of anemia and blood transfusions on flow. With turbulent flow (Fanning equation), the impact of the radius is raised to the fifth power (r^5) as opposed to the fourth power in the Poiseuille equation.

It is important to realize that flow through compressible tubes (blood vessels) is greatly influenced by external pressure surrounding the tubes. Therefore, if a tube is compressed by an external force, the flow will be independent of the pressure gradient along the tube.

Answer: D

Brown SP, Miller WC, Eason JM (2006) *Exercise Physiology; Basis of Human Movement in Health and Disease,* Lippincott Williams & Wilkins, Philadelphia.

Marino P (2007) *The ICU Book,* 3rd edn, Lippincott Williams & Wilkins, Philadelphia, PA, Chapter 1.

3. *Choose the correct physiologic process represented by each of the cardiac pressure-volume loops below.*

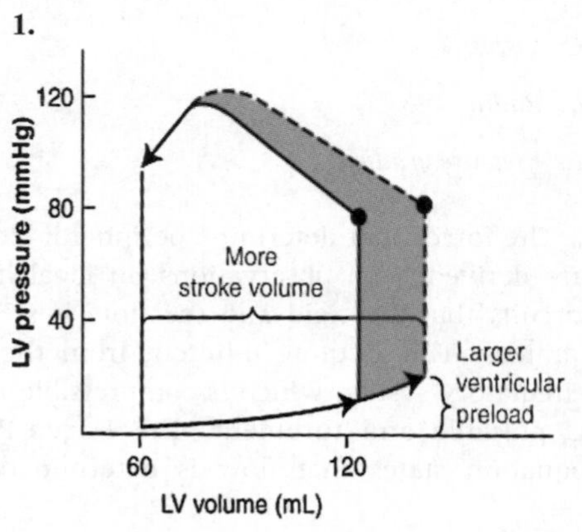

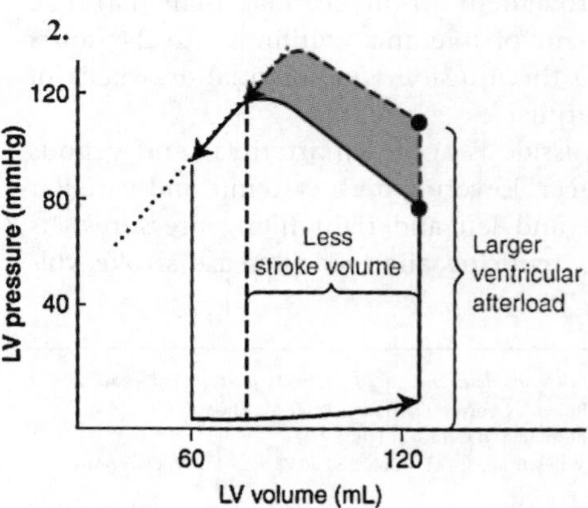

*A. (1) Increased preload, increased stroke volume,
(2) Increased afterload, decreased stroke volume*

*B. (1) Decreased preload, increased stroke volume,
(2) Decreased afterload, increased stroke volume*

*C. (1) Increased preload, decreased stroke volume,
(2) Decreased afterload, increased stroke volume*

*D. (1) Decreased preload, decreased stroke volume,
(2) Increased afterload, decreased stroke volume*

*E. (1) Decreased preload, increased stroke volume,
(2) Increased afterload, decreased stroke volume*

One of the most important factors in determining stroke volume is the extent of cardiac filling during diastole or the end-diastolic volume. This concept is known as the Frank–Starling law of the heart. This law states that, with all other factors equal, the stroke volume will increase as the end-diastolic volume increases. In Figure 1, the ventricular preload or end-diastolic volume (LV volume) is increased, which ultimately increases stroke volume defined by the area under the curve. Notice the LV pressure is not affected. Increased afterload, at constant preload, will have a negative impact on stroke volume. In Figure 2, the ventricular afterload (LV pressure) is increased, which results in a decreased stroke volume, again defined by the area under the curve.

Answer: A

Mohrman D, Heller L (2010) *Cardiovascular Physiology,* 7 edn, McGraw-Hill, New York, Chapter 3.

Shiels HA, White E (2008) The Frank–Starling mechanism in vertebrate cardiac myocytes. *Journal of Experimental Biology* **211** (13), 2005–13.

4. *An 18-year-old patient is admitted to the ICU following a prolonged exploratory laparotomy and lysis of adhesions for a small bowel obstruction. The patient has had minimal urine output throughout the case and is currently hypotensive. Identify the most effective way of promoting end-organ perfusion in this patient.*

A. *Increase arterial pressure (total peripheral resistance) with vasoactive agents*

B. *Decrease sympathetic drive with heavy sedation*

C. *Increase end-diastolic volume with controlled volume resuscitation*

D. *Increase contractility with a positive inotropic agent*

E. *Increase end-systolic volume*

This patient is presumed to be in hypovolemic shock as a result of a prolonged operative procedure with inadequate perioperative fluid resuscitation. The insensible losses of an open abdomen for several hours in addition to significant fluid shifts due to the small bowel obstruction can significantly lower intravascular volume. The low urine output is another clue that this patient would benefit from controlled volume resuscitation.

Starting a vasopressor such as norepinephrine would increase the blood pressure but the effects of increased afterload on the heart and the peripheral vasoconstriction leading to ischemia would be detrimental in this patient. Lowering the sympathetic drive with increased sedation will lead to severe hypotension and worsening shock. Increasing contractility with an inotrope in a hypovolemic patient would add great stress to the heart and still provide inadequate perfusion as a result of low preload. An increase in end-systolic volume would indicate a decreased stroke volume and lower cardiac output and would not promote end-organ perfusion.

$$CO = HR \times SV$$
$$SV = EDV - ESV$$

According to the principle of continuity, the stroke output of the heart is the main determinant of circulatory blood flow. The forces that directly affect the flow are preload, afterload and contractility. According to the Frank–Starling principle, in the normal heart diastolic volume is the principal force that governs the strength of ventricular contraction. This promotes adequate cardiac output and good end-organ perfusion.

Answer: C

Marino P (2007) *The ICU Book,* 3rd edn, Lippincott Williams & Wilkins, Philadelphia, PA, Chapter 12.

Mohrman D, Heller L (2010) *Cardiovascular Physiology,* 7 edn, McGraw-Hill, New York.

5. *Which physiologic process is least likely to increase myocardial oxygen consumption?*

A. *Increasing inotropic support*

B. *A 100% increase in heart rate*

C. *Increasing afterload*

D. *100% increase in end-diastolic volume*

E. *Increasing blood pressure*

Myocardial oxygen consumption (MVO_2) is primarily determined by myocyte contraction. Therefore, factors that increase tension generated by the myocytes, the rate of tension development and the number of cycles per unit time will ultimately increase myocardial oxygen consumption. According to the Law of LaPlace, cardiac wall tension is proportional to the product of intraventricular pressure and the ventricular radius.

Since the MVO_2 is closely related to wall tension, any changes that generate greater intraventricular pressure from increased afterload or inotropic stimulation will result in increased oxygen consumption. Increasing inotropy will result in increased MVO_2 due to the increased rate of tension and the increased magnitude of the tension. Doubling the heart rate will approximately double the MVO_2 due to twice the number of tension cycles per minute. Increased afterload will increase MVO_2 due to increased wall tension. Increased preload or end-diastolic volume does not affect MVO_2 to the same extent. This is because preload is often expressed as ventricular end-diastolic volume and is not directly based on the radius. If we assume the ventricle is a sphere, then:

$$V = {}^4/_3\pi \cdot r^3$$

Therefore

$$r \propto \sqrt[3]{V}$$

Substituting this relationship into the Law of LaPlace

$$T \propto P \cdot \sqrt[3]{V}$$

This relationship illustrates that a 100% increase in ventricular volume will result in only a 26% increase in wall tension. In contrast, a 100% increase in ventricular pressure will result in a 100% increase in wall tension. For this reason, wall tension, and therefore MVO_2, is far less sensitive to changes in ventricular volume than pressure.

Answer: D

Klabunde RE (2005) *Cardiovascular Physiology Concepts*, Lippincott, Williams & Wilkins, Philadelphia, PA.

Rhoades R, Bell DR (2009) *Medical Physiology: Principles for Clinical Medicine*, 3rd edn, Lippincott, Williams & Wilkins, Philadelphia, PA.

6. *A 73-year-old obese man with a past medical history significant for diabetes, hypertension, and peripheral vascular disease undergoes an elective right hemicolectomy. While in the PACU, the patient becomes acutely hypotensive and lethargic requiring immediate intubation. What effects do you expect positive pressure ventilation to have on your patient's cardiac function?*

A. *Increased pleural pressure, increased transmural pressure, increased ventricular afterload*

B. *Decreased pleural pressure, increased transmural pressure, increased ventricular afterload*

C. *Decreased pleural pressure, decreased transmural pressure, decreased ventricular afterload*

D. *Increased pleural pressure, decreased transmural pressure, decreased ventricular afterload*

E. *Increased pleural pressure, increased transmural pressure, decreased ventricular afterload*

This patient has a significant medical history that puts him at high risk of an acute coronary event. Hypotension and decreased mental status clearly indicate the need for immediate intubation. The effects of positive pressure ventilation will have direct effects on this patient's cardiovascular function. Ventricular afterload is a transmural force so it is directly affected by the pleural pressure on the outer surface of the heart. Positive pleural pressures will enhance ventricular emptying by promoting the inward movement of the ventricular wall during systole. In addition, the increased pleural pressure will decrease transmural pressure and decrease ventricular afterload. In this case, the positive pressure ventilation provides cardiac support by "unloading" the left ventricle resulting in increased stroke volume, cardiac output and ultimately better end-organ perfusion.

Answer: D

Marino P (2007) *The ICU Book*, 3rd edn, Lippincott Williams & Wilkins, Philadelphia, PA, Chapter 1.

Solbert P, Wise, RA (2010) Mechanical interaction of respiration and circulation. *Comprehensive Physiology*, 647–56.

7. *Choose the incorrect statement regarding coronary blood flow:*

A. *The blood in the coronary sinus has the lowest oxygen saturation in the entire body*

B. *The relationship between myocardial oxygen demand and coronary blood flow is linear*

C. *The myocardium has no oxygen reserve and relies strictly on very high flow volumes*

D. *Myocardial tissue requires high perfusion pressures in order to maintain constant flow*

E. *Coronary reserve refers to the maximal capacity of the coronary circulation to dilate and increase blood flow to the myocardium*

Myocardial tissue does not always require high perfusion pressures in order to maintain constant flow. The myocardium has the capacity to maintain constant blood flow over a wide range of perfusion pressures. This process is termed autoregulation and it allows the myocardium to be perfused even under low perfusion pressures. All other statements are correct.

Answer: D

Darovic G (2002) Cardiovascular anatomy and physiology, in *Hemodynamic Monitoring, Invasive and Non-invasive Clinical Application*, 3rd edn, WB. Saunders & Co., Philadelphia, PA, Chapter 4, pp. 77–9.

Duncker DJ, Bache RJ (2008) Regulation of coronary blood flow during exercise. *Physiological Reviews* **88** (3), 1009–86.

8. *Following surgical debridement for lower extremity necrotizing fasciitis, a 47-year-old man is admitted to the ICU. A Swan-Ganz catheter was inserted for refractory hypotension. The initial values are CVP = 5 mm Hg, MAP = 50 mm Hg, PCWP = 8 mm Hg, PaO_2 = 60 mm Hg, CO = 4.5 L/min, SVR = 450 dynes·sec/cm^5, and O_2 saturation of 93%. The hemoglobin is 8 g/dL. The most effective intervention to maximize perfusion pressure and oxygen delivery would be which of the following?*

A. *Titrate the FiO_2 to a $SaO_2 > 98\%$*

B. *Transfuse with two units of packed red blood cells*

C. *Fluid bolus with 1 L normal saline*

D. *Titrate the FiO_2 to a $PaO_2 > 80$*

E. *Start a vasopressor*

To maximize the oxygen delivery (DO_2) and perfusion pressure to the vital organs, it is important to determine the factors that directly affect it. According to the formula below, oxygen delivery (DO_2) is dependent on cardiac output (Q), the hemoglobin level (Hb), and the O_2 saturation (SaO_2):

$$DO_2 = Q \times (1.34 \times Hb \times SaO_2 \times 10) + (0.003 \times PaO_2)$$

This patient is likely septic from his infectious process. In addition, the long operation likely included a significant blood loss and fluid shifts so hypovolemic/hemorrhagic shock is likely contributing to this patient's hypotension. The low CVP, low wedge pressure indicates a need for volume replacement. The fact that this patient is anemic as a result of significant blood loss means that transfusing this patient would likely benefit his oxygen-carrying capacity as well as provide volume replacement. Fluid bolus is not inappropriate; however, two units of packed red blood cells would be more appropriate. Titrating the PaO_2 would not add any benefit because, according to the above equation, it contributes very little to the overall oxygen delivery. Starting a vasopressor in a hypovolemic patient is inappropriate at this time and should be reserved for continued hypotension after adequate fluid resuscitation. Titrating the FiO_2 to a saturation of greater than 98% would not be clinically relevant. Although the patient requires better oxygen-carrying capacity, this would be better solved with red blood cell replacement.

Answer: B

Cavazzoni SZ, Dellinger PR (2006) Hemodynamic optimization of sepsis-induced tissue hypoperfusion. *Critical Care* **10** Suppl, 3, S2.

Marino P (2007) *The ICU Book*, 3rd edn, Lippincott Williams & Wilkins, Philadelphia, PA, Chapter 2.

9. *To promote adequate alveolar ventilation, decrease shunting, and ultimately improve oxygenation, the addition of positive end-expiratory pressure (PEEP) in a severely hypoxic patient with ARDS will:*

A. *Limit the increase in residual volume (RV)*

B. *Limit the decrease in expiratory reserve volume (ERV)*

C. *Limit the increase in inspiratory reserve volume (IRV)*

D. *Limit the decrease in tidal volume (TV)*

E. *Increase pCO_2*

Patients with ARDS have a significantly decreased lung compliance, which leads to significant alveolar collapse. This results in decreased surface area for adequate gas exchange and an increased alveolar shunt fraction resulting in hypoventilation and refractory hypoxemia. The minimum volume and pressure of gas necessary to prevent small airway collapse is the critical closing volume (CCV). When CCV exceeds functional residual capacity (FRC), alveolar collapse occurs. The two components of FRC are residual volume (RV) and expiratory reserve volume (ERV).

The role of extrinsic positive end-expiratory pressure (PEEP) in ARDS is to prevent alveolar collapse, promote further alveolar recruitment, and improve oxygenation by limiting the decrease in FRC and maintaining it above the critical closing volume. Therefore, limiting the decrease in ERV will limit the decrease in FRC and keep it above the CCV thus preventing alveolar collapse.

Limiting an increase in the residual volume would keep the FRC below the CCV and promote alveolar collapse. Positive-end expiratory pressure has no effect on inspiratory reserve volume (IRV) or tidal volume (TV) and does not increase pCO_2.

Answer: B

Rimensberger PC, Bryan AC (1999) Measurement of functional residual capacity in the critically ill. Relevance for the assessment of respiratory mechanics during mechanical ventilation. *Intensive Care Medicine* **25** (5), 540–2.

Sidebotham D, McKee A, Gillham M, Levy J (2007) *Cardiothoracic Critical Care*, Butterworth-Heinemann, Philadelphia, PA.

10. *The right atrial tracing below is consistent with:*

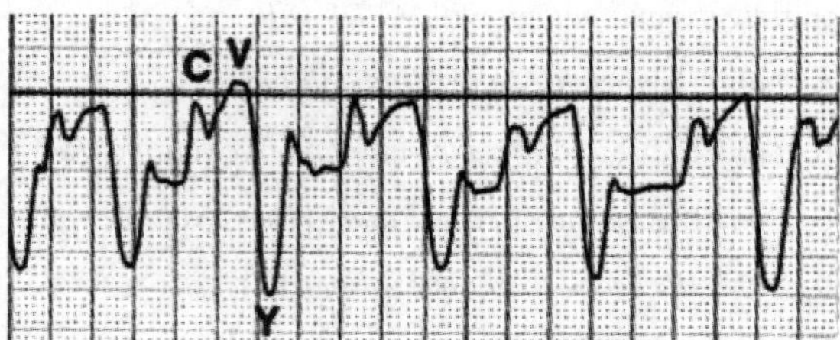

A. *Tricuspid stenosis*

B. *Normal right atrial waveform tracing*

C. *Tricuspid regurgitation*

D. *Constrictive pericarditis*

E. *Mitral stenosis*

The normal jugular venous pulse contains three positive waves. These positive deflections, labeled "a," "c", and "v" occur, respectively, before the carotid upstroke and just after the P wave of the ECG (a wave); simultaneous with the upstroke of the carotid pulse (c wave); and during ventricular systole until the tricuspid valve opens (v wave). The "a" wave is generated by atrial contraction, which actively fills the right ventricle in end-diastole. The "c" wave is caused either by transmission of the carotid arterial impulse through the external and internal jugular veins or by the bulging of the tricuspid valve into the right atrium in early systole. The "v" wave reflects the passive increase in pressure and volume of the right atrium as it fills in late systole and early diastole.

Normally the crests of the "a" and "v" waves are approximately equal in amplitude. The descents or troughs of the jugular venous pulse occur between the "a" and "c" wave ("x" descent), between the "c" and "v" wave ("x′" descent), and between the "v" and "a" wave ("y" descent). The x and x′ descents reflect movement of the lower portion of the right atrium toward the right ventricle during the final phases of ventricular systole. The *y* descent represents the abrupt termination of the downstroke of the v wave during early diastole after the tricuspid valve opens and the right ventricle begins to fill passively. Normally the *y* descent is neither as brisk nor as deep as the *x* descent.

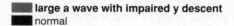

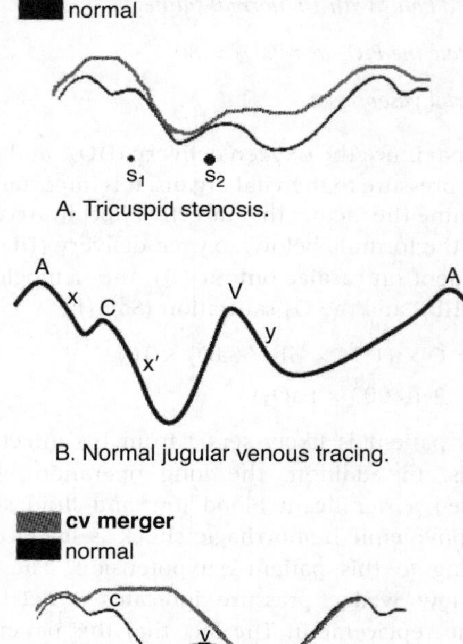

A. Tricuspid stenosis.

B. Normal jugular venous tracing.

C. Tricuspid regurgitation.

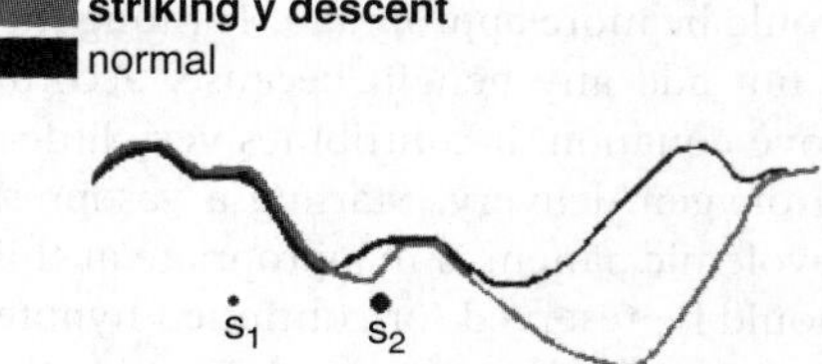

D. Constrictive pericarditis

Answer: C

Hall JB, Schmidt GA, Wood LDH (eds) *Principles of Critical Care*, 3rd edn, McGraw-Hill, New York.

McGee S (2007) *Evidence-based Physical Diagnosis*, 2nd edn, W. B. Saunders & Co., Philadelphia, PA.

Pinsky LE, Wipf JE (n.d.) University of Washington Department of Medicine. *Advanced Physical Diagnosis. Learning and Teaching at the Bedside.* Edition 1, http://depts.washington.edu/physdx/neck/index.html (accessed November 6, 2011).

11. *The addition of PEEP in optimizing ventilatory support in patients with ARDS does all of the following except:*

A. *Increase functional residual capacity (FRC) above the alveolar closing pressure*

B. *Maximize inspiratory alveolar recruitment*

C. *Limit ventilation below the lower inflection point to minimize shear-force injury*

D. *Improve V/Q mismatch*

E. *Increases the mean airway pressure*

The addition of positive-end expiratory pressure (PEEP) in patients who have ARDS has been shown to be beneficial. By maintaining a small positive pressure at the end of expiration, considerable improvement in the arterial PaO_2 can be obtained. The addition of PEEP maintains the functional residual capacity (FRC) above the critical closing volume (CCV) of the alveoli, thus preventing alveolar collapse. It also limits ventilation below the lower inflection point minimizing shear force injury to the alveoli. The prevention of alveolar collapse results in improved V/Q mismatch, decreased shunting, and improved gas exchange. The addition of PEEP in ARDS also allows for lower FiO_2 to be used in maintaining adequate oxygenation.

PEEP maximizes the expiratory alveolar recruitment; it has no effect on the inspiratory portion of ventilatory support.

Answer: B

Gattinoni L, Cairon M, Cressoni M, *et al.* (2006) Lung recruitement in patients with acute respiratory distress syndrome. *New England Journal of Medicine* **354**, 1775–86.

West B (2008) *Pulmonary Pathophysiology—The Essentials*, 8th edn, Lippincott, Williams & Wilkins, Philadelphia, PA.

12. *A 70-year-old man with a history of diabetes, hypertension, coronary artery disease, asthma and long-standing cigarette smoking undergoes an emergency laparotomy and Graham patch for a perforated duodenal ulcer. Following the procedure he develops acute respiratory distress and oxygen saturation of 88%. Blood gas analysis reveals the following:*

pH = 7.43
paO_2 = 55 mm Hg
HCO_3 = 23 mmol/L
pCO_2 = 35 mm Hg

Based on the above results, you would calculate his A-a gradient to be (assuming atmospheric pressure at sea level, water vapor pressure = 47 mm Hg):

A. *8 mm Hg*

B. *15 mm Hg*

C. *30 mm Hg*

D. *52 mm Hg*

E. *61 mm Hg*

The A-a gradient is equal to PAO_2 – PaO_2 (55 from ABG). The PAO_2 can be calculated using the following equation:

$$PaO_2 = FiO_2(P_B - P_{H2O}) - (PaCO_2/RQ)$$
$$= 0.21\,(760 - 47) - (35/0.8)$$
$$PaO_2 = 106 \text{ mm Hg}$$

Therefore, A-a gradient (PaO_2 – PAO_2) = 51 mm Hg.

Answer: D

Marino P (2007) *The ICU Book*, 3rd edn, Lippincott Williams & Wilkins, Philadelphia, PA, Chapter 19.

13. *What is the most likely etiology of his respiratory failure and the appropriate intervention?*

A. *Pulmonary edema, cardiac workup*

B. *Neuromuscular weakness, intubation and reversal of anesthetic*

C. *Pulmonary embolism, systemic anticoagulation*

D. Acute asthma exacerbation, bronchodilators

E. Hypoventilation, pain control

Disorders that cause hypoxemia can be categorized into four groups: hypoventilation, low inspired oxygen, shunting and V/Q mismatch. Although all of these can potentially present with hypoxemia, calculating the alveolar-arterial (A-a) gradient and determining whether administering 100% oxygen is of benefit, can often determine the specific type of hypoxemia and lead to quick and effective treatment.

Acute hypoventilation often presents with an elevated $PaCO_2$ and a normal A-a gradient. This is usually seen in patients with altered mental status due to excessive sedation, narcotic use or residual anesthesia. Since this patient's $PaCO_2$ is low (35 mm Hg), it is not the cause of this patient's hypoxemia.

Low inspired oxygen presents with a low PO_2 and a normal A-a gradient. Since this patient's A-a gradient is elevated, this is unlikely the cause of the hypoxemia.

A V/Q mismatch (pulmonary embolism or acute asthma exacerbation) presents with a normal $PaCO_2$ and an elevated A-a gradient that does correct with administration of 100% oxygen. Since this patient's hypoxemia does not improve after being placed on the nonrebreather mask, it is unlikely that this is the cause.

Shunting (pulmonary edema) presents with a normal $PaCO_2$ and an elevated A-a gradient that does *not* correct with the administration of 100% oxygen. This patient has a normal $PaCO_2$, an elevated A-a gradient and hypoxemia that does not correct with the administration of 100% oxygen. This patient has a pulmonary shunt.

Although an A-a gradient can vary with age and the concentration of inspired oxygen, an A-a gradient of 51 is clearly elevated. This patient has a normal $PaCO_2$ and an elevated A-a gradient that did not improve with 100% oxygen administration therefore a shunt is clearly present. Common causes of shunting include pulmonary edema and pneumonia.

Reviewing this patient's many risk factors for a postoperative myocardial infarction and a decreased left ventricular function makes pulmonary edema the most likely explanation.

Answer: A

Weinberger SE, Cockrill BA, Mandel J (2008) *Principles of Pulmonary Medicine*, 5th edn. W. B. Saunders, Philadelphia, PA.

14. *You are taking care of a morbidly obese patient on a ventilator who is hypotensive and hypoxic. His peak airway pressures and plateau pressures have been slowly rising over the last few days. You decide to place an esophageal balloon catheter. The values are obtained:*

Pplat $= 45$ *cm* H_2O
$\Delta tP = 15$ *cm* H_2O
$\Delta Pes = 5$ *cm* H_2O

What is the likely cause of the increased peak airway pressures and what is your next intervention?

A. Decreased lung compliance, increase PEEP to 25 cm H_2O

B. Decreased lung compliance, high frequency oscillator ventilation

C. Decreased chest wall compliance, increase PEEP to 25 cm H_2O

D. Decreased chest wall compliance, high-frequency oscillator ventilation

E. Decreased lung compliance, bronchodilators

The high plateau pressures in this patient are concerning for worsening lung function or poor chest-wall mechanics due to obesity that don't allow for proper gas exchange. One way to differentiate the major cause of these elevated plateau pressures is to place an esophageal balloon. After placement, measuring the proper pressures on inspiration and expiration reveals that the largest contributing factor to these high pressures is the weight of the chest wall causing poor chest-wall compliance. The small change in esophageal pressures, as compared with the larger change in transpulmonary pressures, indicates poor chest-wall compliance and good lung compliance. It is why the major factor in this patient's high inspiratory pressures is poor chest-wall compliance. The patient is hypotensive, so increasing the PEEP would likely result in further drop in blood pressure. This is why high-frequency oscillator ventilation would likely improve this patient's hypoxemia without affecting the blood pressure.

Answer: D

Talmor D, Sarge T, O'Donnell C, Ritz R (2006) Esophageal and transpulmonary pressures in acute respiratory failure. *Critical Care Medicine* **34** (5), 1389–94.

Valenza F., Chevallard G., Porro GA, Gattinoni L (2007) Static and dynamic components of esophageal and central venous pressure during intra-abdominal hypertension. *Critical Care Medicine* **35** (6), 1575–81.

15. *All of the following cardiovascular changes occur in pregnancy except:*

A. *Increased cardiac output*

B. *Decreased plasma volume*

C. *Increased heart rate*

D. *Decreased systemic vascular resistance*

E. *Increased red blood cell mass – "relative anemia"*

The following cardiovascular changes occur during pregnancy:

- Decreased systemic vascular resistance
- Increased plasma volume
- Increased red blood cell volume
- Increased heart rate
- Increased ventricular distention
- Increased blood pressure
- Increased cardiac output
- Decreased peripheral vascular resistance

Answer: B

DeCherney AH, Nathan L (2007) *Current Diagnosis and Treatment: Obstetrics and Gynecology*, 10th edn, McGraw-Hill, New York, Chapter 7.

Yeomans, ER, Gilstrap, L. C. III. (2005) Physiologic changes in pregnancy and their impact on critical care. *Critical Care Medicine* **33**, 256–8.

16. *Choose the incorrect statement regarding the physiology of the intra-aortic balloon pump:*

A. *Shortened intraventricular contraction phase leads to increased oxygen demand*

B. *The tip of catheter should be between the second and third rib on a chest x-ray*

C. *Early inflation leads to increased afterload and decreased cardiac output*

D. *Early or late deflation leads to a smaller afterload reduction*

E. *Aortic valve insufficiency is a definite contraindication*

Patients who suffer hemodynamic compromise despite medical therapies may benefit from mechanical cardiac support of an intra-aortic balloon pump (IABP). One of the benefits of this device is the decreased oxygen demand of the myocardium as a result of the shortened intraventricular contraction phase. It is of great importance to confirm the proper placement of the balloon catheter with a chest x-ray that shows the tip of the balloon catheter to be 1 to 2 cm below the aortic knob or between the second and third rib. If the balloon is placed too proximal in the aorta, occlusion of the brachiocephalic, left carotid, or left subclavian arteries may occur. If the balloon is too distal, obstruction of the celiac, superior mesenteric, and inferior mesenteric arteries may lead to mesenteric ischemia. The renal arteries may also be occluded, resulting in renal failure.

Additional complications of intra-aortic balloon-pump placement include limb ischemia, aortic dissection, neurologic complications, thrombocytopenia, bleeding, and infection.

The inflation of the balloon catheter should occur at the onset of diastole. This results in increased diastolic pressures that promote perfusion of the myocardium as well as distal organs. If inflation occurs too early it will lead to increased afterload and decreased cardiac output. Deflation should occur at the onset of systole. Early or late deflation will diminish the effects of afterload reduction. One of the definite contraindications to placement of an IABP is the presence of a hemodynamically significant aortic valve insufficiency. This would exacerbate the magnitude of the aortic regurgitation.

Answer: A

Ferguson JJ, Cohen M, Freedman RJ, Stone GW, Joseph DL, Ohman EM (2001) The current practice of intra-aortic balloon counterpulsation: results from the Benchmark Registry. *Journal of American Cardiology* **38**, 1456–62.

Hurwitz, LM., Goodman PC (2005) Intraaortic balloon pump location and aortic dissection. *Am. J. Roentgenology* **184**, 1245–6.

Sidebotham D, McKee A, Gillham M, Levy J (2007) *Cardiothoracic Critical Care,* Butterworth-Heinemann, Philadelphia, PA.

17. *Choose the* ***incorrect*** *statement regarding the West lung zones:*

A. *Zone 1 does not exist under normal physiologic conditions*

B. *In hypovolemic states, zone 1 is converted to zone 2 and zone 3*

C. *V/Q ratio is higher in zone 1 than in zone 3*

D. *Artificial ventilation with excessive PEEP can increase dead space ventilation*

E. *Perfusion and ventilation are better in the bases than the apices of the lungs*

The three West zones of the lung divide the lung into three regions based on the relationship between alveolar pressure (PA), pulmonary arterial pressure (Pa) and pulmonary venous pressure (Pv).

Zone 1 represents alveolar dead space and is due to arterial collapse secondary to increased alveolar pressures (PA > Pa > Pv).

Zone 2 is approximately 3 cm above the heart and represents and represents a zone of pulsatile perfusion (Pa > PA > Pv).

Zone 3 represents the majority of healthy lungs where no external resistance to blood flow exists promoting continuous perfusion of ventilated lungs (Pa > Pv > PA).

Zone 1 does not exist under normal physiologic conditions because pulmonary arterial pressure is higher than alveolar pressure in all parts of the lung. However, when a patient is placed on mechanical ventilation (positive pressure ventilation with PEEP) the alveolar pressure (PA) becomes greater than the pulmonary arterial pressure (Pa) and pulmonary venous pressure (Pv). This represents a conversion of zone 3 to zone 1 and 2 and marks an increase in alveolar dead space. In a hypovolemic state, the pulmonary arterial and venous pressures fall below the alveolar pressures representing a similar conversion of zone 3 to zone 1 and 2. Both perfusion and ventilation are better at the bases than the apices. However, perfusion is better at the bases and ventilation is better at the apices due to gravitational forces.

Answer: B

Lumb A (2000) *Nunn's Applied Respiratory Physiology,* 5 edn, Butterworth-Heinemann, Oxford.

West J, Dollery C, Naimark A (1964) Distribution of blood flow in isolated lung; relation to vascular and alveolar pressures. *Journal of Applied Physiology* **19**, 713–24.

18. *Choose the correct statement regarding clinical implications of cardiopulmonary interactions during mechanical ventilation:*

A. *The decreased transpulmonary pressure and decreased systemic filling pressure is responsible for decreased venous return.*

B. *Right ventricular end-diastolic volume is increased due to increased airway pressure and decreased venous return*

C. *The difference between transpulmonary and systemic filling pressures is the gradient for venous return.*

D. *Patients with severe left ventricular dysfunction may have decreased transmural aortic pressure resulting in decreased cardiac output*

E. *Patients with decreased PCWP usually improve with additional PEEP*

The *increased* transpulmonary pressure and decreased systemic filling pressure is responsible for decreased venous return to the heart resulting in hypotension. This phenomenon is more pronounced in hypovolemic patients and may worsen hypotension in patients with low PCWP.

Right ventricular end-diastolic volume is *decreased* due to the increased transpulmonary pressure and decreased venous return.

Patients with severe left ventricular dysfunction may have decreased transmural aortic pressure resulting in *increased* cardiac output.

Answer: C

Hurford W E (1999) Cardiopulmonary interactions during mechanical ventilation. *International Anesthesiology Clinics* **37** (3), 35–46.

Marino P (2007) *The ICU Book,* 3rd edn, Lippincott Williams & Wilkins, Philadelphia, PA.

19. *The location of optimal PEEP on a volume-pressure curve is:*

A. *Slightly below the lower inflection point*

B. *Slightly above the lower inflection point*

C. *Slightly below the upper inflection point*

D. *Slightly above the upper inflection point*

E. *Cannot be determined on the volume-pressure curve*

In ARDS, patients often have lower compliant lungs that require more pressure to achieve the same volume of ventilation. On a pressure-volume curve, the lower inflection point represents increased pressure necessary to initiate the opening of alveoli and initiate a breath. The upper inflection point represents increased pressures with limited gains in volume. Conventional ventilation often reaches pressures that are above the upper inflection point and below the lower inflection point. Any ventilation above the upper inflection point results in some degree of overdistention and leads to volutrauma. Ventilating below the lower inflection point results in under-recruitment and shear force injury. The ideal mode of ventilation works between the two inflection points eliminating over distention and volutrauma and under-recruitment and shear force injury. Use tidal volumes that are below the upper inflection point and PEEP that is above the lower inflection point.

Answer: B

Lubin MF, Smith RB, Dobson TF, Spell N, Walker HK (2010) *Medical Management of the Surgical Patient: A Textbook of Perioperative Medicine*, 4th edn, Cambridge University Press, Cambridge.

Ward NS, Lin DY, Nelson DL, *et al.* (2002) Successful determination of lower inflection point and maximal compliance in a population of patients with acute respiratory distress syndrome. *Critical Care Medicine* **30** (5), 963–8.

20. *Identify the correct statement regarding the relationship between oxygen delivery and oxygen uptake during a shock state:*

A. *Oxygen uptake is always constant at tissue level due to increased oxygen extraction*

B. *Oxygen uptake at tissue level is always oxygen supply dependent*

C. *Critical oxygen delivery is constant and clinically predictable*

D. *Critical oxygen delivery is the lowest level required to support aerobic metabolism*

E. *Oxygen uptake increases with oxygen delivery in a linear relationship*

As changes in oxygen supply (DO_2) vary, the body's oxygen transport system attempts to maintain a constant delivery of oxygen (VO_2) to the tissues. This is possible due to the body's ability to adjust its level of oxygen extraction. As delivery of oxygen decreases, the extraction ratio will initially increase in a reciprocal manner. This allows for a constant oxygen supply to the tissues. Unfortunately, once the extraction ratio reaches its limit, any additional decrease in oxygen supply will result in an equal decrease of oxygen delivery. At this point, critical oxygen delivery is reached representing the lowest level of oxygen to support aerobic metabolism. After this point, oxygen delivery becomes supply dependent and the rate of aerobic metabolism is directly limited by the oxygen supply. Therefore, oxygen uptake is only constant until it reaches maximal oxygen extraction and becomes oxygen-supply dependent. Oxygen uptake at the tissue level is only oxygen-supply dependent only after the critical oxygen delivery is reached and dysoxia occurs. Unfortunately, identifying the critical oxygen delivery in ICU patients is not possible and is clinically irrelevant.

Answer: D

Marino P (2007) *The ICU Book*, 3rd edn, Lippincott Williams & Wilkins, Philadelphia, PA, Chapter 1.

Schumacker PT, Cain SM (1987) The concept of a critical oxygen delivery. *Intensive Care Medicine* **13**(4), 223–9.

21. *You are caring for a patient in ARDS who exhibits severe bilateral pulmonary infiltrates. The cause for his hypoxia is related to transvascular fluid shifts resulting in interstitial edema. Identify the primary reason for this pathologic process.*

A. *Increased capillary and interstitial hydrostatic pressure gradient*

B. *Increased oncotic reflection coefficient*

C. *Increased capillary and interstitial oncotic pressure gradient*

D. *Increased capillary membrane permeability coefficient*

E. *Increased oncotic pressure differences*

This question refers to the Starling equation which describes the forces that influence the movement of fluid across capillary membranes.

$J_v = K_f([P_c - P_i]) - \sigma[\pi_c - \pi_i]$

P_c = Capillary hydrostatic pressure

P_i = Interstitial hydrostatic pressure

π_c = Capillary oncotic pressure

π_i = Interstitial oncotic pressure

K_f = Permeability coefficient

σ = Reflection coefficient

In ALI/ARDS, the oncotic pressure difference between the capillary and the interstitium is essentially zero due to the membrane damage caused by mediators, which allows for large protein leaks into the interstitum, causing equilibrium. The oncotic pressure difference is zero, so the product with the reflection coefficient is essentially zero. According to this equation only two forces determine the extent of transmembrane fluid flux: the permeability coefficient and the hydrostatic pressure. In this case, the increased permeability coefficient is the major determinant of overwhelming intersitial edema since high hydrostatic pressures are often seen in congestive heart failure and not in ALI/ARDS.

Answer: D

Lewis CA, Martin GS (2004) Understanding and managing fluid balance in patients with acute lung injury. *Current Opinion in Critical Care* **10** (1), 13–17.

Hamid Q, Shannon J, Martin J. (2005) *Physiologic Basis of Respiratory Disease*, B. C. Decker, Hamilton, ON, Canada.

Chapter 2 Cardiopulmonary Resuscitation, Oxygen Delivery, and Shock

Timothy J. Harrison, MS, DO and Mark Cipolle, MD, PhD, FACS, FCCM

1. *All of the following are positive predictors of survival after sudden cardiac arrest except:*

A. *Witnessed cardiac arrest*

B. *Initiation of CPR by bystander*

C. *Initial rhythm of ventricular tachycardia (VT) or ventricular fibrillation (VF)*

D. *Chronic diabetes mellitus*

E. *Early access to external defibrillation*

Significant underlying comorbidities such as prior myocardial ischemia and diabetes have no role in influencing survival rates from sudden cardiac arrest. Survival rates are extremely variable throughout the current literature and can range from 0 to 18%. There are several factors that influence these survival rates. Community education plays a large role in the survival of patients who have undergone a significant cardiac event. Cardiopulmonary resuscitation certification as well as rapid notification of emergency medical services (EMS), and rapid initiation of CPR and defibrillation all contribute to improving survival. Other factors include witnessed versus nonwitnessed cardiac arrest, race, age, sex, and initial VT or VF rhythm. The problem is that only about 20 to 30% of patients have CPR performed during a cardiac arrest. As the length of time increases, the chance of survival significantly falls. Patients who are initially in VT or VF have a two to three times greater chance of survival than patients who initially present in pulseless electrical activity (PEA) arrest.

Answer: D

Cummins RO, Ornato JP, Thies WH, Pepe PE (1991) Improving survival from sudden cardiac arrest: the "chain of survival" concept. A statement for health professionals from the Advanced Cardiac Life Support Subcommittee and the Emergency Cardiac Care Committee, American Heart Association. *Circulation* **83**, 1832–47.

Deutschman C, Neligan P (2010) *Evidence-Based Practice of Critical Care*, W. B. Saunders & Co., Philadelphia, PA.

Zipes D, Hein W (1998) Sudden cardiac death. *Circulation* **98**, 2334–51.

2. *For prehospital VF arrest, compared to lidocaine, amiodarone administration in the field:*

A. *Improves survival to hospital admission*

B. *Decreases the rate of vasopressor use for hypotension*

C. *Decreases use of atropine for treatment of bradycardia*

D. *Improves survival to hospital discharge*

E. *Results in a decrease in ICU days*

Dorian evaluated this question and found more patients receiving amiodarone in the field had a better chance of survival to hospital admission than patients in the lidocaine group (22.8% versus 12.0%, $P = 0.009$). Results showed that there was no significant difference between the two groups with regard to vasopressor usage for hypotension, or atropine usage for bradycardia. Results also revealed that there was no difference in the rates of hospital discharge between the two groups

Surgical Critical Care and Emergency Surgery: Clinical Questions and Answers, First Edition. Edited by Forrest O. Moore, Peter M. Rhee, Samuel A. Tisherman and Gerard J. Fulda.

(5.0% versus 3.0%). The ALIVE trial results did support the 2005 American Heart Association recommendation to use amiodarone as the first-line antiarrhythmic agent in cardiac arrest. The guidelines state that amiodarone should be given as a 300 mg intravenous bolus, followed by one dose of 150 mg intravenously for ventricular fibrillation, paroxysmal ventricular tachycardia, unresponsive to CPR, shock, or vasopressors.

Answer: A

Deutschman C, Neligan P (2010) *Evidence-Based Practice of Critical Care*. WB Saunders & Co., Philadelphia, PA.

Dorian P, Cass D, Schwartz B, *et al.* (2002) Amiodarone as compared with lidocaine for shock-resistant ventricular fibrillation. *New England Journal of Medicine* **346**, 884–90.

3. *All of the following are underlying causes of PEA arrest* ***except****:*

A. *Tension pneumothorax*

B. *Hyperkalemia*

C. *Hypomagnesemia*

D. *Hypothermia*

E. *Cardiac tamponade*

Hypomagnesemia is not commonly associated with PEA arrests. PEA is defined as cardiac electrical activity on the monitor with the absence of a pulse or blood pressure. Recent studies using ultrasound showed evidence of mechanical activity of the heart, however there was not enough antegrade force to produce a palpable pulse or a blood pressure. Medications to treat PEA arrest include epinephrine, and in some cases, atropine. Definitive treatment of PEA involves finding and treating the underlying cause. The causes are commonly referred to as the six "Hs" and the five "Ts". The six "H's" include hypovolemia, hypoxia, hydrogen ion (acidosis), hypo/hyperkalemia, hypoglycemia, and hypothermia. The five "Ts" include toxins, tamponade (cardiac), tension pneumothorax, thrombosis (cardiac or pulmonary), and trauma. Hypomagnesemia manifests as weakness, muscle cramps, increased CNS irritability with tremors, athetosis, nystagmus, and an extensor plantar reflex. Most frequently, hypomagnesemia is associated with torsades de pointes, not PEA.

Answer: C

American Heart Association (2005) Part 7.2: Management of cardiac arrest. *Circulation* **112**, (suppl 1), IV-58–IV-66.

Criner GJ, Barnette RE, D'Alonzo GE (2010) *Critical Care Study Guide, Text and Review*, Springer, New York.

4. *CPR provides approximately what percentage of myocardial blood flow and what percentage of cerebral blood flow?*

A. *10–30% of myocardial blood flow and 30–40% cerebral blood flow*

B. *30–40% of normal myocardial blood flow and 10–30% of cerebral blood flow*

C. *50–60% of myocardial blood flow and cerebral blood flow*

D. *70–80% of myocardial blood flow and cerebral blood flow*

E. *With proper chest compressions, approximately 90% of normal myocardial blood flow and cerebral blood flow*

Despite proper CPR technique, standard closed-chest compressions provide only 10–30% of myocardial blood flow and 30–40% of cerebral blood flow. Most studies have shown that regional organ perfusion, which is achieved during CPR, is considerably less than that achieved during normal sinus rhythm. Previous research in this area has stated that a minimum aortic diastolic pressure of approximately 40 mmHg is needed to have a return of spontaneous circulation. Patients who do survive cardiac arrest typically have a coronary perfusion pressure of greater than 15 mmHg.

Answer: A

Del Guercio LRM, Feins NR, Cohn J, *et al.* (1965) Comparison of blood flow during external and internal cardiac massage in man. *Circulation* **31/32** (suppl. 1), 171.

Kern K (1997) Cardiopulmonary resuscitation physiology. *ACC Current Journal Review* **6**, 11–13.

5. *All of the following are recommended in the 2005 AHA guidelines regarding CPR and sudden cardiac arrest except*

A. *Use a compression to ventilation ratio (C/V ratio) of 30:2*

B. *Initiate chest compressions prior to defibrillation for ventricular fibrillation in sudden cardiac arrest*

C. *Deliver only one shock when attempting defibrillation*

D. *Use high-dose epinephrine after two rounds of unsuccessful defibrillation*

E. *Moderately induced hypothermia in survivors of in-hospital or out-of-hospital cardiac arrest*

The use of high-dose epinephrine has not been shown to improve survival after sudden cardiac arrest. Epinephrine at a dose of 1 mg is still the current recommendation for patients with asystole or PEA arrest. The first new recommendation was to change the old 15:2 C/V ratio to 30:2 in patients of all ages except newborns. This new ratio is based on several studies showing that over time, blood-flow increases with more chest compressions. Performing 15 compressions then two rescue breaths causes the mechanism to be interrupted and decreases blood flow to the tissues. The new 30:2 ratio is thought to reduce hyperventilation of the patient, decrease interruptions of compressions and make it easier for healthcare workers to understand. Compression first versus shock first for ventricular fibrillation in sudden cardiac arrest is based on studies that looked at the interval between the call to the emergency medical services and delivery of the initial shock If the interval was 4–5 minutes or longer, a period of CPR before attempted shock improved survival in patients. One shock versus the three-shock sequence for attempted defibrillation is the latest recommendation. The guidelines state that only one shock of 150 or 200 joules using a biphasic defibrillator or 360 joules of a monophasic defibrillator should be used in these patients. In an effort to decrease transthoracic impedence, a three-shock sequence was used in rapid succession. Because the new biphasic defibrillators have an excellent first shock efficacy, the one-shock method for attempted defibrillation was added to the current guidelines. Also recommended in the 2005 guidelines was the use of hypothermia after cardiac arrest. Brain neurons are extremely sensitive to a reduction in cerebral blood flow, which can cause permanent brain damage in minutes. Two recent trials demonstrated improved survival rates in patients that underwent mild hypothermia as compared to patients who received standard therapy. Both studies also showed an improvement in neurologic function after hypothermia treatment. In several small studies, high-dose epinephrine failed to show any survival benefit in patients that have suffered cardiac arrest.

Answer: D

Deutschman C, Neligan P (2010) *Evidence-Based Practice of Critical Care*, W. B. Saunders & Co., Philadelphia, PA.

Zaritsky A, Morley P (2005) American Heart Association guidelines for cardiopulmonary resuscitation and emergency cardiovascular care. Editorial: The evidence evaluation process for the 2005 International Consensus on Cardiopulmonary Resuscitation and Emergency Cardiovascular Care Science with Treatment Recommendations. *Circulation* **112**, 128–30.

6. *What is the oxygen content (CaO_2) in an ICU patient who has a hemoglobin of 11.0 gm/dl, an oxygen saturation (SaO_2) of 96%, and an arterial oxygen partial pressure of (PaO_2) of 90 mm Hg.*

A. *10 mL/dl*

B. *11 mL/dl*

C. *12 mL/dl*

D. *13 mL/dl*

E. *14 mL/dl*

The oxygen content of the blood can be calculated from knowing the patients hemoglobin, oxygen saturation, and partial pressure of arterial oxygen and the following formula.

$$CaO_2 = (1.3 \times Hb \times SaO_2) + (0.003 \times PaO_2)$$

$$CaO_2 = (1.3 \times 11 \times 0.96) + (0.003 \times 90)$$

$$CaO_2 = (13.72) + (0.27)$$
$$= 13.99 \text{ or } 14 \text{ mL/dl}$$

Answer: E

Marino P (2007). *The ICU Book*, 3rd edn, Lippincott Williams & Wilkins, Philadelphia, PA.

7. *What is the oxygen delivery (DO_2) of an ICU patient with hemoglobin of 10.0 gm/dl; an oxygen saturation of 98% on room air, PaO_2 of 92 mm Hg, and a cardiac output of 4 L/min?*

A. *410 mL/min*

B. *510 mL/min*

C. *521 mL/min*

D. *50.96 ml/min*

E. *610 mL/min*

Oxygen delivery can be calculated knowing the patient's hemoglobin, oxygen saturation, partial pressure of arterial oxygen, and cardiac output and using the following formula.

$$DO_2 = Q \times CaO_2 \text{ or } DO_2 = Q\ ((1.3 \times Hb \times SaO_2) + (0.003 \times PaO_2)) \times 10$$

$$Q = \text{cardiac output, } CaCo_2 = \text{oxygen content of the blood}$$

$$DO_2 = 4 \times ((1.3 \times 10 \times 0.98) + (0.003 \times 92)) \times 10$$

$$DO_2 = 520.6 \text{ or } 521 \text{ mL/min}$$

The equation is multiplied by 10 to convert volumes percent to mL/min. A DO_2 index can be calculated by substituting the cardiac index for the cardiac output, which is the cardiac output divided by the body surface area (BSA).

Answer: C

Marino P (2007) *The ICU Book*, 3rd edn, Lippincott Williams & Wilkins, Philadelphia, PA.

8. *Calculate the oxygen consumption (VO_2) in a ventilated patient in your ICU with a cardiac output of 5 L/min, a Hb of 12.0 gm/dl, PaO_2 90 mmHg, an SaO_2 of 95%, and an SvO_2 of 60%.*

A. *178 mL/min*

B. *278 mL/min*

C. *378 mL/min*

D. *478 mL/min*

E. *578 mL/min*

Venous oxygen consumption, VO_2, can be calculated knowing the patients hemoglobin, oxygen saturation, partial pressure of arterial oxygen, cardiac output and the following formula.

$$VO_2 = \text{Cardiac output} \times \text{oxygen content} \times \text{the difference in oxygen saturation between arterial and venous blood.}$$

$$VO_2 = QL/min \times ((1.3\ mL/g \times Hb\ mL/dl) + (0.003 \times PaO_2)) \times (SaO_2 - SvO_2) \times 10$$

$$VO_2 = 5 \times ((1.3 \times 12.0) + (0.003 \times 90)) \times (0.95 - 0.60) \times 10$$

$$VO_2 = 5 \times 15.87 \times 0.35 \times 10$$

$$VO_2 = 277.7 \text{ mL/min}$$

Answer: B

Marino P (2007) *The ICU Book*, 3rd edn, Lippincott Williams & Wilkins, Philadelphia, PA.

9. *The most effective way of generating ATP is via cellular respiration. The complete cellular respiration of glucose will yield:*

A. *26 ATP*

B. *34 ATP*

C. *36 ATP*

D. *32 ATP*

E. *42 ATP*

At the cellular level, cellular respiration and oxidative phosphorylation are the most efficient way of generating ATP, through a series of oxidation-reduction reactions in which oxygen becomes the final electron acceptor. Thirty-six ATPs are generated via aerobic metabolism during cellular respiration. Anaerobic metabolism converts pyruvate into lactate, which is a very inefficient way to produce ATP. Some books will give the number of ATP as 38; however, two molecules of ATP are consumed during the process, which yields 36 ATP.

Answer: C

Bylund-Fellenius AC, Walker PM, Elander A, Holm S, *et al.* (1981) Energy metabolism in relation to oxygen partial pressure in human skeletal muscle during exercise. *Journal of Biological Chemistry* **200**, 247–55.

Campbell NA, Reece JB (2008) *Biology,* Benjamin Cummings: San Francisco, CA, p. 176.

10. *All of the following shift the oxygen-dissociation curve to the left except:*

A. *Fetal Hb*

B. *Carboxyhemoglobin*

C. *Respiratory alkalosis*

D. *Chronic anemia*

E. *Hypophosphatemia*

The oxygen-dissociation curve is a great tool to help understand how hemoglobin carries and releases oxygen. The sinusoidal curve plots the proportion of saturated hemoglobin on the vertical axis against oxygen tension on the horizontal axis. There are multiple factors that will shift the curve either to the right or to the left. A rightward shift indicates that the hemoglobin has a decreased affinity for oxygen. In other words, it is more difficult for hemoglobin to bind to oxygen but easier for the hemoglobin to release oxygen bound to it. The added effect of this rightward shift increases the partial pressure of oxygen in the tissues where it is mostly needed, such as during strenuous exercise, or various shock states. In contrast, a leftward shift indicates that the hemoglobin has an increased affinity for oxygen, so that the hemoglobin binds oxygen more easily but unloads it more judiciously. Fetal hemoglobin causes a leftward shift of the oxygen-dissociation curve because there is reduced binding of 2,3 DPG to fetal hemoglobin. 2,3 DPG binds best to beta chains of adult hemoglobin. Fetal hemoglobin consists of two alpha chains and two gamma chains. Fetal hemoglobin is therefore less sensitive to the effects of 2,3 DPG, lowering the p50 level and shifting the curve to the left. Hemoglobin binds with carbon monoxide 200–250 times more readily than with oxygen. The presence of just one molecule of carbon monoxide on one of the heme sites causes the oxygen on the other heme sites to bind with greater affinity. This makes it more difficult for the hemoglobin to release the oxygen, shifting the curve to the left. Carbon dioxide affects the oxygen-dissociation curve in two ways; it influences the intracellular pH via the Bohr effect, and there is an accumulation of CO_2, which causes the production of carbamino compounds, which then bind to hemoglobin forming carbaminohemoglobin. Low levels of carbamino compound cause the curve to shift to the right, while higher levels cause a leftward shift. 2,3 DPG is an organophosphate, which is created by erythrocytes during glycolysis. In the presence of diminished peripheral tissue oxygen availability, such as hypoxemia, COPD, anemia, and congestive heart failure, the production of 2,3 DPG is significantly increased. High levels of 2,3 DPG shift the curve to the right, while low levels of 2,3 DPG shift the curve to the left, as seen in conditions such as septic shock, and hypophosphatemia.

Answer: D

Marini JJ, Wheeler AP (2006) *Critical Care Medicine, The Essentials,* Lippincott Williams & Wilkins, Philadelphia, PA.

The Physiology Viva (2003) www.anesthesiamcq.com (accessed April 2, 2011).

Oxygen-Hemoglobin dissociation curve (2011) http://en.wikipedia.org/wiki/Oxygen%E2%80%93hemoglobin_dissociation_curve (accessed March 25, 2011).

11. *The diagnosis of SIRS may include all of the following except:*

A. *A blood pressure of 86/40 mm Hg*

B. *Temperature of 35.6 °C*

C. *Heart rate of 103 beats/minute*

D. *$PaCO_2$ of 27 mm Hg*

E. *WBC of 15.5 × 10^3/microL*

Hypotension is not included in the criteria for the diagnosis of systemic inflammatory response syndrome (SIRS). This is a syndrome characterized by abnormal regulation of various cytokines leading to generalized inflammation, organ dysfunction and eventual organ failure. The definition of SIRS was formalized in 1992 following a consensus statement between the American College of Chest Physicians and the Society of Critical Care Medicine. SIRS was defined as being present when two or more of the following criteria are met:

Temperature: >38 °C or <36 °C
Heart rate: >90 bpm
Respiratory rate >20 breaths/minute or $PaCO_2$ <32 mm Hg
WBC >12 000/microL or <4000/microL

The causes of SIRS can be broken down into infectious causes, which include sepsis, or noninfectious causes, which can include trauma, burns, pancreatitis, hemorrhage and ischemia. Treatment should be directed at fixing the underlying etiology.

Answer: A

Marini JJ, Wheeler AP (2006) *Critical Care Medicine, The Essentials,* Lippincott Williams & Wilkins, Philadelphia, PA.

Marino P (2007) *The ICU Book,* 3rd edn, Lippincott Williams & Wilkins, Philadelphia, PA.

12. *All of the following are consistent with cardiogenic shock except:*

A. *PAOP > 18 mm Hg*

B. *C.I. < 2.2 L/min/m²*

C. *SaO_2 of 86%*

D. *Pulmonary edema*

E. *SVO_2 of 90%*

A SVO_2 of 90% is increased from the normal range of 70 to 75%, which would be consistent with septic shock but not cardiogenic shock. Cardiogenic shock results from either a direct or indirect insult to the heart, leading to a decreased output, and can be further defined as low cardiac output, despite normal ventricular filling pressures. Cardiogenic shock is diagnosed when the cardiac index is less than 2.2 L/min/m^2, and the pulmonary wedge pressure is greater than 18 mm Hg, which excludes answers A and B. The decreased contractility of the left ventricle is the etiology of cardiogenic shock. Because the ejection fraction is reduced, the ventricle tries to compensate by becoming more compliant in an effort to increase stroke volume. After a certain point, the ventricle can no longer work at this level and begins to fail. This failure leads to a significant decrease in cardiac output, which then leads to a buildup of pulmonary edema, an increase in myocardial oxygen consumption, and an increased intrapulmonary shunt. For these reasons, answers C and D are excluded. Progressive cardiac failure would result in a decrease in SVO_2, not an increase.

Answer: E

Marino P (2007) *The ICU Book,* 3rd edn, Lippincott Williams & Wilkins, Philadelphia, PA.

Marini JJ, Wheeler AP (2006) *Critical Care Medicine, The Essentials.* Lippincott Williams & Wilkins, Philadelphia, PA.

13. *All of the following statements regarding* pulsus paradoxus *are true except:*

A. *It is considered a normal variant during the inspiratory phase of respiration*

B. *It has been shown to be a positive predictor of the severity of pericardial tamponade*

C. *A slight increase in blood pressure occurs with inspiration, while a drop in blood pressure is seen during exhalation*

D. *Heart sounds can be auscultated when a radial pulse is not felt during exhalation.*

Pulsus paradoxus is defined as a decrease in systolic blood pressure of greater than 10 mm Hg during the inspiratory phase of the respiratory cycle. It is considered a normal variant during this phase of the respiratory cycle. Under normal conditions, there are several changes in intrathoracic pressure that are transmitted to the heart and great vessels. During inspiration, there is distention of the right ventricle due to increased venous return. This causes the interventricular septum to bulge into the left ventricle, which then causes increased pooling of blood in the expanded lungs, further decreasing return to the left ventricle and decreasing stroke volume of the left ventricle. So this fall in stroke volume of the left ventricle is reflected as a fall in systolic pressure. On clinical examination, you are able to auscultate the heart during inspiration but do lose a signal at the radial artery. *Pulsus paradoxus* has been shown to be a positive predictor of the severity of pericardial tamponade as demonstrated by Curtiss, *et al.* *Pulsus paradoxus* has been linked to several disease processes that can be separated into cardiac, pulmonary and noncardiac/nonpulmlonary causes. Cardiac causes are tamponade, constrictive pericarditis, pericardial effusion, and cardiogenic shock. Pulmonary causes include pulmonary embolism, tension pneumothorax, asthma, and COPD. Noncardiac/nonpulmonary causes include anaphylactic reactions and shock, and obstruction of the superior vena cava.

Answer: C

Curtiss EI, Reddy PS, Uretsky BF, Cecchetti AA (1988) Pulsus paradoxus: definition and relation to the severity of cardiac tamponade. *American Heart Journal* **115** (2), 391–8. PMID 3341174.

Guyton AG (1963) *Circulatory Physiology: Cardiac Output and Its Regulation*, W. B. Saunders, Philadelphia, PA.

14. *Compared to neurogenic shock, spinal shock involves:*

A. *Loss of sensation followed by motor paralysis and gradual recovery of some reflexes*

B. *A distributive type of shock resulting in hypotension and bradycardia that is from disruption of the autonomic pathways within the spinal cord*

C. *A sudden loss of sympathetic stimulation to the blood vessels*

D. *The loss of neurologic function of the spinal cord following a prolonged period of hypotension*

Spinal shock refers to a loss of sensation followed by motor paralysis and eventual recovery of some reflexes. Spinal shock results in an acute flaccidity and loss of reflexes following spinal cord injury and is not due to systemic hypotension. Spinal shock initially presents as a complete loss of cord function. As the shock state improves some primitive reflexes such as the bulbo-cavernosus will return. Spinal shock can occur at any cord level.

Neurogenic shock involves hemodynamic compromise associated with bradycardia and a decreased systemic vascular resistance that typically occurs with injuries above the level of T6. Neurogenic shock is a distributive type of shock which is due to disruption of the sympathetic autonomic pathways within the spinal cord, resulting in hypotension and bradycardia. Treatment consists of volume resuscitation and vasopressors for blood-pressure control, most notably dopamine.

Answer: A

Marini JJ, Wheeler AP (2006) *Critical Care Medicine, The Essentials*. Lippincott Williams & Wilkins, Philadelphia, PA.

Piepmeyer JM, Lehmann KB and Lane JG (1985) Cardiovascular instability following acute cervical spine trauma. *Central Nervous System Trauma* **2**, 153–9.

Neurogenic Shock (2011) http://en.wikipedia.org/wiki/Neurogenic_shock (accessed April 5, 2011).

Spinal Shock (2008) www.wheelessonline.com/ortho/8669 (accessed April 5, 2011).

Chapter 3 Arrhythmias, Acute Coronary Syndromes, and Hypertensive Emergencies

Harrison T. Pitcher, MD and Timothy J. Harrison, DO

1. *The action potential is expressed as the change in cellular membrane voltage over time during depolarization and repolarization of cardiac cells. All of the following are correct regarding the cardiac action potential except:*

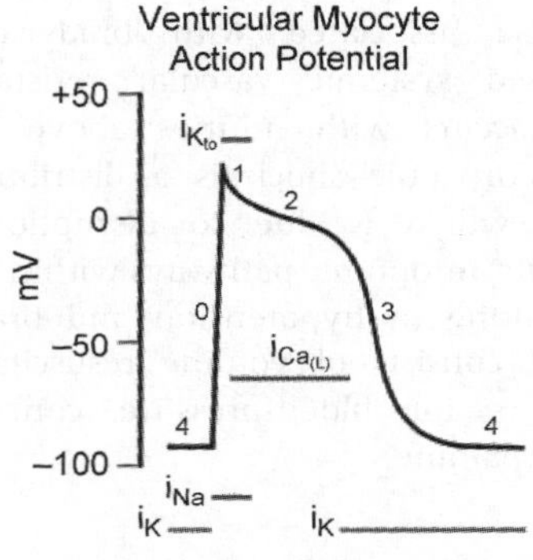

A. *Phase 4 represents the resting membrane potential and is defined as the period from the end of repolarization to the next depolarization*

B. *In phase 3 the membrane conductance to all of the ions remains low and cells are unresponsive to stimuli*

C. *Phase 2 is represented by slow, inward L-type calcium channels and outward movement of potassium through slow, delayed rectifier potassium channels becoming activated*

D. *Phase 1 represents early, transient repolarization due to rapid inactivation of sodium gated channels and activation of outward potassium channels*

E. *The slope of phase 0 helps determine the maximum rate of depolarization of the cell and impulse propagation*

Surgical Critical Care and Emergency Surgery: Clinical Questions and Answers, First Edition. Edited by Forrest O. Moore, Peter M. Rhee, Samuel A. Tisherman and Gerard J. Fulda.

There are two types of cardiac action potentials. The "slow-response" action potentials that make up the pacemaker cells are commonly found in the sinoatrial and atrioventricular nodes and the "fast-response" action potentials are commonly made up of the atrial myocytes, the ventricular myocytes, and the Purkinje cells. There are five phases associated with the cardiac action potential. Phase 0 represents the rapid, depolarization phase, and is characterized by fast sodium ion influx. The slope of phase 0 determines the maximum rate of depolarization of the cell and the impulse propagation. Phase 1 represents early repolarization caused by the rapid inactivation of the sodium channels and the activation of potassium channels moving potassium out of the cell. Phase 1 has a characteristic "notch" on the graph. Phase 2 is the "plateau" phase of the cardiac action potential. The membrane conductance remains relatively low and cells are unresponsive to outside stimuli due to activation of slow, inward L-type calcium channels and outward movement of potassium from the cells through slow, delayed rectifier potassium channels. Phase 3 represents repolarization of the cell, caused by inactivation of the slow gated calcium channels and continued activation of the rectifier potassium channels. It is during this phase of the cardiac action potential that the cells recover the ability to respond to stimuli and regain their "excitability". The relative refractory period can also be associated with Phase 3 of the action potential. This is when a strong stimulus is applied to cells at the end of Phase 3 which encounters other recovered sodium channels thus generating a new action potential. Finally, Phase 4 is noted as the resting membrane potential and is the period from the end of repolarization until the start of depolarization.

Answer: B

Cardiovascular Physiology Concepts (2007) www.cvphysiology.com/Arrhythmias/A010.htm (accessed February 27, 2011).

2. *With regards to the vascular supply to the cardiac conduction system, all of the following are correct except:*

A. The AV node receives dual blood supply from the right coronary artery, and the left anterior descending artery

B. The blood supply to the SA node is from the right coronary artery and the left circumflex artery

C. The blood supply to the anterior fascicle is from the posterior descending artery

D. The blood supply to the Bundle of His and the right bundle branch is from the left anterior descending circulation

E. The posterior fascicle receives its blood supply from the left anterior descending artery and the left circumflex artery

The SA node is located on the superior, lateral surface of the right atrium near the entrance of the superior vena cava. In 60% of cases, the SA node receives its blood supply from the right coronary artery, and 40% of the time from the left circumflex artery. The AV node has a dual blood supply. It receives blood from the posterior descending artery from the right coronary artery and septal branches from the left anterior descending artery. The Bundle of His, and the right bundle branch receives its blood supply from the Left Anterior Descending artery. The Bundle of His protrudes through the central fibrous body and then divides into the left and right bundle branches. The left bundle branch then further divides into the anterior and posterior fascicle. The anterior fascicle receives its blood supply from the left anterior descending artery, the posterior fascicle receives its blood from the left anterior descending artery and the left circumflex artery. The blood supply to the anterior fascicle, a division of the left bundle branch, comes from the left anterior descending artery.

Answer: C

Criner GJ, Barnette RE, D'Alonzo GE (2010) *Critical Care Study Guide, Text and Review.* Springer: New York.

Electric Conduction System of the Heart. http://en.wikipedia.org/wiki/Electrical_conduction_system_of_the_heart (accessed March 1, 2011).

3. *A 21-year-old football player is evaluated for symptomatic tachycardia. He first noticed the symptoms at age 9 while running and has noticed the episodes are becoming more frequent and lasting longer. He denies ever losing consciousness and uses an albuterol inhaler for asthma. He describes atypical chest pain, slight dyspnea, and palpitations. His stress echocardiogram was normal and his baseline EKG is shown here.*

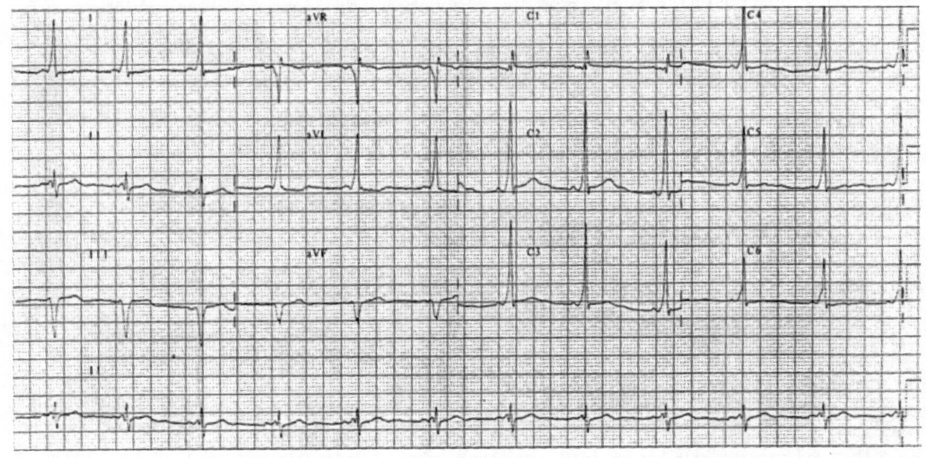

Based upon your patient's symptoms and the EKG findings, your diagnosis is:

A. *First-degree AV block*

B. *Atrial fibrillation with slow ventricular response*

C. *SVT with functional bundle branch block or aberrant conduction*

D. *Wolff–Parkinson–White syndrome*

E. *Mobitz Type II AV block*

Wolff–Parkinson–White syndrome is a pre-excitation syndrome associated with an atrioventricular reentrant tachycardia. The tachycardia is due to an accessory pathway within the conduction system of the heart known as the Bundle of Kent. Certain medications, physical activity, and stress can send the electrical impulse into the accessory Bundle of Kent causing the prior unidirectional block to quickly recover its excitability thus sending the impulse back to reenter the circuit. Most patients remain asymptomatic throughout their lives; however a small percentage of patients becomes symptomatic and progresses to ventricular fibrillation, which then causes sudden death. People who are symptomatic during episodes of tachycardia experience palpitations, dizziness, shortness of breath, and fainting or near-fainting spells. Classic EKG findings include; a short P-R interval (<0.12 s), a wide QRS complex (>0.12 s), slurring of the initial upstroke of the QRS complex (a delta wave), and abnormal T waves indicating problems with repolarization. A classic delta wave can be seen in the precordial leads. Acute treatment in a hypotensive patient involves cardioversion and amiodarone or procainamide in a more stable patient. The definitive treatment for WPW syndrome involves radiofrequency ablation of the accessory pathway.

Answer: D

Marini JJ, Wheeler AP (2006) *Critical Care Medicine, The Essentials*, Lippincott Williams & Wilkins, Philadelphia, PA.

4. *A 40-year-old Asian man with controlled hypertension suddenly collapses while eating. His son promptly initiates CPR. On paramedic arrival he is in ventricular fibrillation and is successfully converted to normal sinus rhythm with external defibrillation. In the emergency room, the EKG shown here was obtained.*

He had a second episode of ventricular fibrillation in the ED and was again successfully defibrillated. Definitive treatment for this patient's diagnosis would be:

A. *Observation*

B. *Isoproterenol*

C. *Quinidine*

D. *Implantable cardiac defibrillator*

E. *Surgical revascularization*

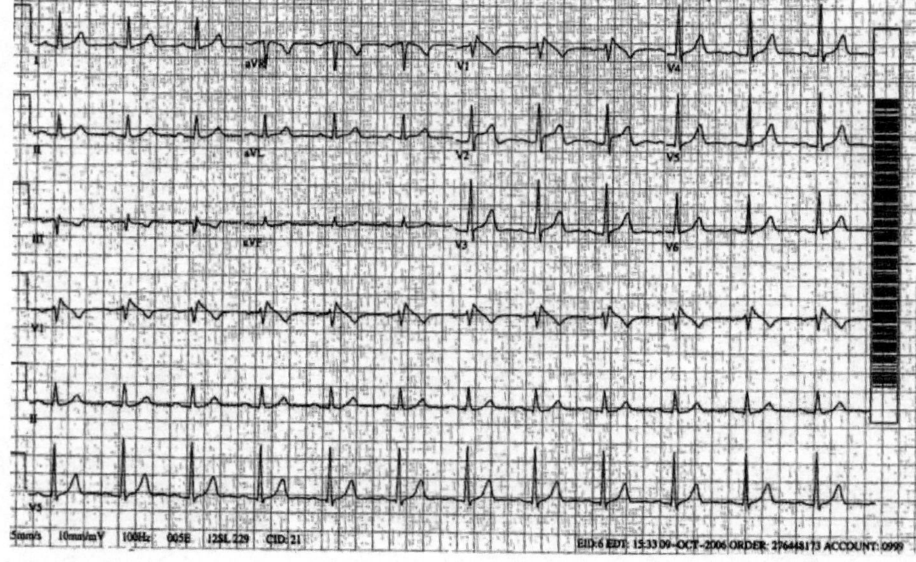

The clinical scenario and classic EKG findings suggest Brugada syndrome. Placement of an implantable cardiac defibrillator is the only definitive for this cardiac pathology. Brugada syndrome has an autosomal dominant pattern of transmission and is characterized by cardiac conduction delays, which can lead to ventricular fibrillation and sudden cardiac death. It is more common in men and Asians. EKG findings typically reveal a right bundle branch block with ST segment elevations in the precordial leads. The pathophysiology is thought to be caused by an alteration in the transmembrane ion currents that together constitute the cardiac action potential. In this case, choice A would not be correct. Even though the patient remains in normal sinus rhythm, the underlying problem has not been fixed, and he would likely revert to ventricular fibrillation. Choice B is an option to help treat ventricular tachycardia storms by augmenting the cardiac L-type channels; however, it is not a definitive treatment. Quinidine is sometimes used because it is a class 1A sodium channel blocker that also blocks the outward potassium channel current (Ito current), which prevents the heart from going into ventricular fibrillation. Surgical revascularization is not an option in these patients. An ICD should be surgically placed, which will then be programmed to fire when it detects an unstable rhythm.

Answer: D

Alings M, Wilde A (1999) "Brugada" syndrome: clinical data and suggested pathophysiological mechanism. *Circulation* **99** (5), 666–73.

5. *A 57-year-old woman is admitted to the ICU after being intubated for respiratory failure following an asthma attack. Several hours after intubation she remains hypotensive. Her EKG is concerning for ST segment elevations in the precordial leads. Troponin is elevated at 0.56 μg/L. Cardiac catheterization demonstrates that her vessels are completely normal. Bedside echocardiogram is done, which reveals an ejection fraction of approximately 25% and significant hypokinesis of the mid and apical segments of the left ventricle. Your diagnosis is:*

A. *Broken heart syndrome*

B. *Myocardial infarction*

C. *Acute pericarditis*

D. *Pulmonary embolism*

E. *Coronary artery vasospasm*

Takotsubo's syndrome or broken heart syndrome is a transient cardiomyopathy that causes significant cardiac depression and closely resembles acute coronary syndromes. This is a typical presentation of a patient with this cardiac disorder; respiratory failure after a significant upper airway problem, EKG changes, with an increase in cardiac enzymes, mimicking acute myocardial infarction. However, when the patient undergoes cardiac catheterization, there is ballooning of the left ventricular and no significant stenotic lesions of the coronary vessels. Researchers believe that this syndrome is caused by stress-induced catecholamine release, with toxicity to and subsequent stunning of the myocardium. Diagnosis is typically by thorough history and physical, EKG changes, most commonly ST segment elevation and T wave inversion, Echocardiogram showing significant wall motion abnormalities, mildly elevated cardiac enzymes, and cardiac angiography ruling out acute cardiac ischemia secondary to occlusion of coronary vessels. Acute coronary syndrome should be the diagnosis until proven otherwise. The prognosis remains excellent and exceeds 95%. Most patients experience a complete recovery in about four to eight weeks and recurrence is less than 3%.

Answer: A

Dorfman TA, Iskandrian AE (2009) Takotsubo cardiomyopathy: State-of-the-art review. *Journal of Nuclear Cardiology* **16** (1), 122–34.

Kawai S, Kitabatake A, Tomoike H (2007) Guidelines for diagnosis of Takotsubo (ampulla) cardiomyopathy. *Circulation Journal* **71** (6), 990–2.

6. *A 76-year-old man comes to the emergency room after his wife states that "he has been falling a lot lately". He is immediately placed on the cardiac monitor and a 12-lead EKG is obtained, which is shown here.*

This EKG represents which of the following?

A. *Complete heart block*

B. *Second degree heart block, Mobitz type II*

C. *Second degree heart block, Mobitz type I (Wenckebach)*

D. *Myocardial infarction*

E. *First degree heart block*

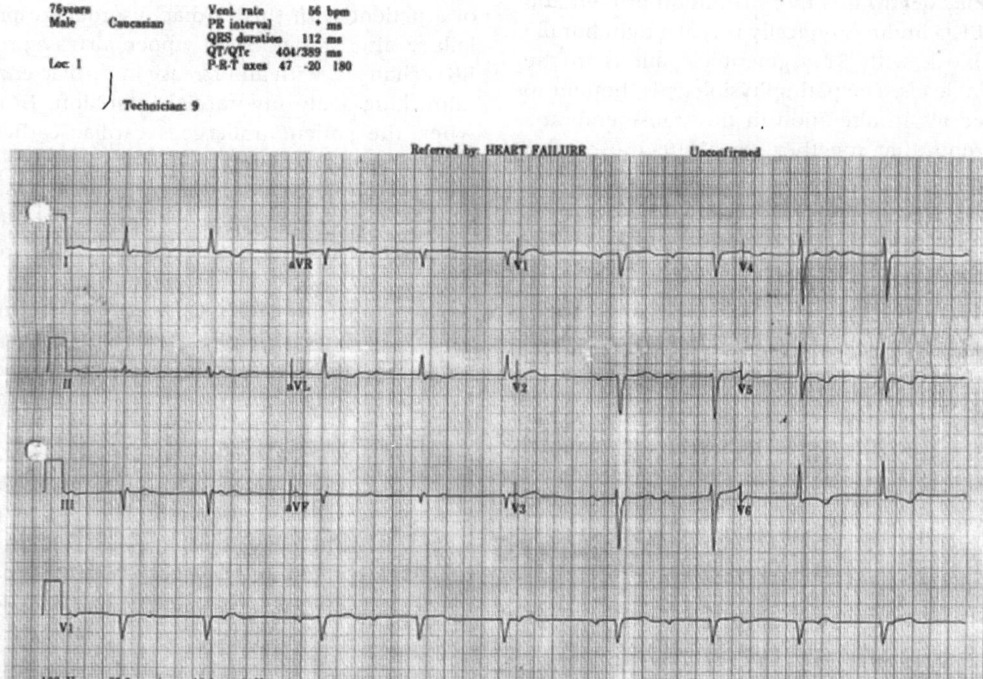

This patient's symptoms are classically seen in the various types of heart blocks. A history of falling, or syncope seems to go along with the physiology behind heart blocks. The EKG findings are characterized by progressive prolongation of the P-R interval on consecutive beats, followed by a dropped QRS complex, followed then by the P-R setting, and the cycle repeating, as shown in the above EKG. Type I second degree AV block is almost always a disease of the AV node. On the other hand, Type II second degree AV block (Mobitz type II) is almost always a disease of the distal conduction system (Bundle of His). On EKG, Mobitz type II is characterized by intermittently non-conducted P waves that do not lengthen or shorten the P-R interval. Mobitz type II AV block can progress to complete heart block leading to sudden cardiac death. First-degree heart block is characterized by a P-R interval greater than 0.2 s, which is not seen in this EKG. The EKG findings of complete heart block, or third-degree heart block, include no concordance between the P waves and the QRS complexes. The most definitive treatment for AV nodal blocks is an implantable pacemaker.

Answer: C

Barold SS, Hayes DL (2001) Second-degree atrioventricular block: a reappraisal. *Mayo Clinical Proceedings* **76** (1), 44–57.

Heart Block, Second Degree (2009) http://emedicine.medscape.com/article/758383-overview (accessed February 26, 2011).

7. *All of the following are true regarding left anterior fascicular block except:*

A. *It is the most common intraventricular conduction defect*

B. *It may mimic left ventricular hypertrophy (LVH) in lead aVL, and mask LVH voltage in leads V5 and V6*

C. *rS complexes can be seen in leads II, III, aVF*

D. *Right axis deviation in the frontal plane (usually >100 degrees)*

E. *Usually see poor R wave progression in leads V1–V3 and deeper S waves in leads V5 and V6*

Left anterior fascicular block is the most common conduction in general and the most common conduction delay seen in acute anterior wall myocardial infarction due to occlusion of the left anterior descending artery. All of the choices seen above are EKG characteristics of LAFB except for choice D. LAFB is classically associated with **left axis deviation** in a frontal plane usually −45 to −90 degrees. There is no specific treatment for the different types of hemiblocks other than diagnosing and treatment the underlying cardiac ischemia. The EKG criteria are as follows:

Left axis deviation (usually −45 to −90 degrees);
rS complexes in leads II, III, aVF;
small q-waves in leads I and/or aVL;
R-peak time in lead aVL >0.04s, often with slurred R wave downstroke;
QRS duration usually <0.12s unless there is coexisting RBBB;
poor R wave progression in leads V1-V3 and deeper S-waves in leads V5 and V6
to note: LAFB may look like LVH in lead aVL, and hide LVH in leads V% and V6.

Answer: D

Raoof S, George L, Saleh A, Sung A (2009) *ACP Manual of Critical Care*, McGraw-Hill, New York.

8. *The main difference between hypertensive emergency and hypertensive urgency is:*

A. *The presence of end-organ damage*

B. *Hypertensive emergencies always have a higher mean arterial pressure*

C. *Hypertensive emergencies are more common in the elderly, African Americans, and twice as high in men than women*

D. *Hypertensive urgency has a higher risk of stroke*

E. *A and C*

The characteristics of both hypertensive emergency and hypertensive urgency are of significant elevations in systolic and diastolic pressure. However, hypertensive emergency is associated with end organ damage and is more common in the elderly, African Americans, and men. The organs most commonly affected are the brain, heart, eyes and kidneys. The goal of hypertensive emergency is to reduce the blood pressure fairly quickly using IV anti-hypertensive medications in a controlled critical care environment. Although the goal of hypertensive urgency is relatively the same, lowering of blood pressure with hypertensive urgency can be done over a longer period of time.

Answer: E

Marik PE, Varon J (2007) Hypertensive crises: challenges and management. *Chest* **131** (6), 1949–62.

9. *Two weeks following a myocardial infarction, 64-year-old man is admitted to the trauma service with multiple rib fractures and a pulmonary contusion. He has a history of alcohol abuse and has been noncompliant with his cardiac medications. On examination he had a pulse of 100 beats/minute, blood pressure 100/70 mm Hg, respirations 20/minute, tenderness and bruising along the right lateral chest wall and no other significant findings. A 12-lead ECG confirms a recent inferior myocardial infarction and an echocardiogram is shown here.*
In view of this finding, which of the following is the most appropriate management for this patient?

A. *Confirmatory cardiac catheterization*

B. *Six months of oral anticoagulation*

C. *Pericardiocentesis*

D. *NSAIDs for six weeks*

E. *Immediate referral to the cardiac surgical service*

The echocardiogram reveals a very large ventricular pseudoaneurysm of the left ventricle

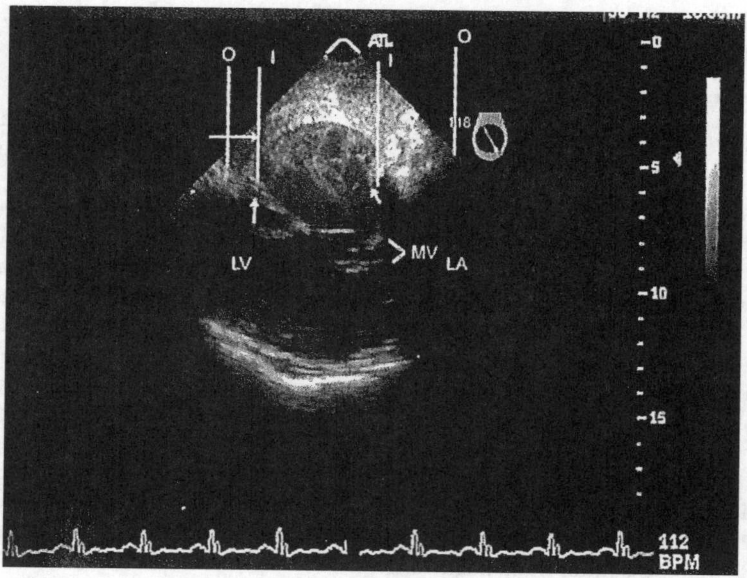

The outer boundary of the pseudoaneurysm is marked by vertical lines O and the communication with the left ventricle by vertical lines l.

A pseudoaneurysm (false aneurysm) results from a free wall rupture of the left ventricle, usually as a result of a previous myocardial infarction. The rupture is contained by overlying pericardium and lacks any organized cardiac structures, unlike a true ventricular aneurysm. The occurrence of free-wall rupture is less than 1%; however the mortality is significant and one-half of the ruptures will result in out-of-hospital sudden deaths. Diagnosis is usually made within six months of infarction. Surgical intervention for large or expanding pseudoaneurysm is recommended when the diagnosis is made. Contrast ventriculography is diagnostic in only 54% of patients versus 97% for 2D echocardiography, therefore answer A is redundant. Pericardiocentesis would be ill advised and NSAIDs possibly increase the chance of free rupture. Although Coumadin is of value in circumstances of left-ventricular clot in the setting of a true left-ventricular aneurysm, it is contraindicated in this setting.

Answer: E

Atik FA, Lytle BW (2007) Surgical Treatment of Post Infarction Left Ventricular Pseudoaneurysm. *The Annals of Thoracic Surgery* **83**, 526–531.

Armstrong WF, Ryan T (2010) *Feigenbaum's Echocardiography*. Lippincott Williams & Wilkins: Philadelphia.

Cohn LH, Edmunds LH (2003) *Cardiac Surgery in the Adult*. The McGraw-Hill Companies: New York.

Califf R, Roe M (2010) *Acute Coronary Syndrome Essentials*. Jones & Bartlett Learning.

Frances C, Romero A, Grady D (1998) Left Ventricular Pseudoaneurysm. *J Am College Cardiology* **32**, 557–561.

Reardon MJ, Carr CL, Diamond A, *et al.* (1997) Ischemic Left Ventricular Free Wall Rupture: prediction, diagnosis and treatment. *Ann Thoracic Surgery* **64**, 1509–1513.

10. *A 39-year-old obese man presents to the emergency room the evening prior to elective hernia surgery with several hours of sudden onset chest pain and shortness of breath. He admits to being anxious concerning the morning surgery. His medications include albuterol, and Lipitor. His pulse is regular and he has a blood pressure of 165/89 mm Hg respiratory rate is 22/minute. He is sitting at the edge of the examining table and states he finds it "easier to breath and feels better" in that position. His electrocardiogram is shown.*

Which of the following options for the care of this patient would be least indicated on the basis of his electrocardiogram and clinical findings?

A. *Cardiac catheterization*

B. *Echocardiogram*

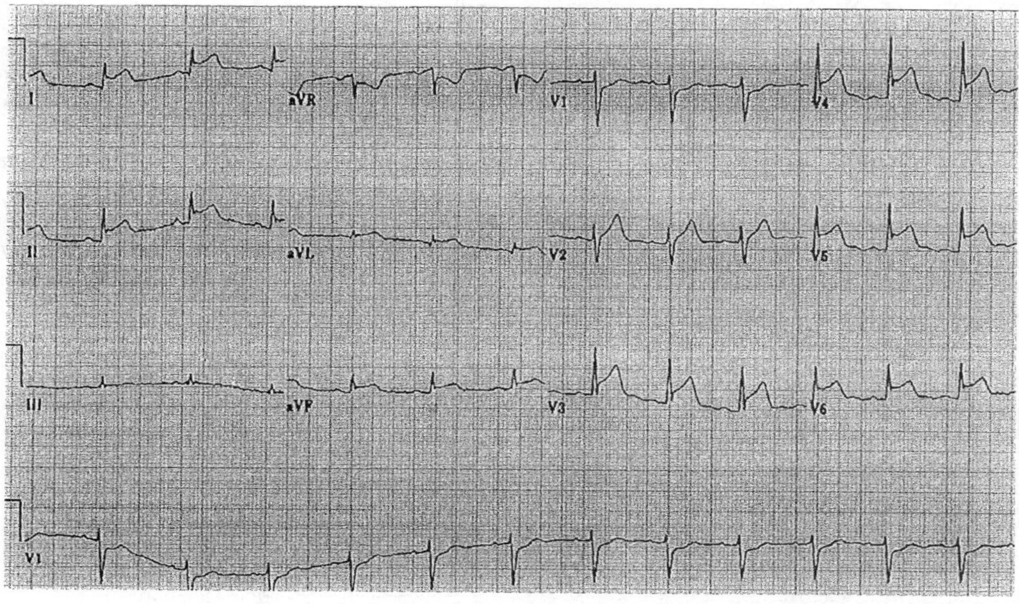

C. *Albuterol*

D. *Thrombolytics*

E. *650 mg of ASA*

The 12 lead reveals ST elevation and diffuse J-point elevation throughout the electrocardiogram (solid arrows) with no localization to coronary artery distribution. There is atrial segment elevation in leads aVR (hollow arrows).

Diffuse ST segment elevation and PR segment elevation in lead aVR strongly support the diagnosis of acute pericarditis. It is important to discern acute pericarditis from an acute myocardial injury. An echocardiogram, in the absence of a prior myocardial infarction, demonstrates normal LV function without wall motion abnormality. An echocardiogram would be appropriate to demonstrate the presence or absence of a pericardial effusion which

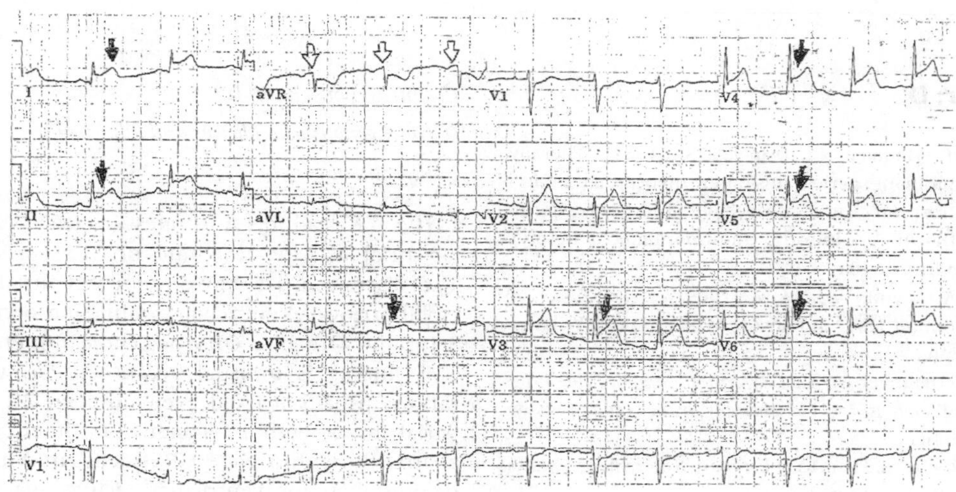

12-lead ECG with arrows showing pericarditis

occurs in up to 30% of patients with acute pericarditis. D would be inappropriate due to the potential of significant morbidity and potentially mortality due to a hemorrhagic pericardial effusion and possible cardiac tamponade that could develop in the setting of thrombolytics given in a patient with acute pericarditis. The most recent published acute coronary syndrome guidelines suggest ASA as the primary therapeutic modality. Indomethacin and corticosteroids have been relegated to refractory cases due to concerns regarding increased coronary vascular resistance, and increased risk of myocardial rupture in the setting of a healing previously unrecognized myocardial infarction. Improvement in chest pain is classic on sitting up and leaning forward in acute pericarditis.

Answer: D

Bermon J, Haffajee CI, Alpert JS (1981) Therapy of Symptomatic pericarditis after myocardial infarction: retrospective and prospective studies of aspirin, indomethacin, prednisone, and spontaneous resolution. *Am Heart J* **101**, 750–753.

Gabrielli A, Layon, AJ, Yu M (2009) *Civetta, Taylor, & Kirby's Critical Care*. Lippincott Williams and Wilkins: Philadelphia.

Parillo JE, Dellinger RD (2008) *Critical Care Medicine Principles of Diagnosis and Management in the Adult*. Mosby: Philadelphia.

Califf R, Roe M (2010) *Acute Coronary Syndrome Essentials*. Jones & Bartlett Learning.

11. *A 72-year-old woman is admitted with nausea and vomiting and a small bowel ileus. She is hypokalemic and mildly hypomagnesemic. Her initial electrocardiogram in the emergency room just prior to transfer is illustrated below.*

Two hours later she complains of retrosternal chest pain relieved by sublingual nitroglycerin. Her daughter states that her mother had been complaining of palpitations for the past three days and has had "heart failure" in the past. Physical examination: heart rate 91 beats/minute and irregular, blood pressure 117/75 mm Hg, respiratory rate 20 breaths/minute, and oxygen saturation of 95% on face mask. Which would be most appropriate?

A. *Synchronized monophasic cardioversion*

B. *Intravenous amiodarone and anticoagulation*

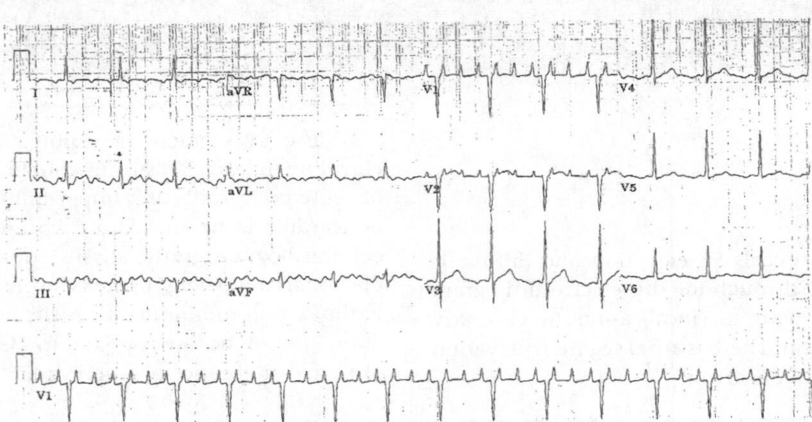

C. *Intravenous ibutilide*

D. *Intravenous beta blocker and diltiazem*

E. *Carotid massage*

The 12 lead demonstrates in lead V1 regular atrial activity at a rate of 275 per minute. The discrete atrial waves represent atrial flutter (solid arrows). Ventricular conduction occurs at a 3:1 ratio with one QRS per three flutter waves. This finding is unusual because the conduction ratio is usually a fixed even number, 2:1 or 4:1. Atrial flutter with 1:1 conduction often conducts aberrantly with a wide QRS tachycardia that can be mistaken for ventricular tachycardia. Typical

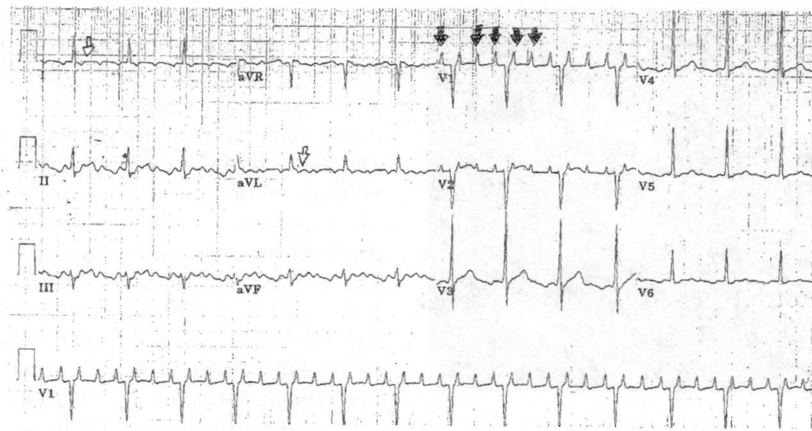

atrial flutter has atrial undulations at a rate of 240–340 a minute. Classically there is flutter morphology with inverted flutter waves lacking an isoelectric base in leads I, II, and aVF with small, positive deflections with a distinct isoelectric baseline in lead V1 as demonstrated in this case. The ECG illustrated demonstrates the baseline artifact in the inferior leads. There are also non-specific ST-T changes (hollow arrows).

This patient is hemodynamically stable and by history has probably been in flutter for at least 72 h prior to admission. Cardioversion should not be performed in patients with a history of atrial flutter greater than 48 h without performing a echocardiogram to rule out the existence of left atrial thrombus with the potential for thromboembolic events. Thrombus may be present in 10% to 34% of patients with atrial flutter after 72 h. Anticoagulation should be initiated for three weeks prior to attempted cardioversion in a relatively stable patient and echocardiography performed. Amiodarone can be used in the setting of ischemic episodes and systolic dysfunction. Although ibutilide has been used in the conversion of atrial flutter, it is recommended that it be avoided in the setting of acute coronary syndromes and electrolyte disturbances such as hypokalemia and decreased serum magnesium, as seen in this patient's history, due to a higher propensity to develop torsades. Beta-blockers are recommended for rate control in atrial flutter, but in conjunction with diltiazem can lead to marked bradycardia and heart block. Carotid massage can unmask flutter waves and help confirm the diagnosis of atrial flutter with 2:1 AV block, but does not convert the arrhythmia; the original ventricular rate resumes upon discontinuation. Therefore of the options listed, the combination of anticoagulation and amiodarone would be the most acceptable under this scenario.

Answer: B

Sidebotham D, Mckee A, Gillhman M, Levy JH (2007) *Cardio Thoracic Critical Care*. Butterworth Heinemann: Philadelphia.

Field J, Gonzales L, Hazinski M (2010) Advanced Cardiac Life Support Manual. American Heart Association.

Parillo JE, Dellinger RD (2008) *Critical Care Medicine Principles of Diagnosis and Management in the Adult*. Mosby: Philadelphia.

Gabrielli A, Layon AJ, Yu M (2009) *Civetta, Taylor & Kirby's Critical Care*. Lippincott Williams and Wilkins: Philadelphia.

Armstrong WF, Ryan T (2010) *Feigenbaum's Echocardiography*. Lippincott Williams & Wilkins: Philadelphia.

12. *One week after colonoscopy, a 65-year-old man complains of increasing fatigue and shortness of breath. Examination reveals BP 110/70 mm Hg, HR 105 beats/minute, marked crackles at both lung bases, and a systolic murmur 4/6 at the base of the heart. An electrocardiogram reveals evidence of recent inferior myocardial infarction. Chest x-ray reveals bilateral pulmonary edema. An echocardiogram is shown.*

Which of the following statements is true in regards to the myocardial complication illustrated?

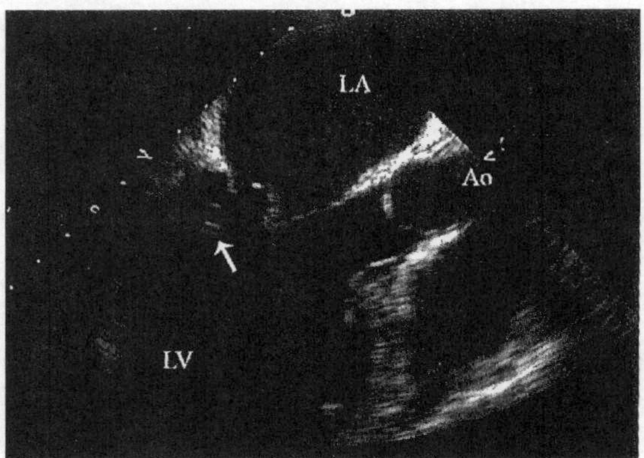

A. The anterolateral papillary muscle is more likely to rupture do to its blood supply

B. Fifty percent of patients have a step up in oxygen content between the right atrium and right ventricle

C. The severity of mitral regurgitation following of acute myocardial infarction is an independent predictor of survival

D. Intra aortic balloon pump utilization is contraindicated due to the risk of significant left ventricular overload

E. Papillary muscle rupture most commonly occurs in the first 24 hours of a significant myocardial infarction

Rupture of the posteromedial papillary muscle represents the majority of the papillary muscle ruptures as it is solely supplied by the posterior descending branch of the right coronary artery. The anterolateral papillary muscle is less likely to rupture having a dual supply from both the diagonal branches of the left anterior descending and circumflex marginal artery branches. In this particular clinical scenario a myocardial infarction was precipitated by the stress of colonoscopy. Papillary muscle rupture should be considered in the differential diagnosis when pulmonary edema develops two to nine days post infarction coinciding with the necrosis of the papillary head. On physical examination, a new apical systolic murmur may be present, audible at the base of the heart, ending prior to S2. A palpable thrill is uncommon. Pulmonary artery catheterization will reveal the presence of a regurgitant left atrial V wave with no evidence of a step up in oxygenation in the right atrium or right ventricle. The echocardiogram reveals prolapse of the posterior mitral leaflet into the left ventricle (the arrow is pointing to the vague outline of the ruptured head of the papillary muscle). There is a significant correlation between mortality and increasing severity of mitral regurgitation on echocardiography in the setting of acute infarction. The acute mitral regurgitation results in a sudden volume overload of the left ventricle. Left ventricular dilation does not have time to develop resulting in abrupt rises in left ventricular end-diastolic and left atrial pressure; subsequently pulmonary hypertension, pulmonary edema, acute right ventricular dysfunction followed by cardiogenic shock. Definitive treatment is expedient surgery, however stabilization requires vasodilating drugs and intra-aortic balloon counter pulsation to promote forward flow.

Answer: C

Cohn LH, Edmunds LH (2003) *Cardiac Surgery in the Adult*. The McGraw-Hill Companies: New York.

Parillo JE, Dellinger RD (2008) *Critical Care Medicine Principles of Diagnosis and Management in the Adult*. Mosby: Philadelphia.

Gabelli A, Layon AJ, Yu M (2009) *Civetta, Taylor & Kirby's Critical Care*. Lippincott Williams and Wilkins: Philadelphia.

Antonio Rosso, et al. (2008) Clinical Outcome after Surgical Correction of Mitral Regurgitation due to Papillary Muscle Rupture. *Circulation* **118**, 1528–1534.

Thompson CR, Buller CE, Sleeper, LA, *et al.* (2000) Cardiogenic Shock due to acute severe mitral regurgitation complicating acute myocardial infarction: a report from the SHOCK Trial Registry. *J A College of Cardiology* **36** (3) (supplement I), 1104–1109.

Tcheng JE, Jacman JD, Nelson CI, *et al.* (1992) Outcome of Patients Substaining Acute Ischemic Mitral Regurgitation during Myocardial Infarction. *Ann Internal Medicine* **117**, 18–24.

Hochman JS, Buller CE, Sleeper, *et al.* (2000) Cardiogenic Shock Complicating Acute Myocardial Infarction: etiologies, management and outcomes: overall findings of the SHOCK Trial Registry. *J Am College of Cardiology* **36**, 1063–1070.

Califf R, Roe M (2010) *Acute Coronary Syndrome Essentials*. Jones and Bartlett Learning.

13. *A 67-year-old man with dementia and severe pancreatitis required chemical restraint to undergo an abdominal CT. On examination he is sedated with a HR 100 beats/minute, BP110/70 mm Hg, and*

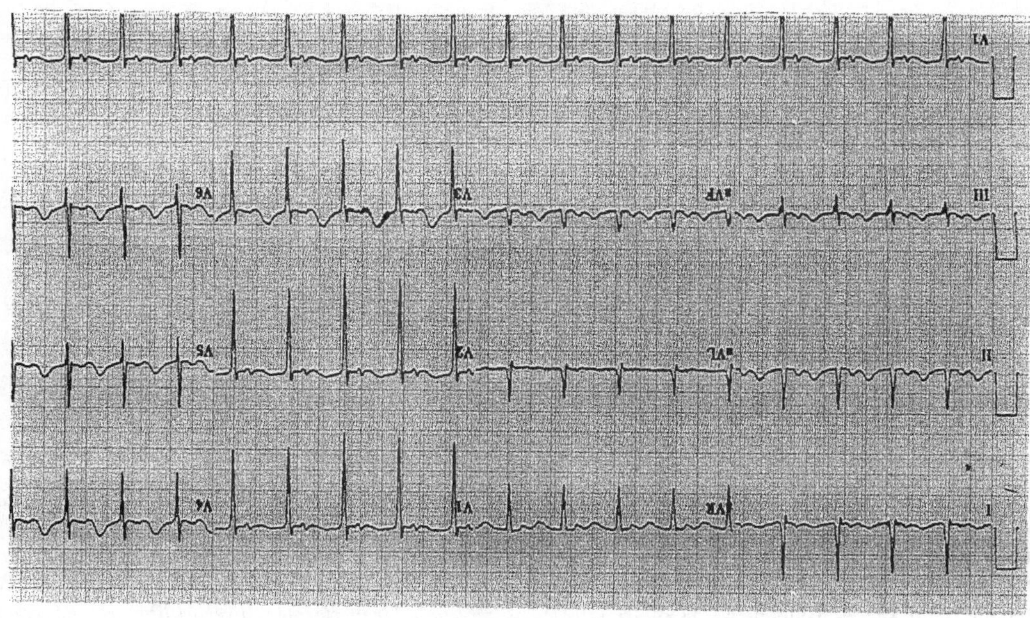

RR 17 breaths/minute. His ionized calcium is 3.2 mg/dl and his serum phosphorus 2.0 mg/dl. His electrocardiogram is illustrated above.

Two days post admission he becomes profoundly hypertensive and the following rhythm strip is generated.

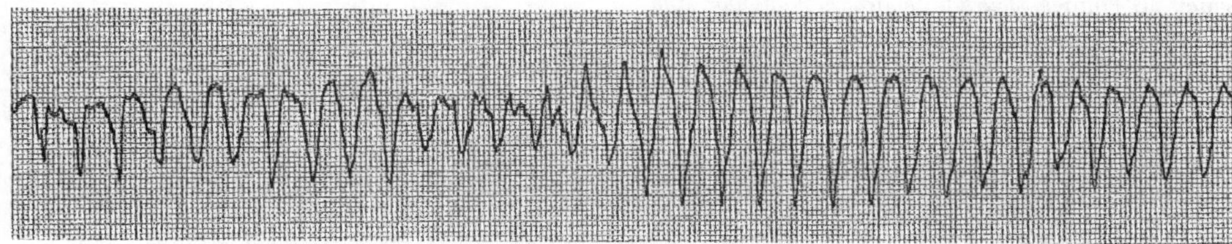

The patient is immediately cardioverted with a return to his baseline rhythm on his monitor and demonstrates a return of his blood pressure to 110/70 mm Hg. Following cardioversion, which agent should be given next?

A. *IV amiodarone*

B. *IV lidocaine*

C. *IV ibutilide*

D. *IV β blocker*

E. *IV magnesium*

The rhythm strip reveals polymorphic ventricular tachycardia consistent with torsades de pointes. The patient was at high risk of developing torsades on the basis of his history and sinus tachycardia on admission. The EKG also revealed a prolonged QT interval where the QT interval is greater than 50% of the R to R interval in lead II.

Polymorphic ventricular tachycardia is poorly tolerated and may degenerate into ventricular fibrillation. In addition to immediate cardioversion, intravenous magnesium (dose of 1–2 gm) should be given over one to two minutes, as well as correction of any underlying electrolyte abnormality. Ibutilide and amiodarone are contraindicated as they worsen QT prolongation. Lidocaine and B-blockers are ineffective.

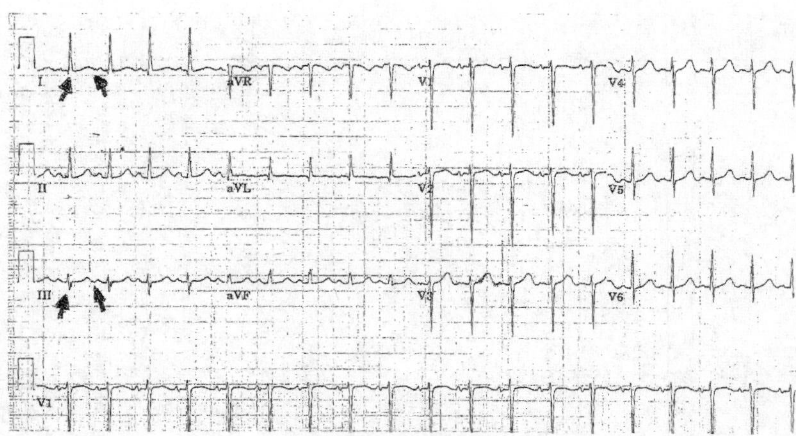

12 lead ECG with solid arrows showing prolonged QT interval

Answer: E

Sidebotham D, Mckee A, Gillham M, Levy JH (2007) *Cardiothoracic Critical Care*. Butterworth Heinemann: Philadelphia.

Parillo JE, Dellinger RD (2008) *Critical Care Medicine: Principles of Diagnosis and Management in the Adult*. Mosby: Philadelphia.

Gabelli A, Layon AJ, Yu M (2009) *Civetta, Taylor & Kirby's Critical Care*. Lippincott Williams and Wilkins: Philadelphia.

Aggerwal R, Prakash O, Medii B (2006) Drug Induced Torsades de Pointes. *Journal of Medical Education and Research* **8** (4), 185–189.

14. *A 58-year-old man develops chest pain on the third postoperative day following emergent sigmoid colon resection for perforated diverticulitis. He has repeated episodes of emesis. The patient becomes progressively more hypotensive, and on examination, a positive Kussmaul's sign. An initial electrocardiogram is performed as illustrated.*

A Swan–Ganz catheter is inserted and the ratio of right atrial pressure to wedge pressure is less than 0.8. A selective right-sided chest lead ECG is carried out as illustrated in the following ECG a few hours later.

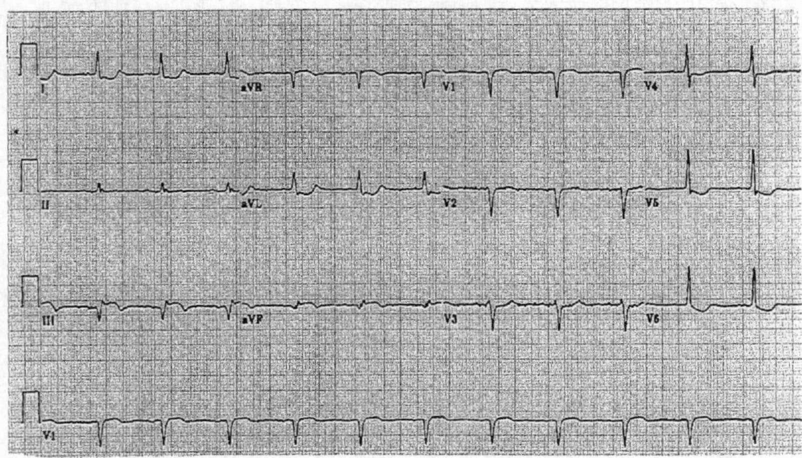

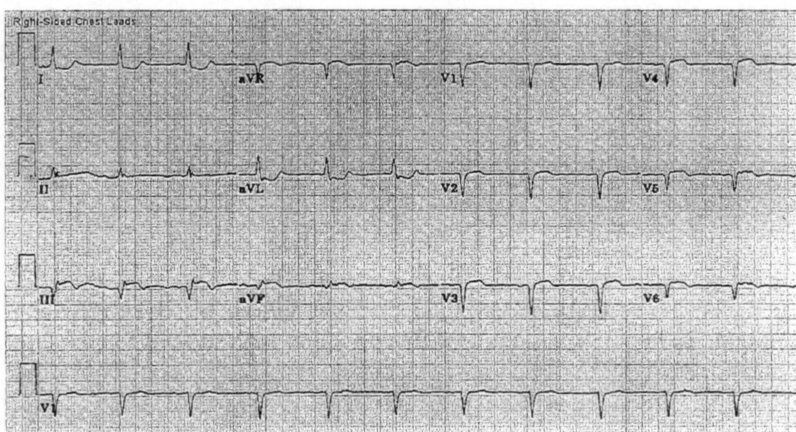

Right-sided chest ECG

Which of the following statements regarding this condition is most correct?

A. *Patients with this type of myocardial infarction complication are older*

B. *Hospital mortality is 25% with defibrillation*

C. *More commonly associated with multi-vessel disease*

D. *Bezold-Jarisch reflex is associated with reperfusion*

E. *The patient should undergo diuresis to relieve his volume overload*

This patient has a significant right-ventricular infarction. Right-ventricular infarct occurs in 30% of inferior infarcts and 10% of anterior infarcts.

The initial 12 lead reveals ST segment elevation and T wave inversion in the inferior leads (solid arrows). There is 1 mm of ST segment elevation in lead V1 (hollow arrows). There is also lateral ST segment depression. These findings represent a concomitant acute right ventricular infarction. Verification can be obtained by performing a right-sided tracing. It is important to assess leads V1-2 for ST segment elevation and R wave prominence, which may reflect a right-ventricular or posterior myocardial infarction.

The right-sided ECG in the following figure reveals inferior Q wave formation (solid arrows) and ST elevation (hollow arrows), which are

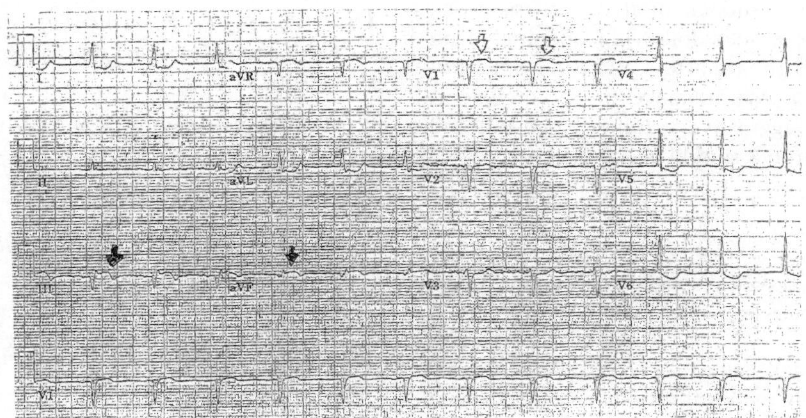

12 lead ECG with arrows inferior MI

indicative of an acute inferior myocardial infarction. ST elevation is present in leads V2-6R, consistent with an acute right-ventricular infarction.

Lim ST, Goldstien JA (2001) RT Ventricular Infarction. *Current Treatment options in Cardiovascular Medicine* **3**, 95–101.

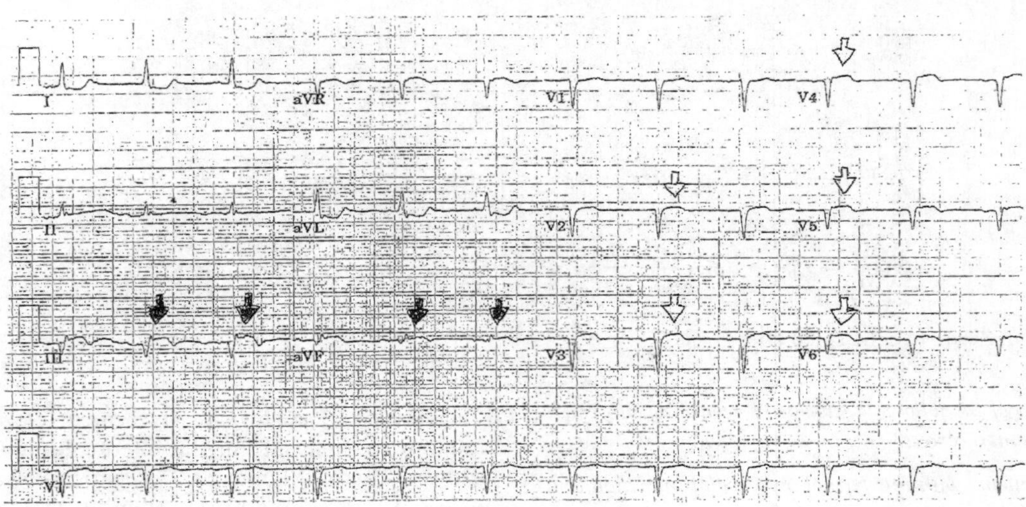

RT sided chest lead ECG

Right ventricular infarction is suggested by the presence of Kussmaul's sign (jugular venous distention on inspiration), in the presence of hypotension with inferior myocardial infarctions. Pulmonary artery catheterization reveals that the right atrial pressure exceeds 10 mm Hg and the ratio of right atrial pressure to wedge pressure is less than 0.8. Treatment requires early reperfusion by mechanical or thrombolytic means. The Bezold–Jarisch reflex is a sudden bradycardia associated with hypotension, seen following opening of an occluded right coronary artery and is a sympatho-inhibitory reflex. Maintenance of RV preload is important with aggressive volume expansion and nitrates and diuretics should be avoided.

Answer: D

Gabelli A, Layon AJ, Yu M (2009) *Civetta, Taylor & Kirby's Critical Care*. Lippincott Williams and Wilkins: Philadelphia.

Jacobs A, Leopold J, Bates E, *et al.* (2003) Cardiogenic Shock caused by RT Ventricular Infarction: A report from the SHOCK Registry. *J Am College of Cardiology* **41**, 1273–1279.

Lim ST, Goldstien JA (2001) RT Ventricular Infarction. *Current Treatment options in Cardiovascular Medicine* **3**, 95–101.

Robalino BD, Whitlow PL, Underwood PA, *et al.* (1989) Electrocardiographic manifestations of RT Ventricular Infarction. *Am Heart J* **118**, 138–144.

Haj, SA, Movahed, A (2000) Right Ventricular Infarction-diagnosis and treatment. *Clinical Cardiology* **23**, 473–482.

15. *Which of the following statements regarding fibrinolytic therapy in acute coronary syndromes is false? Thrombolytics:*

A. *Obtain acute patency rates of 50–60%*

B. *Are indicated in patients with LBBB presenting within 12 hours of symptoms*

C. *Are contraindicated in patients with ischemic stroke within 3 months*

D. *Are relatively contraindicated in severe uncontrolled hypertension on presentation (systolic BP >220 mm Hg or diastolic BP >100 mm Hg)*

E. *Have an associated risk of intracranial hemorrhage of 0.5 to 1.5%*

The limitations of fibrinolytic therapy include acute patency rates of infarct vessels of only 50 to 60%. The incidence of intracranial hemorrhage is 0.5% to 1.5%. The indications for use include: MI with ST-segment elevation or LBBB who present within 12 hours of onset.

Absolute contraindications include:
- Any prior intracranial hemorrhage, trauma, lesion, or neoplasm
- Prior ischemic stroke within 3 months
- Active bleeding

A relative contraindication is uncontrolled hypertension on presentation (systolic BP >180 mm Hg or diastolic BP >110 mm Hg)

Answer: D

Antman EA, Anbe TO, Armstrong PW, *et al.* (2004) ACC/AHA Guidelines for Management of Patients with StElevation Myocardial Infarctions. *J Am College of College of Cardiology* **44**, 671–719.
Parillo JE, Dellinger RD (2008) *Critical Care Medicine: Principles of Diagnosis and Management in the Adult*. Mosby: Philadelphia.
Califf R, Roe M (2010) *Acute Coronary Syndrome Essentials*. Jones and Bartlett Learning.

16. *Which of the following statements concerning the utilization of coronary artery bypass for acute coronary syndrome is false?*

A. *Perioperative mortality for elective CABG three to seven days after acute MI is not increased*

B. *Clopidogrel should be discontinued at least ten days prior to CABG*

C. *Diabetics with multivessel disease and prior PTCA have better outcomes with CABG versus repeat PTCA*

D. *CABG following fibrinolytic therapy leads to reoperation for bleeding in 4%*

E. *Mortality rates for emergent CABG following failed fibrinolytic therapy is 15%*

Plavix should be held for five to seven days prior to CABG to minimize the risk of perioperative bleeding. CABG for patients with preserved LV function who require revascularization can be safely performed within a few days of a STEMI. The other statements are all true.

Answer: B

The BARI (Bypass Angioplasty Revasculization Investigation) Investigators (2000) Seven Year Outcome by Treatment. *J Am College of Cardiology* **35**, 1122–1129.
Califf R, Roe M (2010) *Acute Coronary Syndrome Essentials*. Jones and Bartlett Learning.
Parillo IE, Dellinger RD (2008) *Critical Care Medicine: Pirinciples of Diagnosis and Management in the Adult*. Mosby: Philadelphia.

17. *A 73-year-old man undergoes a right hemicolectomy. He has a history of hypertension and hyperlipidemia. Forty-eight hours after the procedure, he complains of epigastric discomfort. An electrocardiogram is performed and is illustrated below.*

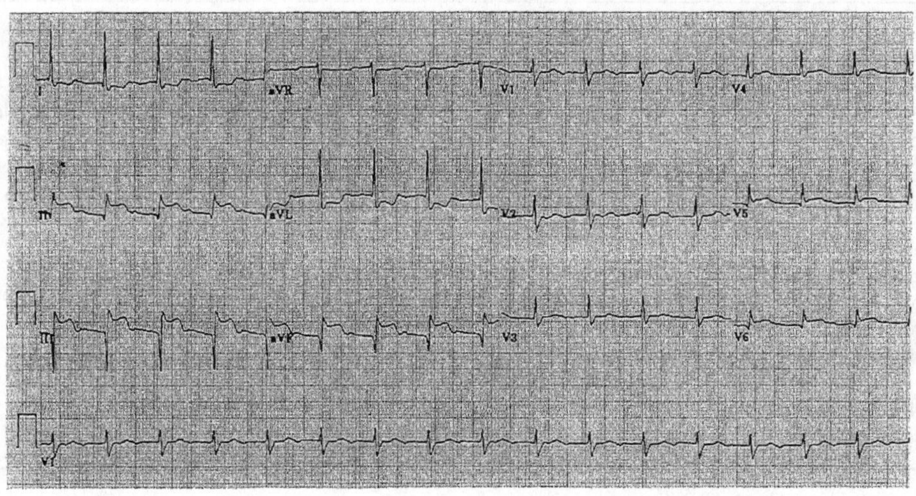

He is treated conservatively but seventy-two hours later is noted to have a new pan-systolic murmur and a palpable thrill along the left sternal border. An echocardiogram is performed as illustrated below.

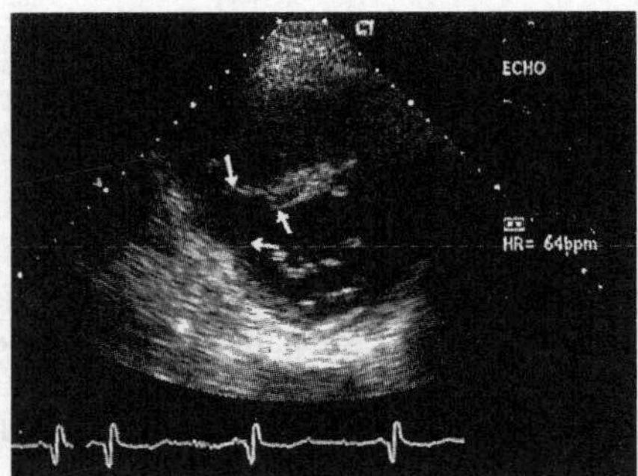

Of the following statements concerning the clinical scenario depicted above, which is correct?

A. Most commonly occurs with inferior-posterior myocardial infarctions

B. If pulmonary artery catheterization were performed you would expect a prominent v-wave in the pulmonary capillary wedge pressure tracing

C. This complication is found in 5% to 6% of acute myocardial infarctions

D. The expected mortality would be 40% to 60% with medical therapy, and is equivalent to surgical intervention at one year

E. Survival is worse with inferior posterior infarctions compared to anterior infarctions

The patient has a postmyocardial infarction VSD, which complicates 0.5 to 2% of acute myocardial infarctions, occurring two to five days following the event. Patients are older with multi-vessel disease. Rupture of the interventricular septum is more common with anterior myocardial infarctions because the septum is supplied by the septal perforating branches of the left anterior descending artery. Evidence of the septal necrosis is heralded by a pan-systolic murmur at left sternal border indicating a significant VSD. Diagnosis is confirmed by two-dimensional echocardiography combined with Doppler flow studies. The echocardiogram illustrated in the figure demonstrates an inferior septal defect with thinning of portions of the necrotic septal wall (arrows). Pulmonary artery catheterization with oximetry demonstrates a greater than 5 to 7% step-up in oxygenation between the right atrium and ventricle. There is an absence of V waves in the pulmonary artery wedge pressure tracing, which differentiate a ventricular septal defect from a papillary muscle rupture. VSD is the cause of death in 5% of all fatal myocardial infarctions. The SHOCK study revealed that twenty-five percent of patients die in the first 24 hours and 50% at one week with a 90% in-hospital mortality rate when there is associated cardiogenic shock. The survival for inferior-posterior or right ventricular associated ventricular septal defects is worse than for those with anterior myocardial infarctions.

High Risk	Intermediate Risk	Low Risk
At least one feature must be present:	No high-risk features but must have one of the following:	No high- or intermediate-risk features but may have any of the following:
• Prolonged (>20 min) ongoing rest pain	• Prolonged (>20 min) rest angina, now resolved, with moderate or high likelihood of coronary heart disease	• New-onset angina or progressive CCS class III–IV angina without prolonged (>20 min) chest pain but with moderate or high likelihood of coronary heart disease
• Angina at rest with dynamic ST-depression ≥0.5 mm or new bundle branch block	• Rest angina (<20 min) relieved with rest or sublingual nitroglycerin	
• Angina with new or worsening MR murmur	• Angina with dynamic T-wave changes >2.0 mm or abnormal O-waves	
• Angina with new or worsening rales, or pulmonary edema	• Angina use hospitalization	

High Risk	Intermediate Risk	Low Risk
• Angina with hypotension, bradycardia, or tachycardia	• Prior MI or CABG	• Normal or unchanged ECG during chest discomfort
• Age ≥75 years	• Peripheral vascular disease or cerebrovascular disease	
• Elevated cardiac troponins (>0.1 ng/mL)	• Slightly elevated cardiac troponins (>0.01 ng/mL but <0.1 ng/mL)	• Cardiac markers not elevated
• Sustained ventricular tachycardia	• Age >70 years	

Answer: E

Gabelli A, Layon AJ, Yu M (2009) *Civetta, Taylor & Kirby's Critical Care*. Lippincott, Williams and Wilkins: Phildelphia.

Armstrong WF, Ryann T (2010) *Feigenbaum's Echocardiography*. Williams & Wilkins: Lipipncott.

Topaz O, Taylor AL (1992) Interventricular Septal rupture complicating acute myocardial infarction: from path physiologic features to the role of invasive and non invasive diagnostic modalities in current management. *Am J Med* **93**, 683–688.

Blanche C, Khan SS, Choux A, Metloff JM (1994) Post Infarction Ventricular Septal Defect in the elderly: analysis and results. *Ann Thoracic Surg* **57**, 91–98.

Levey R et al. Prognosis in Rupture of Ventricular infarct and the role of early Surgical Intervention. *Am J.*

18. *All of the following represent features associated with non-ST elevated-acute coronary syndromes with high risk for short-term death or non-fatal myocardial infarction except:*

A. *Age greater than 75*

B. *Angina with elevated T waves greater than 2.0 mm or abnormal Q-waves*

C. *Angina with new or worsening mitral regurgitation*

D. *Sustained ventricular tachycardia*

E. *Prolonged (>20 min) ongoing chest pain*

The updated ACC/AHA guidelines recommend risk-category classification for NSTE-ACS patients to serve as a basis for initial management decisions. Recommendations range from immediate angiography, GP IIb/IIIa inhibitors, or PCI for high-risk patients to outpatient management for low-risk patient. These are based on the risk for short-term death or nonfatal myocardial infarctions. Risk prediction scores use determinants of low, intermediate and high risk as illustrated in the following table.

Answer: B

Anderson JL, et al (2007) ACC/AHA Guidelines for the Management of Patients with Unstable Anginainon-st Elevation Myocardial Infarction. *J Am College Cardiology* **50**, 5652–726.

Wright SR, et al (2011) ACCF/AHA Focused Update Incorporated into the ACC/AHA 2007 Guidelines for Management of Patients with UnstablelNon St Elevated Myocardial Infarction. *J Am College Cardiology* **57**, 215–367.

Califf R, Roe M (2010) *Acute Coronary Syndrome Essentials*. Jones and Bartlett Learning.

19. *A 69-year-old man on postoperative day 3 following a small bowel resection for ischemia, demonstrates ST changes on a routine electrocardiogram. The patient has not voiced complaints and cardiac enzymes are drawn. That evening the patient suddenly demonstrates the following rhythm after being found unresponsive.*
The blood pressure is 50/20 mm Hg and no pulse is detected. Cardioversion is immediately attempted without success and repeated cycles of CPR and epinephrine is alternated with vasopressin followed by repeat cardioversion. The rhythm remains unchanged.

What would be the next most appropriate management step in this setting?

A. *IV procainamide*

B. *IV magnesium*

C. *IV lidocaine*

D. *IV amiodarone*

E. *IV bretylium tosylate*

Ventricular fibrillation (VF) occurs within the first four hours following a MI in 4% of patients. VF

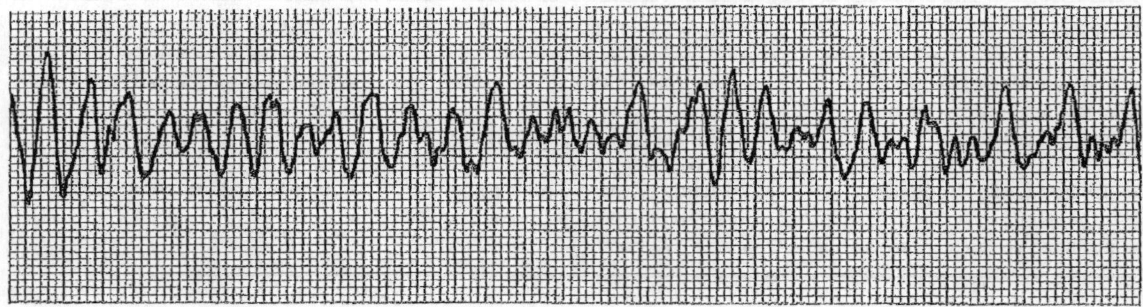

can usually be cardioverted within the first minute but is less than 25% successful when initiated after 4 minutes. Current ACLS guidelines for witnessed arrest recommend immediate unsynchronized defibrillation at 200 J monophasic followed by resumption of CPR for 2 minutes or five cycles. Epinephrine 1 mg IV push every 3 to 5 minutes or vasopressin 40 U IV once, for persistent VF. After five cycles of CPR, if the patient persists in VF, another shock should be delivered. If VF persists, amiodarone (300 mg or 5 mg/kg, IV bolus) should be given. Procainamide is an option for intermittent or recurrent VF but is not recommended acutely due to its long administration time. Magnesium (1–2 gm IV bolus over 5 min) would be recommended for torsades de pointes. Lidocaine has no short-term or long-term efficacy in cardiac arrest while amiodarone has demonstrated increased survival to hospital admission compared to lidocaine. Bretylium tosylate is no longer recommended for use in cardiac arrest.

Answer: D

Gabelli A. Layon AJ, YU M (2009) *Civetta, Taylor & Kirby's Critical Care*. Lippincott, Williams and Wilkins: Philadelphia.

Sidenbotham D, Mckee A, Gillham M, Levy JH (2007) *Cardio Thoracic Critical Care*. Butterworth Heinemann: Philadelphia.

Field J, Gonzales L, Hazinski M (2010) *Advanced Cardiac Life Support*. American Heart Association.

20. *From the list of hemodynamic findings below, match the post-myocardial infarction complication:*

A. *Increased RAP; RAP/PCWP ratio>0.8; decreased CO*

B. *Decreased BP; decreased CO; increased PCWP; increased SVR*

C. *Increased PCWP (prominent V-wave may be seen); CO decreased*

D. *Decreased BP; paradoxical pulse; RAP approximates PCWP; decreased CO; prominent X descent on CVP*

E. *Oxygen step-up from RA to RV/PA. Increased left-to-right shunting with increased pulmonary blood flow results in falsely elevated CO*

1 *Acute mitral regurgitation*

2 *Cardiac tamponade*

3 *Acute ventricular septal defect*

4 *Right ventricular infarct*

5 *Cardiogenic shock*

As per the discussions listed in the answer sections for questions 9, 12, 14, 17 it is important to recognize the hemodynamic variations that exist between the different surgical complications associated with acute myocardial infarctions do to the variation required in their management.

Answer: 1. C., 2. D., 3. E., 4. A., 5. B

Gabelli A, Layon AJ, Yu M (2009) *Civetta, Taylor & Kirby's Critical Care*. Lippincott, Butterworth Heinemann: Philadelphia.

Sidenbotham D, Mckee A, Gillham M, Levy JH (2007) *Cardio Thoracic Critical Care*. Butterworth Heinemann: Philadelphia.

Parrillo JE, Dellinger RP (2008) *Critical Care Medicine: Principles of Diagnosis and Management in the Adult*. Mosby: Philadelphia.

Chapter 4 Sepsis and the Inflammatory Response to Injury

Juan C. Duchesne, MD, FACS, FCCP and Marquinn D. Duke, MD

1. *Which of the following treatments has been shown in a large randomized, multicenter trial to reduce mortality in patients with septic shock?*

A. *Intravenous (IV) immunoglobulin*

B. *IV hydrocortisone*

C. *IV Pentastarch*

D. *Renal Replacement Therapy (RRT)*

E. *Drotrecogin alfa (activated)*

Recombinant human activated protein C, or drotrecogin alfa (activated), is the only FDA-approved treatment for reducing mortality in patients with severe sepsis and a high risk of death. In a large, randomized, placebo controlled trial of patients with severe sepsis (PROWESS trial), drotrecogin alfa administered as a continuous IV infusion at 24 μg/kg/h for 96 hours resulted in a 19.4% relative risk reduction in the risk of death. This survival benefit was even more pronounced in patients with more than one organ dysfunction or APACHE II score of 24 or greater. The other choices have shown anecdotal evidence of efficacy, but have not shown statistically significant benefit in randomized trials.

Answer: E

Bernard GR, Vincent JL, Laterre PF, *et al.* (2001) Recombinant human protein C Worldwide Evaluation in Severe Sepsis (Prowess) Study Group. Efficacy and safety of recombinant human activated protein C for severe sepsis. *New England Journal of Medicine* **344**, 699–709.

Surgical Critical Care and Emergency Surgery: Clinical Questions and Answers, First Edition. Edited by Forrest O. Moore, Peter M. Rhee, Samuel A. Tisherman and Gerard J. Fulda.

2. *A 67-year-old man with a history of chronic obstructive pulmonary disease (COPD), hypertension, and chronic renal failure is admitted to the ICU with community-acquired pneumonia. His treatment includes broad-spectrum antibiotics, corticosteroids, and inhaled β2 stimulants. Due to a severe ileus and gastric intolerance, total parenteral nutrition is commenced. The patient's temperature normalizes after the third day in ICU, and his oxygenation improves. However, on the ninth hospital day he develops a fever with an increase in the peripheral leukocyte count. Antibiotics are stopped and blood, urine, and sputum cultures are performed. Candida krusei is isolated from a single blood culture, and 60 000 CFU/mL of* C. krusei *is isolated from the urine. Which of the following is the most appropriate next step in the management of this patient?*

A. *Remove, culture, and replace all vascular catheters*

B. *Remove, culture, and replace all vascular catheters and begin intravenous (IV) fluconazole*

C. *Remove, culture, and replace all vascular catheters and begin an echinocandin*

D. *Remove, culture, and replace all vascular catheters; replace urinary catheter; and begin amphotericin bladder irrigations*

E. *Repeat the blood and urine cultures and observe the patient*

The risk factors for Candida intravascular infection include use of broad-spectrum antibiotics, total parenteral nutrition, and immunosuppressive therapy. A single positive blood culture is highly predictive of systemic Candida infection, so it should never be considered a contaminant. The initial treatment of Candida infections includes removal of all possible foci of infection, including removal of intravascular lines. Candidemia may resolve spontaneously after removal of intravascular catheters. However, evidence increasingly suggests that metastatic foci of infection may develop in some patients even after catheter removal and may manifest as endophthalmitis, endocarditis, arthritis, or meningitis. Therefore, all critically ill patients with candidemia should be regarded as having a systemic infection and should be treated accordingly. Fluconazole and amphotericin demonstrate similar effectiveness in treating candidemia in patients without neutropenia and without major immunodeficiency. However, both *in vitro* and clinical data have demonstrated *C. krusei* to be intrinsically resistant to fluconazole. Prolonged bladder catheterization in the critically ill patient is often accompanied by the appearance of candiduria. Candiduria usually reflects catheter colonization; however, rarely, Candida species may cause cystitis and/or retrograde renal parenchymal infection. The management of asymptomatic candiduria in the catheterized patient, in whom no suspicion of renal candidiasis or renal obstruction exists, requires change of the indwelling catheter only, followed by observation. No data suggest that amphotericin B bladder irrigations prevent infections in colonized patients. Echinocandins can also be used to treat *C. Krusei.* It covers a broad range and can be used against Candida. It cannot be used in pregnancy and needs adjustment in liver disease. Its efficacy is equal to amphotericin B but it has fewer side effects.

Answer: C

Denning DW (2003) Echinocandin drugs. *Lancet* **362** (9390), 1142–51.

3. *All of the following are components of early goal-directed therapy (EGDT) in patients with severe sepsis/septic shock except*

A. *IV fluid resuscitation targeting CVP 8 to 12 cm H_2O*

B. *IV vasodilator infusion to maintain MAP < 90 mm Hg*

C. *IV vasopressor infusion to maintain MAP > 65 mm Hg*

D. *Transfusion of packed RBCs to achieve hematocrit > 35% if venous oxygen saturation (Svo2) < 70%*

E. *Placement of a central venous line able to continuously monitor Svo2*

Therapy targeting a specific blood pressure and oxygen delivery has been tried unsuccessfully in many critical care diseases. However, goal-directed therapy, directed by continuous measurement of central Svo2, has been shown to reduce mortality of patients with severe sepsis when initiated early in their hospital course. The initiation and continuation of EGDT in the ED for 6 hours resulted in a 16% absolute and 34% relative reduction in hospital mortality (46.5% versus 30.5%) as compared with standard care. EGDT patients received protocolized care consisting of the following: (1) placement of a central venous line able to continuously monitor Svo2; (2) IV volume resuscitation using crystalloids or colloids to achieve a CVP of 8 to 12 cm H_2O; and (3) initiation of vasopressor agents to maintain MAP greater than 65 mm Hg or vasodilator agents to maintain MAP less than 90 mm Hg. Once the patient reached a CVP of 8 to 12 cm H_2O and MAP of 65 to 90 mm Hg, care was directed using Svo2. Patients with Svo2 less than 70% were transfused with packed RBCs to achieve hematocrit values above 30%. If the hematocrit was above 30% but the Svo2 remained below 70%, dobutamine infusion was initiated.

Answer: D

Rivers E, Nguyen B, Havstad S, *et al.* (2001) Early Goal-Directed Therapy Collaborative Group. Early goal-directed therapy in the treatment of severe sepsis and septic shock. *New England Journal of Medicine* **345**, 1368–77.

4. *Which of the following is true of vasopressin in septic shock?*

A. *Continuous infusion at low doses improves 28-day overall mortality*

B. *Continuous infusion at low doses improves mortality in patients with severe septic shock*

C. *Continuous infusion at low doses increases cardiac output*

D. *Continuous infusion at low doses reduces the catecholamine infusion requirement*

E. *Is the first line vasopressor for septic shock*

Vasopressin is a peptide synthesized in the hypothalamus and released from the posterior pituitary. Vasopressin produces a wide range of physiologic effects, including blood-pressure maintenance. Acting through vascular V1-receptors, the endogenous hormone directly induces vasoconstriction in hypotensive patients but does not significantly alter vascular smooth muscle constriction in humans with normal blood pressure. Landry and colleagues demonstrated that patients with septic shock had inappropriately low levels of serum vasopressin compared with patients with cardiogenic shock, who had normal or elevated levels. In addition, they demonstrated that supplementing a low-dose infusion of vasopressin in septic shock patients allowed for the reduction or removal of the other catecholamine vasopressors. This was seen despite a reduction in cardiac output. Although these results were duplicated in subsequent studies, none evaluated outcomes such as length of stay or mortality until recently. A randomized double-blind study comparing vasopressin versus norepinephrine for the treatment of septic shock demonstrated no difference in 28-day mortality between the two treatment groups. Subgroup analysis of patients with severe septic shock, defined as requiring 15 μg/min of norepinephrine or its equivalent, also did not demonstrate a mortality benefit. However, patients with less severe septic shock (requiring 5–15 μg/min of norepinephrine) experienced a trend toward lower mortality when treated with low-dose (0.01–0.03 U/min) vasopressin.

Answer: D

Gordon AC, Hébert PC, Cooper DJ, *et al.* (2008) Vasopressin versus norepinephrine infusion in patients with septic shock. *New England Journal of Medicine* **358**, 877–87.

Landry DW, Levin HR, Gallant EM, *et al.* (1997) Vasopressin deficiency contributes to the vasodilation of septic shock. *Circulation* **95**, 1122–5.

5. *All of the following are principles of antibiotic prophylaxis to prevent surgical site infection except:*

A. *Administer intravenous (IV) antibiotics within one hour of incision time*

B. *Select an antibiotic with a spectrum of activity against pathogens likely to be encountered during surgery*

C. *Discontinue antibiotics 48 hours postoperatively*

D. *Intraoperatively redose cephalosporin prophylactic antibiotics every two half-lives for long procedures*

E. *Antibiotics should not be administered after the wound is closed unless there is suspicion of contamination*

As a result of a forum held by National Surgical Infection Prevention project leaders, consensus was reached regarding antibiotic selection, timing, and duration for select types of surgery. It is recommended that IV antibiotics used to prevent surgical site infection should be given within one hour before surgery and should not be used for more than 24 hours postoperatively. In addition, prophylactic antibiotics should be selected for various procedures based on pathogens likely to be encountered. Redosing of antibiotics (not only cephalosporins) during surgery is recommended for long procedures or for patients with blood loss or a large amount of fluid administration. Antibiotics should not be administered after the wound is closed unless there is suspicion of contamination, at which point the duration of therapy should not exceed 24 hours.

Answer: C

Bratzler DW, Houck PM (2004) Antimicrobial prophylaxis for surgery: an advisory statement from the National Surgical Infection Project. *Clinical Infectious Diseases* **38**, 1706–15.

6. *All of the following can decrease the rate of surgical site infection in the colorectal surgical patient except*

A. *IV antibiotic administration preoperatively*

B. *Oral antibiotic bowel preparation*

C. *Postoperative prophylactic antibiotics*

D. *Targeting Escherichia coli and* Bacteroides fragilis *with prophylactic antibiotics*

E. *Thorough and complete mechanical bowel preparation*

It is estimated that 20% of patients undergoing intra-abdominal procedures will develop a surgical site infection, and in elective colorectal resections, this incidence is reported to be as high as 26%. To reduce surgical site infection in colorectal surgery, IV antibiotics should be administered preoperatively and as close to the time of incision as possible. In colorectal surgery, *E. coli* and *B. fragilis* are the target pathogens. Systemic antibiotics after wound closure have not been shown to reduce surgical site infection rates. Prolonged postoperative administration increases cost, produces resistance, and will cause antibiotic-associated morbidity. Each patient must have a thorough and complete mechanical bowel preparation. When properly given, oral antibiotics have been shown to reduce surgical site infections.

Answer: C

Fry DE (2005) The truth is in the dialogue. Surgical Infection Society–Europe Semmelweis Lecture. Surgical Infection Society–Europe. *Surg Infect (Larchmt)*. **6** (1), 19–25.

Smith RL, Bohl JK, McElearney ST, *et al.* (2004) Wound infection after elective colorectal resection. *Annals of Surgery* **239**, 599–608.

Questions 7 and 8 refer to the following case.

A 70-year-old man presents to the emergency department with a 2-day history of fever, chills, cough, and right-sided pleuritic chest pain. On the day of admission, the patient's family noted that he was more lethargic and dizzy and was falling frequently. The patient's vital signs are: temperature, 101.5 °F; heart rate, 120 bpm; respiratory rate, 30 breaths/min; blood pressure, 70/35 mm Hg; and oxygen saturation as measured by pulse oximetry, 80% without oxygen supplementation. A chest radiograph shows a right lower lobe infiltrate.

7. *This patient's condition can best be defined as which of the following?*

A. *Multi-organ dysfunction syndrome (MODS)*

B. *Sepsis*

C. *Septic shock*

D. *Severe sepsis*

E. *Systemic inflammatory response syndrome (SIRS)*

8. *What is the first step in the initial management of this patient?*

A. *Antibiotic therapy*

B. *β-Blocker therapy to control heart rate*

C. *Intravenous (IV) fluid resuscitation*

D. *Supplemental oxygen and airway management*

E. *Vasopressor therapy with dopamine*

The patient fulfills criteria for severe sepsis, defined as sepsis with evidence of organ dysfunction, hypoperfusion, or hypotension. SIRS is defined as an inflammatory response to insult manifested by two of the following: temperature greater than 38 °C (100.4 °F) or less than 36 °C (96.8 °F), heart rate greater than 90 bpm, respiratory rate greater than 20 breaths/min, and white blood cell count greater that 12 × 103/μL, less than 4 × 103/μL, or 10% bands. A diagnosis of sepsis is given if infection is present in addition to meeting criteria for SIRS. Septic shock includes sepsis-induced hypotension (despite fluid resuscitation) along with evidence of hypoperfusion. MODS is the presence of altered organ function such that hemostasis cannot be maintained without intervention. This patient's lack of fluid resuscitation classifies him as having severe sepsis rather than septic shock.

The initial evaluation of any critically ill patient in shock should include assessing and establishing an airway, evaluating breathing (which includes consideration of mechanical ventilator support), and restoring adequate circulation. Adequate oxygenation should be ensured with a goal of achieving an arterial oxygen saturation of 90% or greater.

Answers: D, D

Bone RC, Balk RA, Cerra FB, *et al.* (1992) Definition for sepsis and organ failure and guidelines for the use of innovative therapies in sepsis. The ACCP/SCCM Consensus Conference Committee. American College of Chest Physicians/Society of Critical Care Medicine. *Chest* **101**, 1644–55.

Holmes CL, Walley KR (2003) The evaluation and management of shock. *Clinical Chest Medicine* **24**, 775–89.

9. *Which of the following is an indication for using corticosteroids in septic shock?*

A. Acute respiratory distress syndrome (ARDS)

B. Necrotizing pneumonia

C. Peritonitis

D. Sepsis responding well to fluid resuscitation

E. Vasopressor-dependent septic shock

An inappropriate cortisol response is common in patients with septic shock. Low-dose IV corticosteroids (hydrocortisone 200–300 mg/day) are recommended in patients with vasopressor-dependent septic shock. However, steroids should not be used in the absence of vasopressor requirement. Higher doses of corticosteroids have been shown to be harmful in severe sepsis. The use of adrenal function tests to guide decisions on corticosteroid therapy is considered a reasonable approach. An absolute incremental increase of 9 μg/dL at 30 or 60 minutes after administration of 250 μg of corticotropin was found as the best cutoff value to distinguish between adequate adrenal response (responders) and relative adrenal insufficiency (nonresponders). Another approach is to use IV dexamethasone 4 mg every 6 hours until a low-dose corticotropin stimulation test can be performed; dexamethasone does not interfere with the cortisol assay but will interfere with adrenal axis response. Corticosteroids may then be continued in nonresponders and discontinued in responders. While the Meduri protocol has been advocated for treatment of ARDS, patients must have no demonstrable infection for its recommended use. This includes undrained abscesses, disseminated fungal infections, and septic shock.

Answer: E

Rivers EP, Gaspari M, Saad GA, *et al.* (2001) Adrenal insufficiency in high-risk surgical ICU patients. *Chest* **119**, 889–96.

Annane D, Sebille V, Troche G, *et al.* (2000) A 3-level prognostic classification in septic shock based on cortisol levels and cortisol response to corticotropin. *Journal of the American Medical Association* **283**, 1038–45.

10. *Which one of the following represents an absolute contraindication to the use of drotrecogin alfa (activated) in septic shock patients?*

A. International normalized ratio (INR) of 1.9

B. Platelet count of 75 000 cells/μL

C. Hemorrhagic CVA two months ago

D. Lumbar puncture four hours ago

E. Post-trauma splenectomy seven days ago

In addition to anti-inflammatory properties, activated protein C also possesses anticoagulant and profibrinolytic properties, and, not unexpectedly, these properties increase the risk of bleeding in patients receiving drotrecogin alfa (activated). In the PROWESS trial, bleeding was the only adverse effect of administration of drotrecogin alfa (activated). Serious bleeding, defined as intracranial hemorrhage, life-threatening bleed, or bleeding that required administration of 3 U of packed RBCs on two consecutive days, occurred in 3.5% of patients receiving drotrecogin alfa (activated) as compared with 2% of those receiving placebo. This increased risk occurred primarily during the peri-infusion period. Any bleeding event during the 28-day study period also occurred more frequently in patients receiving drotrecogin alfa (activated) (24.9% versus 17.7% with placebo). rhAPC should not be given to any patient with a recent history (within three months) of hemorrhagic stroke due to the risk of intracranial hemorrhage. Post-hoc analysis of PROWESS trial data found that increased bleeding was associated with a platelet count that fell below 30 000 cells/μL and/or INR that rose above 3.0.1. As such, both represent relative contraindications to administration of rhAPC; the case patient has adequate platelets and an acceptable INR for rhAPC. Uncomplicated bedside procedures (such as lumbar puncture) are not contraindications to rhAPC therapy; rhAPC should be discontinued for two hours prior to the procedure and restarted once hemostasis is achieved.

Answer: C

Bernard GR, Vincent JL, Laterre P, *et al.* (2001) Recombinant human protein C Worldwide Evaluation in Severe Sepsis (Prowess) Study Group. Efficacy and safety of recombinant human activated protein C for severe sepsis. *New England Journal of Medicine* **344**, 699–709.

Dellinger RP, Levy MM, Carlet JM, *et al.* (2008) Surviving Sepsis Campaign: international guidelines for management of severe septic shock: 2008. *Critical Care Medicine* **36** (1), 296–327.

11. *Which of the following cytokines is/are pyrogenic?*

A. *IL-2*

B. *IL-4*

C. *IL-5*

D. *IL-12*

E. *TNF*

In response to stress, the host resets various set points in an attempt to maintain homeostasis. Neuroendocrine changes in this process may be manifested by fever. IL-1, IL-6 and TNF all stimulate PGE_2 synthesis. PGE_2 directly affects the hypothalamus and increases the hypothalamic temperature set point resulting in fever. In addition, PGE_2 stimulates vasoconstriction and shivering, both of which increase body core temperature and contribute to the fever. Of the choices available, only TNF is pyrogenic.

Answer: E

Mulholland MW, Lillemoe KD, Doherty G, *et al.* (2010) *Greenfield's Surgery: Scientific Principles and Practice*, Lippincott Williams & Wilkins, Philadelphia, PA.

12. *The major cause of vasodilation in sepsis appears to be mediated by:*

A. *ATP-sensitive potassium channels in smooth muscle*

B. *ATP-sensitive calcium channels in smooth muscle*

C. *l-arginine*

D. *Interruption of sympathetic afferents endings*

E. *None of the above*

The endothelium is an endocrine organ, capable of regulating the function of the microcirculation. The most important compound produced is nitric oxide (NO), an endogenous vasodilator. Its major effects are to cause local vasodilatation and inhibition of platelet aggregation. Nitric oxide is produced from l-arginine by nitric oxide synthetase (NOS), and its actions are mediated by cGMP. NO is an essential to the normal functioning of the vascular system. There are two forms of the enzyme nitric oxide synthetase, a constitutive form, produced as part of the normal regulatory mechanisms, and an inducible form, whose production appears to be pathologic. Inducible NOS (iNOS) is an offshoot of the inflammatory response, by TNF and other cytokines. It results in massive production of nitric oxide, causing widespread vasodilatation (due to loss of vasomotor tone) and hypotension, which is hyporeactive to adrenergic agents.

Nitric oxide has a physiological antagonist, endothelin-1, a potent vasoconstrictor whose circulating level is increased in cardiogenic shock and following severe trauma.

The major cause of vasodilation in sepsis appears to be mediated by ATP-sensitive potassium channels in smooth muscle. The result of activation is increased permeability of vascular smooth muscle cells to potassium, and hyperpolarization of the cell membranes, preventing muscle contraction, leading to vasodilation.

In addition to potassium channels and inducible nitric oxide, there is a relative deficiency of vasopressin in early sepsis, the cause and significance of which is unknown.

Answer: A

Jackson WF (2000) Ion channels and vascular tone. *Hypertension* **35**(1 Pt 2), 173–8.

Landry DW, Levin HR, Gallant EM, *et al.* (1997) Vasopressin deficiency contributes to the vasodilation of septic shock. *Circulation* **95**, 1122–5.

13. *The natural defense against infection includes all of the following except:*

A. *Macrophages*

B. T and B lymphocytes

C. Platelets and coagulation factors

D. Appearance of proinflammatory and anti-inflammatory mediators in the systemic circulation

E. All of the above

The natural defense of the body to an infection, or other assault, involves a number of cellular and humoral factors. They include B and T lymphocytes, macrophages, neutrophils, platelets, tumor necrosis factor (TNF), interleukins, the coagulation factors, and probably several other products. There are five rather distinct phases that describe how these biological products work together to overcome the assault and, paradoxically, how they can interact to cause SIRS and MODS.

First phase: the local response
An infection, injury, burn, or similar process can initiate a response that causes the release of various proinflammatory mediators in the immediate area of involvement.

Second phase: the early systemic response
If the initial injury or insult is severe enough, the proinflammatory and anti-inflammatory mediators can appear in the systemic circulation. This may occur by direct entry into the bloodstream in the case of massive trauma, by spillover from the local site in the event of a severe infection, or by other means.

Third phase: proinflammatory excess
In some patients, control of the proinflammatory process does not occur, and there is a systemic reaction that can include hypotension, tachycardia, and abnormal body temperature. These are the early findings of SIRS.

Fourth phase: excessive immunosuppressive response
In some patients who survive an initial massive infection or other inflammatory process, there may be a compensatory, but excessive, anti-inflammatory response that results in immunosuppression. This may explain the increased susceptibility to infection in patients with severe burns, trauma, hemorrhage, or pancreatitis.

Fifth phase: transition to MODS
This phase indicates that there has been an overwhelming and inappropriate bodily response to the biological insult. It can take varied forms, including persistently elevated levels of proinflammatory mediators, whereby mortality is due to overwhelming inflammation and organ failure. This has been found in patients with SIRS and MODS.

Answer: E

Bone RC (1996) Immunologic dissonance: a continuing evolution in our understanding of the systemic inflammatory response syndrome (SIRS) and the multiple organ dysfunction syndrome (MODS). *Annals of Internal Medicine* **125** (8), 680–7.

14. *Diagnostic criteria for sepsis include:*

A. Heart rate 96 beats/minute

B. Temperature of 36.5 °C (97.7 °F)

C. Respiratory rate 18 breaths/minute

D. Leukocyte count between 5 000 and 11 000 cells/mm^3

E. Platelet count 90 000/mm^3

The American College of Chest Physicians (ACCP) and the Society of Critical Care Medicine (SCCM) have developed definitions for sepsis and its sequelae. Infection is defined as the invasion of a normally sterile host tissue by micro-organisms or the inflammatory response of a host to an infection. Bacteremia is defined as the presence of viable bacteria in the blood.

Sepsis is defined as a systemic inflammatory response arising from infection, leading to widespread tissue injury and manifested by two or more of the following conditions:
• hyperthermia (temperature greater than 38 °C [100.4 °F])
• hypothermia (temperature less than 36 °C [96.8 °F])
• tachycardia (heart rate greater than 90 beats per minute in adults)
• tachypnea (respiratory rate greater than 20 breaths per minute)
• hyperventilation (partial pressure of carbon dioxide [$PaCO_2$] less than 32 mm Hg)

- leukocytosis (leukocyte count greater than 12 000 cells per mm^3)
- leukopenia (leukocyte count less than 4000 cells per mm^3)

The recognition that noninfectious conditions may also produce a systemic response complicated by tissue injury led researchers to recommend use of the term systemic inflammatory response syndrome (SIRS). This term emphasizes that infection is not the exclusive cause of physiologic changes. The inflammatory response of the host is very important in determining the severity of the illness.

Systemic inflammatory response syndrome is an uncontrolled inflammation in response to an insult to the body or an ongoing process that can result in end-organ damage and multisystem failure.

In an acutely ill patient, altered organ function in more than one major organ constitutes multiple organ dysfunction syndrome (MODS). Organ dysfunction is characterized by various laboratory and clinical assessments, such as:

- a ratio of arterial oxygen tension to fraction of inspired oxygen of 280 or less
- the presence of a metabolic acidosis
- oliguria (urinary output of less than 0.5 mL/kg of body weight for at least one hour in a patient with a urinary catheter in place)
- an acute alteration in mental status.

Answer: A

Levy MM, Fink MP, Marshall JC, *et al.* (2003) SCCM/ESICM/ACCP/ATS/SIS international sepsis definitions conference. *Intensive Care Medicine* **29**, 530–8.

15. *The role of the coagulation system in the sepsis-induced inflammatory cascade includes*

A. *Up regulating fibrinolysis*

B. *Blocking further inflammation*

C. *Down regulating the anticoagulant system*

D. *Up regulation of Protein C production*

E. *Up regulaton of Protein S production*

The coagulation system plays an important role in the sepsis-induced inflammatory cascade. Coagulation is activated by the inflammatory reaction to tissue injury and is activated independent of the type of microbe (e.g., gram-positive and gram-negative bacteria, viruses, fungi, or parasites). Increased coagulation contributes to mortality in sepsis by down regulating fibrinolysis and the anticoagulant systems. The collaboration between clotting and inflammation, which works to wall off damaged and infected tissues, is an important host survival strategy. Coagulation induced by inflammation can in turn contribute to further inflammation. A key to determining survival in sepsis is to limit the damage while retaining the benefits of localized clotting and controlled clearance of pathogens.

A continuum of coagulopathy in sepsis has been suggested, extending from the appearance of mild coagulation abnormalities prior to the onset of any clinical signs of severe sepsis to consumption of anticoagulant proteins and suppression of the fibrinolytic system. Depletion of anticoagulant and fibrinolytic factors contributes to the microvascular deposition of fibrin that is associated with organ dysfunction. Coagulation abnormalities in sepsis contribute significantly to organ dysfunction and death.

Answer: C

Cinel I, Opal SM (2009) Molecular biology of inflammation and sepsis: a primer. *Critical Care Medicine* **37** (1), 291–304.

Wheeler AP (2007) Recent developments in the diagnosis and management of severe sepsis. *Chest* **132**, 1967–76.

16. *The common manifestations of sepsis are seen in all of the following organ systems except:*

A. *Skeletal*

B. *Endocrine*

C. *Skin*

D. *Central nervous*

E. *Gastrointestinal*

The manifestations of sepsis may be seen in the cardiovascular, pulmonary, central nervous, renal, gastrointestinal, and hematologic systems of the body (most frequently in the lungs and circulatory system). The skeletal system does not manifest signs of sepsis.

Cardiovascular

Hypotension and tachycardia are the most common cardiovasculiar manifestations. In addition, the left and right ventricles are dilated, ejection fractions are often depressed, and the Frank–Starling and diastolic pressure-volume relationships are altered.

Prior to hypotension the patient is usually hyperdynamic. As shock develops, SVR drops precipitously while cardiac output continues to increase. In the later phases of shock, cardiac output declines, which exacerbates the effects of hypoperfusion and allows lactate to accumulate.

Pulmonary

Tachypnea, with a respiratory rate of more than 20 breaths per minute, is often the earliest pulmonary sign of sepsis, occurring before hypoxemia. As sepsis continues, marked respiratory alkalosis often ensues; $PaCO_2$ may be 30 mm Hg or less.

Central nervous system

Altered mental status may be the most common and most overlooked manifestation of sepsis. This causes elderly patients to be at particularly high risk. Early changes include withdrawal, confusion, irritability, or agitation.

Renal

The renal manifestations of sepsis include oliguria and azotemia. The urinary excretion of sodium may be markedly reduced (less than 20 mEq/L), and urinary osmolality may be increased (greater than 450 mOsm/kg). Protracted oliguria may lead to acute tubular necrosis or renal failure.

Gastrointestinal

Impaired motility is the most common gastrointestinal problem. Stress ulceration is another common problem. There is some evidence that stress ulcers are less likely to develop when patients are given adequate fluid resuscitation, although this has not been proven conclusively.

Hepatic

Large but transient elevations in serum transaminase levels may follow an episode of severe shock or hypoxemia.

Hematologic

Leukocytosis, usually accompanied by a shift to the left, is common in sepsis. Multifactorial anemia is seen in late-stage sepsis. Decreased maturity and/or survival of red blood cells may contribute to anemia. Thrombocytopenia and coagulation abnormalities (elevated prothrombin or partial thromboplastin times) are often seen in sepsis.

Answer: A

Dellinger RP, Levy MM, Carlet J, *et al.* (2008) Surviving sepsis campaign: international guidelines for management of severe sepsis and septic shock. *Intensive Care Medicine* **34** (1), 17–60. Summary retrieved from National Guideline Clearinghouse at http://www.guideline.gov/summary/summary.aspx?doc_id=12231 (accessed April 6, 2009).

Rivers E, Nguyen B, Havstad S, *et al.* (2001) Early Goal-Directed Therapy Collaborative Group. Early goal-directed therapy in the treatment of severe sepsis and septic shock. *New England Journal of Medicine* **345**, 1368–77.

17. *Altered mental status is a common manifestation of sepsis. An early sign of this change may be*

A. *Irritability*

B. *Disorientation*

C. *Polyneuropathy*

D. *Nonfocal manifestations*

E. *Seizures*

Altered mental status may be the most common and most overlooked manifestation of sepsis. This causes elderly patients to be at particularly high risk. Early changes include withdrawal, confusion, irritability, or agitation. In patients with severe infection, one may see disorientation, lethargy, seizures, or frank obtundation.

Eventually, symptoms and signs of encephalopathy, including nonfocal neurologic manifestations, may be seen, and some patients may become comatose. In addition, evidence of polyneuropathy, including impaired deep tendon reflexes, muscle weakness, and wasting, may be present.

Answer: B

Cunha BA (1998) *Infectious Diseases in Critical Care Medicine*, New York, NY: Marcel Dekker.

Ely EW, Kleinpell RM, Goyette RE (2003) Advances in the understanding of clinical manifestations and therapy of severe sepsis: an update for critical care nurses. *American Journal of Critical Care* **12**, 120–35.

18. *Which agent is preferred to restore blood pressure and perfusion in a patient with septic shock after volume replacement?*

A. *Dobutamine infusion*

B. *Norepinephrine infusion*

C. *Intermittent phenylephrine*

D. *Low dose vasopressin*

E. *Low dose dopamine*

Vasopressors may be required to restore adequate blood pressure and perfusion. Norepinephrine or dopamine are considered first-choice vasopressor agents to correct hypotension in septic shock. Norepinephrine appears to be more effective at reversing hypotension than dopamine, but there are concerns that many of the biological effects of dopamine might cause harm to patients in septic shock. Low-dose dopamine should not be used for renal protection.

If these agents do not provide mean arterial pressure of ≥65 mm Hg, vasopressin may be added to the norepinephrine and administered at an infusion rate of 0.03 units/min. Vasopressin should not be administered as the initial agent in septic shock. Phenylephrine can also be used to increase blood pressure, especially if a tachyarrhythmia is present, but should not be administered as the initial vasopressor. Intravenous preparations should be administered only by properly trained individuals familiar with its use.

Inotropic therapy may involve the use of dobutamine if the cardiac output remains low. If dobutamine is used, it should be combined with the vasopressors. All patients requiring vasopressors should have an arterial line placed as soon as practically possible.

Answer: B

Dellinger RP, Levy MM, Carlet JM, *et al.* (2008) Surviving sepsis campaign: international guidelines for management of severe sepsis and septic shock *Intensive Care Medicine* **34** (1), 17–60. Summary retrieved from National Guideline Clearinghouse at www.guideline.gov/summary/summary.aspx?doc_id=12231 (accessed April 6, 2009).

19. *Diagnostic criteria for SIRS in children include:*

A. *Temperature of 36.5 °C*

B. *Leukocyte count that is either elevated or depressed for the child's age*

C. *Tachycardia greater than 1 standard deviation above normal for the child's age*

D. *Mean respiratory rate greater than 1 standard deviation above normal for the child's age*

E. *Leukocyte count that is either elevated or depressed independent of child's age*

The panel's definition of SIRS for children includes the presence of at least two of the following criteria (one of which must be abnormal temperature or leukocyte count):

• Core temperature greater than 38.5 °C or less than 36 °C (measured by rectal, bladder, oral, or central catheter probe). Hypothermia may indicate serious infection (especially in infants).

• Tachycardia greater than 2 standard deviations above normal for the child's age in the absence of external stimulus; or unexplained persistent elevation over a four-hour time period; or, for children younger than one year of age, bradychardia (as defined by the panel); or unexplained persistent depression over a 30-minute time period. Bradychardia is not a sign of SIRS in older children but may be a sign in the newborn.

• Mean respiratory rate greater than two standard deviations above normal for the child's age or mechanical ventilation.

• Leukocyte count that is either elevated or depressed for the child's age; or greater than 10% immature neutrophils.

Answer: B

Goldstein B, Giroir B (2005) Randolph International pediatric sepsis consensus conference: definitions for sepsis and organ dysfunction in pediatrics. *Pediatric Critical Care Medicine* **6** (1), 2–8.

20. *A major cause of sepsis among hospitalized severely ill patients is*

A. *Malignancy*

B. *Hyperglycemia*

C. *Intestinal ulceration*

D. *Nosocomial infection*

E. *Gastrointestinal bleeding*

Factors considered important in the development of sepsis include: inappropriate broad-spectrum antibiotic therapy; immunosuppressive treatments, such as cancer chemotherapy; invasive procedures; transplantations; fungal organisms; burns or other trauma; anatomic obstruction; intestinal ulceration; age extremes; and progressive clinical conditions, such as malignancy, diabetes, or AIDS.

Nosocomial infections are a major cause of sepsis among severely ill patients. Increased risk of nosocomial infection is associated with the presence of underlying chronic disease, alteration in host defenses, prolonged hospital stay, and the presence of invasive catheters or monitoring devices. Pulmonary, urinary tract, gastrointestinal, and wound infections predominate. In hospitalized adult patients, the etiology of sepsis has shifted from being predominantly gram-negative nosocomial infections (*Escherichia coli*, Klebsiella, Enterobacter species, and *Pseudomonas aeruginosa*) to gram-positive infections (*Staphylococcus aureus*, *Streptococcus pneumoniae*, and *Streptococcus pyogenes*). The incidence of sepsis caused by gram-positive infections has increased by 26.3% per year since the early 1980s. Multidrug-resistant pathogens, such as *S. aureus*, now account for more than half of all sepsis cases. *S. aureus* is singly responsible for 40% of ventilator-associated pneumonia episodes and most cases of nosocomial pneumonia. Group B Streptococcus is a leading cause of neonatal sepsis in the United States.

The risk of catheter-related sepsis is increased when the IV catheter is placed in a central vein, particularly if the catheter remains in place longer than three to five days or if the catheter is used for blood sampling. Full sterile barrier precautions, strict protocols for catheter care, and prompt removal of the catheter when it is no longer needed are recommended to prevent infectious complications.

Urinary catheters left in the bladder longer than two weeks often cause infection. Therefore, increased surveillance for signs of urinary tract infections when catheters remain in place beyond a few days is necessary.

Answer: D

Martin GS, Mannino DM, Eaton S (2003) The epidemiology of sepsis in the United States from 1979 through 2000. *New England Journal of Medicine* **348** (16), 1546–54.

National Nosocomial Infections Surveillance System. National Nosocomial Infections Surveillance (NNIS) System Report, data summary from January 1992 through June 2004, issued October 2004 (2004) *American Journal of Infection Control* **32** (8), 470–85.

Chapter 5 Hemodynamic and Respiratory Monitoring

Christopher S. Nelson, MD, Jeffrey P. Coughenour, MD, and Stephen L. Barnes, MD, FACS

1. *An 18-year-old boy involved in a motor-vehicle collision is admitted with multiple orthopedic injuries and requires intubation. A right internal jugular central venous catheter is placed to assist in volume resuscitation and hemodynamic monitoring. The phlebostatic axis is correctly identified and the catheter is connected properly. When is the proper time during a normal breath cycle to accurately measure intravascular pressure?*

A. *End of expiration*

B. *During a sustained breath hold*

C. *End of inspiration*

D. *Measurement is unaffected by timing during the normal breath cycle*

E. *Plateau pressure*

The phlebostatic axis corresponds to the position of the right and left atrium with the patient in the supine position. Intravascular pressure (the pressure in the vessel lumen relative to atmospheric pressure) is the vascular pressure measured at bedside. Transmural pressure is the difference between the intravascular and extravascular pressures. Changes in thoracic pressure can cause a discrepancy between intravascular and transmural pressures. Intravascular pressures should be equivalent to transmural pressures when the extravascular pressure is zero or at the end of expiration.

Answer: A

Kee LL, Simonson JS, Stotts NA, *et al.* (1993) Echocardiographic determination of valid zero reference levels in supine and lateral positions. *American Journal of Critical Care* **2**, 72–80.

Marino P (2007) *The ICU Book*, 3rd edn, Lippincott Williams & Wilkins, Philadelphia, PA.

Surgical Critical Care and Emergency Surgery: Clinical Questions and Answers, First Edition. Edited by Forrest O. Moore, Peter M. Rhee, Samuel A. Tisherman and Gerard J. Fulda.

2. *A 76-year-old woman, is admitted to the ICU following a Hartmann's procedure for complicated diverticulitis. A pulmonary artery catheter is placed through the right internal jugular vein to assist in hemodynamic monitoring and resuscitation. To ensure an accurate venous pressure tracing, the pulmonary artery catheter tip should lie in which West lung zone?*

A. *Zone I*

B. *Zone II*

C. *Zone III*

D. *Zone IV*

E. *Anatomic location of placement does not affect reading*

Multiple conditions may exist that can adversely affect the accuracy of the wedge pressure as a measure of left atrial pressure. If the pressure in the surrounding alveoli exceeds capillary (venous)

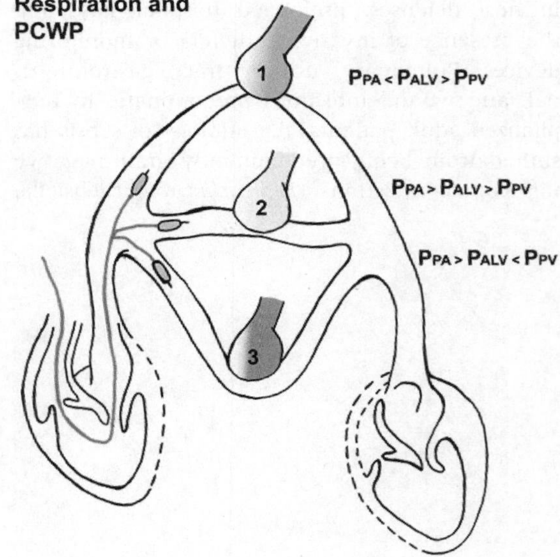

pressure, the pressure at the tip of the pulmonary artery catheter may reflect the alveolar pressure more than the pressure in the left atrium. Wedge pressure is a reflection of left atrial pressure only when the tip of the catheter is located in West zone 3 of the lung. Other conditions that may affect accuracy include: catheter tip position, PEEP, aortic insufficiency, a noncompliant ventricle, and respiratory failure.

Answer: C

Marino P (2007) *The ICU Book,* 3rd edn, Lippincott Williams & Wilkins, Philadelphia, PA.

Mathews L (2007) Paradigm shift in hemodynamic monitoring. *The Internet Journal of Anesthesiology* **11**, 1–2.

Oquin R, Marini JJ (1983) Pulmonary artery occlusion pressure: clinical physiology, measurement, and interpretation. *American Review of Respiratory Disorders* **128**, 319.

3. *A pulmonary artery catheter uses the thermodilution principle for determining cardiac output. A number of factors can affect the accuracy of these readings. Which cardiac valvular abnormality may produce a falsely depressed cardiac output reading?*

A. *Tricuspid regurgitation*

B. *Tricuspid stenosis*

C. *Mitral prolapse*

D. *Aortic regurgitation*

E. *Aortic stenosis*

Thermodilution is an indicator-dilution method of measuring blood flow. This method is based on the premise that, when an indicator substance is added to circulating blood, the rate of blood flow is inversely proportional to the change in concentration of the indicator over time. This can either be a dye (dye-dilution method) or a fluid with a different temperature than blood (thermodilution method). Using a pulmonary artery catheter, cold fluid mixes in the right heart chambers and the cooled blood is ejected into the pulmonary artery and flows past the thermistor on the distal end of the catheter. The thermistor records the change in blood temperature with time. This information is sent to an electronic device that records and displays a temperature time curve. The area under the curve is inversely proportional to the rate of blood flow in the pulmonary artery, and this flow is equivalent to the cardiac output. Tricuspid regurgitation causes the cold indicator fluid to be recycled back and forth across the tricuspid valve. This produces a prolonged, low-amplitude thermodilution curve, thus tricuspid regurgitation produces a falsely low thermodilution cardiac output. Aortic regurgitation, aortic stenosis and mitral prolapse are left sided heart abnormalities that will not affect the thermodilutional method. Similarly, tricuspid stenosis will still allow a steady rate of flow across the valve and will not affect thermodilution.

Answer: A

Konishi T, Nakamura Y, Morii I, *et al.* (1992) Comparison of thermodilution and Fick methods for measurement of cardiac output in tricuspid regurgitation. *American Journal of Cardiology* **70** (4), 538–9.

Marino P (2007) *The ICU Book,* 3rd edn, Lippincott Williams & Wilkins, Philadelphia, PA.

4. *A 69-year-old man with known benign prostatic hypertrophy (BPH) and poorly-controlled non-insulin dependent diabetes mellitus is admitted to the ICU in septic shock secondary to a urinary source. A right subclavian central venous catheter is inserted and a left radial arterial line is placed.*

Resuscitation is most accurately guided by which value derived from intra-arterial cannulation?

A. *Systolic pressure*

B. *Diastolic pressure*

C. *Mean arterial pressure*

D. *Pulse pressure*

E. *Frequent hemoglobin and hematocrit sampling*

The contour of an arterial pressure waveform changes as the pressure moves away from the proximal aorta. As the pressure wave moves toward the periphery, the systolic pressure gradually increases and the systolic portion of the waveform narrows. The systolic pressure can increase by as much as 20 mm Hg. The increase in peak systolic pressure is offset by the narrowing of the systolic pressure wave so that the mean arterial pressure remains unchanged, therefore, mean arterial pressure is a more accurate measure of central aortic pressure. Amplification of the systolic pressure is particularly prominent when the arteries are noncompliant. Because a large proportion of patients in the ICU are elderly with comorbid conditions, systolic pressure amplification is probably commonplace in the ICU.

Answer: C

Marino P (2007) *The ICU Book,* 3rd edn, Lippincott Williams & Wilkins, Philadelphia, PA.

Martin C, Saux P, Papazian L, Gouin F (2001) Long-term arterial cannulation in ICU patients using the radial artery or dorsalis pedis artery. *Chest* **119**, 901–6.

Nichols WW, O'Rourke MF (1990) *McDonald's Blood Flow in Arteries,* 3rd edn, Arnold, London.

5. *A 63-year-old woman has an extended ICU course secondary to inability to wean from the ventilator following a right upper lobe lobectomy performed for adenocarcinoma of the lung. Her blood glucose levels have been well controlled without the use of exogenous insulin, in a range from 140–180 mg/dl. Spot glucose checks over the previous 18 hours reveal an increasing hyperglycemia and the nurse notifies you of a temperature of 39.1 °C. A right subclavian central venous catheter is identified as having a 2 cm rim of surrounding erythema at the insertion site, which was not present on physical examination 24 hours prior. Blood, urine, and sputum cultures are sent to pathology, the foley catheter is changed, peripheral IV access is established and the central venous catheter is removed and sent for gram-stain and culture.*

Suspecting a catheter-related bloodstream infection (CRBSI), the most likely organism to be identified on gram-stain and culture will be:

A. *Escherichia coli*

B. *Staphylococcus epidermidis*

C. *Enterococcus faecalis*

D. *Pseudomonus aeriginosus*

E. *Candida albicans*

CRBSIs usually manifest as an unexpected fever in a patient who has had an indwelling vascular catheter longer than 48 hours. In this condition, the same pathogenic organism is found on the catheter tip and in the systemic circulation. Common routes of CRBSI include: 1) microbes enter the internal lumen through break points in the infusion system, such as stopcocks and catheter hubs. 2) microbes on the skin can migrate along the subcutaneous tract created by the catheter. 3) microorganisms in circulating blood can become entrapped in the fibrin meshwork that surrounds the intravascular portion of the indwelling catheter. The organisms involved in catheter-related septicemia are most commonly: *Staphylococcus epidermidis* (27%), *Staphylococcus aureus* (24%), *Candida* species (17%), *Klebsiella* or *Enterobacter* (11%), *Serratia* (5%), *Enterococcus* (5%), and others (8%).

Answer: B

Leonidu L, Gogos C (2010) Catheter-related bloodstream infections: catheter management according to pathogen. *International Journal of Antimicrobial Agents* **36** (Suppl. 2), S26–32.

Marino P (2007) *The ICU Book,* 3rd edn, Lippincott Williams & Wilkins, Philadelphia, PA.

Norwood S, Ruby A, Civetta J, Cortes V (1991) Catheter-related infections and associated septicemia. *Chest* **99** (4), 968–75.

6. *Gastric tonometry is a novel method that has been introduced in an attempt to identify earlier and more accurate methods for recognizing tissue hypo-perfusion. The basis of this is hypothesized by splanchnic hypoperfusion being a prelude to multi-organ failure and that oxygen deficits at the gastric mucosa will produce a local acidosis and then be recognized and therapy instituted. All of the following may affect gastric tonometry except:*

A. *Gastric acid secretion*

B. *Systemic acid-base balance*

C. *Arterial bicarbonate*

D. *Mechanical ventilation*

E. *Zollinger–Ellison syndrome*

Gastric tonometry uses an indirect measurement of the pH in gastric mucosa to evaluate the adequacy of tissue oxygenation (oxygen deficits produce a local acidosis). The tonometer is a CO_2-permeable silicone balloon affixed to the distal end of a standard 16 Fr. nasogastric tube. The balloon is placed in the stomach and partially filled with saline and left in place for 30 minutes. The

CO_2 in the adjacent mucosa eventually equilibrates between the tissues and the saline in the balloon. The pCO_2 in the saline approximates the pCO_2 in the gastric mucosa. The pH calculation also requires a measure of tissue bicarbonate, and the bicarbonate concentration in an arterial blood sample is used for this purpose. Acid secretion in the stomach is a confounding variable that must be eliminated when using gastric mucosal pH as a marker of tissue oxygenation. Systemic acid-base disorders can also influence the pH of the gastric mucosa; of particular concern is metabolic acidosis. The use of arterial bicarbonate as a measure of mucosal bicarbonate is problematic because the two are not equivalent in low-flow states. Mechanical ventilation in and of itself will not affect tonometry readings given a normal acid-base status. Zollinger–Ellsion syndrome creates inappropriate amounts of acid production and will decrease the gastric pH resulting in a false reading.

Answer: D

Gutierrez G., Brown SD (1995) Gastric tonometry: a new monitoring modality in the intensive care unit. *Journal Intensive Care Medicine* **10** (1), 34–44.

Gutierrez G, Palizas F, Goglio G, *et al.* (1992) Gastric intramucosal pH as a therapeutic index of tissue oxygenation in critically ill patients. *Lancet* **339**, 195–9.

Marino P. (2007) *The ICU Book,* 3rd edn, Lippincott Williams & Wilkins, Philadelphia, PA.

7. *A 56-year-old man is admitted to the ICU following an elective hemi-thyroidectomy for papillary thyroid cancer. He experiences an acute asthma exacerbation and is intubated, however the patient's oxygen saturation continues to decline and he ultimately becomes pulseless and expires despite aggressive resuscitation attempts. Post-mortem examination reveals the endotracheal tube tube to be placed within the lumen of the esophagus.*

All of the following are reliable indicators of tracheal intubation except:

A. *CO_2 excretion color detector*

B. *Capnometry*

C. *Squeeze bulb syringe*

D. *Fogging of endotracheal tube*

E. *Flexible bronchoscopy*

Although useful, traditional methods for confirming the endotracheal placement of the tube have limited reliability. These include stethoscopic audibility and symmetry of breath sounds, direct visualization of the cords, ease of insufflation and recovery of tidal volume, tidal fogging and clearing of the endotracheal tube, palpation of tube in larynx, loss of voice, coughing and expulsion of airway secretions, expansion of upper chest and failure of the abdomen to progressively distend during gas delivery. To improve reliability and speed of placement, the phasic detection of CO_2 during expiration by capnography and capnometry can be used. CO_2 detection and measurement by these methods can occasionally and transiently be misleading. Minimal CO_2 is evolved or expelled during shock or circulatory arrest and some CO_2 may be liberated initially after esophageal intubation from gas trapped in the gastric pouch. However, this concentration falls rapidly as serial tidal volumes are delivered. When compressed, a large-capacity squeeze bulb affixed to the endotracheal tube will fail to fill easily if the tube is in the collapsible esophagus.

Answer: D

Littlewood K, Durbin CG Jr (2001) Evidence-based airway management. *Respiratory Care* **46** (12), 1392–405.

Marini JJ, Wheeler AP (2006) *Critical Care Medicine, The Essentials*. Lippincott Williams & Wilkins, Philadelphia, PA, (third edn).

8. *A 72-year-old man is admitted to the ICU after undergoing emergent laparotomy for perforated viscus. A central venous catheter and arterial line are placed and volume resuscitation is goal-directed to ensure adequate tissue perfusion. The factor least responsible for increasing oxygen delivery to tissues is:*

A. *Hemoglobin (Hgb)*

B. *Stroke volume*

C. *Oxygen saturation (SaO_2)*

D. *Partial pressure of arterial oxygen (PaO_2)*

E. *Heart rate*

Volume resuscitation should ideally be driven by the principle of correcting inadequate oxygen delivery to the end organs. The quantity of oxygen that moves into, or out of, the blood depends on three factors: (1) the amount of dissolved oxygen (PO_2); (2) the amount of oxygen combined with hemoglobin (%$HgbO_2$); and (3) the strength with which the hemoglobin binds oxygen (Hgb-O_2 affinity). The volume (ml) of oxygen contained in 100 ml of blood is defined as the arterial oxygen content or CaO_2. Oxygen delivery (DO_2) is the volume of oxygen presented to the tissues in one minute, expressed in the equation: DO_2 = cardiac output × (1.34 × Hgb × SaO_2) + (0.003 × PaO_2) or DO_2 (ml/min/m_2) = CaO_2 × CO where CaO_2 = (1.34 × Hgb × SaO_2) + (0.003 × PaO_2) and CO is cardiac output (stroke volume × heart rate). 1.34 is the amount of oxygen bound to each gram of hemoglobin and PaO_2 times 0.003 represents the dissolved hemoglobin in the blood. Under normal atmospheric pressure, the PaO_2 is very small and often ignored. Once the oxygen content is maximized, the largest increase in the delivery of oxygen is achieved through increasing cardiac output. Resuscitation can therefore be optimized by understanding the oxygen delivery equation along with the variables that can be manipulated by the practitioner.

Answer: D

Bock A, Field H, Adair G (1924) Oxygen and carbon dioxide dissociation curves of human blood. *Journal of Biologic Chemistry* **59**, 353–78.

Parrillo J, Dellinger R (2008) *Critical Care Medicine: Principles of Diagnosis and Management in the Adult*, 3rd edn, Mosby/Elsevier, Philadelphia, PA.

Russell JA, Phang PT (1994) The oxygen delivery/consumption controversy. Approaches to management of the critically ill. *American Journal of Respiratory Critical Care Medicine* **149**, 533.

9. *A 22-year-old man undergoes a splenectomy for a positive focused abdominal sonography of trauma (FAST) and class 4 hemorrhagic shock following a motor-vehicle collision. A left subclavian central venous catheter and arterial line are placed intraoperatively. The patient is admitted to the SICU for postoperative resuscitation and monitoring. Urine output is monitored along with central venous pressure and fluid resuscitation is guided accordingly. Stroke volume and stroke volume variability are measured through the arterial line. The stroke volume variability corresponding to adequate intravascular volume status is:*

A. 10%

B. 20%

C. 40%

D. 60%

E. Cannot be accurately assessed

Stroke volume variability (SVV) has been shown repeatedly to be a reliable predictor of fluid responsiveness. It is calculated from percentage changes in stroke volume (SV) during the ventilator cycle. Calculation of SV by pulse contour technology is based on the contribution of pulse pressure to SV being proportional to the standard deviation of arterial pulse pressure. In order to determine SV, the influences of vascular resistance and compliance on SV are considered using manually entered patient data and pulse wave analysis. SVV values of less than 15% are an indication of euvolemia. Numbers greater than 15% shows a larger percentage change between strokes and are thus thought to be an indicator of hypovolemia and may benefit from a fluid challenge.

Answer: A

Hofer CK, Senn A, Weiber L, Zollinger A. (2008) Assessment of stroke volume variation for prediction of fluid responsiveness using the modified FloTrac and PiCCOplus system. *Critical Care* **12**(3), R82.

De Backer D, Heenan S, Piagnerelli M, Koch M, Vincent J. (2005) Pulse pressure variations to predict fluid responsiveness: influence of tidal volume. *Intensive Care Medicine* **31**, 517–23.

10. *When inserting a pulmonary artery catheter, as the catheter is advanced from the right ventricle into the pulmonary artery, which of the following pressures being recorded from the catheter changes the most?*

A. Diastolic pressure

B. Systolic pressure

C. Mean pressure

D. Central venous pressure

E. All change equally

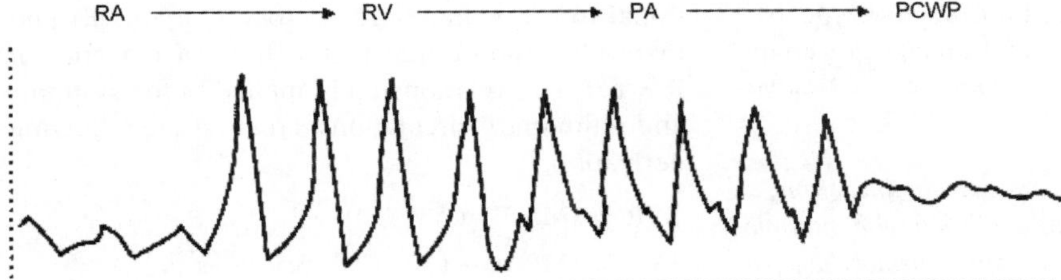

When the catheter is inserted via the right internal jugular vein (RIJ), the balloon is inflated 15 cm from the point of neck entry. From the RIJ approach, the RA is entered at approximately 25 cm, the RV at approximately 30 cm, and the PA at approximately 40 cm; the PCWP can be identified at approximately 45 cm. As a rule of thumb, the catheter tip should not require advancement of more than 20 cm beyond its current position before encountering the next vascular compartment. Coiling within the right ventricle and misdirection of the catheter should be suspected after reaching 45 to 50 cm and the appropriate PA waveform is not encountered. Fluoroscopy can be a helpful adjunct in difficult cases and is especially worthwhile to consider before attempting an insertion from the femoral site.

Answer: A

Marini JJ, Wheeler AP (2006) *Critical Care Medicine, The Essentials*. Lippincott Williams & Wilkins, Philadelphia, PA, (third edn).

Iberti TJ, Fischer EP, Leibowitz AB, Panacek EA, Silverstein JH, Albertson TE (1990) A multicenter study of physicians' knowledge of the pulmonary artery catheter. Pulmonary Artery Catheter Study Group. *JAMA* **264** (22), 2928–32.

Rhodes A, Cusack RJ, Newman PJ, Grounds RM (2002) A randomized, controlled trial of the pulmonary artery catheter in critically ill patients. *Intensive Care Medicine* **28** (3), 256–64.

11. *Which of the following are needed to calculate oxygen delivery from the data obtained using a pulmonary artery catheter?*

A. *Cardiac output, hemoglobin, arterial O_2 Saturation, arterial pO_2*

B. *Stroke volume, hemoglobin, pulmonary artery pO_2, arterial saturation*

C. *Arterial pO_2, pulmonary artery pO_2, arterial saturation, cardiac output*

D. *Pulmonary artery saturation, arterial saturation, cardiac output, oxygen consumption*

E. *None of the above*

Tissues attempt to extract the amount of oxygen required to maintain aerobic metabolism, thus mixed-venous O_2 tension falls when O_2 delivery (the product of cardiac output and arterial O_2 content) becomes insufficient for tissue needs. As a primary determinant of O_2 delivery, cardiac output measurements often prove helpful during selection of the appropriate PEEP level for the patient with life-threatening hypoxemia. Depression of venous return may nullify any beneficial effect of improved pulmonary gas exchange on O_2 tissue delivery. A rational goal of resuscitative therapy in severe sepsis and shock is to restore balance between O_2 delivery and demand, and boosting cardiac output is fundamental to such an approach. Aggressive goal-oriented resuscitation in the earliest phase of management appears to improve mortality in septic patients, whereas the literature is inconclusive as to which patients in other clinical settings benefit from raising cardiac output to normal or supranormal values.

Answer: A

Marini JJ, Wheeler AP (2006) *Critical Care Medicine, The Essentials*. Lippincott Williams & Wilkins, Philadelphia, PA.

Iberti TJ, Fischer EP, Leibowitz AB, Panacek EA, Silverstein JH, Albertson TE (1990) *A multicenter study of physicians' knowledge of the pulmonary artery catheter. Pulmonary Artery Catheter Study Group. JAMA* **264** (22), 2928–32.

Rhodes A, Cusack RJ, Newman PJ, Grounds RM (2002) A randomized, controlled trial of the pulmonary artery catheter in critically ill patients. *Intensive Care Medicine* **28** (3), 256–64.

12. and 13. *The following data are obtained from a 45-year-old man s/p motor vehicle collision with multiple orthopedic fractures, a small subdural hemorrhage, a grade 3 splenic laceration and multiple skin abrasions: height 60 inches, weight 140 lbs, body surface area (BSA) 1.5 m^2, temperature 37.5 °C, heart rate (HR) 114, mean arterial pressure (MAP) 60, pulmonary artery pressure (PAP) 40/20, pulmonary capillary wedge pressure (PCWP 18, central venous pressure (CVP) 10, cardiac output (CO) 4 L/min, Hgb 10.0, FiO$_2$ 80%, pH 7.39, pCO$_2$ 40 mm Hg, pO$_2$ 70 mm Hg, SaO$_2$ 95%, mixed venous oxygen saturation (MVO$_2$) 75%. Assume 1.34 ml of O$_2$ per gram Hgb at 100% saturation.*

12. *Systemic vascular resistance:*

A. *Is a measurement obtained directly from the pulmonary artery catheter*

B. *Can be calculated by (MAP − PCWP/CO) × 80*

C. *Can be calculated by (SAP − PCWP/CO) × 80*

D. *Can be calculated by (SAP − PCWP/MAP) × 80*

E. *Can be calculated by (MAP − CVP/CO) × 80*

13. *What is the systemic vascular resistance (dyne sec/cm^5) of the patient in question?*

A. *840*

B. *1000*

C. *1300*

D. *1900*

E. *2200*

A major component of afterload is the resistance to ventricular outflow in the aorta and large, proximal arteries. The total hydraulic force that opposes pulsatile flow is known as impedance. This force is a combination of 2 forces: A force that opposes the rate of change in flow, *compliance* and a force that opposes mean or volumetric flow, *resistance*. Vascular resistance is derived by assuming that hydraulic resistance is analogous to electrical resistance. Ohm's law predicts that resistance to flow of an electric current(R) is directly proportional to the voltage drop across a circuit (E) and inversely proportional to the flow of current (I); R = E/I. This relationship is applied to the systemic and pulmonary circulations, creating the following derivations:

SVR = (MAP − CVP/CO)

PVR = (MPAP − LAP/CO)

Answers: 12 E, 13 B

Harvey S, Harrison DA, Singer M (2005) Assessment of the clinical effectiveness of pulmonary artery catheters in management of patients in intensive care (PAC-Man): A randomized controlled trial. PAC-Man study collaboration. *Lancet* **366**, 472–7.

Marino P. (2007) *The ICU Book*, 3rd edn, Lippincott Williams & Wilkins, Philadelphia, PA.

Iberti TJ, Fischer EP, Leibowitz AB, Panacek EA, Silverstein JH, Albertson TE (1990) *A multicenter study of physicians' knowledge of the pulmonary artery catheter. Pulmonary Artery Catheter Study Group. JAMA* **264** (22), 2928–32.

14. *A 67-year-old man is an unrestrained passenger in a rollover motor vehicle collision and suffers multiple injuries including a subdural hemorrhage without mass effect, a grade 3 liver laceration without active extravasation per CT imaging, and multiple orthopedic extremity fractures. He is intubated for a decreased GCS of 7 and admitted to the intensive care unit for further resuscitation. His vital signs are HR 135 beats/minute, BP 105/75 mm Hg. Upon family arrival they inform you that the patient has had a previous right pneumonectomy for invasive lung cancer and an unknown abnormal heart rhythm. Cardiac output monitoring may be accomplished by all of the following except:*

A. *Esophageal doppler*

B. *Trans-esophageal echocardiography*

C. *Pulmonary artery catheter*

D. *Pulse contour waveform analysis*

E. *Trans-thoracic echocardiography*

Relative contraindications to placement of a pulmonary artery cathertization include: tricuspid or pulmonary stenosis, right atrial or ventricular mass, previous pnuemonectomy, cyanotic heart disease,

LBBB, and latex allergy. Noninvasive investigation of cardiac performance is warranted in such patients. The esophageal doppler technique is based on measurement of blood flow velocity in the descending aorta by means of a doppler transducer (4 MHz continuous or 5 MHz pulsed wave, according to the type of device) at the tip of a flexible probe. Measurement of stroke volume using esophageal doppler is derived from the well established principles of stroke volume measurement in the left ventricular outflow tract using transthoracic echo and doppler. Calculation of SV by pulse contour technology is based on the contribution of pulse pressure to SV being proportional to the standard deviation of arterial pulse pressure.

Answer: C

Berton C, Cholley B (2002) Equipment review: new techniques for cardiac output measurement—oesophageal Doppler, Fick principle using carbon dioxide, and pulse contour analysis. *Critical Care* **6** (3), 216–21.

Chittock DR, Dhingra VK, Ronco JJ (2004) Severity of illness and risk of death associated with pulmonary artery catheter use. *Critical Care Medicine* **32** (4), 911–15.

15. *A 64-year-old man is admitted to the SICU following a segmental small bowel resection for ischemia related to a CHF exacerbation and subsequent low flow state. The patient has a pulmonary artery catheter placed along with an arterial line. He undergoes successful resection and has a temporary abdominal dressing in place for a planned second look operation. The normalization of which of the following is most consistent with successful fluid resuscitation?*

A. *Hemoglobin*

B. *Lactate*

C. *Basic natriuretic peptide*

D. *Serum* CO_2

E. *Serum creatinine*

Blood lactate levels help determine whether oxygen delivery is adequate for the needs of aerobic metabolism. Adding lactate determinations to oxygen transport monitoring provides a more complete assessment of tissue oxygen balance. In one study, patients were randomly allocated to two groups. In the lactate group, treatment was guided by serial lactate levels with the objective to decrease lactate by 20% or more from the admission value every 2 hours for the initial 8 hours of ICU stay. In the control group, the treatment team had no knowledge of lactate levels (except for the admission value) during this period. In the lactate group, sequential organ failure assessment (SOFA) scores were lower between 9 and 72 hours, inotropes were discontinued earlier, and patients were weaned from mechanical ventilation and discharged from the ICU earlier. Lactate-guided therapy significantly reduced hospital mortality when adjusting for predefined risk factors.

Answer B

Jansen T, Bommel J, Schoonderbeek F, *et al.* (2010) Early lactate-guided therapy in intensive care unit patients: a multicenter, open-label, randomized controlled trial. *American Journal of Respiratory and Critical Care Medicine* **182** (6), 752–61.

Husain FA, Martin MJ, Mullenix PS, *et al.* (2003) Serum lactate and base deficit as predictors of mortality and morbidity. *American Journal of Surgery* **185** (5), 485–91.

Rivers E, Nguyen B, Havstad S (2001) Early goal directed therapy in the treatment of severe sepsis and septic shock. New England Journal of Medicine **345** (19), 1368–77.

16. *Several factors cause peripheral pulse oximetry monitors to lose accuracy. All of the following are examples of these factors except?*

A. *Sickle cell anemia*

B. *Acute blood loss anemia*

C. *Carboxyhemoglobin and methemoglobin*

D. *Motion*

E. *Ambient light*

Sickle-cell anemia, causing deformation of hemoglobin and decreasing flow through the microcirculation, may cause an overestimation of readings. The clinical significance of these readings is often downplayed in most studies. Acute blood-loss anemia, by itself, seems to have no affect on oximetry readings. Most peripheral sensors use two wavelengths of light: those associated with oxygenated and deoxygenated hemoglobin. The presence of carboxyhemoglobin and methemoglobin, which have differing specific wavelengths, cause an overestimation of oxygen saturation. Motion artifact has long been a reason for inaccuracy with peripheral sensors, and despite several attempts at correction, this remains a common cause for alarms that are not associated with actual patient decline. Other causes of pulse oximetry inaccuracy include methylene blue, indocyanine green, indigo carmine (low readings), and black, blue, or green nail polish.

Answer: B

Barker SH, Tremper KK, Hyatt J (1989) Effects of methemoglobinemia on pulse oximetry and mixed-venous oximetry. *Anesthesiology* **70**, 112.

Jay GD, Hughes L, Renzi FP (1994) Pulse oximetry is accurate in acute anemia from hemorrhage. *Annals of Emergency Medicine* **24**, 32.

Ortiz FO, Aldrich TK, Nagel RL, *et al.* (1999) Accuracy of pulse oximetry in sickle cell disease. *American Journal of Respiratory Critical Care Medicine* **159**, 447.

17. *A 64-year-old man with diabetes mellitus, peripheral vascular disease, chronic obstructive pulmonary disease, and coronary artery disease with an 80-pack per year history of smoking is admitted to the SICU with sepsis from a presumed infection in his right lower extremity. A guillotine amputation is performed below-the-knee with application of a negative pressure dressing. The patient is begun on IV fluid resuscitation and IV antimicrobials. A central venous catheter is placed to monitor CVP and guide fluid resuscitation. Multiple attempts at arterial line cannulation are unsuccessful and finally a left femoral artery catheter is successful placed. In relation to placement of an arterial line catheter, all of the following occur as the distance from the heart increases except:*

A. *The waveform narrows*

B. *The dicrotic notch becomes smaller*

C. *The systolic pressure rises*

D. *The diastolic pressure rises*

E. *The pulse pressure rises*

The placement of arterial catheters permits reliable and continuous monitoring of arterial pressure and easy repeated blood sampling. Analysis of the arterial pulse pressure curve also may have other applications, including assessment of fluid responsiveness and estimation of cardiac output. The appearance of arterial pressure waves will vary according to the site at which the artery is cannulated. As the arterial pressure wave is conducted away from the heart multiple effects can be observed: (1) the wave appears narrower; (2) the dicrotic notch becomes smaller; (3) the perceived systolic and pulse pressure rise and the perceived diastolic pressure falls. The pulse pressure increases from the core to the periphery. The smaller the diameter of the artery, the more the systolic pressure is overestimated.

Answer: D

De Backer D, Heenen S, Piagnerelli M, *et al.* (2005) Pulse pressure variations to predict volume responsiveness: Influence of tidal volume. *Intensive Care Medicine* **31** (4), 517–23.

Martin C, Saux P, Papazian L, Gouin F (2001) Long Term Arterial cannulation in ICU patients using the radial artery or the dorsalis pedis artery. *Chest* **119** (3), 901–6.

Parrillo J, Dellinger R. (2008) *Critical Care Medicine: Principles of Diagnosis and Management in the Adult.* 3rd edn. Mosby/Elsevier, Philadelphia, PA.

18. *A 15-year-old girl is injured in a motor vehicle collision and is intubated on scene secondary to decreased GCS. She suffers a grade 2 splenic laceration, a grade 1 liver laceration, multiple pelvic fractures, a right femur fracture, a small left occipital subdural hematoma without mass lesion effect and multiple right-sided nondisplaced rib fractures. An external fixation device is used on both the pelvis and femur fractures to provide stabilization. She is hemodynamically stable with a HR of 96 beats/minute, BP 110/75 mm Hg, SaO_2 100% with a set respiratory rate of 14 on pressure control ventilation. She is admitted to the SICU for further resuscitation. A right radial artery catheter is placed along with a right subclavian vein triple lumen catheter. CVP is transduced to help guide fluid resuscitation. All of the following can induce variability of CVP interpretation except:*

A. *Body position*

B. *Changes in thoracic pressure*

C. *Spontaneous variations*

D. *Manometer pressures*

E. *Internal jugular versus subclavian vein insertion site*

CVP is identical to right atrial pressure and to right ventricular end diastolic pressure. It is thus equivalent to the right-sided filling pressure. Analysis of the CVP waveform can provide some interesting information. Typically the ***a*** wave is greater than or equal to the ***v*** wave in the CVP tracing of a normal person. The presence of a large ***y*** descent indicates restriction of right ventricular filling; this can be due to intrinsic stiffness of the ventricular wall or occur in a ventricle that is excessively volume loaded. In either case, further volume loading is unlikely to change cardiac output. Loss of the ***x*** and ***y*** descent argues strongly for tamponade, whereas the presence of a prominent ***y*** descent argues against tamponade. The ***x*** and ***y*** descents are lost in tamponade because the pericardial fluid keeps the pressure inside the pericardium constant. Patients who have no inspiratory fall in CVP are on the flat part of their cardiac function curve and will not respond to fluids whereas patients who have an inspiratory fall in CVP are on the ascending part of the cardiac function curve and may or may not respond to fluids.

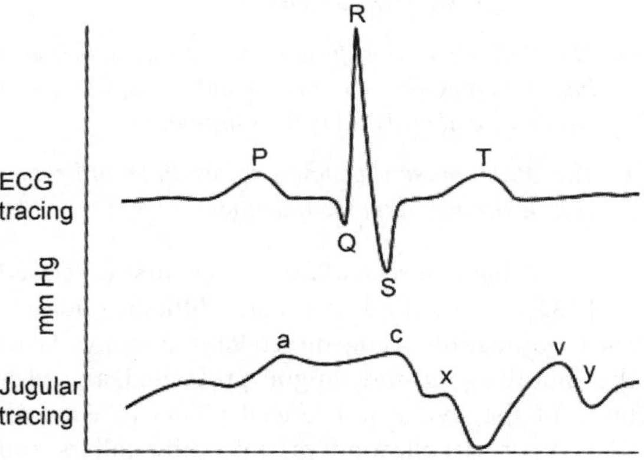

Central venous pressure waveforms.

Source: Reproduced from http://www.healthsystem.virginia.edu/internet/anesthesiology-elective/cardiac/cvpwave.cfm by permission of the University of Virginia School of Medicine.

- **a wave**: This wave is due to the increased atrial pressure during right atrial contraction. It correlates with the P wave on an EKG.
- **c wave**: This wave is caused by a slight elevation of the tricuspid valve into the right atrium during early ventricular contraction. It correlates with the end of the QRS segment on an EKG.
- **x descent**: This wave is probably caused by the downward movement of the ventricle during systolic contraction. It occurs before the T wave on an EKG.
- **v wave**: This wave arises from the pressure produced when the blood filling the right atrium comes up against a closed tricuspid valve. It occurs as the T wave is ending on an EKG.
- **y descent**: This wave is produced by the tricuspid valve opening in diastole with blood flowing into the right ventricle. It occurs before the P wave on an EKG.

Answer: E

Cook DJ, Simel DJ (1996) The rational clinical examination: does this patient have abnormal central venous pressure? *Journal of the American Medical Association* **275** (8), 630–4.

Joynt G, Gomersall C, Buckley T, Oh T, Young R, Freebairn R (1996) Comparison of intra-thoracic and intra-abdominal measurements of central venous pressure. *Lancet* **347** (9009), 1155–7.

Magder S (2006) Central venous pressure monitoring. *Current Opinion in Critical Care* **12** (3), 219–27.

Chapter 6 Airway Management, Anesthesia, and Perioperative Management

Jeffrey P. Coughenour, MD, FACS and Stephen L. Barnes, MD, FACS

1. *A 55-year-old man is admitted to the ICU with blunt chest trauma and multiple rib fractures. The patient develops progressive hypoxemia. Prior to medication administration to facilitate endotracheal intubation, what factors predict difficulty of bag-mask ventilation?*

A. *Body mass index*

B. *Lack of dentation*

C. *Age*

D. *History of snoring or sleep apnea*

E. *All of the above*

Effective oxygenation and ventilation may be difficult or impossible in some patients. Langeron and colleagues described several factors predictive of difficult or ineffective bag-mask ventilation: Age >55, body mass index >26 kg/m^2, beard, lack of teeth, and a history of snoring. Difficult bag-mask ventilation was also associated with difficult endotracheal intubation. Clinicians should be aware of these easily identifiable factors as they prepare personnel and equipment for airway management procedures, and should be familiar with failed airway alternatives. Use of a laryngeal mask airway (LMA), fiber-optic equipment, or surgical airway methods may be required.

Answer: E

Langeron O, Masso E, Huraux C (2000) Prediction of difficult mask ventilation. *Anesthesiology* **92**, 1229.

Surgical Critical Care and Emergency Surgery: Clinical Questions and Answers, First Edition. Edited by Forrest O. Moore, Peter M. Rhee, Samuel A. Tisherman and Gerard J. Fulda.

2. *Concerning the Mallampati classification of upper airway assessment, which of the following is correct?*

A. *Mallampati first described four classifications of airway visualization to predict difficulty of direct laryngoscopy*

B. *Modifications to the original Mallampati classification simplified its clinical application*

C. *The classification method is accurately predictive of difficult airway management*

D. *The Mallampati classification, while useful, carries a high false-positive rate and should be supplemented with a careful oral and neck examination*

E. *The Mallampati classification has little utilization outside the operating room setting*

The Mallampati classification was first described in 1985 as a method to predict difficult endotracheal intubation using direct laryngoscopy. With the mouth open and tongue protruded, the visibility of the uvula and faucial pillars is assessed. Class I, or visualization of the entire pillars and uvula, correlates with full visualization of the larynx and vocal cords. Class II is an approximate 50% view of these same structures. Class III, in which only the base of the uvula can be seen, suggests a partial view of the larynx but no visualization of the true vocal cords. Class IV was not a part of the original evaluation scheme; it was subsequently added to describe patients that could not be intubated with direct laryngoscopy. Modifications of the original classification scheme added physical characteristics or degree of medical illness in an attempt to improve accuracy. Unfortunately, these complex algorithms appear to result in high false-positive rates of predicting difficulty (as high as 50% in some series). Other factors to consider beyond basic upper airway assessment include cervical spine mobility, dentation, thyromental distance, and a history of previous difficult endotracheal intubation.

Answer: D

Mallampati SR, Gatt SP, Gugino LD, *et al.* (1985) A clinical sign to predict difficult tracheal intubation: a prospective study. *Canadian Anaesthetists Society Journal* **32**, 429.

El-Ganzouri AR, McCarthy RJ, Tuman KJ, *et al.* (1996) Preoperative airway assessment predictive value of a multivariate risk index. *Anesthesia and Analgesia* **82**, 1197.

3. *A 47-year-old man with an unremarkable past medical history is referred to you for right groin pain. Exam reveals a mildly painful, reducible inguinal hernia. Prior to surgery, what perioperative testing (if any) is indicated?*

A. No testing is indicated

B. CBC, electrolyte panel, and urinalysis

C. CBC only

D. 12-lead EKG, chest radiograph

E. Electrolytes and evaluation of renal function

Many surgeons, anesthesiologists, and certainly administrators believe perioperative testing is one way to avoid unnecessary complications during surgical procedures. In fact, nearly 50–60% of perioperative tests could be eliminated without additional risk to patients or providers. When a careful history and physical suggest no underlying medical conditions, no testing is indicated for patients younger than 40 years of age. In patients above 40, selected studies may be beneficial, and are listed as follows: if patient age >40, CBC; >50, BUN/creatinine and 12-lead EKG; >60, chest radiograph and electrolytes. In 2007, the American Heart Association published perioperative testing guidelines based on a patient's underlying functional status. This represents the most comprehensive, evidence-based guide to risk assessment for non-cardiac surgery.

Answer: C

Macpherson DS (1993) Preoperative lab testing: should any tests be routine before surgery? *Medical Clinics of North America* **77**, 289–308.

Perioperative Medical Therapy (2007) ACC/AHA 2007 Guidelines on Perioperative Cardiovascular Evalution and Care for Noncardiac Surgery: Executive Summary. *Circulation* **116**, 1971–96.

4. *A 25-year-old man is found down in the street. There is no obvious trauma on rapid assessment. He is minimally responsive as paramedics prepare to intubate him for airway protection. The natural cardiovascular response to direct laryngoscopy is:*

A. Hypertension and bradycardia

B. Hypertension and tachycardia

C. Hypotension and tachycardia

D. Hypotension and bradycardia

E. No significant cardiovascular response is expected

The upper airway contains significant innervation from both the sympathetic and parasympathetic systems. During laryngoscopy, proprioceptors at the tongue base stimulate catecholamine release, leading to hypertension and tachycardia. Receptors in the larynx and trachea may also contribute. These physiologic changes may also lead to increased myocardial oxygen use and peripheral oxygen consumption; both detrimental effects that may increase morbidity or mortality in patients with post-traumatic shock or traumatic brain injury.

Answer: B

Hassan HG, El-Sharkawy TY, Renck H, *et al.* (1991) Hemodynamic and catecholamine responses to laryngoscopy with vs. without endotracheal intubation. *Acta Anaesthesiologia Scandanavica* **35**, 442.

Shribman AJ, Smith G, Achola KJ (1987) Cardiovascular and catecholamine responses to laryngoscopy with and without tracheal intubation. *British Journal of Anaesthesia* **59**, 295.

5. *After intubating the patient in the previous question, a colorimetric carbon dioxide detection device is used to confirm tube placement. Situations which may render this method ineffective and unreliable include all of the following except:*

A. *Persistent shock with a pH <7.0*

B. *Significant antacid use*

C. *Diminished pulmonary blood flow*

D. *Cardiopulmonary arrest*

E. *Ingestion of carbonated beverages*

Qualitative colorimetic carbon dioxide detection devices are often employed in the pre-hospital environment because of their low cost and durability. Assuming carbon dioxide is detected after ventilation of the airway, several things can alter accuracy of these devices. Acid-base disorders, while affecting the patient's overall physiology, should not have an effect on the device itself. Antacids convert sodium bicarbonate to carbon dioxide in the stomach and may create a false-positive result. Diminished pulmonary blood flow means diminished alveolar gas exchange, and thus lower amounts of CO_2 available for detection. Acute pulmonary embolus, cardiopulmonary arrest, or profound shock with hypoperfusion may render the device useless. Large amounts of carbonated beverages contain high amounts of carbon dioxide and can also provide false assurance about a misplaced tube. The astute clinician employs several methods to confirm correct tube placement and will avoid potentially devastating consequences.

Answer: A

Sum Ping ST, Mehta MP, Symreng T (1991) Reliability of capnography in identifying esophageal intubation with carbonated beverage or antacid in the stomach. *Anesthesia and Analgesia* **73**, 333.

Falk JL, Rackow EC, Weil MH (1994) End-tidal carbon dioxide concentration during cardiopulmonary resuscitation. *New England Journal of Medicine* **12**, 413.

6. *A 58-year-old man suffers a distal tibia fracture in a motorcycle crash and is admitted to the orthopedic service. Three days later the orthopedic surgeon planning operative repair stops you in the lounge to ask if beta-blocker therapy would be beneficial. Your response should be:*

A. *Beta-blocker therapy has been proven to reduce risk in patients of all ages undergoing non-cardiac surgery*

B. *Beta-blocker therapy only benefits patients over 65, and is therefore not indicated*

C. *While the evidence is not definitive, it strongly supports beta-blocker therapy as early as possible before an intermediate-risk operation*

D. *This patient is low risk, thus beta-blocker therapy is not indicated*

E. *This patient is high risk, the operation should be delayed until the patient completes at least five (5) days of perioperative beta-blockade therapy*

Recent randomized trials have failed to reproduce the initial favorable results supporting the use of beta-blocker therapy in noncardiac surgery. Many studies lack adequate power but, when taken as a whole, the recommendations continue to "strongly suggest" benefit. Specifically, a reduction in perioperative ischemia, MI, and death may be seen in patients with known coronary artery disease. Therapy should be initiated days to weeks prior to planned operations, and long-acting beta-blockade agents may hold additional benefit over shorter acting alternatives. Orthopedic surgical procedures fall in the intermediate risk category.

Answer: C

Juul AB, Wetterslev J, Gluud C, *et al.* (2006) Effect of perioperative beta blockade in patients with diabetes undergoing major non-cardiac surgery: randomized placebo controlled, blinded multicentre trial. *British Medical Journal* **332**, 1482.

Perioperative Medical Therapy, ACC/AHA (2007) Guidelines on perioperative cardiovascular evaluation and care for noncardiac surgery: executive summary. *Circulation* **116**, 1971–96.

Redelmeier D, Scales D, Kopp A (2005) Beta blockers for elective surgery in elderly patients: population based, retrospective cohort study. *British Medical Journal* **331**, 932.

7. *An elderly woman falls from standing height and suffers a traumatic brain injury. While she has known coronary artery disease, she has not required stent placement or bypass surgery. On hospital day 6, she complains* *of chest pain and has ECG changes consistent with an acute MI. After moving to the ICU, she quickly deteriorates and suffers cardiac arrest. Her home medication list, which was never restarted, consisted of aspirin, atorvastatin, warfarin, and lisinopril. Which medication is most likely related to her acute cardiac event?*

A. Aspirin

B. Atorvastatin

C. Warfarin

D. Lisinopril

E. Aspirin and warfarin

By an incompletely understood mechanism, statin use in the perioperative or injury phase relays a protective effect (plaque stabilization is the most widely accepted theory). Hindler and colleagues, through a meta-analysis, demonstrated a 44% reduction in mortality. Other investigators demonstrated postoperative statin withdrawal was an independent predictor of myonecrosis. Complications began to manifest in patients as early as four (4) days after drug cessation, thus statins should be resumed as early as possible after operation or injury. In contrast, management of the other medications listed is often driven by surgeon or institutional practice, as little evidence exists to guide decision making. Antiplatelet agents are usually held for two weeks after a TBI, warfarin use may depend on the extent or location of injury, and ACE-inhibitors should be tailored to the patient's hemodynamic and renal function assessment following injury.

Answer: B

Hindler K. Shaw AD, Samuels J, Fulton S, *et al.* (2006) Improved postoperative outcomes associated with preoperative statin therapy. *Anesthesiology* **105**, 1260–72.

Le Manach Y, Godet G, Coriat P, *et al.* (2007) The impact of postoperative discontinuation or continuation of chronic statin therapy on cardiac outcome after major vascular surgery. *Anesthesia and Analgesia* **104**, 1326–33.

8. *Regarding the perioperative use of pulmonary artery catheters, which is correct?*

A. No benefit to routine use

B. Controlled trials show equivocal results

C. Some studies suggest potential harm

D. All of the above

E. None of the above

While pulmonary artery (PA) catheters provide advanced hemodynamic measures, clinicians may or may not possess the expertise to interpret and correctly act on the information to maximize patient benefit. Catheters should be reserved for high-risk patients. Controlled trials have shown equivocal results and the last citation showed potential harm. There is a growing amount of literature to support the use of continuous cardiac output evaluation using peripheral arterial catheters and/or ultrasound evaluation of vena cava size and respiratory variation as alternatives to assess volume status and responsiveness in the ICU setting. Utilization of a PA catheter should be guided by provider skill and institutional practice.

Answer: D

American Society of Anesthesiologists Task Force on Pulmonary Artery Catheterization (2003) Practice guidelines for pulmonary artery catheterization: an updated report by the American Society of Anesthesiologists Task Force on Pulmonary Artery Catheterization. *Anesthesiology* **99**, 988–1014.

Tote SP, Grounds RM (206) Performing perioperative optimization of the high-risk surgical patient. *British Journal of Anaesthesiology* **97**, 4–11.

Connors AF Jr, Speroff T, Dawson NV, *et al.* (1996) The effectiveness of right heart catheterization in the initial care of critically ill patients. SUPPORT Investigators, *Journal of the American Medical Association* **276**, 889–97.

9. *The critical care fellow has ordered an echocardiogram to evaluate the left ventricular function of a 69-year-old man admitted to your ICU for "medical optimization" before a right hemicolectomy for a cecal mass. The family relays a significant history of coronary disease. He is often short of breath after walking back from the mailbox, but improves with rest and is stable on his home antihypertensives and diuretics. In this situation, the echo is:*

A. Indicated and likely to yield information to guide care

B. Indicated but unlikely to yield information to guide care

C. Not indicated for this patient

D. *Not indicated, but the patient's condition mandates intraoperative use of a pulmonary artery catheter*

E. *Not indicated, regardless of functional assessment*

This clinical scenario describes a patient with stable heart failure. Patients with dyspnea of unknown origin or those with previous heart failure *and* new or worsening dyspnea (or other significant clinical change) should undergo preoperative evaluation of left ventricular (LV) function. If studies were preformed within 12 months of the planned operative date, new testing may not be necessary. Those without symptoms, even if there is a known history of CAD and/or heart failure, do not need mandated LV function assessment prior to proceeding to surgery (Class IIa and IIb evidence).

Answer: C

Fleisher LA, Beckman JA, Brown KA, *et al.* (2007) Recommendations for perioperative noninvasive evaluation of left ventricular function, ACC/AHA 2007 guidelines on perioperative cardiovascular evaluation and care for noncardiac surgery: executive summary. *Circulation* **116**, 1971–96.

10. *A 24-year-old woman is 15 weeks pregnant. She comes to the emergency department with a 36-hour history of abdominal pain and is diagnosed with appendicitis. You spend considerable time discussing the treatment plan with the anesthesiologist because of your extensive review of the literature regarding airway management in pregnant patients. All of the following are true except:*

A. *Higher complication rates, but no change in mortality*

B. *Relaxation of bronchial smooth muscle and relaxation of the upper esophageal sphincter*

C. *Functional residual capacity is decreased*

D. *Baseline oxygen consumption is increased, causing higher risk for hypoxemia*

E. *None of the above—all statements are correct*

Failed intubation may occur eight times as often as in the non-pregnant population. Mortality has also been reported as 13–15 times higher, often associated with general anesthesia and the inability to place an airway. Increased levels of circulating progesterone cause relaxation of bronchial smooth muscle and minute ventilation is increased. Despite these favorable changes, the pregnant patient is at high risk for developing hypoxemia during intubation. Functional residual capacity is decreased, because of the gravid uterus, and this effect progresses as the fetus grows. Baseline oxygen consumption is also increased. Progesterone also slows gastric motility and relaxes the upper esophageal sphincter, making the pregnant patient prone to aspiration. Early oxygenation, assurance of gastric decompression, proper patient positioning, and thorough preoperative assessment are necessary to minimize potential complications.

Answer: A

Rasmussen GE, Malinow AM (1994) Toward reducing maternal mortality: the problem airway in obstetrics. *International Anesthiology Clinics* **32**, 83.

Rizk NW, Kalassian KG, Gilligan T, *et al.* (1996) Obstetric complications in pulmonary and critical care medicine. *Chest* **110**, 791.

11. *As the associate medical director for your hospital's air ambulance program, the chief flight nurse has asked you to review the pharmacologic guidelines for airway management in brain injured patients. After review of the protocol and existing literature, which drug are you going to suggest be used during rapid-sequence induction of patients with a traumatic brain injury?*

A. *Midazolam*

B. *Propofol*

C. *Etomidate*

D. *Both A. and B.*

E. *All of the above*

While each induction agent is acceptable, midazolam and propofol possess certain effects that make them less desirable in the specific clinical setting of traumatic brain injury. At the standard induction dose of 0.2 mg/kg, midazolam can cause moderate hypotension, decreasing blood pressure an average of 15–25%. Propofol causes a similar decrease in mean arterial pressure, thus decreasing cerebral perfusion pressure and potentially causing secondary brain injury. Etomidate is a good alternative, especially for the hemodynamically unstable, as it has little if any cardiovascular effect. Single induction doses have been associated with decreased plasma cortisol levels, but the clinical significance of this effect is difficult to define outside the setting of septic shock. Ketamine is another good alternative, with few adverse hemodynamic effects and historical concerns of ICP elevation unfounded in contemporary literature.

Answer: C

Nordt SP, Clark RF (1997) Midazolam: a review of therapeutic uses and toxicity. *Journal of Emergency Medicine* **15** (3), 357–65.

Steiner LA, Johnston AJ, Chatfield DA, *et al.* (2003) The effects of large-dose propofol on cerebrovascular pressure autoregulation in head-injured patients. *Anesthesia and Analgesia* **97** (2), 572–6.

Zed PJ, Abu-Laban RB, Harrison DW (2006) Intubating conditions and hemodynamic effects of etomidate for rapid sequence intubation in the emergency department: an observational cohort study. *Academic Emergency Medicine* **13** (4), 378–83.

12. *A 45-year-old man is scheduled to undergo an open ventral herniorrhaphy 12 months after damage-control surgery for a grade 4 liver injury. He smokes 1 to 2 packs per day, takes two agents to control his hypertension, and uses an assist device for ambulation. The correct American Society of Anesthesiologists (ASA) classification for this patient and this operation is:*

A. 2

B. 2E

C. 3

D. 3E

E. 4

The American Society of Anesthesiologists (originally the American Society of Anesthetists) developed this simple scale to describe the degree of a patient's medical illness. The numeric system was designed to ease communication between providers, provide a common language for documentation, and ease data abstraction for research. Because of variation among providers, it should not be used as the sole determinant of patient status and is not meant to act as an evaluation of perioperative risk.

ASA 1: Healthy patient; excludes extremes of age, good exercise tolerance.

ASA 2: Mild systemic disease, well controlled disease of one body system without functional limitations; controlled hypertension, smoking without COPD, mild obesity, pregnancy.

ASA 3: Severe systemic disease, controlled disease of more than one body system or one major system, often with some degree of functional limitation; no immediate danger of death; controlled congestive heart failure (CHF), poorly controlled hypertension, morbid obesity, etc.

ASA 4: Severe systemic disease, at least one severe disease that is poorly controlled or at end stage; possible risk of death; unstable angina, symptomatic COPD, symptomatic CHF, hepatorenal failure.

ASA 5: Moribund patients not expected to survive >24 hours without surgery; imminent risk of death; multiorgan failure, sepsis syndrome with hemodynamic instability, hypothermia, coagulopathy.

ASA 6: Brain dead patients undergoing organ or tissue procurement procedures for transplantation.

An "E" is added to any case designated emergent.

Answer: C

ASA Physical Status Classification System, American Society of Anesthesiologists, available at www.asahq.org (accessed September 25, 2010).

Haynes SR, Lawler PG (1995) An assessment of the consistency of ASA physical status classification allocation. *Anaesthesia* **50**(3), 195–9.

13. *A patient with extremity fractures and an open abdomen develops sudden hypoxemia. A chest radiograph shows a new right lower lobar collapse. Propofol is selected to facilitate flexible bronchoscopy and directed bronchoalveolar lavage. Concerning the use of propofol in the ICU, which of the following statements is incorrect?*

A. ASA guidelines recommend only anesthesia providers utilize propofol, even in the ICU setting

B. Propofol can have rapid, dose-dependent variations in sedation/anesthetic affect

C. *Because bronchoscopy is a minimally invasive procedure, the surgeon performing bronchoscopy can safely direct propofol dosing, administration, and monitoring by the ICU nursing staff*

D. *Myocardial depression and hypotension are known side effects*

E. *None of the above—all are correct statements*

Propofol is a general anesthetic agent, and is preferably administered by an anesthesia provider, however qualified non-anesthesia personnel can safely use the drug in the critical-care setting. Propofol is used to facilitate airway management or other invasive procedures, but rapid variations in sedation/anesthetic depth and hemodynamic alterations make adequate preparation vital to assure optimal outcomes. After a careful history, physical examination, and review of current medications and allergies, physiologic parameters should be continuously monitored (heart rate, blood pressure, oxygenation, and ventilation). A single provider, not involved in the planned procedure, should direct the administration of sedative agents and monitor for potential complications. Proficiency in life saving (or sustaining) maneuvers for common complications (hypoventilation, hypoxemia, hypotension) is necessary, and the provider should remain in this role throughout the procedure and recovery period.

Answer: C

American Society of Anesthesiologists, Statement on Safe Use of Propofol, available at www.asahq.org (accessed September 20, 2010).

14. *In the previous question, propofol was used by the ICU team during an endoscopic procedure to clear an acute lobar collapse. During the procedure, the patient would not awaken or move purposefully. Shortly after completion, he slowly returned to his baseline mental state, responding appropriately and following commands. There were no hemodynamic complications. What type of sedation did this patient receive?*

A. *Minimal sedation*

B. *Moderate sedation*

C. *Deep sedation*

D. *Conscious sedation*

E. *General anesthesia*

The defining lines of levels of sedation and analgesia in the ICU can be blurred, especially when patients may have differing responses to medications. Patients may go "deeper" than intended, thus necessitating preparedness to deal with potential complications. Generally accepted definitions are as follows:

Minimal sedation—anxiolysis, the patient maintains a normal response to questions; airway patency, adequate ventilation, and hemodynamics are not affected.

Moderate sedation—normal, purposeful response to verbal or light tactile stimulus; airway patency, adequate ventilation, and hemodynamics are unlikely to be affected.

Deep sedation—purposeful response only after repeated verbal or painful stimulus; airway patency and adequate ventilation may be an issue, hemodynamics usually preserved.

General anesthesia—loss of consciousness, no purposeful response; airway maneuvers are likely required, ventilation likely needs assistance, hemodynamics may require attention.

Answer: E

American Society of Anesthesiologists. Continuum of Depth of Sedation: Definition of General Anesthesia and Levels of Sedation/Analgesia, available at www.asahq.org (accessed September 20, 2010).

15. *About one week ago, a young man was thrown from a car and suffered blunt chest trauma with severe pulmonary contusions. He was originally admitted to a community hospital, and has now been transferred to your ICU with suspected ventilator-associated pneumonia. He has been started on antimicrobials and methyprednisolone for suspected critical-illness related corticosteroid insufficiency. Ventilation and oxygenation became increasingly difficult, so the team initiated neuromuscular blockade and prone positioning. Concerning the use of neuromuscular blockade agents in the ICU, which of the following is incorrect?*

A. Indications include facilitation of mechanical ventilation, managing increased ICP, treatment of muscle spasms, and decreasing oxygen consumption

B. Patients requiring external cooling for fevers ≥40 °C may benefit from NMBAs

C. Patients should be monitored clinically and by TOF (train-of-four) testing, with the goal of one or two twitches

D. There is no correlation between corticosteroids and NMBAs in the development of polyneuropathy

E. Development of tachyphylaxis to one NMBA is not a contraindication to trying a second agent, assuming NMB is still required

Neuromuscular blockade in the ICU may be required for the most severely ill or injured. Assurance of adequate sedation and analgesia is a prerequisite prior to initiation of NMBAs. Commonly accepted indications include attempts to improve ventilation/oxygenation, treating persistent ICP elevations, muscle spasms associated with tetanus, seizures, or drug overdose, and decreasing elevated oxygen consumption. Attempts to externally cool significantly febrile patients may produce shivering, and thus increase oxygen consumption—NMBAs can be employed to counteract this effect. Clinical assessment and train-of-four testing are required. The goal is to use as little agent as possible while maintaining one or two twitches. Daily interruptions and resuming NMBAs only in patients with continued indications is best. Several neuromuscular blockade agents have been implicated in the development of diffuse muscle weakness, fiber atrophy, and occasionally myonecrosis. An association with steroid administration exists, with the incidence of myopathy as high as 30% in patients also receiving corticosteroids. It does appear safe to try another NMBA when patients development tachyphylaxis. Despite relatively safe utilization guidelines, it remains in the patient's best interest to minimize the dose and duration of therapy.

	Cisatracurium (Nimbex)	Pancuronium (Pavulon)	Vecuronium (Norcuron)	Rocuronium (Zemuron)
Initial dose (mg/kg)	0.1–0.2	0.06–0.1	0.08–0.1	0.6–1
Duration (min)	45–60	90–100	35–45	30
Infusion described	Yes	Yes	Yes	Yes
Infusion dose (μg/kg/min)	2.5–3	1–2	0.8–1.2	10–12
Recovery (min)	90	120–180	45–60	20–30
% Renal excretion	Hofmann elimination	45–70	50	33
Renal failure	No change	Increased effect	Increased effect	Minimal
% Biliary excretion	Hofmann elimination	10–15	35–50	<75
Hepatic failure	Minimal to no change	Mild increased effect	Variable, mild	Moderate
Active metabolites	No	Yes, 3-OH and 17-OH pancuronium	Yes, 3-desacetyl-vecuronium	No
Histamine release hypotension	No	No	No	No
Vagal block tachycardia	No	Yes	No	At higher doses
Ganglionic blockade hypotension	No	No	No	No

Source: Adapted from Table 1, Clinical practice guidelines for sustained neuromuscular blockade in the adult critically ill patient. *Critical Care Medicine* 2002; **30**, 142–56.

Answer: D

Murray MJ, Cowen J, DeBlock H, *et al.* (2002) Clinical practice guidelines for sustained neuromuscular blockade in the adult critically ill patient. *Critical Care Medicine* **30**, 142–56.

16. *An emergency medicine faculty member at your institution requires cholecystectomy for recent gallstone-associated pancreatitis. He is taking a beta-blocker and calcium-channel blocker for hypertension. His perioperative evaluation did not reveal any hypertensive complications. In the pre-op holding area his blood pressure is 180/118. You should:*

A. *Cancel the case, admit the patient for parenteral antihypertensive therapy*

B. *Cancel the case, reschedule only after the patient has seen his primary care physician*

C. *Proceed only after administering parenteral beta-blockade*

D. *Proceed after a discussion with the patient and anesthesia team, understanding the patient would likely benefit most from undergoing the operation (and avoiding recurrent pancreatitis) and making subtle adjustments to his chronic antihypertensive therapy as warranted*

E. *Make no changes to his medication regimen, the hypertension is probably related to pain*

This case describes a patient with long-standing hypertension, who has a fairly urgent (although not emergent) reason for an operation. This is not a hypertensive urgency/emergency, thus admission is not warranted. Patients with significant hypertension (SBP ≥180 mm Hg or DBP ≥110 mm Hg) require careful assessment of the risks and benefits of proceeding with any planned operation. Additional adjustment of chronic therapy may benefit patients prior to proceeding. This decision is likely made on a case-by-case basis, with one randomized trial showing no benefit to delaying operations in patients without end-organ damage. As a general rule, antihypertensive medications should be continued to the operative date and resumed as soon as deemed safe. Exceptions include ACE inhibitors and angiotensin receptor antagonists, where perioperative volume depletion may exacerbate the risk of renal dysfunction. Sudden decreases in chronically elevated blood pressure, as in choice c, may have unintended consequences such as diminished myocardial perfusion, increasing the risk for ischemia.

Answer: D

Fleisher LA, Beckman JA, Brown KA, *et al.* (2007) Disease-Specific Approaches–Hypertension, ACC/AHA 2007 guidelines on perioperative cardiovascular evaluation and care for noncardiac surgery: executive summary. *Circulation* **116**, 1971–96.

Weksler N, Klein M, Szendro G, *et al.* (2003) The dilemma of immediate preoperative hypertension: to treat and operate, or to postpone surgery? *Journal of Clinical Anesthesia* **15**, 179–83.

17. *The charge nurse frantically calls you to the ICU. The residents have appropriately sedated a patient with progressive pulmonary insufficiency, but have thus far been unable to intubate him. After three failed attempts at direct laryngoscopy, the next maneuver may be:*

A. *Change to a different blade and reattempt direct laryngoscopy*

B. *Consider placing a laryngeal mask airway (LMA) as a rescue device*

C. *Obtain a bougie and attempt blind passage into the trachea*

D. *Attempt fiber-optic intubation using a flexible bronchoscope*

E. *All of the above*

When unable to intubate, call for help. Next follow your institution's difficult airway algorithm, to direct a stepwise approach to achieve endotracheal intubation. Simple maneuvers, such as repositioning the head or neck, or obtaining a larger blade may be enough. A floppy epiglottis may require switching from a curved MacIntosh blade to a straight Miller blade. Several rescue devices are commercially available. The LMA is probably the most popular in the hospital setting. While it does not provide a definitive airway, it can enable oxygenation and ventilation while more advanced equipment is mobilized. As a last resort, a tube exchanger or bougie can be passed blindly, feeling for ridges of the tracheal rings as it passes distally. This has a surprisingly high success rate in some studies. Fiberoptic intubation is also an alternative, but often requires time to gather equipment and a considerable amount of skill. It would not be the best option in an unprepared, emergent setting. Remember, all these maneuvers assume you are able to ventilate and oxygenate the patient with a bag-valve mask.

Answer: E

Berkow LC, Greenberg RS, Kan KH, *et al.* (2009) Need for emergency surgical airway reduced by a comprehensive difficult airway program. *Anesthesia and Analgesia* **109** (6), 1860–9.

Combes X, Jabre P, Margenet A, *et al.* (2011) Unanticipated difficult airway management in the prehospital emergency setting: prospective validation of an algorithm. *Anesthesiology* **114** (1), 105–10.

18. *In the patient scenario above, you are trying to find a fiber-optic laryngoscope or bronchoscope to assist with intubation when the resident informs you the patient continues to desaturate. You ask if he is able to move any air with the bag-valve mask. The answer is "no!" Your next maneuver is:*

A. Proceed with cricothyroidotomy

B. Administer additional sedative agents

C. Perform trans-tracheal jet ventilation

D. Proceed with percutaneous tracheostomy

E. Proceed with open tracheostomy

The difficult airway algorithm has converted to a failed airway management scenario when providers are unable to adequately oxygenate or ventilate the patient using a bag-valve mask. The patient is about to die—you need to act now! Cricothyroidotomy is the procedure of choice. Trans-tracheal jet ventilation is an option in pediatric patients, but practically is seldom used, and therefore would be very difficult. While percutaneous tracheostomy can be performed successfully in an emergency situation, cricothyroidotomy is still the surgical airway procedure of choice given the readily identifiable anatomy and short distance from skin to tracheal lumen.

Answer: A

Latto IP, Stacey M, Mecklenburgh J, Vaughan RS (2002) Survey of the use of the gum elastic bougie in clinical practice. *Anaesthesia* **57**, 379–84.

American Society of Anesthesiologists Task Force on Management of the Difficult Airway (2003) Practice guidelines for management of the difficult airway: an updated report by the American Society of Anesthesiologists Task Force on Management of the Difficult Airway. *Anesthesiology* **98**, 1269–77.

19. *An elderly patient with known peripheral vascular disease requires a percutaneous intervention for acute lower extremity ischemia. This fails and the vascular team plans a formal bypass operation with fasciotomies. The patient has an implantable cardiac defibrillator (ICD). Concerning the perioperative care of implantable devices, which of the following is correct?*

A. Electromagnetic interference can be interpreted as ventricular tachycardia or fibrillation

B. Interrogation is recommended within 1 month of major operations

C. If cardioversion is required with a disabled device, paddles should be placed in the standard anterior and left apical position

D. Magnets only temporarily disable implantable device function while in place

E. Regardless of the manufacturer, ICDs respond to magnets the same way

Implantable pacemakers and defibrillators are affected by electromagnetic interference, often from intra-operative electrocautery. The interference causes abnormal signals that can be interpreted as tachy-arrythmias, causing devices to fire unnecessarily. Because devices and modes have specific interpretation and therapeutic algorithms, interrogation is recommended within 3–6 months of operations likely to require significant amounts of electrocautery. Devices are safely placed into an asynchronous mode during the operation. If emergent cardioversion is required, paddles should be placed in an anterior-posterior position, to direct current away from device leads. Magnets can also be placed over implantable devices to disable various functions but results are specific to the manufacturer and device. Some stop the antitachycardia function only while the magnet is in place, others permanently disable the device, making re-evaluation after the surgery necessary. A practice guideline has been published by the American Society of Anesthesiologists to assist practitioners.

Answer: A

American Society of Anesthesiologists Task Force on Perioperative Management of Patients with Cardiac Rhythm Management Devices (2005) Practice advisory for the perioperative management of patients with cardiac rhythm management devices: pacemakers and implantable cardioverter-defibrillators: a report by the American Society of Anesthesiologists Task Force on Perioperative Management of Patients with Cardiac Rhythm Management Devices. *Anesthesiology* **103**, 186–98.

20. *The orthopedic surgeons have called you to the operating theater to assist in the resuscitation of a pelvic fracture patient. The patient was injured 2 days ago, and while undergoing fixation of a sacral fracture, developed significant hemorrhage. An ABG shows a pH of 7.2 and a base deficit of 8. The last patient temperature was 95 °F and hemoglobin sent just prior to you being called was 10.6. There is obvious ongoing bleeding from the presacral venous plexus. What resuscitation strategy would you recommend?*

A. *2 U FFP and two U packed red blood cells, prepare two more units of each product*

B. *Begin lactated ringers at a "wide-open" rate, and begin packed red blood cells after 2 L have been infused*

C. *Two U packed red blood cells only and reassess lab values assuming hemorrhage control is obtained*

D. *Activate the institution's massive transfusion policy, as this patient already demonstrates several risk factors of increased mortality related to acute blood loss anemia*

E. *Given the hemoglobin of 10.6, no transfusion is currently required*

Resuscitation with the early use of blood and blood products with minimization of crystalloid volume seems to hold promise in correcting physiologic abnormalities early and limiting complications. Contemporary research from the United States Armed Forces identified five physiologic factors that reliably predict the need for massive transfusion, commonly defined as a transfusion requirement of 10 units of packed red blood cells during the initial 24 hours of care. Although employing a damage-control resuscitation" strategy is necessary in a minority of civilian trauma patients, the triggers are applicable to the perioperative management of ICU patients undergoing major operations. Coagulopathy (INR >1.5) present on admission is a marker of severe injury. Degree of coagulopathy and mortality carry a linear correlation. Next, a base deficit of >6 confirms cellular hypoperfusion, which may be present despite a normal blood pressure. A temperature of <96 °F is associated with an increased mortality. The key to hypothermia is prevention. Hemoglobin levels of <11 gm/dl are likely caused by acute blood loss anemia. The ICU population may manifest other causes and clinicians should balance the correlation with increased mortality with literature supporting a more restrictive transfusion policy in patients without ongoing blood loss. Lastly, hypotension from blood loss represents late class III or class IV shock, and requires aggressive hemostasis and return of normal cellular perfusion.

Answer: D

Cotton BA, Au BK, Nunez TC, *et al.* (2009) Predefined massive transfusion protocols are associated with a reduction in organ failure and postinjury complications. *Journal of Trauma* **66**, 41–9.

Duchesne JC, Islam TM, Stuke L, *et al.* (2009) Hemostatic Resuscitation during surgery improves survival in patients with traumatic-induced coagulopathy. *Journal of Trauma* **67**, 33–9.

21. *Concerning management of anticoagulation and antiplatelet medication prior to elective surgery, which of the following is correct?*

A. *Antiplatelet agents should be discontinued in all patients 7–10 days prior to operation*

B. *Generally speaking, patients on chronic aspirin therapy for cerebrovascular or coronary events should not have therapy withheld*

C. *Operations with a risk for confined space hemorrhage (CNS, spine, ocular) do not carry special considerations when compared to other elective surgical operations*

D. *Patients with recent PCI and stent placement can have therapy withheld 1–2 weeks after the procedure*

E. *Warfarin should be held for three days prior to a planned surgical intervention*

Platelet activity returns to normal levels in most patients 7–10 days after discontinuation of antiplatelet therapy. Stopping antiplatelet agents to minimize bleeding risk is generally accepted and safe. Special situations exist in two groups: those on chronic aspirin therapy for cerebrovascular or coronary events, and those recently undergoing percutaneous interventions with stent placement. Patients on chronic therapy should not have therapy withheld unless the risk of bleeding complications (CNS, spine, and ocular—confined space hemorrhage). outweighs that of thrombotic events. Recent PCI patients require combination aspirin and clopidogrel therapy for a recommended 2–4 weeks, and should have elective procedures delayed for 1–3 months. Warfarin should be held for 5–7 days prior to the planned procedure, with heparin used in the perioperative period for high-risk patients.

Answer: B

Backman SB, Bondy RM, Deschamps A, *et al.* (2005) Perioperative considerations for anesthesia. In: Souba WW, Fink MP, Jurkovich GJ, *et al.* (eds) *ACS Surgery: Principles and Practice*. WebMD Inc.: New York, NY.

22. *Issues related to hyperglycemia in the perioperative period include all of the following except:*

A. *Impaired phagocytosis*

B. *Increased incidence of wound complications*

C. *Enhanced production of catecholamines, glucagon, and insulin*

D. *Infectious complications are common among poorly controlled diabetics undergoing surgery*

E. *Hypoglycemia associated with intensive insulin therapy is not clearly related to increased mortality*

Several physiologic changes occur during surgery in patients with diabetes. Hyperglycemia retards phagocytic function of PMNs, and may contribute to poor collagen synthesis, thus wound complications and infection are common. Hormones elevated during the stress response include catecholamines, growth hormone, cortisol, and glucagon. In contrast, insulin production is depressed. Intensive insulin therapy has become common practice in the ICU. What is less clear, however, is the role of hypoglycemia in patient outcome. While target levels have been relaxed from the initial 80–110 mg/dL range, conflicting literature exists about the impact of hypoglycemia episodes and mortality. Patients undergoing minor procedures should likely receive all or 50% of their home dose prior to operation, assuming a quick return to oral intake. Patients poorly controlled or those with major operations are best managed on continuous insulin infusions until the stress response abates and home regimens can be resumed with reasonable control.

Answer: C

Lawrence RM, Walter RM (1995) Diabetes mellitus. In: Lubin MF, Walker HK, Smith RB III (eds) *Medical Management of the Surgical Patient, Third Edition.* J. B. Lippincott Company, Philadelphia, PA, pp. 317–21.

Mowery NT, Guillamondegui OD, Gunter OL, *et al.* (2010) Severe hypoglycemia while on intensive insulin therapy is not an independent predictor of death after trauma. *Journal of Trauma* **68** (2), 342–7.

23. *A 28-year-old woman is shot in the abdomen. Prior to moving to the operating room for celiotomy, she relates a history of inflammatory bowel disease and prednisone 20 mg daily as her current therapy. Before anesthesia induction, you should:*

A. *Administer cosyntropin 250 mcg IV and draw a cortisol level*

B. *Presume HPA-axis suppression and administer 100 mg hydrocortisone IV now*

C. *Presume HPA-axis suppression and administer 10 mg hydrocortisone IM now*

D. *Not administer any additional steroid but resume her home medication dose as soon as possible*

E. *Not administer additional steroid, and hold her home dose to minimize wound complications*

The perioperative evaluation and management of patients on chronic exogenous steroid therapy remains controversial, with little literature to guide practice. In general, patients on more than 20 mg per day for at least three weeks should be considered to have a suppressed hypothalamic-pituitary-adrenal (HPA) axis. Symptoms are extremely vague, and may include nausea, anorexia, weakness, and fatigue. For elective operations, consider performance of a cortisol-stimulation test by administering cosyntropin 250 mcg IV/IM. A rise of ≥9 mg/dL from baseline indicates a positive response. For major emergency cases, administer hydrocortisone 100 mg before anesthesia induction and 100 mg every 8 hours for at least 24 hours. Moderate stress procedures should receive 100 mg once. Minor procedures done under local anesthesia or MAC likely do not require additional therapy—continuing maintenance doses are often adequate. Supplemental steroids should then be tapered rapidly to avoid immunosuppression, altered wound healing, or other complications.

Answer: B

Zalolga GP, Marik P (2001) Hypothalamic-pituitary-adrenal insufficiency. *Critical Care Clinics* **17**, 25–41.

Salem M, Tainsh RE Jr, Bromberg J *et al.* (1994) Perioperative glucocorticoid coverage—A reassessment 42 Years after emergence of a problem. *Annals of Surgery* 1994; **219**, 416–25.

24. *A 73-year-old man with advanced COPD and an 80-pack-year history of smoking is admitted to the ICU with an acute COPD exacerbation following inguinal hernia repair. Attempts to improve oxygenation through noninvasive measures are unsuccessful. A decision to orally intubate the patient is made. All of the following physical exam findings are predictive of a difficult orotracheal intubation except:*

A. *Invisibility of faucial pillars, soft palate, uvula*

B. *Mentohyoid distance > three finger breadths*

C. *Restricted TM joint excursion*

D. *Restricted excusion of atlanto-occipital joint*

E. *Excessive facial hair or beard*

In a minority of critically ill patients, even a well trained practitioner familiar with conventional intubation techniques will experience difficulty. This is particularly important for patients with acute hypoxemia, acidosis, or hemodynamic instability. Certain physical features predicting difficulty include: (1) non-visibility of key oropharyngeal landmarks, (2) poor atlanto-occipital joint mobility, (3) short mentohyoid distance (<3 finger breaths), (4) mentohyoid distance <6 cm, and (5) restricted TM joint excursion (maximal oral aperture less than three vertical breadths in the sagital midline).. While the presence of excess facial hair or a beard is often omitted from airway evaluation, it may result in difficulty obtaining a seal during bag-valve mask ventilation. Numerous techniques are available to aid in securing the difficult airway.

Answer: B

Marini JJ, and Wheeler AP (2006) Airway Intubation. In: Marini J. J. and Wheeler A. P. (eds) *Critical Care Medicine*, 3rd edn. Lippincott Williams & Wilkins, Philadelphia, PA.

25. *Ten days after a MVC, a 2-year-old boy is persistently cognitively impaired from diffuse axonal injury. The patient remains on mechanical ventilation through an orally placed endotracheal tube while the trauma team schedules a tracheostomy. Tracheostomy has many benefits over translaryngeal intubation for long-term mechanical ventilation, which may include all of the following except:*

A. *Secretion removal*

B. *Decreased airway resistance*

C. *Patient comfort and decreased sedation/analgesia requirements*

D. *Fewer acute and long-term airway complications*

E. *Decreased incidence of ventilator-associated pneumonia*

Tracheostomy improves comfort and potentially allows patients to eat, talk, and ambulate. Secretion management is much easier, and airway resistance, anatomic dead space, and laryngeal injury are minimized. However, tracheostomies have the highest associated risk of serious complications including bleeding, stenosis, dysphagia, and aspiration after decannulation. Conventional methods of tracheostomy should be performed in an operating theatre, however when clinician comfort and anatomic landmarks are favorable, percutaneous tracheostomy in the ICU is a safe alternative.

Answer: D

Littlewood K, Durbin CG Jr. (2002) Evidence-based airway management. *Respiratory Care* **47** (6), 696; author reply 696–9.

Livingston, DH (2000) Prevention of ventilator-associated pneumonia. *American Journal of Surgery* **179**, 12S7S.

Chapter 7 Acute Respiratory Failure and Mechanical Ventilation

Lewis J. Kaplan, MD, FACS, FCCM, FCCP and Adrian A. Maung, MD, FACS

1. *In the immediate postoperative setting, noninvasive ventilation has been demonstrated to be most effective at:*

A. *Reversing atelectasis*

B. *Decreasing laryngeal edema*

C. *Improving cardiac performance*

D. *Reducing inspiratory stridor*

E. *Decreasing wheezing*

By applying positive pressure ventilation, noninvasive ventilation (NIV) is able to augment a patient's native respiratory efforts, overcoming critical closing pressures and volumes, better match regional time constant variations and therefore move the zero-pressure point more proximal in the airway. These effects help reverse atelectasis and therefore NIV has been used to great effect in the immediate post-operative setting in the PACU as well as on the general ward. NIV has no effect on laryngeal edema, inspiratory stridor or wheezing. NIV may augment cardiac performance by reversing hypoxic pulmonary vasoconstriction, but this is not universally observed, even in those with hypoxemia that is reversed, nor in those with atelectasis that is effectively treated with NIV.

Answer: A

Jaber S, Chanques G, Jung B (2010) Postoperative noninvasive ventilation. *Anesthesiology* **112** (2), 453–61.

Papadakos PJ, Karcz M, Lachmann B (2010) Mechanical ventilation in trauma. *Current Opinion in Anaesthesiology* **23** (2), 228–32.

Surgical Critical Care and Emergency Surgery: Clinical Questions and Answers, First Edition. Edited by Forrest O. Moore, Peter M. Rhee, Samuel A. Tisherman and Gerard J. Fulda.

2. *A 72-year-old, non-obese woman undergoes a laparoscopic ventral hernia repair without incident. She is extubated in the OR but is found to be hypoxic, hypercarbic and acidotic in the PACU requiring reintubation. The most likely cause of her acute respiratory failure is:*

A. *Acute pulmonary edema from volume overload*

B. *Post-operative hemorrhage*

C. *Carbon dioxide gas embolism*

D. *Inadequate neuromuscular blocker reversal*

E. *Abdominal compartment syndrome*

Inadequate reversal of neuromuscular blocking (NMB) agents is an important cause for acute respiratory failure in the PACU, although it is less likely than intrinsic pulmonary disorders—an unlikely event in this healthy 72-year-old woman. The likelihood of NMB reversal inadequacy is increased in the elderly, the clinically severely obese, patients with hypoperfusion, and those whose procedure occurs more rapidly than anticipated after receiving a long-acting NMB agent. Uneventful OR cases are uncommonly associated with pulmonary edema in the relatively young, but are more frequently observed in those with preexisting significant cardiopulmonary disease. While a patient with obesity is likely to have pulmonary HTN, pulmonary edema is still less likely than inadequate NMB agent reversal. Post-op hemorrhage is uncommonly associated with hypercarbia, and CO_2 embolism generally occurs while the abdomen in insufflated with CO_2—not after desufflation. Similarly, ventral hernia repair that is performed laparoscopically is unlikely to result in abdominal compartment syndrome as patients who are suitable for a laparoscopic repair generally do not demonstrate significant loss of domain.

Answer: D

Cobb WS, Fleishman HA, Kercher KW, Matthews BD, Heniford BT (2005) Gas embolism during laparoscopic cholecystectomy. *Journal of Laparoendoscopic and Advanced Surgical Techniques. Part A.* **15** (4), 387–90.

Lee PJ, MacLennan A, Naughton NN, O'Reilly M (2003) An analysis of reintubations from a quality assurance database of 152 000 cases. *Journal of Clinical Anesthesia.* **15** (8), 575–81.

3. *A 19-year-old man undergoes an uneventful laparoscopic appendectomy for microperforated appendicitis. The case goes more quickly than anticipated and he is transferred to the PACU still intubated. He is then extubated with a train-of-four of 4/4 twitches and shortly thereafter develops stridor as well as hypoxia despite vigorous respiratory efforts and gas movement. A portable CXR is most likely to demonstrate:*

A. *Westermark sign*

B. *Pneumothorax*

C. *Pulmonary edema*

D. *Diffuse atelectasis*

E. *Clear lung fields*

This patient is demonstrating the classic presentation of negative pressure pulmonary edema. It primarily occurs in young, muscular patients who are able to move large volumes of gas using significant muscular effort. Hypoxia is common as is stridor as the patient tries to move gas through partly opposed cords. Westermark sign is consistent with pulmonary embolus and is inconsistent with this presentation. Pneumothorax should demonstrate asymmetric breath sounds. Atelectasis should demonstrate decreased air movement, especially at the bases in the postoperative patient, and a normal CXR would be unexpected in a patient with hypoxemia.

Answer: C

Krodel DJ, Bittner EA, Abdulnour R, *et al.* (2010) Case scenario: acute postoperative negative pressure pulmonary edema. *Anesthesiology* **113** (1), 200–7.

4. *A 56-year-old man undergoes an urgent sigmoid colectomy and Hartmann's prouch for perforated diverticulitis eight hours prior. Due to a history of coronary disease he is monitored using telemetry. The patient has the acute onset of tachycardia to 146 beats/minute and an ECG strip demonstrates p waves with three different morphologies. His respiratory rate is 34 breaths/minute, BP is 146/88 mm Hg with a S_aO_2 of 94% on 40% O_2 by FM. The most appropriate and effective therapy for this condition is:*

A. *Furosemide 40 mg IVP and KVO IVF*

B. *100% oxygen via non-rebreather mask*

C. *BiPAP at 15/7 cm H_2O and FIO_2 100%*

D. *Amiodarone 150 mg IVP bolus*

E. *Intubation and mechanical ventilation*

An ECG trace with tachycardia demonstrating p waves of three different morphologies is termed multifocal atrial tachycardia (MAT). MAT is unique among atrial dysrhythmias in that is it strongly associated with impending acute respiratory failure and as such represents a stress rhythm. Therapy hinges on addressing the patient's elevated work of breathing by providing immediate endotracheal intubation and mechanical ventilation. None of the other therapies provides definitive management and do not address the underlying cause of MAT. BiPAP does provide some ventilatory support but is in general inadequate at relieving the patient of all of the work of breathing.

Answer: E

Biggs FD, Lefrak SS, Kleiger RE, *et al.* (1977) Disturbances of rhythm in chronic lung disease. *Heart and Lung* **6** (2), 256–61.

5. *A 77-year-old woman is involved in a MVC with rollover. She arrives on 100% by nonrebreather with a $SaO_2 = 96\%$. Her respirations are shallow and labored. She has a past medical history remarkable for COPD. Her CXR demonstrates rib fractures on the left of 2 through 7. The most appropriate step to manage her respiratory status is:*

A. *Nebulized albuterol and atrovent*

B. *Morphine bolus and PCA pump*

C. Bolus and scheduled IV ketorolac

D. Fursoemide 40 mg IVP and Q day

E. Paravertebral block placement

Rib fracture management hinges on adequate analgesia to support coughing, deep breathing and maintenance of ventilation of the segments of lung that are contused and underlie the fractured ribs. Inadequate ventilatory efforts lead to widespread atelectasis and eventually an unsupportable work of breathing. One must also balance analgesia with sedative effects of analgesic medications. In particular, this patient has COPD and may be more sensitive to reductions in respiratory drive with the potential for significant CO_2 retention and respiratory acidosis. Thus, an analgesic method that minimizes sedation is ideal, and placing a paravertebral block meets those needs. Ketorolac can do so as well but is generally an add-on medication to an opioid or block-based regimen, as NSAIDs are generally inadequate as stand-alone agents for multiple rib fracture management, and are generally contraindicated with those at high risk for hemorrhage. Inhaled agents designed to manage bronchoconstriction are useful adjuncts but not primary therapy for rib fracture management and diuresis is generally inappropriate immediately after acute injury because patients generally need fluid resuscitation to support macro- and microcirculatory oxygen delivery.

Answer: E

Bulger EM, Edwards T, Klotz P, Jurkovich GJ (2004) Epidural analgesia improves outcome after multiple rib fractures. *Surgery* **136** (2), 426–30.

Mohta M, Verma P, Saxena AK, *et al.* (2009) Prospective, randomized comparison of continuous thoracic epidural and thoracic paravertebral infusion in patients with unilateral multiple fractured ribs—a pilot study. *Journal of Trauma-Injury Infection and Critical Care* **66** (4), 1096–101.

6. *A 42-year-old man remains in the SICU on post-injury day 2 after a fall from 20 feet. He sustained multiple axial skeletal injuries, a grade III splenic laceration (nonoperative management) and a small left-sided SDH. Since admission he has received 10 L crystalloids and two units of packed cells. He is sedated and mechanically ventilated on AC/VCV and you are called for slowly rising peak airway pressures without a change in other parameters or SaO_2; he is readily suctioned for moderately bloody secretions. His INR is 2.2 and his urine output has decreased from 70 ml/hour to 18 ml/hour. The next most appropriate step in management is:*

A. Magnesium sulphate 4 gm IVP

B. N-acetyl cysteine prior to suctioning

C. Neuromuscular blockade

D. Bladder pressure measurement

E. Change to pressure control ventilation

The clinician must frequently assess rising peak airway pressures. In this scenario, slowly rising pressures indicate a different process than those that rise acutely. The bloody secretions provide a clue that the patient is likely coagulopathic. Given his multiple injuries he is likely to need large-volume fluid resuscitation and clotting factor dilution. He is at risk for failure of nonoperative management of his splenic laceration as well. Each of these factors can lead to an increase in intra-abdominal pressure from visceral edema, hemorrhage, as well as acute ascites formation. Measuring the intra-abdominal pressure using the bladder pressure to assess for intra-abdominal HTN and the abdominal compartment syndrome would readily assess for this possibility. The lack of change in other ventilator parameters is also suggestive of a process that is external to the pulmonary circuit. Thus, magnesium sulphate for bronchodilatation, as well as n-acetyl cysteine for mucolysis, will not address the underlying condition. Neuromuscular blockade may mask the underlying cause and should be used with caution. Changing the ventilator mode will also not address the intra-abdominal HTN.

Answer: D

Lui F, Sangosanya A, Kaplan LJ (2007) Abdominal compartment syndrome: clinical aspects and monitoring. In: Guest ED, Siegel, *Critical Care Clinics*, Elsevier Inc., Amsterdam; **23**, 415–33.

7. *A 68-year-old woman remains intubated and ventilated on POD 6 after a ruptured AAA repair. She is febrile to 101.8 F, tachycardic to 104 beats/minute, but not hypotensive. She has thick yellow secretions. A CXR demonstrates bibasilar atelectasis. Her WBC is 9.4 × 10^3/microL with 72% neutrophils. The next most appropriate step is management is to:*

A. *Begin empiric vancomycin and piperacillin-tazobactam*

B. *Obtain an urgent CT scan of the abdomen and pelvic*

C. *Obtain a bronchoalveolar lavage*

D. *Administer acetaminophen and a cooling blanket*

E. *Send stool sample for C. difficile*

This patient's presentation may be consistent with new onset pneumonia while mechanically ventilated including fever, tachycardia, yellow secretions, and >4 days of mechanical ventilation. However, the CXR does not describe a new infiltrate. Therefore, the diagnosis of ventilator associated pneumonia (VAP) is not clear. Current data identifies that the invasive diagnosis of pneumonia is more cost effective than an empiric therapeutic course of antimicrobial management. Therefore, the best choice is to perform a flexible bronchoscopy and bronchoalveolar lavage to investigate for airway inflammation and to obtain a specimen for culture. This method allows one to culture directly from the involved airway segment, and to avoid culturing tracheal secretions that may be colonized with bacteria resident in the omnipresent biofilm that accompanies indwelling devices.

Answer: C

Porzecanski I, Bowton DL (2006) Diagnosis and treatment of ventilator-associated pneumonia. *Chest.* **130** (2), 597–604.

Fagon JY (2006) Diagnosis and treatment of ventilator-associated pneumonia: fiberoptic bronchoscopy with bronchoalveolar lavage is essential. *Seminars in Respiratory and Critical Care Medicine* **27** (1), 34–44.

8. *Which of the following interventions will prolong the inspiratory time in volume-cycled ventilation:*

A. *Decreasing the respiratory rate*

B. *Increasing the PEEP*

C. *Changing to a square waveform*

D. *Decreasing the flow rate*

E. *Neuromuscular blockade*

Prolonging the inspiratory time (Ti) in volume-cycled ventilation (VCV) may be accomplished by any of the following interventions: increasing the tidal volume (increased time to deliver more gas), decreasing the flow rate (longer time to deliver the same volume of gas), or changing to a decelerating waveform (progressive decrease in gas flow requires a longer tome to deliver the same volume of gas). Neuromuscular blockade, increased PEEP and a change in respiratory rate will not alter the Ti at all. Changing to a square waveform will provide a constant gas flow and will shorten Ti. Thus, the only intervention that will prolong Ti is decreasing the flow rate.

Answer: D

Bailey H, Kaplan LJ (2009) Mechanical ventilation. In: Hedges J, Roberts J (2009) *Clinical Procedures in Emergency Medicine*, 5th edn, WB Saunders, Philadelphia, PA, pp. 138–59.

9. *A 72-year-old patient remains ventilated after a low anterior resection for malignancy. On body weight and habitus appropriate AC/VCV, the patient remains hypoxic. Which of the following interventions is most likely to improve oxygenation?*

A. *Decrease in peak airway pressure*

B. *Increase in expiratory time*

C. *Increase in mean airway pressure*

D. *Increase in respiratory rate*

E. *Increase in dead space: tidal volume*

Oxygenation most closely correlates with mean airway pressure and is a reflection of the area under the curve described by the gas-flow waveform. Decreasing peak airway pressure will not change pO_2. Increases in expiratory time may increase CO_2 clearance if the patient has difficulty with expiratory flow (as in COPD) as may an increase in respiratory rate if minute ventilation is inadequate. An increase in the dead space to tidal volume ratio is associated with an increase in pCO_2 and a decrease in pO_2 and when it approaches 70% it generally indicates an unsupportable work of breathing.

Answer: C

Bailey H, Kaplan LJ (2009) Mechanical ventilation. In: Hedges J, Roberts J (2009) *Clinical Procedures in Emergency Medicine,* 5th edn, W. B. Saunders, Philadelphia, PA, pp. 138–59.

10. *A 24-year-old man is S/P MVC with persistent large volume air leaks via bilateral chest tubes placed for the management of traumatic pneumothoraces. He is currently managed on AC/VCV with a delivered VT of 750 mL and recovered volume of 400 mL. Which is the next most appropriate intervention?*

A. *Initiation of high-frequency oscillation ventilation*

B. *Increase in delivered tidal volume on AC/VCV*

C. *VATS for stapled lung repair using bovine pericardium*

D. *Initiation of extracorporeal membrane oxygenation*

E. *Change to inverse ratio pressure control ventilation*

This patient demonstrates a parenchymal-pleural fistula (PPF) with a net loss of 350 cc of tidal volume out through the chest tubes. The management of such injuries relies in part on excluding a fistula from a major bronchus (bronchopleural fistula; BPF) that would prompt surgical repair. Once a major bronchial disruption is excluded, one may manage the PPF by reducing peak airway pressure and minimizing intratidal shear forces. One effective management strategy is to change from AC/VCV to high-frequency oscillation ventilation, a strategy that uses very small quantities of gas delivered at a very high frequency by a driving pressure to create a central column of standing gas that moves by laminar flow in major airways, and more turbulent but relatively static waves in more distal airways. Gas returns more proximally along the lateral aspects of the central jet of high-frequency and small-volume machine-delivered gas. In this way HFOV is more effective at oxygenation than it is CO_2 clearance. The small volumes and the lack of intratidal shear help PFF to heal. Increasing the delivered tidal volume, or prolonging the inspiratory time as in inverse ratio PCV will drive more gas out through the PFF and impede healing. ECMO is not supported for this condition as first-line therapy (but may serve as a bridge), and VATS is generally not indicated as there are typically multiple areas of leak that are not amenable to surgical stapling. Another useful technique is simultaneous independent lung ventilation that allows the clinician to use two different modes of ventilation and very different airway pressures and gas flow rates in the case of a unilateral PPF.

Answer: A

Cheatham ML, Promes JT (2006) Independent lung ventilation in the management of traumatic bronchopleural fistula. *American Surgeon* **72** (6), 530–3.

Ha DV, Johnson D (2004) High frequency oscillatory ventilation in the management of a high output bronchopleural fistula: a case report. *Canadian Journal of Anaesthesia* **51** (1), 78–83.

11. *A 54-year-old patient is s/p abdominal wall reconstruction and is changed from AC/VCV to airway pressure release ventilation (APRV) for hypoxemic rescue. Which of the following observations is expected?*

A. *Lower mean airway pressures*

B. *Increased need for sedation for comfort*

C. *Uncoupling of oxygenation and ventilation*

D. *Increased minute ventilation requirement*

E. *Higher central venous pressures*

Airway pressure release ventilation (APRV) is a modified form of high-pressure CPAP that is periodically turned off for a very short time to allow gas egress and CO_2 clearance. It is a superior recruitment mode and relies on a significant increase in mean airway pressure to match regional time constant variations, recruit atelectatic alveoli, and improve oxygenation. Airway pressure release ventilation's effect on p_aO_2 may occur independent from its effect on CO_2 clearance, and maximal change in CO_2 often lags behind the maximal change in pO_2; in this way oxygenation and ventilation are uncoupled. Airway pressure release ventilation generally requires less sedation, is more efficient than traditional AC/VCV and requires lower minute ventilation for equivalent CO_2 clearance. Due to the effects of abrogation of hypoxic pulmonary vasconstriction and the subsequent reduction in downstream pressures, the measured CVP typically decreases.

Answer: C

Bailey H, Kaplan LJ (2009) Mechanical ventilation. In: Hedges J. and Roberts J. (2009) *Clinical Procedures in Emergency Medicine,* 5th edn, WB Saunders, Philadelphia, PA, pp. 138–59.

Kaplan LJ, Bailey H, Formosa V (2001) APRV increases cardiac performance in patients with acute lung injury/adult respiratory distress syndrome. *Critical Care* **5** (4), 221–6.

12. *A 62-year-old woman is immediately s/p right hepatic lobectomy for malignancy. She sustained a large volume blood loss and was resuscitated and therefore left on mechanical ventilation. She is placed on the same ventilator settings that were used in the OR. Which of the following findings is expected before the patient begins to take spontaneous breaths?*

A. *Higher* p_aCO_2

B. *Higher* p_aO_2

C. *Auto-PEEP*

D. *Decreased inspiratory time*

E. *Increased expiratory time*

Intraoperative ventilator settings generally reflect neuromuscular blockade or deep sedation as well as the reduction in metabolic rate that accompanies inhalational or intravenous general anesthesia. Thus, the minute ventilation required for maintaining a normal CO_2 clearance will be less than that required in the SICU where the patient generally has a normal or elevated metabolic rate by comparison to that present in the OR under anesthesia. Thus, if the patient is placed on the same settings used in the OR, only a higher pCO_2 is expected before spontaneous respiratory efforts may adjust the minute ventilation to meet CO_2 production needs.

Answer: A

Bailey H, Kaplan LJ (2009) Mechanical Ventilation. In: Hedges J, Roberts J (eds) Clinical Procedures in Emergency Medicine, 5th edn, WB Saunders, Philadelphia, PA, pp. 138–59.

13. *You are called to the bedside of a patient on body weight and habitus appropriate AC/VCV settings with high peak airway pressures; she is POD 2 after a Hartmann's procedure for perforated diverticulitis.* SaO_2 *is 97% on* FIO_2 *of 0.4. The most appropriate investigation is:*

A. *Pulmonary artery catheter assessment*

B. *Lower inflection point assessment*

C. *Pressure versus volume tracing assessment*

D. *Flow versus time tracing assessment*

E. *CT scan to assess for pulmonary embolus*

High peak airway pressures on a body weight and habitus appropriate AC/VCV setting may be a reflection of increased airway resistance, or in appropriate gas delivery for the volume of available lung. The latter may be especially true in the patient with perforated diverticulitis who may have received significant fluid resuscitation to help manage her peritonitis associated capillary leak syndrome. Thus, some evaluation of how gas delivery is being received by the patient's lung is appropriate. Bedside assessment may be readily accomplished by using the dynamic pressure-volume curve and assessing for increases in airway pressure without a corresponding increase in pulmonary volume producing a characteristic curve trace known as the "bird's beak phenomenon" that reflects alveolar overdistension. Placing a pulmonary artery catheter will not help in investigating peak airway pressures, nor will a CT to evaluate for pulmonary embolus be appropriate in the absence of hypoxemia. The flow over time trace is useful to assess for auto-PEEP.

Determination of the lower inflection point in the dynamic or static pressure volume curve assesses for inadequate PEEP, not the presence or absence of alveolar overdistension.

Answer: C

Pestana D, Hernandez-Gancedo C, Royo C, *et al.* (2005) Pressure-volume curve variations after a recruitment manoeuvre in acute lung injury/ARDS patients: implications for the understanding of the inflection points of the curve. *European Journal of Anaesthesiology* **22** (3), 175–80.

Vieillard-Baron A, Jardin F (2003) The issue of dynamic hyperinflation in acute respiratory distress syndrome patients. *European Respiratory Journal—Supplement* **42**, 43s–47s.

14. *A 35-year-old man is post injury day two following a collision with an automobile and remains mechanically ventilated on inverse-ratio pressure control ventilation for the management of severe bilateral pulmonary contusions. He is hemodynamically appropriate on low-dose norepinephrine. He has the following ABG: 7.18/P_aCO_2: 63/P_aO_2: 72 on AC 8/PCV 30/Ti 4.0/80%/PEEP: +10, decelerating waveform. The next most appropriate intervention is:*

A. *CT scan to rule out pulmonary embolus*

B. *D_5W+75 mEq/L $NaHCO_3$ at maintenance rate*

C. *Increase in AC rate to 12 breaths/minute*

D. *Decrease PEEP to 5 cm H_2O pressure*

E. *Decrease inspiratory time (T_i) to 3.2 seconds*

This patient demonstrates a respiratory acidosis and is only marginally oxygenated on high-level airway pressure ventilator settings to manage his severe bilateral pulmonary contusions. This would suggest that his ventilator settings may be optimally adjusted for his pulmonary mechanics, and he requires pressor support to help mange pulmonary flow. In such circumstances, allowing the patient to have a higher than normal pCO_2 provided there is adequate oxygenation may be ideal to avoid inducing ventilator-induced lung injury in an effort to clear additional CO_2. This strategy is termed "permissive hypercapnia" and may require buffering of the associated respiratory acidosis as suggested by using a sodium bicarbonate containing infusion. There is no need to perform a CT scan for pulmonary embolus as the underlying cause of respiratory failure is identified as pulmonary contusion. Increasing the respiratory rate in fixed inspiratory time PCV will decrease CO_2 clearance and increase pCO_2. Decreasing PEEP will move the zero pressure point more distally and lead to worsened oxygenation. Decreasing the inspiratory time may increase CO_2 clearance by increasing the available expiratory time but will also decrease oxygenation and is counterproductive.

Answer: B

Hemmila MR, Napolitano LM (2006) Severe respiratory failure: advanced treatment options. *Critical Care Medicine* **34** (9 Suppl.), S278–90.

15. *A 68-year-old clinically severely obese woman is two days s/p a extensive head and neck resection with radial forearm free flap and tracheostomy. While in the SICU she becomes agitated and her tracheostomy is dislodged. She is acutely hypoxic. The most appropriate management is:*

A. *Initiation of heliox (80/20) therapy*

B. *Oral endotracheal intubation*

C. *Tracheostomy tube replacement*

D. *100% O_2 via tracheostomy mask*

E. *Nebulized albuterol and IV furosemide*

The standard and safe approach to a dislodged tracheostomy tube prior to a well-formed track forming (generally POD 7) is to place a standard oral endotracheal tube to secure airway control. The surgeon's finger may need to cover the trachesotomy site to help keep the orally placed tube from egressing via the tracheotomy site. Once the airway is secured from above, the tracheostomy tube may be safely replaced in a controlled fashion. Many surgeons will place tracheal stay sutures to facilitate pulling up on the trachea and easing replacement should the tube become dislodged. In this case, the patient's body habitus will likely render replacement via the stoma site more difficult, especially since her neck was dissected and many planes that would help guide the tube into the trachea have been disturbed—increasing the likelihood of extratracheal placement. Heliox has some role in reducing airway gas passage in patients with stidor. 100% O_2 via tracheostomy mask requires a tube to be present to be efficacious, and albuterol and a diuretic are not effective management strategies for a dislodged tracheostomy tube.

Answer: B

Barbetti JK, Nichol AD, Choate KR, *et al.* (2009) Prospective observational study of postoperative complications after percutaneous dilatational or surgical tracheostomy in critically ill patients. *Critical Care and Resuscitation* **11** (4), 244–9.

Colman KL, Mandell DL, Simons JP (2010) Impact of stoma maturation on pediatric tracheostomy-related complications. *Archives of Otolaryngology Head and Neck Surgery* **136** (5), 471–4.

Engels PT, Bagshaw SM, Meier M, Brindley PG (2009) Tracheostomy: from insertion to decannulation. *Canadian Journal of Surgery* **52** (5), 427–33.

16. *A 16-year-old patient is shot in the left chest, arrives with agonal vital signs, undergoes a transverse thoracotomy for resuscitation, and undergoes nonanatomic lingual resection, repair of a thoracic aortic tangential injury and a left-ventricle and right-ventricle laceration, as well as a nonanatomic right middle lobe resection. On attempts at closure, he becomes tachycardia and hypotensive. The next most appropriate step in management is:*

A. *Exploratory laparotomy for abdominal decompression*

B. *Intraoperative mannitol for diuresis*

C. *Intraoperative CVVH for solute and water removal*

D. *Thoracic closure with pressor agent BP support*

E. *Thoracic packing and open chest management*

Compartment syndrome is not limited to an extremity or the abdomen as it may also occur in the chest. Treatment paradigms are similar in that the cavity to be closed is instead temporarily expanded to allow for visceral edema. While more often described after cardiac surgery, thoracic compartment syndrome is also reported after extensive thoracic injury. While abdominal decompression addresses abdominal compartment syndrome and may address refractory intracranial HTN as well, it does not as effectively address thoracic pressures as does leaving the chest open. Diuresis is not acutely effective in reducing visceral edema immediately after injury and is generally contraindicated during resuscitation from hemorrhagic shock. Similarly renal support therapies are ineffective and not supported during resuscitation for total body salt and water removal. Pressor support is inappropriate when a simple maneuver, leaving the chest open, will more directly support perfusion without increasing myocardial consumption of oxygen.

Answer: E

Kaplan LJ, Trooskin SZ, Santora TA (1996) Thoracic compartment syndrome. *Journal of Trauma* **40** (2), 291–3.

Rizzo AG. Sample GA (2003) Thoracic compartment syndrome secondary to a thoracic procedure: a case report. *Chest* **124** (3), 1164–8.

17. *A 32-year-old woman is admitted to the burn ICU with 60% Total BSA third-degree burns to the torso and lower extremities including a circumferential chest burn. She is intubated in the ED and placed on pressure control ventilation with settings of AC 12/PCV 20/T_i 2.0 sec/FIO_2 100%/+5 generating a VT of 550 mL with an initial ABG = 7.41/42/350. Twelve hours later, after fluid resuscitation, her resultant tidal volumes are in the 200s and a subsequent ABG = 7.20/60/280. Over the next six hours, she requires a progressive increase in PC to recover the desired tidal volume. Bladder pressure is 10 mm Hg. Chest x-ray is clear. The next step in management should be to:*

A. *Change to volume cycled ventilation*

B. *Increased pressure control*

C. *Increase PEEP to 10 cm H_2O pressure*

D. *Bilateral thoracic escharotomies*

E. *Decompressive laparotomy*

Full-thickness circumferential burns over the torso can result in significant compromise of chest wall movement and hinder ventilation. This is manifested either with decreasing tidal volumes in pressure-cycled ventilation (and increasing pCO_2) or increasing peak airway pressures in volume-cycled ventilation (with high airway pressure limited gas delivery and rising pCO_2). The definitive treatment is to incise the thick eschar that is limiting chest-wall excursion. Abdominal compartment syndrome may present similarly but would be associated with an elevated bladder pressure and an attributable organ failure. Increasing PEEP, increasing the pressure control limit, and changing to volume-cycle ventilation will not address the circumferential thoracic eschar.

Answer: D

Foot C, Host D, Campher D, *et al.* (2008) Moulage in high-fidelity simulation-a chest wall burn escharotomy model for visual realism and as an educational tool. *Simulation in Healthcare: The Journal of The Society for Medical Simulation* **3** (3), 183–5.

Orgill DP, Piccolo N (2009) Escharotomy and decompressive therapies in burns. *Journal of Burn Care and Research* **30** (5), 759–68.

18. *A 54-year-old, 70 kg man is POD #2 following an orthotopic hepatic transplantation. He has been maintained on AC/VCV and has just completed a 30-minute spontaneous breathing trial on pressure support of 5 cm H_2O and PEEP of 5 cm H_2O pressure with the following parameters obtained: negative inspiratory force 15 cm H_2O pressure, minute ventilation 12 L/minute, SaO_2 at completion 95% on FIO_2 0.4, and a respiratory rate that started at 16 breaths/minute and ended at 24 breaths/minute with a spontaneous tidal volume of 500 mL. He is net negative by 1200 mL over the last 12 hours. The next most appropriate course of action is to:*

A. *Resume the prior AC/VCV settings*

B. *Extubate to 40% O_2 via face mask*

C. *Repeat the trial 12 hours later*

D. *Change to flow-by and reevaluate*

E. *Obtain a CXR to rule out pulmonary edema*

This question assesses the appropriate determinants for safe extubation. Weaning parameters are commonly obtained but perhaps the most useful is the rapid shallow breathing index (RSBI; aka. Tobin index) obtained by dividing the frequency of respiration by the tidal volume. Here the RSBI is 24 breaths/min divided by 0.5 L yielding an index of 48; an index less than 105 is generally believed to be supportive of the ability of a patient to support their own work of breathing without mechanical ventilatory support. Since negative inspiratory force is effort dependent its validity is readily questioned. In this case, the NIF is less than 25 (normal value) and would mitigate against extubation. However, the acceptable total minute ventilation, respiratory rate, oxygen saturation, and net negative fluid balance, and the low RSBI readily supports extubation. Repeating the trial, changing to flow-by or obtaining a CXR are all argued against by the excellent spontaneous breathing trial performance.

Answer: B

Lessard MR, Brochard LJ (1996) Weaning from ventilatory support. *Clinics in Chest Medicine* **17** (3), 475–89.

19. *Which statement regarding non-invasive positive pressure ventilation (NIPPV) is most accurate?*

A. *Level I evidence in patients with COPD exacerbations*

B. *Level I evidence in post-op patients to prevent reintubation*

C. *NIPPV is ineffective in cardiogenic pulmonary edema patients*

D. *NIPPV can provide patients a mandatory respiratory rate*

E. *NIPPV effectively clears secretions in cystic fibrosis patients*

NIPPV utilizes pressure-cycled modes that assist respiration and provide a PEEP equivalent to help retard alveolar collapse and assist in alveolar recruitment. The clinician sets the amount of pressure during inspiration and expiration while the patient controls the respiratory rate and inspiratory and expiratory times. Level I evidence supports the use of NIPPV in patients with COPD exacerbations, maintaining extubation in COPD patients and as an adjunct in treatment of cardiogenic pulmonary edema. Its use in postoperative patients is not as well defined, although CPAP by helmet has been demonstrated to be effective in managing atelectasis. Two multicenter randomized trials have failed to show benefit in established respiratory distress although other smaller trials have demonstrated some benefit. Only negative pressure ventilation has been proven effective in enhancing expectoration of secretions in the cystic fibrosis patient population.

Answer: A

Jhanji S, Pearse RM (2009) The use of early intervention to prevent postoperative complications. *Current Opinion in Critical Care* **15** (4), 349–54.

Osthoff M, Leuppi JD (2010) Management of chronic obstructive pulmonary disease patients after hospitalization for acute exacerbation. *Respiration* **79** (3), 255–61.

20. *Contraindications for noninvasive positive pressure ventilation (NIPPV) include:*

A. Hemodynamic instability

B. Excessive secretions

C. Inability to protect the airway

D. Respiratory arrest

E. All of the above

Contraindications for NIPPV include inability to protect the airway, respiratory arrest, hemodynamic instability, agitation, uncooperative patient, excessive secretions or significant upper GI bleeding. There is a theoretical but unproven concern regarding the use of NIPPV in patients with recent upper GI anastomosis.

Answer: E

Jaber S, Chanques G, Jung B (2010) Postoperative noninvasive ventilation. *Anesthesiology* **112** (2), 453–61.

Papadakos PJ, Karcz M, Lachmann B (2010) Mechanical ventilation in trauma. *Current Opinion in Anaesthesiology* **23** (2), 228–32.

Chapter 8 Infectious Disease

Charles Kung Chao Hu, MD, Heather Dolman, MD, and Patrick McGann, MD

1. *A 65-year-old is POD #4 following left hemicolectomy with colostomy and Hartmann's pouch due to perforated diverticulitis with peritonitis. His postoperative course is complicated by ARDS and he remains febrile on antibiotics. Temperature 38.6 °C, heart rate 110 beats/minute, and blood pressure 132/74 mm Hg. Blood cultures grew ESBL (extended-spectrum β lactamase) Escherichia coli. The appropriate antibiotic regimen for this organism is:*

A. *Piperacillin-tazobactam*

B. *Vancomycin*

C. *Cefepime*

D. *Cefoxitin*

E. *Meropenem*

There is concern for increasing antimicrobial resistance in the ICU. ESBL (extended-spectrum β lactamase) resistance is noted in gram-negative bacteria, especially in high-risk groups including those greater than 60-years-old, or where there has been previous in-hospital antibiotic use, emergency surgery, ICU admission, and in patients requiring mechanical ventilation. ESBLs are enzymes that break down the β-lactam ring. Piperacillin-tazobactam, cefepime, cefoxitin, and meropenem are all β-lactam antibiotics. Vancomycin only covers gram-positive organisms. Carbapenems are much more resistant to beta lactamses than the other beta lactams. Treatment for ESBL gram-negative bacilli infections is carbapenems, thus meropenem is the answer.

Answer: E

Clark NM, Patterson J, Lynch JP, *et al.* (2003) Antimicrobial resistance among gram-negative organisms in the intensive care unit. *Current Opinions in Critical Care* **9**, 413–23.

Harris AD, McGregor JC, Johnson JA, *et al.* (2007) Risk factors for colonization with extended-spectrum β-lactamase-producing bacteria and intensive care unit admission. *Emerging Infectious Diseases* **13** (8), 1144–9.

2. *A 33-year-old HIV positive woman is s/p I & D of a left deltoid abscess with cellulitis from active intravenous drug use. Cultures from the abscess were positive for MRSA with the following susceptibility panel: clindamycin-susceptible, erythromycin-resistant, D zone test positive. She was on preoperative vancomycin. The appropriate outpatient antibiotic is:*

A. *Vancomycin*

B. *Clindamycin*

C. *Daptomycin*

D. *TMP-SMX (trimethoprim – sulfamethoxazole)*

E. *Penicillin*

Antimicrobial resistance continues to be a global concern. Clindamycin-susceptible, erythromycin-resistant *Staphylococcus aureus* can become clindamycin resistant. One should be concerned when the susceptibility panel has clindamycin-susceptible, erythromycin-resistant results for MRSA, since resistance to clindamycin *in vivo* may be present. To confirm susceptibility, a D-test (disk test) should be performed. A D-test will determine if the strain of MRSA is inducible to develop clindamycin resistance. Antibiotics are recommended for abscesses in those with cellulitis and comorbidities. An active intravenous drug use patient does not need IV antibiotics (vancomycin, daptomycin) at home because of the risk catheter infection. Previous exposure to vancomycin may cause daptomycin resistance. Penicillin will not treat MRSA. The appropriate antibiotic for community-acquired clindamycin-resistant MRSA is TMP-SMX.

Surgical Critical Care and Emergency Surgery: Clinical Questions and Answers, First Edition. Edited by Forrest O. Moore, Peter M. Rhee, Samuel A. Tisherman and Gerard J. Fulda.

Answer: D

Levin TP, Suh B, Axelrod P, *et al.* (2005) Potential clindamycin resistance in clindamycin-susceptible, erythromycin-resistance Staphylococcus aureus: Report of a clinical failure. *Antimicrobial Agents and Chemotherapy* **49** (3), 1222–4.

Liu C, Bayer A, Cosgrove SE, *et al.* (2011) Clinical practice guidelines by the Infectious Diseases Society of America for the treatment of methicillin-resistant Staphylococcus aureus infections in adults and children. *Clinical Infectious Diseases* **52**, 1–38.

3. *A 52-year-old is hospital day #3, s/p MVC. He is critically ill and has developed ARDS. Temperature 38.2°C, white count 15.4 × 10^3/microL. A ventilator-associated pneumonia (VAP) may be diagnosed from all the following except:*

A. *Deep endotracheal aspirate*

B. *BAL (bronchial alveolar lavage) with quantitative cultures of >10^4 cfu/mL*

C. *PBS (protective brush specimen) with quantitative cultures of >10^3 cfu/mL*

D. *Sputum gram stain with mixed flora*

E. *Chest x-ray with new infiltrate*

Diagnosis of VAP (ventilator-associated pneumonia) involves clinical suspicion, new infiltrate on chest x-ray, purulent sputum, fever or hypothermia, leukocytosis or leukopenia, and hypoxia. This is augmented by lower respiratory tract cultures including deep entotracheal aspirate, BAL of >10^4 cfu/mL, or PBS of >10^3 cfu/mL. After 48 hours, sputum from an endotracheal tube is likely to be contaminated with oral flora; if there is not a single dominate organism on a gram stain the diagnosis of VAP should be questioned. Additionally, mixed flora suggest a contaminated specimen which is not indicative of a VAP.

Answer: D

American Thoracic Society and the Infectious Diseases Society of America (2005) Guidelines for the management of adults with hospital-acquired, ventilator-associated, and healthcare-associated pneumonia. *American Journal of Respiratory Critical Care Medicine* **171**, 388–416.

Valencia M, Torres A (2009) Ventilator-associated pneumonia. *Current Opinions in Critical Care* **15**, 30–5.

4. *A 58-year-old remains in critical condition following omental patch repair of perforated duodenal ulcer. He is in septic shock, on dopamine, norepinephrine, and vasopressin with a MAP of 50 mm Hg. An echocardiogram reveals hyperdynamic LVEF, with adequate filling pressures. The next step should be:*

A. *Add phenylephrine*

B. *Bolus one liter normal saline*

C. *An ACTH stimulation test should be performed before administration of steroids*

D. *Hydrocortisone should be given at a dose less than or equal to 300mg/d*

E. *Give indomethacin*

This patient is in septic shock, nonresponsive to vasopressors. Based on echocardiogram, the patient is volume replete. He is most likely adrenally insufficient with an inadequate response to vasopressors. Adding more vasopressors or fluid will not help this patient. Indomethacin has no role in septic shock or in adrenal insufficiency. The Surviving Sepsis campaign has outlined recommendations for steroid use in septic shock including: addition of hydrocortisone when hypotension does not respond to vasopressors; an ACTH stimulation test prior to steroid administration is not necessary and the interpretation of the results remain controversial; hydrocortisone should be given at a dose less than or equal to 300 mg per day; steroids should be weaned when vasopressors are no longer needed; and consider adding fludrocortisone.

Answer: D

Dellinger RP, Levy MM, Carlet JM, *et al.* (2008) Surviving sepsis campaign: International guidelines for management of severe sepsis and septic shock: 2008. *Critical Care Medicine* **36** (1), 296–327.

Marik PE (2009) Critical illness-related corticosteroid insufficiency. *Chest* **135**, 181–93.

5. *A 62-year-old woman is POD #6 after colon resection for ischemic colitis. She is on the ventilator and remains febrile. Her white count is 15.2 × 10^3/microL on TPN via a newly placed PICC. The patient was previously in septic shock and steroids are currently being weaned.*

Urine cultures grew Candida glabrata. The appropriate antifungal is:

A. *Fluconazole*

B. *Traconazole*

C. *Micafungin*

D. *Voriconazole*

E. *No treatment necessary*

Candidiasis diagnosis and treatment can be difficult. Risk factors for systemic infection include antibiotic use, Candida from other sites, central lines, TPN, and immunosuppressive use. *C. glabrata* has high rates of resistance to triazoles (fluconazole, itraconazole, voriconazole) in the ICU. Due to this patient's increased risk factors and urine with *C. glabrata*, the appropriate treatment is micafungin.

Answer: C

Guery BP, Arendrup MC, Auzinger G, *et al.* (2009a) Management of invasive candidiasis and candidemia in adult non-neutropenic intensive care unit patients: Part I. Epidemiology and diagnosis. *Intensive Care Medicine* **35**, 55–62.

Guery BP, Arendrup MC, Auzinger G, *et al.* (2009b) Management of invasive candidiasis and candidemia in adult non-neutropenic intensive care unit patients: Part II. Treatment. *Intensive Care Medicine* **35**, 206–14.

Pappas PG, Kauffman CA, Andes D, *et al.* (2009) Clinical practice guidelines for the management of candidiasis: 2009 update by the Infectious Diseases Society of America. *Clinical Infectious Diseases* **48**, 503–35.

6. *A 42-year-old man suffers a severe traumatic brain injury after motor vehicle collision. He remains intubated on mechanical ventilation, in septic shock with shock liver, on pressors and requiring CRRT for renal failure. His APACHE II score is 32. Use of Xigris (drotrecogin alfa-activated recombinant protein C) would be* ***absolutely*** *contraindicated in this patient if:*

A. *Creatinine clearance is less than or equal to 20 mL per minute*

B. *The right femur is fractured*

C. *He is s/p colectomy*

D. *He has a subarachnoid hemorrhage*

E. *The platelets are 55 × 10^3/microL*

The Surviving Sepsis Campaign has outlined recommendations for Xigris (drotrecogin alfa) in septic shock with multiple organ failure, high risk of death, and no contraindications. If the APACHE II score is less than 20 with only one organ dysfunction, then no differences in outcomes are seen with Xigris use and it is not recommended. Severe sepsis causes immunological reaction that is pro-inflammatory and prothrombotic. Activated protein C (drotrecogin alfa) inhibits the process. Contraindications to drotrecogin alfa include trauma with increased risk of life threatening bleeding, active internal bleeding, hemorrhagic stroke within 3 months, platelets less than 30,000 per mm^3, and bleeding diathesis; thus the best answer is D.

Answer: D

Dellinger RP, Levy MM, Carlet JM, *et al.* (2008) Surviving sepsis campaign: International guidelines for management of severe sepsis and septic shock: 2008. *Critical Care Medicine* **36** (1), 296–327.

Gentry CA, Gross KB, Sud B, Drevets DA (2009) Adverse outcomes associated with the use of drotrecogin alfa (activated) in patients with severe sepsis and baseline bleeding precautions. *Critical Care Medicine* **37** (1), 19–25.

7. *All of the following are SCIP (surgical care improvement project) measures except:*

A. *Prophylactic antibiotics within one hour of surgical incision*

B. *Prophylactic antibiotics discontinued within 24 hours*

C. *Immediate postoperative normothermia for all surgical patients*

D. *Morning postoperative blood glucose level less than 200 mg/dL in cardiac patients*

E. *Prophylactic vancomycin within two hours of surgical incision*

SCIP was developed in 2002 by the Centers of Medicaid and Medicare to reduce surgical site infections, decrease length of stay, and reduce cost and mortality. Surgical care infection prevention performance measures include prophylactic antibiotics within one hour of surgical incision, two hours if vancomycin; the appropriate antibiotic for the surgical procedure; discontinuation of prophylactic antibiotics in 24 hours of surgery end time; postoperative normothermia in colorectal patients; and morning blood glucose less than 200 mg/dL in cardiac patients. Other SCIP measures include DVT prophylaxis and perioperative beta blockade in patients on beta blockade prior to admission. Currently, normothermia is a SCIP measure only in colorectal patients.

Answer: C

Kirby JP, Mazuski JE (2009) Prevention of surgical site infection. *Surgical Clinics of North America* **89**, 365–89.

Stulberg JJ, Delaney CP, Neuhauser DV, *et al.* (2010) Adherence to surgical care improvement project measures and the association with postoperative infections. *Journal of the American Medical Association* **303** (24), 2479–85.

8. *A 55-year-old woman with necrotizing fasciitis of the buttocks and thighs is in the ICU in septic shock. Immediate therapy includes all of the following except:*

A. *Aggressive debridement*

B. *Broad-spectrum antibiotics*

C. *Coverage for Streptococcus pyogenes*

D. *Clindamycin for endotoxin production*

E. *Hyperbaric oxygen therapy*

Appropriate therapy for necrotizing fasciitis includes: aggressive debridement, broad-spectrum antibiotics, treatment of pathogens including *Streptococcus pyogenes*, use of clindamycin (a protein synthesis inhibitor against toxin production), and physiologic support. The data for the use of hyperbaric oxygen therapy demonstrates variable results and based on current evidence should not be used.

Answer: E

Anaya DA, Dellinger EP (2007) Necrotizing soft-tissue infection: Diagnosis and management. *Clinical Infectious Diseases* **44**, 705–10.

May AK, Stafford RE, Bulger EM, *et al.* (2009) Treatment of complicated skin and soft tissue infections. *Surgical Infections* **10** (5), 467–99.

9. *All of the following decrease central venous line infections except:*

A. *Use of the subclavian site*

B. *Scheduled line changes*

C. *Removing catheters when no longer needed*

D. *Maximum sterile barrier precautions with insertion*

E. *Antimicrobial impregnated catheter usage*

Catheter-related blood stream infections (CR-BSI) cause significant morbidity and mortality. Minimizing CR-BSI is important to improve patient outcomes. Guidelines have been created to prevent intravascular catheter infections. Prevention strategies include the following: use of the subclavian site, nonscheduled line changes, removing catheters when no longer needed, and maximum sterile barrier precautions with insertion. Antimicrobial-impregnated catheters can be used to reduce catheter related infections when the above efforts fail to satisfactorily reduce infection rates. Scheduled line changes may increase the incidence of infection, thus (b) is the correct answer.

Answer: B

McGee DC, Gould MK (2003) Preventing complications of central venous catheterization. *New England Journal of Medicine* **348** (12), 1123–33.

Mermel LA, Farr BM, Sherertz RJ, *et al.* (2001) Guidelines for the management of intravascular catheter-related infections. *Clinical Infectious Diseases* **32,** 1249–72.

O'Grady NP, Alexander M, Dellinger EP (2002) Guidelines for prevention of intravascular catheter-related infections. *Clinical Infectious Diseases* **35**, 1281–307.

10. *A 72-year-old is s/p open abdominal aortic aneurysm repair, in septic shock with a white count of 42 × 10^3/microL and a temperature of 38.4 °C. He is on empiric antibiotics and has no bowel function. He is Clostridium difficile positive by PCR. The appropriate antibiotic regimen is:*

A. *Oral metronidazole only*

B. *Oral vancomycin only*

C. *Oral metronidazole and oral vancomycin*

D. IV metronidazole and rectal vancomycin

E. IV vancomycin and oral vancomycin

There are risk factors for infectious *C. difficile* diarrhea including previous antibiotic use, hospitalization, and increased age. Fever and very high white counts may accompany the abdominal pain. Rarely, diarrhea may be absent due to paralytic ileus. *C. difficile* diarrhea varies in severity (mild, moderate, and severe) and treatment depends on severity. Two or more of the following indicates severe disease: age greater than 60, temperature greater than 38.3 °C, white count greater than 15 000 cells/mm^3, and albumin less than 2.5 mg/dL. This patient has a severe infection based on his increased age, WBC, and fever. The optimal treatment for severe infection is oral vancomycin. Since this patient does not have bowel function, IV metronidazole will provide appropriate concentration in the colonocytes for treatment of *C. difficile* diarrhea. Addition of oral vancomycin or metronidazole could benefit if the drug would reach the site of infection—the colon. Some data exists regarding the use of rectal administration of vancomycin (intraluminal). Thus the answer is D.

Answer: D

Bartlett JG, Gerding DN (2008) Clinical recognition and diagnosis of clostridium difficile infection. *Clinical Infectious Diseases* **46**, S12–18.

Gerding DN, Muto CA, Owens RC Jr., *et al.* (2008) Treatment of clostridium difficile infection. *Clinical Infectious Diseases* **46**, S32–42.

11. *An 18-year-old boy arrives to the trauma bay in traumatic shock after sustaining multiple gunshot wounds to the abdomen. He is taken immediately to the operating room where injuries to his stomach and small bowel are repaired. A temporary abdominal wound closure is placed. His abdomen was subsequently washed out twice and closed after bowel edema subsided.*

The patient has been on the ventilator for ten days now since admission and has been developing persistent fevers despite broad spectrum antibiotic coverage and continual surveillance of cultures. You noted that in the patient's subsequent abdominal washouts, everything looked clean. He has been on TPN since his ileus has not resolved.

What do you do next in terms of antibiotic treatments?

A. Continue with current regiment of antibiotics and await cultures

B. Continue with current regiment of antibiotics and add fungal coverage

C. Change antibiotics to cover gram negatives only and await cultures

D. Change antibiotics to cover MRSA only and add fungal coverage

E. Discontinue all previous antibiotics and start fungal coverage

This patient is at risk for developing tertiary peritonitis. In addition, he has risk factors for fungal infection: open abdomen, shock, TPN, gastric perforation, prior antibiotic treatments. With persistent fevers and lack of new culture results, starting an antifungal agent is the correct regiment. Fungal cultures can take two to three weeks to become positive. Common organisms in patients with tertiary peritonitis are Enterobacter, Enterococcus, Candida, and *Staphylococcus epidermidis*. Candida infection is associated with 60–70% mortality.

Answer: B

Christou NV, Barie PS, Dellinger RP, *et al.* (1993) Surgical Infection Society intraabdomianl infection study: Prospective evaluation of management techniques and outcomes. *Archives of Surgery* **128**, 193–8.

Wacha H, Hau T, Dittmer R, Ohmann R (1999) Risk factors associated with intraabdominal infections: a prospective multicenter study. Peritonitis Study Group. *Langenbecks Archives of Surgery* **384**, 24–32.

12a. *A 58-year-old woman with no past medical history suffered pulmonary contusions and rib fractures after falling down a flight of stairs. She has been in the SICU for about six days now with marginal pulmonary status. On hospital day 3, she developed fevers and the morning CXR showed developing infiltrates not seen on previous x-rays. You are concerned with nosocomial pneumonia in this patient. Which organism is a typical pathogen in this scenario?*

A. Methicillin-sensitive Staphylococcus aureus

B. Haemophilus influenza

C. *Pseudomonas aeruginosa*

D. *Acinetobacter baumannii*

E. *Klebsiella pneumonia*

This patient is moderate-to-high risk of developing pneumonia due to her marginal pulmonary mechanics as a result of her injuries. Hospital-acquired pneumonia (HAP) is defined as pneumonia occurring more than 48 hours after admission, excluding any at time of admission. Early-onset HAP ($<$ 4 days) is presumed to be caused by gram-positive organisms, typically MSSA and *Streptococcus pneumonia*.

Answer: A

12b. *In the above scenario, which organism would you consider antibiotic coverage when pneumonia is suspected on hospital day 6?*

A. *Streptococcus pneumonia*

B. *MSSA*

C. *MRSA*

D. *Beta-hemolytic Streptococcus*

E. *Staphylococcus epidermidis*

Late-onset HAP occurs more than four days after admission and is typically caused by gram-negative organisms and MRSA. Risk factors are prior use of antibiotics, history of chronic lung disease, mechanical ventilation $>$3 days, and history of corticosteroid therapy. Patients who receive early and adequate antibiotic therapy have the lowest mortality rates.

Answer: C

NNIS (1999) National Nosocomial Infections Surveillance (NNIS) System report, data summary from January 1990–May 1999, issued June 1999. *Am J Infect Control* **27** (6), 520–32.

Rello J, Ollendorf DA, Oster G, *et al.* (2002) Epidemiology and outcomes of ventilator-associated pneumonia in a large US database. *Chest* **122** (6), 2115–21.

13. *If the patient in question 12 was intubated on hospital day 2 and develops VAP, how long would you continue antibiotic treatment if the inciting organism is found to be MRSA? Pseudomonas aeruginosa?*

A. *MRSA 8 days, Pseudomonas 8 days*

B. *MRSA 8 days, Pseudomonas 14 days*

C. *MRSA 14 days, Pseudomonas 14 days*

D. *MRSA 14 days, Pseudomonas 21 days*

E. *MRSA 21 days, Pseudomonas 21 days*

The length of treatment for VAP has been a controversial topic. Historical data suggests 7–10 days of treatment for routine organisms and 14–21 days for multi-drug resistant organisms. Recent trials suggest shorter duration of therapy should be tailored to seven or eight days of therapy with no difference in the recurrence rate as compared to longer duration therapies, unless the inciting organism is caused by nonfermenting gram-negative bacilli such as Pseudomonas. Patients with these infections should have a longer duration of treatment. Chastre demonstrated a successful approach to these two scenarios; 8 days for generally sensitive organisms and 15 days for more resistant organisms.

Answer: B

Chastre J, Wolff M, Fagon JY, *et al.* (2003) Comparison of 8 versus 15 days of antibiotic therapy for ventilator-associated pneumonia in adults: a randomized trial. *Journal of the American Medical Association* **290**, 2588.

Ibrahim EH, Ward S, Sherman G, *et al.* (2004) Experience with a clinical guidelines for the treatment of ventilator-associated pneumonia. *Critical Care Medicine* **32**, 1109.

14. *A 57-year-old man is POD #5 s/p renal transplant and he develops fevers of 101.5°F. You are concerned about nosocomial urinary tract infection and cultures have been taken. In addition to removing or replacing the catheter, what would you do next?*

A. *Start broad-spectrum antibiotics and an antifungal, ultrasound the transplant kidney*

B. *Start broad-spectrum antibiotics, await fungal cultures*

C. *Await bacterial and fungal cultures*

D. *Start broad spectrum antibiotics while awaiting cultures, ultrasound the transplant kidney*

E. *Start broad spectrum antibiotics with antifungal coverage, remove the kidney*

Nosocomial UTI is one of the most common infections in the hospital and duration of catheterization is the most common etiology. *E. coli* is the most common organism. In long-term catheterizations, polymicrobial organisms predominate and may include: Klebsiella, Pseudomonas, Enterococcus, or Staphylococcus. Diagnosis is based on cultures (quantitative greater than 10^5 CFU/ml when available) and the presence of white blood cells in the urine. Initial treatment is removal or replacement of the catheter. Candida is a common isolate in the ICU, however for neutropenic and immune-suppressed patients, aggressive treatment is warranted, especially against disseminated candidiasis. Nonalbican species can occur in 20–30% of isolates. Invasive candidiasis can occur in up to 5–10% of solid organ transplants, such as *Candida tropicalis, Candida parapsilosis, Candida glabrata*, and *Candida krusie*. For Candida in the urine, either fluconazole or amphotericin B should be used depending on the sensitivity. High-risk patients can be treated with the echinocandin class of antifungals, such as caspofungin, micafungin, and anidulafungin, which has a high sensitivity to these invasive Candida organisms. Imaging studies are obtained to rule out obstructive causes.

Answer: A

Platt R, Polk BF, Murdock B, *et al.* (1982) Mortality associated with nosocomial urinary tract infections. *New England Journal Medicine* **307**, 637.

Singh N (2000) Infections in solid organ transplant recipients. *Current Opinions in Infectious Disorders* **13**, 343–7.

15. *In systemic inflammatory response syndrome (SIRS), which of the following is NOT true?*

A. *Occurs only by infectious insults*

B. *Occurs from hypo-perfusion*

C. *Occurs continuously even after controlling the initial insult*

D. *Organ dysfunction can occur with variability*

E. *Starts with activation of the immune response*

Systemic inflammatory response syndrome can occur through noninfectious causes such as trauma, toxins, ARDS, pancreatitis, abdominal compartment syndrome, and excessive resuscitation. Neutrophils and macrophages are activated through inflammatory mediators such as tumor necrosis factor (TNF), and interleukin-6 (IL-6). Oxygen radicals are released causing damage to the basement membranes of endothelial cells. The end result is capillary leak and subsequent tissue destruction.

Answer: A

American College of Chest Physicians/Society of Critical Care Medicine Consensus Conference (1992) Definitions for sepsis and organ failure and guidelines for the use of innovative therapies in sepsis. *Critical Care Medicine* **20**, 864.

Marshall J, Sweeny D (1990) Microbial infection and the septic response in critical surgical illness. *Archives of Surgery* **125**, 17.

16. *A 29-year-old woman is a restrained passenger involved in a motor vehicle crash in which she was rear ended. She was brought to the emergency room with complaints of abdominal pain. A computed tomography scan of the abdomen was unremarkable for acute traumatic injury. With continual pain, you admit her for observation. The next morning, her abdominal pain is worsened and her exam showed a very tender abdomen. Her vitals are as follows: temperature 101.8°F, HR 130 beats/minute, SBP 90/60 mm Hg, RR 35 breaths/minute, and O_2 saturation 95% on 2L NC. Given her change in status, you repeated the CT scan of the abdomen which shows large amounts of intra-abdominal fluid.*

Which of the following is inadequate therapy in the management of this patient?

A. *Fluid resuscitation with normal saline, gentamicin/clindamycin, exploratory laparotomy*

B. *Fluid resuscitation with normal saline, exploratory laparotomy, imipenem*

C. *Fluid resuscitation with lactated Ringers, vancomycin/metronidazole, exploratory laparotomy*

D. *Fluid resuscitation with blood products if needed, piperacillin/tazobactam, diagnostic laparoscopy*

E. *Fluid resuscitation with lactated Ringers, levofloxacin/metronidazole, exploratory laparotomy*

Surgical infection is defined as infection that should be controlled with surgical intervention. For intra-abdominal sources of infection, early source control is critical in determining outcome. Antibiotics also play a crucial role. Selection of agents is based on activity against *Staphylococcus aureus*, enteric gram negative bacilli, and anaerobes including *Bacteroides fragilis*. Combination therapy with aminoglycosides, clindamycin, and metronidazole, or monotherapy with carbapenems has been shown to be effective in randomized trials. Choice C is incorrect because the antibiotic selection does not cover enteric gram negative organisms. Resuscitation with normal saline, lactated ringers, or blood products are crucial for maintaining volume. The choice of laparoscopy is dependent on the skill set of the operating surgeon.

Answer: C

Montgomery RS, Wilson SE (1996) Intraabdominal abscess: image guided diagnosis and therapy. *Clinical Infectious Diseases* **23**, 28.

Nathens AB, Rotstein OD (1994) Therapeutic options in peritonitis. *Surgical Clinics of North America* **74**, 677.

17. *In the previous scenario, given adequate source-control, how long would you continue the antibiotic that is chosen to treat the intra-abdominal infection?*

A. *48 hours*

B. *4–7 days*

C. *10–12 days*

D. *14 days*

E. *21 days*

The consensus paper published from the Surgical Infection Society and the Infectious Diseases Society of America recommends antimicrobial therapy should be limited to four to seven days, unless it is difficult to achieve adequate source control. Prolonged therapy with broad-spectrum antibiotics carries increased risks for the development of resistant organisms, drug toxicities, and superinfections, particularly *Clostridium difficile*. Duration of therapy should be guided by resolution of infection as evidenced by normalization of clinical signs.

Answer: B

Hedrick TL, Evans HL, Smith RL, *et al.* (2006) Can we define the ideal duration of antibiotic therapy? *Surgical Infections* **7**, 419–32.

Solomkin JS, Mazuski JE, Bradley JS, *et al.* (2010) Diagnosis and management of complicated intra-abdominal infection in adults and children: guidelines by the Surgical Infection Society and the Infectious Diseases Society of America. *Clinical Infectious Diseases* **50**, 133–64.

18. *What is the most common pathogen related to central venous line (CVL) infections in the ICU in the USA?*

A. *VRE*

B. *E. coli*

C. *Coagulase-negative S. aureus*

D. *MRSA*

E. *Klebsiella*

Coagulase-negative Staphylococcus infections are now the most common CVL-related infection in the USA (37%). The three most common gram-positive pathogens are coagulase-negative *S. aureus*, MRSA, and Enterococcus. The most common gram negative pathogens are *E. coli*, *P. aeruginosa*, Enterobacter, and Klebsiella.

Answer: C

CDC (1999) National Nosocomial Infections Surveillance (NNIS) System report, data summary from January 1990–May 1999, issued June 1999. *American Journal of Infection Control* **27**, 520–32.

Mermel LA, Allon M, Bouza E, *et al.* (2009) Clinical Practice Guidelines for the Diagnosis and Management of Intravascular Catheter-Related Infection: 2009 Update by the Infectious Diseases Society of America. *Clinical Infectious Diseases* **49**, 1–45.

19. *Which maneuver will most significantly reduce the incidence of pulmonary aspiration in the ventilated patient?*

A. *Deep suctioning*

B. *Sterile suctioning*

C. *Assisted cough*

D. Head-of-bed elevation

E. Chest percussions

In 1997, the CDC published guidelines for preventing aspiration pneumonia and in 2003, the CDC Healthcare Infection Control Practices Advisory Committee recommended elevating the HOB between 30-45 degrees unless contraindicated. As recently as 2006, the Society for Critical Care Medicine Outcomes Task Force endorsed HOB elevation as a method to reduce aspiration pneumonia.

Answer: D

Luna C, Vujacich P, Niederman M, *et al.* (1997) Impact of BAL data on the therapy and outcome of ventilator-associated pneumonia. *Chest* **111**, 676–85.

Orozco-Levi M, Torres A, Ferrer M, *et al.* (1995) Semirecumbent position protects from pulmonary aspiration but not completely from gastroesophageal reflux in mechanically ventilated patients. *American Journal of Respiratory Critical Care Medicine* **152**, 1387–90.

20. *What is the percent reduction in the incidence of VAP if the measure in question 19 is initiated in the first 24 hours?*

A. 5% reduction in incidence of VAP

B. 20% reduction in incidence of VAP

C. 40% reduction in the incidence of VAP

D. 60% reduction in the incidence of VAP

E. 80% reduction in the incidence of VAP

Elevation of HOB, if initiated in the first 24 hours of admission, may reduce the incidence of VAP by up to 67%. As a part of the prophylaxis bundle in the ICU, implementation of this policy has decreased the morbidity and mortality of the ventilated patient. Oral care has been shown to decrease the incidence of VAP by 63%. These measures along with sedation interruption and ventilator weaning trials all help to significantly reduce the incidence of VAP in the ICU.

Answer: D

Kollef MH (1993) Ventilator-associated pneumonia: a multivariate analysis. *Journal of the American Medical Association* **270**, 1965–70.

Orozco-Levi M, Torres A, Ferrer M, *et al.* (1995) Semirecumbent position protects from pulmonary aspiration but not completely from gastroesophageal reflux in mechanically ventilated patients. *American Journal of Respiratory Critical Care Medicine* **152**, 1387–90.

21. *Empiric therapy for VAP should cover all of the following except:*

A. Streptococcus pneumoniae

B. Haemophilus influenzae

C. VRE

D. Methicillin-resistent Staphylococcus aureus

E. Moraxella catarrhalis

The most common pathogens for VAP, when risk factors for multi-drug resistant organisms are not present, are *Streptococcus, Haemophilus, MSSA,* and *Moraxella* species. Appropriate initial antibiotics are quinolones, ceftriaxone, or ampicillin/sulbactam. VRE is not a common pathogen for initial treatment. It is mainly born out of selection from antibiotic administration.

When the possibility of MDR exists, treatment should be expanded to include *Pseudomonas aeriginosa, Enterobacter, Serratia, Klebsiella, Stenotrophomonas maltophilia,* and MRSA. Appropriate antibiotic choices are vancomycin or linezolid for MRSA, and pipercillin-tazobactam (beta-lactam/beta lactamase inhibitor), fluoroquinolones or aminoglycosides (gentamicin or tobramicin) for Pseudomonas coverage. Sulfamethoxazole/trimethoprim is the treatment of choice for Stenotrophomonas.

Answer: C

American Thoracic Society (2005) Guidelines for management of adults with hospital-acquired, ventilator associated pneumonia, and health-care associated pneumonia. *American Journal of Respiratory Critical Care Medicine* **171**, 388–416.

Kollef MH (1993) Ventilator-associated pneumonia: a multivariate analysis. *Journal of the American Medical Association* **270**, 1965–70.

Chapter 9 Pharmacology and Antibiotics

Michelle Strong, MD, PhD

1. *Which one of the following is not an expected adverse effect related to the use of propofol sedation in the ICU?*

A. *Hypotension*

B. *Hyperlipidemia*

C. *Atrial arrhythmias*

D. *Supraventricular tachycardia*

E. *Green urine*

Propofol is known to commonly cause bradycardia, decreased cardiac output and hypotension as adverse cardiovascular effects. Atrial arrhythmias, ventricular tachycardia and cardiac arrest have been described, but the cause is not known. Hyperlipidemia occurs with an incidence of 3 to 10% and is associated with use of propofol for an extended period of time. Green urine has also been reported with the use of propofol. Green urinary discoloration has been reported after both short-term and prolonged therapy. It is known that propofol can have effects on atrioventricular node conduction. Propofol has been shown to have a direct concentration-dependent inhibitory effect on the cardiac conduction system in isolated rabbit heart. There have been instances of termination of supraventricular tachycardia (SVT) and suppression of premature atrial contractions during propofol anesthesia in children and adults. Propofol has not been related with supraventricular tachycardia in adults when used for ICU sedation. Strict aseptic technique is required for the administration of propofol, due to previously reported bacterial contamination of the product.

Surgical Critical Care and Emergency Surgery: Clinical Questions and Answers, First Edition. Edited by Forrest O. Moore, Peter M. Rhee, Samuel A. Tisherman and Gerard J. Fulda.

Answer: D

Blakely SA, Hixson-Wallace JA (200) Clinical significance of rare and benign side effects: propofol and green urine. *Pharmacotherapy* **20**, 1120–2.

Kannan S, Sherwood N (2002) Termination of supraventricular tachycardia by propofol. *British Journal of Anaesthesia* **88**, 874–5.

Medical Economics Company, Inc. (2002) *Physician's Desk Reference*, 56th edn, Medical Economics Company, Inc., Montvale, NJ, pp. 667–73.

2. *A 70-year-old man has been admitted to the ICU after colectomy because of his history of end-stage renal disease, respiratory failure and pain management. The procedure was uncomplicated and the patient is extubated 2 hours after admission to the ICU. On examination, the patient's RR is 18 breaths/min, and he rates his pain on a 0–10 scale as 7. He is currently doing well receiving oxygen at 4 L/min by nasal cannula.*

Which one of the following analgesics for postoperative pain management is most appropriate for this patient?

A. *Fentanyl*

B. *Morphine*

C. *Oxycodone*

D. *Hydromorphone*

E. *Meperidine*

Morphine should be used cautiously. Morphine metabolites can accumulate increasing therapeutic and adverse effects in patients with renal failure. Both parent and metabolite can be removed with dialysis. Hydromorphone should be used cautiously and the dose adjusted as appropriate in patients with renal failure. The 3-glucuronide metabolite of hydrodromorphone can accumulate and cause neuro-excitatory effects in these patients.

The parent drug can be removed by dialysis, but metabolite accumulation remains a risk. Oxycodone should not be used in patients in renal failure. Metabolites and oxycodone itself can accumulate causing toxic and CNS-depressant effects. There is no data on oxycodone and its metabolites' removal with dialysis. Meperidine should not be used. Metabolites can accumulate causing increased risk of adverse effects. There are few data on meperidine and its metabolites in dialysis. Fentanyl appears safe, but dose adjustment is necessary. There are no active metabolites to have added risk of adverse effects. Use some caution because fentanyl is poorly dialyzable.

Answer: A

Davison SN (2003) Pain in hemodialysis patients: prevalence, cause, severity, and management. *American Journal of Kidney Disorders* **42**, 1239–47.

Foral PA, Ineck JR, Nystrom KK (2007) Oxycodone accumulation in a hemodialysis patient. *Southern Medical Journal*; **100**, 212–14.

Kurella M (2003) Analgesia in patients with ESRD: A review of available evidence. *American Journal of Kidney Disorder* **42**, 217–28.

3. *Which one of the following best describes the clinical antibacterial spectrum of tigecycline?*

A. *Gram-positive bacteria*

B. *Gram-negative bacteria*

C. *Gram-positive + gram-negative bacteria + anaerobes*

D. *Gram-positive + gram-negative bacteria*

E. *Gram-negative bacteria + anaerobes*

Tigecycline is a glycylcycline antibacterial drug for IV infusion. It is a broad-spectrum antibiotic that has been approved for treatment of infections caused by Gram-positive bacteria, gram-negative bacteria, and anaerobic bacteria. Current clinical indications include complicated skin infections caused by *Escherichia coli, Enterococcus faecalis, Staphylococcus aureus,* Streptococcus and *Bacteroides fragilis.* Tigecycline is also indicated for complicated intra-abdominal infections caused by resistant Gram-negative bacteria, Gram-positive bacteria, and anaerobic bacteria. Tigecycline was found to have *in vivo* activity for intra-abdominal infections for the following bacteria: Citrobacter, Enterobacter, *E. coli,* Klebsiella, and *E. faecalis* (vancomycin-susceptible strains only), *S. aureus* (MSSA only), *Streptococcus,* bacteroides, *Clostridium perfringes,* and Peptostreptococcus.

Answer: C

Garrison MW, Neumiller JJ, Setter SM (2005) Tigecycline: an investigational glycycline antimicrobial with activity against resistant Gram-positive organisms. *Clinical Therapeutics* **27**, 12–22.

4. *A 64-year-old woman was on continuous electrocardiographic monitoring because of a history of coronary artery disease following an open cholecystectomy. On postoperative day 1, she developed nausea and vomiting. She was treated with multiple doses of an antiemetic. She had a rhythm strip showing QT-prolongation and then torsade de pointes. She was successfully resuscitated.*

Which one of the following antiemetics was most likely used to treat her nausea and vomiting?

A. *Famotidine*

B. *Prochlorperazine*

C. *Metoclopramide*

D. *Ondansetron*

E. *Dexamethasone*

A number of drugs can lead to QT prolongation and torsade de pointes. Phenothiazines, such as prochlorperazine, used for nausea and vomiting have the potential of prolonging the QT interval. Droperidol may also cause QT prolongation. Fortunately, it rarely produces this phenomenon at recommended doses. Ondansetron (serotonin antagonist) and metoclopramide (antidopaminergic and antiserotonergic) are *not* known to cause QT prolongation. H2 blockers and steroids are also *not* known to cause QT prolongation.

Postoperative nausea and vomiting are often multifactorial in origin. Drugs, physical stimuli, or emotional stress can cause the release of neurotransmitters that stimulate serotoninergic (5-HT3), dopaminergic (d2), histaminergic (H1), and muscarinic (M1) receptors. The vomiting center, rather than a discrete area, is a neural network comprised of the chemoreceptor trigger zone, area postrema, and nucleus tractus solitarius.

Phenothiazines and butyrophenones act on D2, H1, and M1 receptors. Benzamides, such as metoclopramide and domperidone, affect 5-HT3 and 5-HT4 receptors; scopolamine is an M1-receptor antagonist; and diphenhydramine and cyclizine are H1-antagonists. Specific 5-HT3-receptor antagonists, such as ondansetron and granisetron, represent the most recently developed class of antiemetics.

Answer: B

Sung YF (1996) Risks and benefits of drugs used in the management of postoperative nausea and vomiting. *Drug Safety* **14**, 181–97.

Yap GY, Camm AJ (2003) Drug induced QT prolongation and torsades de pointes. *Heart* 89, 1363–72.

5. *A 53-year-old woman who weighs 100 kg and is 5 ft tall fell down several stairs and sustained an anterior right hip dislocation. Her past medical history was positive for chronic alcoholism. She underwent operative reduction. Preoperatively, her blood urea nitrogen is 32 mg/dl, serum creatinine is 3.3 mg/dL, serum glucose was 155 mg/dL, asparate amiontransaminase 315 U/L, and international normalized ratio (INR) was 1.4. The following day, she developed sudden onset of shortness of breath. Pulmonary embolism diagnosis was made. Enoxaparin 100 mg q 12 h subcutaneously was begun.*

Which one of the following statements about the current enoxaparin dose is most correct?

A. *She is excessively anticoagulated, because dosing should be based on ideal body, not actual body weight*

B. *She is inadequately anticoagulated, because of morbid obesity and increased volume of distribution*

C. *She is inadequately anticoagulated, because of hepatic dysfunction*

D. *She is excessively anticoagulated, because of renal dysfunction*

E. *She is inadequately anticoagulated, because of increased cytochrome P450 activity*

Low-molecular-weight heparins (LMWHs) do not undergo hepatic metabolism and primarily undergo renal elimination. Thus, answer C is not correct. Generally, dosing of LMWH is based on **actual body weight**. However, if a patient weighs more than 140 kg (this patient is only 100 kg), using standard dosing may cause excessive anticoagulation. This patient is likely to be over anticoagulated from LMWH accumulation due to her renal dysfunction, not from excessive LMWH dose.

The primary advantages of LMWH, compared with unfractionated heparin (UFH), are better bioavailability and consistency of action. Dose-independent renal clearance of LMWHs results in predictable antithrombotic activity; thus, anticoagulation monitoring is typically not needed.

Answer: D

Hirsch J, Warkentin TE, Shaughnessy SG, *et al.* (2001) Heparin and low-molecular-weight heparin: Mechanisms of action, pharmacokinetics, dosing, monitoring, efficacy, and safety. *Chest* **119**, 64S–94S.

6. *A 52-year-old woman with diabetes was treated 10 days ago for a urinary tract infection by the medical service. She was readmitted 3 days ago with diarrhea, abdominal pain and fever. She had stool samples sent for Clostridium difficile toxin and then was started empirically on Flagyl 500 mg orally every 8 hours. She was transferred to the ICU for confusion, hypotension, abdominal distention, and continued severe diarrhea.*

All of the following would be appropriate treatment considerations except:

A. *Vancomycin PO*

B. *Surgical consultation*

C. *Intravenous immunoglobulin*

D. *Tigecycline IV*

E. *Vancomycin IV*

Clostridium difficile infection (CDI) has become more refractory to standard therapy. Recent data showed severe refractory CDI successfully treated with tigecycline. Oral vancomycin is now advocated as the therapy of choice for severe CDI. Vancomycin administered intravenously does not reach therapeutic levels in the colonic lumen. Metronidazole, administered either orally or intravenously, only reaches low therapeutic levels in the colon. Therefore, even a slightly elevated minimal inhibitory concentration (MIC) of *C. difficile* for metronidazole may lead to therapy failure. Recently, *C. difficile* was reported to have low MIC values for tigecycline.

Because *C. difficile* colitis is a toxin-mediated disease, it has been assumed that immune globulin acts by binding and neutralizing toxin. Off-label use of pooled IVIG from healthy donors has been used in cases of severe refractory *C. difficile* infection and in patients with recurrent disease.

Surgical management should be considered in patients with severe CDI who fail to respond to medical therapy or have signs of systemic toxicity, organ failure, or peritonitis.

Answer: E

Herpers BJ, Vlaminckx B, Burkhardt O, *et al.* (2009) Intravenous Tigecycline as adjunctive or alternative therapy for severe refractory Clostridium difficile infection. *Clinical Infectious Diseases* **48**, 1732–5.

McPherson S, Rees CJ, Ellis R, *et al.* (2006) Intravenous immunoglobulin for the treatment of severe, refractory and recurrent Clostridium difficile diarrhea. *Diseases of the Colon and Rectum* **49**, 640–645.

Synnott K, Mealy K, Merry C, *et al.* (1998) Timing of surgery for fulminating pseudomembranous colitis. *British Journal of Surgery* **85**, 229–31.

7. *Which one of the following statements is* not *true in reference to the use of vasopressin in septic shock?*

A. *Septic shock is associated with a relative vasopressin deficiency*

B. *Low-dose (0.01 to 0.04 U/min) vasopressin infusion increases plasma vasopressin levels, increases mean arterial blood pressure, and reduces the required dose of catecholamine vasopressors (i.e. norepinephrine)*

C. *Vasopressin decreases mortality of patients who have septic shock*

D. *The most likely mechanism of action of vasopressin in septic shock is binding to the V1a receptor causing vasoconstriction*

E. *Low-dose vasopressin infusion appears safe for the treatment of septic shock*

Vasopressin is an endogenous hormone secreted from the posterior pituitary. Normally, plasma vasopressin concentrations in humans are <4 pg/ml. Hypotension is the most potent stimulus to vasopressin secretion. In cardiogenic shock and severe hemorrhagic shock, vasopressin concentrations increase to >20 pg/ml and 100 to 1000 pg/ml, respectively. In septic shock, there is a relative vasopressin deficiency. In recent studies in septic shock patients, vasopressin levels are low and patients developed a relative vasopressin deficiency. Vasopressin exerts its effects through interaction with vasopressin receptors. V1a receptors are located on smooth muscle cells and are responsible for vasoconstriction. In multiple studies in septic shock patients, low dose vasopressin (0.01 to 0.04 U/min) increased plasma vasopressin concentrations to 100 pg/ml, increased mean arterial blood pressure, caused no change or decrease in heart rate, reduced the required dose of catecholamines (such as norepinephrine) needed. However, the studies have shown no significant difference in overall mortality. In the only large randomized controlled trial of vasopressin (VASST), there were no safety concerns.

Answer: C

Dunser MW, Mayr AJ, Ulmer H, *et al.* (2003) Arginine vasopressin in advanced vasodilatory shock: A randomized, prospective, controlled study. *Circulation* **107**, 2313–19.

Russell JA, Walley KR, Singer J, *et al.* (2008) Vasopressin versus norepinephrine infusion in patients with septic shock. *New England Journal of Medicine* **358**, 877–87.

8. *Which one of the following statements is NOT true as it relates to the use of benzodiazepines in the ICU for sedation?*

A. *Benzodiazepines have anxiolytic, sedative-hypnotic, muscle relaxant, and anticonvulsant properties*

B. *Benzodiazepines are effectively removed with hemodialysis, which is recommended for management of overdose*

C. *The mechanism of action of benzodiazepines is to modulate the subunits of the gamma amino butyric acid ($GABA_A$) receptor*

D. *Midazolam has rapid onset of action and a short half-life of 1.5 to 3.5 hours*

E. *When used for prolonged periods, the solvent used for lorazepam infusion has been reported to cause acute tubular necrosis and lactic acidosis*

The benzodiazepines are the most common sedative medications used in the ICU. They have anxiolytic, sedative-hypnotic, muscle relaxant and anticonvulsant properties. Their mechanism of action is to modulate the benzodiazepine receptor (subunits of $GABA_A$ receptor). The binding of benzodiazepines to the $GABA_A$ receptor increases the affinity of GABA and its receptor, thereby increasing the opening frequency of $GABA_A$ receptor. As a consequence of this, benzodiazepines potentiate GABAergic neurotransmission. Most benzodiazepines are metabolized by the liver and the metabolites are excreted by the kidneys. Thus, benzodiazepines are *not* effectively removed by hemodialysis. Midazolam is a short-acting benzodiazepine that has a half-life between 1.5 and 3.5 hours. Midazolam has properties that make it useful for continuous infusion because it has a rapid onset of effects, it is potent, and patients are usually awakened rapidly after discontinuation of the infusion. Midazolam elimination may be decreased in critically ill patients with low albumin, decreased renal function, or obesity. Lorazepam is recommended in the ICU for patients requiring sedation for longer than 24 hours. However, the solvent used for lorazepam infusion contains propylene glycol and with prolonged use or high dosage has been reported to cause acute tubular necrosis, lactic acidosis and a hyperosmolar state.

Flumazenil is used as an antidote in the treatment of benzodiazepine overdoses. It reverses the effects of benzodiazepines by competitive inhibition at the benzodiazepine binding site on the $GABA_A$ receptor.

Answer: B

Murray MJ, Oyen LJ, Browne WT (2008) Use of sedative, analgesics, and neuromuscular blockers. In: Parrillo JE, Dellinger RP (eds) *Critical Care Medicine*: Principles of Diagnosis and Management in the Adult, 3rd edn, Mosby, Philadelphia, PA, pp. 327–42.

9. *Which one of the following is the correct mechanism of action of dexmedetomidine?*

A. *It has been proposed to act as a sodium channel blocker*

B. *It inhibits dopamine-mediated neurotransmission in the cerebrum and basal ganglia*

C. *It acts to modulate subunits of the $GABA_A$ receptor in the limbic system of the brain*

D. *It acts by binding to α_2-adrenoreceptors located in the locus coeruleus, subsequently releasing norepinephrine and decreasing sympathetic activity*

E. *Its effects are mediated by the activation of the μ_1 receptor*

Dexmedetomidine is a new sedative agent that acts by binding to α_2-adrenoreceptors located in the locus coeruleus with an affinity of 1620:1 compared with the affinity of the α_1-receptor. At this site, it releases norepinephrine and decreases sympathetic activity. It has sedative, analgesic and amnestic properties.

Answer: D

Murray MJ, Oyen LJ, Browne WT (2008) Use of sedative, analgesics, and neuromuscular blockers. In Parrillo JE and Dellinger RP (eds) *Critical Care Medicine: Principles of Diagnosis and Management in the Adult,* 3rd edn, Mosby, Philadelphia, PA, pp. 327–42.

10. *Which one of the following definitions of pharmacokinetic and pharmacodynamic principles in the critically ill patient is incorrect?*

A. *Drug absorption is altered by gut wall edema, changes in gastric or intestinal blood flow, concurrent administration of enteral nutrition and incomplete oral medication dissolution.*

B. *Volume of distribution is altered by fluid shifts, hypoalbuminemia, and mechanical ventilation.*

C. *Metabolic clearance by the liver, mostly via the cytochrome P450 system, may be compromised in the critically ill patient by decreases in hepatic blood flow, intracellular oxygen tension and cofactor availability.*

D. *Alterations in renal function increase the half-life of medications cleared via the kidney and result in accumulation of drugs or their metabolites.*

E. *The response to antibiotics that have time-dependent killing pharmacodynamics would be improved by administering a higher dose of drug to increase the area under the inhibitory curve.*

Critically ill patients have alterations in both pharmacokinetics and pharmacodynamics of medications. Pharmacokinetics characterizes what the body does to a drug—the absorption, distribution, metabolism and elimination of the drug. Pharmacodynamics is what the drug does to the body and describes the relationship between the concentration of drug at the site of action and the clinical response observed. Many factors affect drug absorption, distribution and clearance in the critically ill patient. Failure to recognize these variations may result in unpredictable serum concentrations that may lead to therapeutic failure or drug toxicity. Drug absorption is altered by gut wall edema and stasis, changes in gastric and intestinal blood flow, concurrent medications and therapies such as enteral nutrition and incomplete disintegration or dissolution of oral medications. The volume of distribution describes the relationship between the amount of drug in the body and concentration in the plasma. Fluid shifts, particularly after fluid resuscitation, and protein binding changes that occur during critical illness alter drug distribution. Plasma protein concentrations may change significantly during critical illness and may affect the volume of distribution by altering the amount of the active unbound or free drug. Metabolic clearance by the liver is the predominant route of drug detoxification and elimination. With hepatic dysfunction that may occur in the critically ill patient, drug clearance may be decreased secondary to reduced hepatic blood flow, decreased hepatocellular enzyme activity or decreased bile flow. A common pathway for drug metabolism is the cyctochrome P_{450} system. Critical illness may compromise this system by decreasing hepatic blood flow, intracellular oxygen or cofactor availability. Antibiotics are usually categorized as having either concentration dependent or time-dependent killing. The activity of concentration-dependent antibiotics increases as the peak serum concentrations of drug increase. Time-dependent antibiotics kill at the same rate regardless of the peak serum concentration that is attained above the MIC (minimum inhibitory concentration). Thus, an increase in dose is **not** associated with improved AUIC (area under the inhibitory concentration curve). Instead, increasing dosing frequency would improve antibiotic killing.

Answer: E

Devlin JW, Barletta JF (2008) Principles of drug dosing in critically ill patients. In Parrillo JE and Dellinger RP (eds) *Critical Care Medicine: Principles of Diagnosis and Management in the Adult*, 3rd edn, Mosby, Philadelphia, PA, pp. 343–76.

11. *Antibiotic resistance is a world crisis. Most nosocomial outbreaks caused by antibiotic-resistant micro-organisms have occurred in patients hospitalized in an ICU. Which of the following statements is an incorrect principle of antimicrobial therapy?*

A. *Fever without other indications of infection should mandate antimicrobial therapy in an ICU patient*

B. *Unless antimicrobial therapy is being given for surgical prophylaxis, gram-stain smears, cultures and other appropriate diagnostic tests should be obtained prior to starting antimicrobial therapy for treatment of presumed infection in an ICU patient*

C. *The need for continued antimicrobial therapy should be reassessed daily. If diagnostic studies are negative after 72 hours and the patient is not exhibiting signs of sepsis, antibiotic therapy should be discontinued*

D. *Surgical antimicrobial prophylaxis should not extend beyond 24 hours postoperatively*

E. *If cultures identify the infecting micro-organism(s), therapy should be modified to the most narrow-spectrum drug(s) likely to be effective*

Antimicrobials are widely misused and overused. Methods of controlling antimicrobial use include restricted formularies, policies on clinical microbiology laboratory on reporting of susceptibility testing, and automatic stop orders for surgical prophylaxis. Several principles can reduce unnecessary antimicrobial therapy and improve the use of the drugs that are given. Fever without indications of infection should *not* mandate automatically beginning antimicrobial therapy in an ICU patient. Fever is not uncommon in the postoperative patient, especially in the early postoperative period. Appropriate cultures should be obtained and empiric antibiotics started if indicated, especially if the patient is exhibiting signs and symptoms consistent with sepsis. The need for continued antibiotic therapy should be reassessed **daily** and if diagnostic tests are negative in 48–72 hours without signs of sepsis, antimicrobial therapy should be stopped. Surgical antimicrobial *prophylaxis* should not extend beyond 24 hours postoperatively and, in most cases, can be limited to one postoperative dose. If cultures identify the infecting micro-organism or micro-organisms, antimicrobial therapy should be modified as soon as possible to the most narrow-spectrum drug or drugs likely to be effective.

Answer: A

Dellit TH, Owens RC, McGowan Jr JE, *et al.* (2007) Infectious Diseases Society of America and the Society of Healthcare Epidemiology of America guidelines for developing and institutional program to enhance stewardship. *Clinical Infectious Diseases* **44**, 159–77.

Maki DG, Crnich CJ, Safdar N (2008) Nosocomial infection in the intensive care unit. In Parrillo JE and Dellinger RP (eds) *Critical Care Medicine: Principles of Diagnosis and Management in the Adult,* 3rd edn, Mosby, Philadelphia, PA, pp. 1003–69.

12. *A 76-year-old obese woman (100 kg) with diabetes and a history of methicillin-resistant staph aureus (MRSA) soft-tissue skin infection develops ventilator-associated pneumonia following sigmoid colon resection with colostomy and Hartmann's procedure for perforation from diverticulitis. Broncho-alveolar lavage gram-stain shows many gram-positive cocci.*

From microbial sensitivity, pharmacokinetic and pharmacodynamic perspectives, which one of the following antimicrobial agents is likely to give optimal empiric treatment?

A. *Cefepime 1 gm IV q 12 hours*

B. *Vancomycin 1 gm IV q 12 hours*

C. *Linezolid 600 mg IV q 12 hours*

D. *Daptomycin 500 mg IV q 24 hours*

E. *Quinupristin/dalfopristin 500 mg IV q 12 hours*

This patient is at increased risk for, and likely has, a MRSA ventilator-associated pneumonia (VAP). Cefepime has activity against most Gram-negative bacilli, but poor activity against methicillin-resistant *S. aureus* and *enterococci*. Vancomycin is still the standard antibiotic for the treatment of nosocomial pneumonia. Vancomycin has *very poor lung tissue penetration.* Thus, among the choices listed, vancomycin would may *not* be the best choice. Specifically, the dose suggested here is not likely to result in adequate lung penetration. There are great concerns about the inactivation of daptomycin by pulmonary surfactants and thus it is not recommended for treatment of MRSA pneumonia. Linezolid has been shown in several studies to have excellent lung penetration. Quinupristin-dalfopristin (Synercid) is bactericidal for clindamycin-susceptible isolates of MRSA. However, clinical response rates of MRSA pneumonia were only 19% for quinupristin-dalfopristin when compared with a 40% response rate for vancomycin.

Answer: C

American Thoracic Society/Infectious Diseases Society of America (2005) Guidelines for the management of adults with hospital-acquired, ventilator-associated, and health care-associated pneumonia. *American Journal of Respiratory Critical Care Medicine* **171**, 388–416.

13. *Which one of the following statements related to fluoroquinolones is incorrect:*

A. *Fluoroquinolones are bactericidal agents that act by interfering with DNA gyrase, thus impairing DNA synthesis, repair and transcription resulting in bacterial cell lysis*

B. *Similar to β-lactams, fluoroquinolones kill in a time-dependent manner*

C. *Fluoroquinolones penetrate well into secretions and inflammatory cells within the lung and may achieve concentrations that may exceed plasma concentrations*

D. *Fluoroquinolones are highly bioavailable with oral administration reaching similar concentrations via oral and intravenous administration*

E. *Fluoroquinolones, in comparison to other antibiotic classes, rank among the highest for risk of causing C. difficile colitis*

Fluoroquinolones are bactericidal agents that act by interfering with DNA gyrase. They impair DNA synthesis, repair and transcription, resulting in bacterial cell lysis. *Unlike* β-lactams, fluoroquinolones kill in a *concentration-dependent* manner related to the Cmax:MIC (concentration maximum: minimum inhibitory concentration) and the AUC:MIC (area under the curve: minimum inhibitory concentration) of drug concentration relative to organism susceptibility. Features of quinolones make them well suited for treatment of respiratory infections. They penetrate well into secretions and inflammatory cells within the lung. Pulmonary concentrations may exceed plasma concentrations. In addition, quinolones are nearly 100% bioavailable with oral administration. The high bioavailability of these agents permits easy transition from intravenous to oral therapy. *C. difficile*-associated diarrhea (CDAD) has been associated with fluoroquinolones, just like with almost all antibiotics. When compared to other antibiotics, however, the risk of CDAD was found to be 2.5 times greater.

Answer: B

Mehlhorn AJ, Brown DA (2007) Safety concerns with fluoroquinolones. *Annals of Pharmacotherapy* **41**, 1859–66.

Owens RC, Ambrose P (2005) Antimicrobial safety: focus on fluoroquinolones. *Clinical Infectious Diseases* **41**, S144–517.

14. *A 65-year-old man has been in the ICU for one week following an open cholecystecomy secondary to gangrenous cholecystitis with bacteremia. Intravenous ceftazidime was started empirically perioperatively. The blood culture was positive for* Escherichia coli *sensitive to ceftazidime, cefepime, and meropenem, but resistant to aztreonam and piperacillin.*

On day 2 of treatment, the patient continues to have fever and tachycardia. Which one of the following interventions is the best antimicrobial treatment strategy for this patient?

A. Discontinue ceftazidime, and start cefepime

B. Add gentamicin

C. Add fluoroquinolone

D. Discontinue ceftazidime, and start meropenem

E. Continue ceftazidime and add fluconazole

Despite the susceptibility results, the organism is not actually sensitive to ceftazidime. Ceftazidime is a potent inducer of chromosomal β-lactamase expression. Extended spectrum β-lactamases (ESBLs) are plasmid-mediated enzymes that inactivate all β-lactam antibiotics, except for cephamycins (cefoxitin) and carbapenems. Detection of ESBLs is often difficult. Some microbiology laboratories do not employ reliable methods, which may result in false susceptible reporting of ESBL strains to cefotaxime, ceftazidime and ceftriaxone. Cefepime, a fourth-generation cephalosporin, does not appear to induce this type of chromosomal-mediated resistance to the same degree as ceftazidime, but is susceptible to the action of ESBLs. Most ESBLs also co-express resistance to other agents including aminoglycosides and fluoroquinolones.

Carbapenems (specifically meropenem) are the most effective agents against ESBLs. An ESBL E-test should be performed for this isolate, and the patient should be started on meropenem pending the results.

Answer: D

Pfaller MA, Segreti J (2006) Overview of the epidemiological profile and laboratory detection of extended-spectrum beta-lactamases. *Clinical Infectious Disorders* **42**, S153–S163.

The next paragraph relates to questions 15 and 16.

An 18-year-old boy sustained multiple gunshot wounds to the abdomen. He underwent multiple laparotomies with resection of multiple enterotomies and delayed abdominal closure. He received antibiotic prophylaxis with cefoxitin for his laparotomies. On post-op day 10, he developed pneumonia. He had a bronchoaveolar lavage that grew P. aeruginosa.

15. *Which one of the following antimicrobial medications would be least likely to successfully treat this patient?*

A. Levaquin 750 mg IV q 24 hr

B. Piperacillin/tazobactam 4.5 gm IV q 6 hr

C. Ceftriaxone 1 gm IV q 24 hr

D. Meropenem 500 mg IV q 6 hr

E. Amakacin 15 mg/kg IV q24 hr

16. *How long should this patient receive treatment for this micro-organism?*

A. 5 days

B. 10 days

C. *8 days*

D. *12 days*

E. *14 days*

P. aeruginosa is a ubiquitous, avirulent opportunist organism. Its virulence is enhanced in critically ill patients. Therapy is complicated by both intrinsic and acquired resistance to a diverse spectrum of antimicrobials. Although antibiotic resistance in gram-negative bacilli may occur by means of several mechanisms, one that provides a foundation for understanding resistance is related to β-lactamase production in gram-negative organisms. These enzymes can be divided into categories of type I and non-type I enzymes. Type I β-lactamases are chromosomally mediated, with production controlled by the *ampC* gene. The micro-organisms that produce these enzymes are Serratia, *P. aeruginosa,* Acinetobacter, Citrobacter and Enterobacter. The mnemonic "SPACE bugs" may be used to remember these organisms. Nosocomial infections of lung, skin, urine or blood are caused by one of these pathogens 20% of the time. The four classes of antibiotics that have the most predictable stability in the presence of the Type I β-lactamases are aminoglycosides, carbapenems, fluoroquinolones, and fourth generation cephalosporins (i.e., cefepime). Type I β-lactamases have an affinity for cephalosporins and thus, third-generation cephalosporins are *not* stable in the presence of these enzymes (i.e., ceftriaxone). In addition, β-lactamase inhibitors, clavulanic acid, sulbactam and tazobactam also lack stability against these enzymes; however, tazobactam is the most likely to resist their destruction. Thus, piperacillin/tazobactam is effective against this micro-organism and is considered an antipseudomonal penicillin.

Answers: 15: C, 16: E

Godke J, Karam G (2008) Principles governing antimicrobial therapy in the intensive care unit. In Parrillo JE and Dellinger RP (eds) *Critical Care Medicine: Principles of Diagnosis and Management in the Adult,* 3rd edn, Mosby, Philadelphia, PA, pp. 1071–88.

Chastre J, Wolff M, Fagon JY, *et al.* (2003) Comparison of 8 vs. 15 days of antibiotic therapy for ventilator-associated pneumonia in adults: a randomized trial. *Journal of the American Medical Association* **290**, 2588–98.

17. *A 53-year-old previously healthy man underwent sigmoid resection and Hartmann procedure for perforated sigmoid diverticulitis. On postop day 10, he developed sepsis. Blood, sputum, and urine cultures were obtained. The ICU sepsis bundle, which included fluconazole 200 mg IV q 24 hours, was ordered. This patient had previously received fluconazole for Candida in his sputum and urine. Two other patients in this ICU have* C. glabrata.

Which one of the following would be the best antifungal treatment for this patient?

A. *Continue with the current fluconazole as provided in the sepsis bundle*

B. *Increase the dose of fluconazole to 400 mg IV q 24 hrs*

C. *Change the fluconazole to voriconazole 5 mg/kg IV q 12 hrs*

D. *Change the fluconazole to caspofungin 70 mg IV initially, then 50 mg IV q 24 hr*

E. *Change out his Foley catheter and hold antifungal therapy*

Although *C. albicans* is the most common pathogen in oropharyngeal and cutaneous candidiasis, non-*albicans* species of Candida are increasingly frequent causes of invasive candidiasis. Candidemia may be treated initially with fluconazole, voriconazole, amphotericin B or a candin (e.g. caspofungin). In critically ill and hemodynamically unstable patients, amphotericin B lipid preparation or candins are preferred because of their broader spectrum of activity and more rapid onset of action. Because of their greater safety, candins are increasingly viewed as initial agents of choice. Bloodstream isolates of *C. albicans, C. tropicalis* and *C. parapsilosis* are generally susceptible to fluconazole and amphotericin B. Isolates of *C. glabrata* and *C. krusei* will often be resistant to fluconazole. In immunocompetent patients a history of azole use and an increased incidence of *C. glabrata* and *C. krusei* in the same ICU (such as in the example given above in this patient) will decrease the likelihood of azoles eradicating the candidemia.

Answer: D

Ostrosky-Zeichner L, Rex JH (2008) Antifungal and antiviral therapy. In Parrillo JE and Dellinger RP (eds) *Critical Care Medicine: Principles of Diagnosis and Management in the Adult,* 3rd edn, Mosby, Philadelphia, PA, pp. 1089–109.

18. *A 43-year-old diabetic woman who is found to have a fever of 39.0°C and blood pressure 81/43 mm Hg 18 hours after exploratory laparotomy for lysis of adhesions. She is transferred to the ICU and her examination is notable for acute distress with erythema and bullous lesions near the surgical wound. Aspiration of one of the lesions reveals numerous white blood cells with Gram-positive cocci in chains. What is the antibiotic that would be most helpful in reducing toxin production in this patient?*

A. *Clindamycin*

B. *Ciprofloxacin*

C. *Aztreonam*

D. *Cefepime*

E. *Gentamicin*

Necrotizing soft tissue infection is an uncommon, severe infection that causes necrosis of the subcutaneous tissue and fascia with sparing of the underlying muscle. Two types, based on microbiology, are described. In type I, at least one anaerobic species is isolated along with one or more facultative anaerobes and members of Enterobacteriaceae. In type II, group A streptococci (GAS) are generally isolated alone (also known as hemolytic streptococcal gangrene). Predisposing factors include blunt and penetrating trauma, varicella infection, intravenous drug abuse, surgical procedures, childbirth, and possibly nonsteroidal anti-inflammatory drug use, but necrotizing soft tissue infections may occur in the absence of an obvious portal of entry. Type II necrotizing fasciitis is commonly associated with Streptococcal toxic shock syndrome. The involved area is extremely painful, erythematous, and edematous. Infection spreads widely in deep fascial planes with relative sparing of the overlying skin and therefore may be unrecognized. This form of necrotizing fasciitis is present in approximately 50% of cases of streptococcal toxic shock syndrome. The skin becomes dusky and bullae develop. Streptococci can usually be cultured from the fluid in the early bullae or from blood. Mortality from this infection is high. Treatment consists of penicillin and clindamycin. Intravenous immunoglobulin administration may also be considered.

Recent studies suggest clindamycin is superior to penicillin in the treatment of necrotizing fasciitis due to GAS. Penicillin failure is probably due to a reduction in bacterial expression of critical penicillin binding proteins during the stationary growth phase of these bacteria. Clindamycin is likely more effective because it is not affected by inoculum size or stage of growth, suppresses toxin production, facilitates phagocytosis of *S. pyogenes* by inhibiting M-protein synthesis, suppresses production of regulatory elements controlling cell wall synthesis, and has a long post antibiotic effect.

Answer: A

Sarani B, Strong M, Pascual J, *et al.* (2009) Necrotizing fasciitis: current concepts and review of the literature. *Journal of the American College of Surgeons* **208**, 279–88.

19. *Which one of the following statements related to vasopressors used in the ICU is incorrect:*

A. *Dobutamine is an inotropic agent and sympathomimetic. Its mechanism of action is via selective stimulation of β1-adrenergic receptors.*

B. *Epinephrine is an inotropic agent and endogenous catecholamine. Its mechanism of action is via stimulation of both α and β adrenergic receptors.*

C. *Milrinone is inotropic agent and phosphodiesterase 3 inhibitor. It prevents the breakdown of cyclic adenosine monophosphate (cAMP) in muscle and leads to increased Ca^{+2} ions in proximity to contractile fibers of cardiac muscle. It also has significant vasodilatory effects and some chronotropic effect.*

D. *Norepinephrine is a direct-acting sympathomimetic. Its mechanism of action is via stimulation of both α and β-adrenergic receptors. It has significant inotropic and vasoconstrictor effects and minimal chronotropic effects.*

E. *Phenylephrine is a synthetic sympathomimetic. Its mechanism of action is primarily via stimulation of β adrenergic receptors. It has significant chronotropic and inotropic effects and vasodilation.*

Dobutamine is an inotropic agent and synthetic catecholamine. Its mechanism of action is via the stimulation of β1-adrenergic receptors. It has 3+ inotropic effect, 2+ chronotropic effect and 1+ vasodilatory effects. Epinephrine is an inotropic agent and endogenous catecholamine. Its mechanism of action is to stimulate both α and β adrenergic receptors. It has 4+ inotropic effect, 4+ chronotropic effect,and 4+ vasoconstriction. Milrinone is an inotropic agent. It is a phosphodiesterase 3 inhibitor that potentiates the effectof cyclic adenosine monophosphate (cAMP) by preventing the breakdown of cAMP in muscle leading to increased Ca^{+2} ions in proximity to contractile fibers of cardiac muscle. Milrinone also enhances relaxation of the left ventricle by increasing Ca^{2+}-ATPase activity on the cardiac sarcoplasmic reticulum. This increases calcium ion uptake. It has positive inotropic, vasodilating and minimal chronotropic effects. It is used in the management of heart failure typically when conventional treatment with vasodilators and diuretics has proven insufficient. Norepinephrine is an adrenergic agent and endogenous catecholamine. Its mechanism of action is via stimulation of both α and β-adrenergic receptors (primarily α). It has 2+ inotropic effect, minimal chronotropic effect, 4+ vasoconstriction. Phenylephrine is a pure vasoconstrictor (pure α-adrenergic agonist) without direct cardiac effect. It may cause reflex bradycardia. Isoproterenol is a synthetic sympathomimetic agent with primarily β adrenergic effects. It has large (4+) chronotropic effect, 4+ inotropic effect, and 3+ vasodilation.

Answer: E

Gonzalez ER, Kannewurf BS, Hess ML (2000) Inotropic therapy and the critically ill patient. In: Grenvik A, Ayres SM, Holbrook PR, *et al.* (eds) 4th ed. *Textbook of Critical Care*, WB Saunders, Philadelphia, PA, 4th edn, pp. 1123–30.

Chapter 10 Transfusion, Hemostasis and Coagulation

Stacy Shackelford, MD, FACS and Kenji Inaba, MD, FRCSC, FACS

1. *A 45-year-old man was admitted to the ICU five days ago after a motorcycle crash in which he suffered a severe left pulmonary contusion, pneumothorax, cardiac contusion, humerus fracture, clavicle fracture, and brachial plexus injury. Blood pressure is stable. He is currently undergoing a spontaneous breathing trial. The patient's hemoglobin is 8.1 g/dL, platelets 30 000/mm^3, prothrombin time 18 s, and partial thromboplastin time 42 s.*

Which blood products should be transfused at this time?

A. *Red blood cells, platelets, and fresh-frozen plasma*

B. *Red blood cells and platelets*

C. *Red blood cells*

D. *Platelets*

E. *No blood products*

In this stable trauma patient without evidence of active bleeding, no blood products are needed at this time. A restrictive transfusion strategy maintaining hemoglobin at 7.0–9.0 g/dL has been shown to be as effective as a liberal transfusion strategy maintaining hemoglobin concentration at 10.0–12.0 g/dL. For those with an APACHE II score ≤ 20, 30-day mortality is significantly less with a restrictive strategy.

In the absence of clinical bleeding, FFP transfusion has been association with increased mortality and an increased incidence of acute lung injury.

Evidence to support prophylactic platelet transfusion in critically ill patients without active bleeding is conflicting. Several authors have recommended avoidance of prophylactic platelet transfusion altogether, while others have recommended thresholds ranging from 10 000/mm^3 to 100 000/mm^3 for patients at risk of bleeding.

Answer: E

Hébert P, Wells B, Blajchman M, *et al.* (1999) A multicenter, randomized, controlled clinical trial of transfusion requirements in critical care. *New England Journal of Medicine* **340** (6), 409–17.

MacLennan S, Williamson L. (2006) Risks of fresh frozen plasma and platelets. *Journal of Trauma* **60** (6 Suppl.), S46–S50.

Napolitano L, Kurek S, Luchette F (2009) Clinical practice guideline: Red blood cell transfusion in adult trauma and critical care. *Critical Care Medicine* **37** (11), 3124–57.

2. *A 23-year-old man was involved in a bicycle-versus-auto accident, sustaining a large, complex laceration to the right anterior tibial region. No other injuries were identified. Dorsal pedal and posterior pedal pulses were normal. Admission laboratory studies showed a hemoglobin of 11.3 g/dL, platelet count 210 000/mm^3, prothrombin time of 12.8 s, and activated partial thromboplastin time of 65 s. He was scheduled for irrigation and debridement in the operating room. After 3 h, the wound, which initially manifested mild hemorrhage, developed ongoing bleeding, which saturated through multiple dressings. The bleeding was not able to be controlled with direct pressure. Dorsal pedal and posterior tibial pulses remained intact.*

Which one of the following is the most likely etiology of this patient's bleeding?

A. *Disseminated intravascular coagulation*

B. *Hemophilia A*

C. *Hypothermia*

Surgical Critical Care and Emergency Surgery: Clinical Questions and Answers, First Edition. Edited by Forrest O. Moore, Peter M. Rhee, Samuel A. Tisherman and Gerard J. Fulda.

D. Von Willebrand disease

E. Arterial injury

Hemophilia may present as excessive bleeding after trauma or surgery; frequently the bleeding is delayed. Patients with mild or moderate hemophilia A have a factor VIII level that is 1–50% of normal. These patients may have no history of spontaneous bleeding into joints or soft tissues, yet may develop significant bleeding complications after trauma or surgery. Laboratory abnormalities in hemophilia are characterized by a normal prothrombin time, variable prolongation of partial thromboplastin time, and a normal platelet count. The diagnosis can be confirmed with a Factor VIII assay and treated with concentrated Factor VIII. Hemophilia B (Factor IX deficiency) has a similar presentation and treatment.

Bleeding associated with invasive procedures in patients with clotting factor deficiencies is commonly delayed, and may present as large subcutaneous or soft tissue hematomas. In contrast, platelet defects including Von Willebrand disease are typically characterized by spontaneous mucocutaneous bleeding and epistaxis, or immediate bleeding and diffuse oozing at the surgical site.

Disseminated intravascular coagulation may occur after severe trauma, however this patient's injury was not extensive and he had an elevated partial thromboplastin time at presentation.

Arterial injury is unlikely given the delayed presentation of bleeding and normal distal pulses.

Answer: B

Goldman G, Holoborodska Y, Oldenburg J, *et al.* (2010) Perioperative management and outcome of general and abdominal surgery in hemophiliacs. *American Journal of Surgery* **199**, 702–7.

Cohen, A (1995) Treatment of inherited coagulation disorders. *American Journal of Medicine* **99**, 675–82.

3. *A 33-year-old man is undergoing exploratory laparotomy for a gunshot wound to the liver with massive hemorrhage and hemorrhagic shock. Rapid thrombelastography (TEG) demonstrates a prolonged activated clotting time (ACT), prolonged K time, decreased angle (TEG α) and normal maximum amplitude (MA).*

Using goal-directed component replacement based on the above rapid TEG results, this patient should receive:

A. Fresh frozen plasma

B. Platelets

C. Fresh frozen plasma and platelets

D. Amicar

E. Cryoprecipitate

Thrombelastography has been used as a guide to blood product replacement for acutely bleeding patients, and has been studied as an alternative to ratio-based mass transfusion protocols. TEG offers the advantage of real-time point of care testing of coagulation function in whole blood.

A rapid TEG differs from conventional TEG because tissue factor is added to the whole blood specimen, resulting in a rapid reaction and subsequent analysis.

The R value, which is recorded as activated clotting time (ACT) in the rapid TEG specimen, reflects clotting factor activation and the time to onset of clot formation. A deficiency of clotting factors will result in a prolonged ACT, which can be treated by FFP transfusion.

The K value is the interval from the beginning of clot formation to a fixed level of clot firmness measured at a standard 20 mm amplitude and reflects the activity of thrombin to cleave fibrinogen. Similarly, the α angle reflects the rate of clot formation and is another measure of fibrinogen activity. A prolonged K value and a decreased α angle represent a fibrinogen deficit which can be treated by transfusion of FFP or cryoprecipitate.

The maximum amplitude (MA) measures the final clot strength, reflecting the end result of platelet-fibrin interaction. If the MA is decreased after transfusion of FFP, then platelet transfusion should be considered.

The patient described has a prolonged ACT as well as prolonged K time and decreased α angle. This is best treated by FFP transfusion to replace both the clotting factor deficiency and fibrinogen deficiency. If the K time remains prolonged after correction of the ACT, then cryoprecipitate can be given.

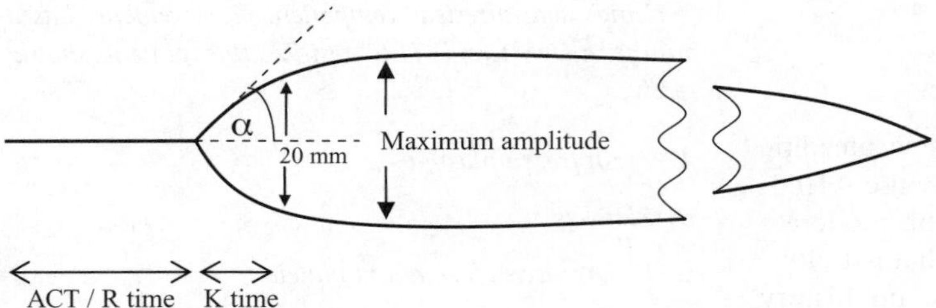

Answer: A

Johansson P, Stensball J (2010) Hemostatic resuscitation for massive bleeding: the paradigm of plasma and platelets—a review of the current literature. *Transfusion* **50**, 701–10.

Kashuk J, Moore E, Sawyer M, *et al.* (2010) Postinjury coagulopathy management, goal directed resuscitation via POC thrombelastography. *Annals of Surgery* **251** (4), 604–14.

4. *A 68-year-old woman is admitted to the surgical intensive care unit after a fall down five stairs where she sustained a right femoral neck fracture. She is scheduled for urgent pinning of the femoral neck fracture. The patient's home medications include warfarin which she takes for atrial fibrillation. On admission, her laboratory tests show Hg 10.4 g/dL, Hct 32%, platelet count 155 000/mm^3, prothrombin time 32 s, INR 3.1, and activated thromboplastin time 33 seconds. Six units of FFP are ordered to reverse her anticoagulation. After transfusion of two units FFP, the patient complains of shortness of breath, and develops a fever of 38.5 °C, heart rate of 115 beats per minute, and SaO_2 85%. Respiratory status deteriorates rapidly, requiring intubation and mechanical ventilation. A chest X-ray was obtained that demonstrates diffuse bilateral infiltrates. CVP is 10 mm Hg.*

What is the most appropriate intervention?

A. *Administer diuretics*

B. *Administer corticosteroids*

C. *Administer heparin bolus followed by continuous infusion*

D. *Administer antibiotics*

E. *Aggressive respiratory support*

Transfusion associated acute lung injury (TRALI) is a serious complication of transfusion defined as hypoxia ($PaO_2/FiO_2 \leq 300$ or $SpO_2 < 90\%$), bilateral infiltrates on chest X-ray, and pulmonary artery occlusion pressure ≤18 mm Hg or no clinical evidence of left atrial hypertension. Additional criteria include: acute lung injury developing during or within six hours of transfusion, no acute lung injury present before transfusion, or a clinical course suggesting that worsening of acute lung injury resulted from transfusion. Symptoms include dypsnea, hypotension and fever. TRALI is associated with transfusion of all blood products, including plasma.

The treatment of TRALI is supportive, and includes measures to avoid worsening of lung injury and a restrictive transfusion policy.

The differential diagnosis of respiratory distress during or after transfusion includes TRALI, transfusion associated circulatory overload (TACO), anaphylactic reaction, and bacterial contamination of blood products. The patient presented is unlikely to have TACO as evidenced by associated fever and relatively low CVP. Early fever, hypoxia, and pulmonary infiltrates associated with transfusion are most typical of TRALI.

Answer: E

Benson A, Moss M, Silliman C (2009) Transfusion-related acute lung injury (TRALI): a clinical review with emphasis on the critically ill. *British Journal of Haematology* **147**, 431–43.

Insunza A, Romon I, Gonzalez-Ponte ML, *et al.* (2004) Implementation of a strategy to prevent TRALI in a regional blood center. *Transfusion Medicine* **14**, 157–64.

5. *A 22-year-old man sustained a gunshot wound to the right upper quadrant. He arrives in the emergency department 20 minutes after injury. Blood pressure is 70/0 mm Hg, heart rate 140 beats per minute. Focused*

Abdominal Sonography for Trauma (FAST) is positive for intra-abdominal hemorrhage and the patient is taken directly to the operating room. In the operating room, he is found to have a laceration of the right lobe of the liver and inferior vena cava with ongoing massive hemorrhage.

Current evidence most strongly supports the following approach to blood component therapy:

A. *Early use of Factor VIIa*

B. *Goal directed component transfusion based on PT/PTT and platelet count*

C. *Avoidance of uncrossmatched blood transfusion*

D. *Transfusion of blood components in a fixed ratio*

E. *Minimizing transfusion of fresh frozen plasma*

Multiple retrospective studies of patients receiving massive transfusion have shown a survival advantage for patients who received a high ratio of FFP:PRBC during initial resuscitation. Studies originating from the military and civilian experience have recommended a ratio approaching 1:1:1 FFP:PRBC:platelet transfusion.

Retrospective studies of massive transfusion have been criticized for a potential survival bias where the patients who survived longer were able to receive more FFP. Nevertheless, despite the flaws in study design and the retrospective nature of the data, massive transfusion protocols targeting a high ratio of FFP:PRBC including the use of immediately available prethawed plasma have consistently demonstrated improved survival in trauma patients.

Routine use of Factor VIIa has not demonstrated a decrease in mortality, although subpopulations of coagulopathic patients may benefit. Component therapy based on traditional lab results will result in a marked delay in administration of FFP and platelets and likely does not accurately reflect in vivo clotting activity. Although crossmatched blood is preferable to minimize the risk of transfusion reaction, initial resuscitation with uncrossmatched or type specific blood may be necessary.

Answer: D

Borgman M, Spinella P, Perkins J, *et al.* (2007) The ratio of blood products transfused affects mortality in patients receiving massive transfusions at a combat support hospital. *Journal of Trauma* **63**, 805–13.

Holcomb J, Wade C, Michalek J, *et al.* (2008) Increased plasma and platelet to red blood cell ratios improves outcome in 466 massively transfused civilian trauma patients. *Annals of Surgery* **248** (3), 447–58.

6. *Liberal transfusion of packed red blood cells in stable ICU patients is associated with:*

A. *Improved oxygen consumption*

B. *Increased incidence of nosocomial pneumonia*

C. *Decreased incidence of acute respiratory distress syndrome (ARDS)*

D. *Decreased mortality*

E. *Decreased incidence of multiorgan failure*

Accumulating evidence has increasingly highlighted the risks and lack of efficacy of red blood cell transfusion.

Although traditionally used to improve oxygen delivery, multiple studies have failed to demonstrate an improvement in end organ oxygen consumption with red blood cell transfusion. This may be partially explained by the decreased deformability and adverse microcirculatory effects of stored red blood cells.

Risks associated with red blood cell transfusion include fluid overload, fever, acute transfusion reaction, increased rate of multi-organ failure, increased infection rates, transfusion-associated immunomodulation, human error with incorrect blood administration, TRALI, and viral transmission.

A liberal transfusion strategy, when compared to a restrictive red blood cell transfusion strategy, has not been shown to improve survival.

Answer: B

Hebert P, Wells G, Blajchman M, *et al.* (1999) A multicenter, randomized, controlled clinical trial of transfusion requirements in critical care. *New England Journal of Medicine* **340** (6), 409–17.

Napolitano L, Kurek S, Luchette F (2009) Clinical practice guideline: red blood cell transfusion in adult trauma and critical care. *Critical Care Medicine* **37**, 3124–57.

7. *A hospital's massive transfusion protocol should be immediately activated for which of the following patients?*

A. *A 63-year-old man with grade IV liver laceration who has received 4 units of packed red blood cells over the last 12 hours in the intensive care unit.*

B. *A 23-year-old man with a gunshot wound to the right chest, who had 500cc of blood drained on initial chest tube placement.*

C. *A 31-year-old man with gunshot wound to the epigastrium who has fluid on abdominal ultrasound and has received 8 units of uncrossmatched blood for hypotension in the emergency department.*

D. *A 55-year-old man with grade IV splenic laceration and active contrast extravasation on abdominal CT scan.*

E. *A 71-year-old woman taking warfarin for atrial fibrillation who sustained a loss of consciousness after falling down a flight of stairs.*

Massive transfusion protocols have been successfully implemented in major trauma centers and have demonstrated an improvement in trauma outcomes in several studies. The purpose of a massive transfusion protocol is to provide blood products to massively bleeding patients in an immediate and sustained manner.

The rationale is based on retrospective studies that have demonstrated improved survival for massive transfusion patients who received a high ratio of FFP:PRBC transfused. Massive transfusion has been variably defined as ≥10 units PRBC in the first 6–24 hours.

There are no uniformly accepted criteria for activating a massive transfusion protocol. Clinical factors associated with massive transfusion are systolic blood pressure ≤90 mm Hg, heart rate ≥120 beats per minute, penetrating mechanism, and positive fluid on abdominal ultrasound. Emergency department transfusion of uncrossmatched PRBC is also associated with massive transfusion. Alternatively, protocols can be initiated when a threshold of 6–10 PRBC has been transfused to ensure subsequent transfusion of one unit of FFP for each unit PRBC.

Transfusion of FFP in patients who receive <10 units PRBC has been shown to increase ARDS, MSOF, and infectious complications without improving survival. Therefore overly aggressive or premature activation of a massive transfusion protocol should be avoided. Of the above patients, only patient C has a clear indication for initiation of massive transfusion protocol.

Answer: C

Inaba K, Branco B, Rhee P, *et al.* (2010) Impact of plasma transfusion in trauma patients who do not require massive transfusion. *Journal of the American College of Surgeons* **210**, 957–65.

Nunez T, Voskresensky I, Dossett L, *et al.* (2009) Early prediction of massive transfusion in trauma: simple as ABC (assessment of blood consumption)? *Journal Trauma.* **66** (2), 346–52.

Nunez T, Young P, Holcomb J, Cotton B (2010) Creation, implementation, and maturation of a massive transfusion protocol for the exsanguinating trauma patient. *Journal of Trauma* **68** (6), 1498–505.

8. *Which of the following is true regarding platelets in massive transfusion?*

A. *Platelets should be transfused empirically in a high ratio*

B. *Platelet transfusion is unnecessary in a massive transfusion if sufficient FFP is transfused*

C. *Apheresis platelets are more effective than pooled donor platelets*

D. *Platelet transfusion should only be given for actively bleeding patients with a platelet count less than 50 000/mm^3*

E. *Apheresis platelets are associated with an increased rate of bacterial contamination compared to pooled donor platelets*

Multiple retrospective studies have demonstrated improved survival for trauma patients who received a high ratio of platelets to packed red blood cells during massive transfusion of ≥10 units PRBC in the first 24 hours. Although defined variably in different studies, a high ratio of platelets to PRBC is approximately one unit of apheresis platelets for every 6–10 units PRBC transfused. During a massive transfusion, a high ratio platelet transfusion should be maintained without delay for clinical laboratory results to confirm low platelet counts.

One unit of apheresis platelets is obtained from a single donor, while pooled platelets are combined from six to eight donors. As a result, pooled platelets have a higher risk of bacterial contamination as well as viral transmission, however there is no difference in transfusion related lung injury, and no study has definitely compared outcomes between apheresis and pooled donor platelets in trauma patients.

Answer: A

Inaba K, Lustenberger T, Rhee P, *et al.* (2011) The impact of platelet transfusion in massively transfused trauma patients. *Journal of the American College of Surgeons* **211**, 573–9.

Zink K, Sambasivan C, Holcomb J, *et al.* (2009) A high ratio of plasma and platelets to packed red blood cells in the first six hours of massive transfusion improves outcomes in a large multicenter study. *American Journal of Surgeons* **197**, 565–70.

9. *A 35-year-old man is admitted to the intensive care unit following an emergency splenectomy and nephrectomy for injuries sustained in a motorcycle crash. He required a total of 12 units packed red blood cells intraoperatively. What electrolyte abnormality is most likely to occur?*

A. *Hypokalemia*

B. *Hyperkalemia*

C. *Hypocalcemia*

D. *Hypomagnesemia*

E. *Respiratory acidosis*

Hypocalcemia is the most common abnormality associated with massive transfusion, occurring in 94% of patients receiving a massive blood transfusion. Stored blood is anticoagulated with citrate, which binds calcium and causes hypocalcemia after rapid blood transfusion. Complications of hypocalcemia include prolonged QT, decreased myocardial contractility, hypotension, muscle tremors, pulseless electrical activity and ventricular fibrillation.

Hyper and hypokalemia are both common electrolyte abnormalities following massive transfusion, occurring in 22% and 18% of patients respectively. The potassium concentration of plasma increases in stored blood, becoming higher with increased duration of PRBC storage. Rapid transfusion through a central venous catheter has been associated with cardiac arrest in vulnerable populations, including critically ill adults.

Hypomagnesemia may be caused by dilution as well as the binding of magnesium to citrate.

Acidosis occurs in approximately 80% of massive transfusion patients, however is most commonly metabolic acidosis.

Answer: C

Sihler K, Napolitano L (2010) Complications of massive transfusion. *Chest* **137**, 209–20.

Wilson R, Binkley L, Sabo F, *et al.* (1992) Electrolyte and acid-base changes with massive blood transfusions. *The American Journal of Surgery* **58** (9), 535–44.

10. *A 26-year-old previously healthy woman is admitted to the surgical ICU after appendectomy for perforated appendicitis with diffuse peritonitis. She was extubated in the operating room, but required reintubation in the post anesthesia care unit for progressive shortness of breath and hypoxia. Chest X-ray demonstrates diffuse bilateral infiltrates. On the first postoperative day, platelet count is 75 000/mm^3, PT 19 seconds, PTT 50 s, and oozing is noted from IV sites as well as with endotracheal suction. Which of the following test results would confirm the diagnosis of disseminated intravascular coagulation?*

A. *Decreased antithrombin level*

B. *Elevated fibrin degradation products*

C. *Increased bleeding time*

D. *Elevated fibrinogen level*

E. *Decreased D-dimer*

Disseminated intravascular coagulation (DIC) is characterized by widespread microvascular thrombosis with activation of the coagulation system and impaired protein synthesis leading to exhaustion of clotting factors and platelets. The end result is organ failure and profuse bleeding from various sites. Disseminated intravascular coagulation is always associated with an underlying condition that triggers diffuse activation of coagulation, most commonly sepsis, trauma with soft tissue injury, head injury, fat embolism, cancer, amniotic fluid embolism, toxins, immunologic disorders, or transfusion reaction.

There is no single laboratory test that can confirm or rule out a diagnosis of disseminated intravascular coagulation. A combination of tests in a patient with an appropriate clinical condition can be used to make the diagnosis. A DIC scoring system was shown in two studies to have a sensitivity and specificity of approximately 95% for the diagnosis of DIC. When calculating the DIC score, a low platelet count, elevated fibrin degradation products or D-dimer, prolonged prothrombin time, and low fibrinogen level were found to be consistent with a diagnosis of DIC.

Answer: B

Levi M (2007) Disseminated intravascular coagulation. *Critical Care Medicine* **35** (9), 2191–5.

Taylor F, Toh C, Hoots W, *et al.* (2001) Towards definition, clinical and laboratory criteria, and a scoring system for disseminated intravascular coagulation. *Journal of Thrombosis and Haemostasis* **86**, 1327–30.

11. *A 61-year-old woman with a history of aortic stenosis and chronic renal insufficiency underwent aortic valve replacement. Unfractionated heparin was started 6 hours after surgery and warfarin was started on post-operative day 3. On day 7, she developed pain in the right lower extremity. Examination demonstrated a cool extremity with absent distal pulses. Platelet count fell from 220 000/mm³ on day 4 to 90 000/mm³ on day 7, and creatinine increased from 1.8 mg/dL on day 4 to 2.9 mg/dL on day 7. She was taken to the operating room where she underwent thrombectomy of the right femoral artery. Intraoperatively, extensive white clot was present in the superficial femoral artery.*

Which therapeutic option is most appropriate at this time?

A. *Discontinue unfractionated heparin and start argatroban*

B. *Discontinue unfractionated heparin and start enoxaparin*

C. *Discontinue unfractionated heparin and start lepirudin*

D. *Increase unfractionated heparin*

E. *Discontinue anticoagulation*

The patient has heparin-induced thrombocytopenia (HIT) type II. Heparin-induced thrombocytopenia is a life-threatening disorder, which occurs after exposure to unfractionated or less commonly low molecular weight heparin. Type I HIT is characterized by a mild decrease in platelet counts occurring after 1 to 4 days of heparin therapy. It is nonimmune mediated and follows a benign course, which does not require treatment. Type II HIT usually occurs after 5 to 10 days of heparin therapy and is caused by antibodies against the heparin-platelet factor 4 complex. Heparin-induced thrombocytopenia can occur much sooner in patients who received prior heparin within 100 days. Orthopedic and cardiac surgery patients are at a particularly high risk. Thrombotic complications occur in 20 to 50% of patients.

Thrrombocytopenia is common in the critically ill, and diagnosis of HIT can be difficult. Laboratory confirmation includes immunoassay for the detection of PF4-heparin antibodies and a confirmatory functional assay measuring serotonin release from activated platelets. Delays in obtaining test results mean that clinical decisions must be made on the basis of clinical suspicion. The most consistent clinical findings of HIT are a platelet fall of more than 50% from baseline, onset on day 5 to 10, thrombosis or skin necrosis, and no other cause for the thrombocytopenia.

The thrombus associated with HIT has been described as "white clot" with predominantly fibrin platelet aggregates and few red blood cells.

Treatment of HIT includes discontinuation of all sources of heparin and if anticoagulation is clinically warranted, use of a direct thrombin inhibitor such as lepirudin, argatroban, or bivalirudin. Lepirudin requires renal clearance and may be best avoided in renal insufficiency, therefore treatment with argatroban is the best answer in this case.

Answer: A

Arepally G, Ortel T (2006) Heparin-induced thrombocytopenia. *New England Journal of Medicine* **355** (8), 809–17.

Warkentin T (2004) Heparin-induced thrombocytopenia, diagnosis and management. *Circulation* **110**, e454–e458.

12. *A 55-year-old homeless man is admitted to the ICU after being found down in a local park. He is lethargic, hypoxic, mildly hypotensive, and tachycardic. Chest X-ray demonstrates multiple right rib fractures with a large right pleural effusion. Laboratory data include white blood cell count 15 000/mm^3, hemoglobin 9 g/dL, platelet count 90 000/mm^3, prothrombin time 13 s, partial thromboplastin time 35 s, sodium 145 meq/L, blood urea nitrogen 140 mg/dL, and creatinine 8 mg/dL. Prolonged bleeding is noted from venipuncture sites.*

Which therapy should be administered prior to chest tube placement?

A. *Conjugated estrogens*

B. *Platelet transfusion*

C. *Fresh frozen plasma*

D. *Desmopressin acetate*

E. *Hemodialysis*

This patient is profoundly uremic with clinical evidence of bleeding. Bleeding in uremic patients is complicated by platelet dysfunction and is characterized by mucocutaneous bleeding and bleeding in response to injury or invasive procedures. Prothrombin time and partial thromboplastin time may be normal, and platelet counts are normal to slightly low. Bleeding from surgical procedures may be difficult to control.

Desmopressin acetate (dDAVP) at a dose of 0.3–0.4 μg/kg intravenously or subcutaneously is the simplest and least toxic way to improve platelet function acutely in the uremic patient. Desmopressin acts by increasing the release of Factor VIII and von Willebrand factor from the endothelium and will cause improvement in bleeding time within one hour. Unfortunately, the effect is short lived, lasting 4 to 24 hours, and tachyphylaxis frequently develops after a second dose, limiting its use.

Cryoprecipitate is a source of Factor VIII and fibrinogen and may be used for acute bleeding episodes, however the response may be unpredictable in uremic patients. Cryoprecipitate should have a rapid effect within the first hour, lasting 4–24 h.

Hemodialysis can correct the bleeding time in uremic patients, but is time consuming and may acutely prolong bleeding through platelet activation on artificial surfaces. More prolonged control of bleeding in uremic patients can be achieved with conjugated estrogens, with peak control reached after five to seven days.

If the effusion is found to be a hemothorax, or if there is alternative evidence of ongoing bleeding, a platelet transfusion should be given.

Answer: D

Hedges S, Dehoney S, Hooper J, *et al.* (2007) Evidence-based treatment recommendations for uremic bleeding. *Nature Clinical Practice Nephrology* **3** (3), 138–53.

Mannucci P, Remuzzi G, Pusineri F, *et al.* (1983) Deamino-8-d-arginine vasopressin shortens the bleeding time in uremia. *New England Journal of Medicine* **308** (1), 8–12.

13. *A 58-year-old man sustained a fracture of the right humerus when he fell from a ladder. His past medical history is significant for coronary artery disease for which he underwent coronary stenting of the left anterior descending artery with a drug eluting stent 3 months ago. His current medications include aspirin and clopidogrel. He does not have any other injuries. Surgical fixation of the humerus fracture is required.*

What is the best perioperative management of his platelet inhibitors?

A. *Stop aspirin and clopidogrel for seven days, then proceed with surgery*

B. *Continue aspirin, stop clopidogrel for seven days, then proceed with surgery*

C. *Stop clopidogrel and aspirin for five days, continue a short acting IV antiplatelet agent until four hours before surgery*

D. *Transfuse platelets and proceed with immediate surgery*

E. *Stop aspirin and clopidogrel, for 5 days, then proceed with surgery*

The combination of aspirin and clopidogrel is commonly used following coronary stent placement. Placement of drug eluting stents has become increasingly common, and current recommendations are to continue dual antiplatelet therapy for 1 year following stent placement. A bare metal stent requires six weeks of dual antiplatelet therapy.

Premature interruption in antiplatelet therapy is associated with a high risk of stent thrombosis with a resultant 64% rate of death or myocardial infarction.

Perioperative management of antiplatelet agents is based on balancing the risk of surgical bleeding with the risk of stent thrombosis. In this situation, it is important to know the indication for stenting, the date of implant, the type of stent used, as well as the proposed duration of current antiplatelet therapy. Drug eluting stents placed within one year are at high risk for thrombosis. When possible, surgery should be delayed until after the recommended period of dual antiplatelet therapy.

If urgent surgery must be performed, the risk and consequences of surgical bleeding must be assessed. For procedures with a low bleeding risk, dual antiplatelet agents should be continued through the surgery. For moderate and high bleeding risk procedures, the patient may be converted to a short-acting intravenous antiplatelet agent such as tirofiban or abciximab; 4–6 hours after stopping the infusion, platelet inhibition will decrease by 50% and bleeding time will return to normal.

Answer: C

Lecompte T, Hardy J. (2006) Antiplatelet agents and perioperative bleeding. *Canadian Journal of Anesthesiology* **53** (6), s103–112.

Savonitto S, D'Urbano M, Caracciolo M, *et al.* (2010) Urgent surgery in patients with a recently implanted coronary drug-eluting stent: a phase II study of "bridging" antiplatelet therapy with tirofiban during temporary withdrawal of clopidogrel. *British Journal of Anaesthesiology* **104** (3), 285–91.

14. *A 71-year-old woman taking warfarin for chronic atrial fibrillation arrives in the emergency department after a fall down a flight of stairs at home. A scalp hematoma is present on the left side. She is confused, mumbling, and unable to follow commands, but withdraws to pain in all extremities.*

What is the most important intervention to improve her survival?

A. *Rapid neurosurgical evaluation*

B. *Rapid administration of recombinant Factor VIIa*

C. *Rapid evaluation, head CT, and plasma transfusion*

D. *Rapid administration of vitamin K*

E. *Early admission to a neuro intensive care unit*

A protocol for the rapid evaluation, diagnosis, and treatment of anticoagulated trauma patients has been shown to significantly reduce the mortality of warfarin anticoagulated trauma patients with intracranial hemorrhage.

According to the protocol, all warfarin anticoagulated patients at risk for intracranial injury are triaged for immediate evaluation by an emergency room physician and emergent head CT is obtained. Simultaneously, the blood bank is notified to thaw two units universal donor plasma followed by two units of type specific plasma. An immediate read of the head CT is completed. FFP and vitamin K are immediately given for any positive head CT.

This protocol for rapid evaluation and treatment of warfarin associated intracerebral hemorrhage resulted in a reduction in mortality from 48% to 10%.

Answer: C

Ivascu F, Howells G, Junn F, *et al.* (2005) Rapid warfarin reversal in anticoagulated patients with traumatic intracranial hemorrhage reduces hemorrhage progression and mortality. *Journal of Trauma* **59** (5), 1131–9.

15. *Which of the following is true regarding the use of recombinant Factor VIIa in trauma patients?*

A. *Factor VIIa may be administered in place of fresh frozen plasma to correct the coagulopathy of trauma.*

B. *Treatment with Factor VIIa is associated with an increase in thrombotic complications.*

C. *The use of Factor VIIa is cost effective for the treatment of trauma patients.*

D. *Treatment with Factor VIIa results in a significant reduction in mortality in severely injured trauma patients.*

E. *Treatment with Factor VIIa results in a significant reduction in red blood cell transfusion in severely injured trauma patients.*

Although recombinant Factor VIIa has been used extensively off-label to correct coagulopathy in multiple situations, the only FDA approved use for Factor VIIa is for hemophiliacs with known antibodies to Factor VIII.

Two randomized controlled trials demonstrated a significant decrease in red blood cell transfusions for patients with severe blunt trauma, with a trend toward decreased transfusion in penetrating trauma. Neither study demonstrated a survival advantage with the use of Factor VIIa. The studies did not show any increase in thrombotic complications with the use of Factor VIIa.

The high cost of recombinant Factor VIIa with lack of proven benefit in trauma patients argues against routine use in trauma patients.

Answer: E

Boffard K, Riou B, Warren B, *et al.* (2005) Recombinant Factor VIIa as adjunctive therapy for bleeding control in severely injured trauma patients: two parallel randomized, placebo-controlled, double-blind clinical trials. *Journal of Trauma* **59** (1), 8–18.

Goodnough L, Shander A. (2007) Recombinant factor VIIa: safety and efficacy. *Current Opinion in Hematology* **14**, 504–9.

Hauser C, Boffard K, Dutton R, *et al.* (2010) Results of the CONTROL trial: efficacy and safety of recombinant activated Factor VII in the management of refractory traumatic hemorrhage. *Journal of Trauma* **69** (3), 489–500.

16. *An 18-year-old boy is admitted to the surgical ICU after a gunshot wound to the chest, right thoracotomy and right upper lobe non-anatomic lobectomy for bleeding near the pulmonary hilum. A wound to the thoracic spine was difficult to control and was packed with sponges. He received 12 units of packed red blood cells, 10 units of fresh frozen plasma, and 1 unit of apheresis platelets in the operating room. Vital signs: BP 100/60 mm Hg, HR 120 beats/min, temperature 32.5 °C. Laboratory studies: hemoglobin 8.5 g/dL, platelets 100 000/mm^3, prothrombin time 14 s, partial thromboplastin time 40 s. Chest tube output is 300 mL for the first hour in the ICU.*

What is the most appropriate treatment for his bleeding?

A. *Transfuse FFP*

B. *Transfuse platelets*

C. *Transfuse cryoprecipitate*

D. *External warming*

E. *Return to the operating room*

Immediately following surgical control of bleeding and massive resuscitation, aggressive resuscitation must continue addressing all potential causes of bleeding.

Clotting factor and platelet deficiencies can be addressed early during resuscitation by maintaining a high ratio of FFP and platelets to red blood cell transfusion, followed by ongoing correction of coagulation abnormalities when laboratory results become available. In this patient, a platelet count of 100 000/mm^3 and slightly prolonged PT and PTT demonstrate adequate platelets and clotting factors.

Notably, the patient is severely hypothermic. Hypothermia <35 °C has been shown to be a strong independent risk factor for mortality in trauma patients. Mortality increases progressively with increasing severity of hypothermia. Hypothermia contributes to coagulopathy through platelet and clotting factor dysfunction. Clotting assays performed in the laboratory are warmed to 35 °C, and may not represent the patient's actual clotting activity in vivo.

If bleeding continues after aggressive warming and correction of clotting abnormalities, the patient must return to the operating room without further delay.

Answer: D

Brohi K, Cohen M, Davenport R. (2007) Acute coagulopathy of trauma: mechanism, identification, and effect. *Current Opinion in Critical Care* **13**, 680–5.

Inaba K, Teixeira P, Rhee P, *et al.* (2009) Mortality impact of hypothermia after cavitary explorations in trauma. *World Journal of Surgery* **33** (4), 864–9.

17. *A 29-year-old man was involved in a motorcycle crash. He now has a distended abdomen that is diffusely tender. Blood pressure is 80/60 mm Hg.*

What fluid should be administered?

A. *Lactated ringers*

B. *Hypertonic saline*

C. *O positive blood*

D. *Type specific blood*

E. Crossmatched blood

The described patient has hemoperitoneum and should be taken to the operating room for control of any surgically correctable sources of bleeding. Crystalloid resuscitation should be minimized and O negative or if unavailable, O positive blood transfused without delay. If uncrossmatched blood resources are limited, O negative blood is reserved for woman of child-bearing age to avoid the risk of Rh isoimmunization, while O positive or negative blood is used for men and women beyond child-bearing age. O positive blood has been shown to be safe for transfusion in hemorrhaging trauma patients, with a very low rate of transfusion reaction.

Advantages of using uncrossmatched type O blood include immediate availability before type specific blood becomes available and avoidance of errors in multi-casualty situations. The safety of type O blood has been improved by prescreening donor blood for anti-A and anti-B antibodies which can lead to hemolysis of native red blood cells.

Answer: C

Dutton R, Shih D, Edelman B, *et al.* (2005) Safety of uncrossmatched type-O red cells for resuscitation from hemorrhagic shock. *Journal of Trauma* **59** (6), 1445–9.

Sihler K, Napolitano L (2009) Massive transfusion: new insights. *Chest* **136** (6), 1654–67.

Chapter 11 Analgesia and Sedation

Juan C. Duchesne, MD, FACS, FCCP and Marquinn D. Duke, MD

1. *What physiologic abnormality is associated with an increased risk of analgesic toxicity?*

A. *Hypocalcemia*

B. *Hypokalemia*

C. *Hypomagnesemia*

D. *Hyponatremia*

E. *Hypoproteinemia*

Patients with hypoproteinemia have less of the drug bound to proteins, leaving more of the drug free. This, in turn, causes an increase in active drug levels. The elevated drug level increases the possibility of drug toxicity. Neither hypocalcemia, hypokalemia, hypomagnesemia, nor hyponatremia affect the binding of the drug. Therefore, their serum levels are less likely to affect the toxicity of the drug.

Answer: E

Power, BM, Forbes, AM, van Heerden, PV, *et al.* (1998) Pharmacokinetics of drugs in critically ill adults. *Clinical Pharmacokinetics* **34**, 25–56.

Sakata, RK. (2010) Analgesia and sedation in intensive care unit. *Revista Brasileira de Anestesiologia* **60** (6), 648–58.

Stevens, DS, Edwards, WT (1999) Management of pain in intensive care settings. Surgical Clinics of North America **79**, 371–86.

2. *A 42-year-old man is undergoing a laparoscopic bilateral inguinal hernia repair. The anesthesiologist induces the patient with propofol. Propofol works through which mechanism?*

A. *Alpha-2 adrenergic agonist*

B. *Alpha-2 adrenergic antagonist*

C. *GABA (gamma-aminobutyric acid) agonist*

D. *GABA (gamma-aminobutyric acid) antagonist*

E. *mu receptor antagonist*

Benzodiazepines (e.g. midazolam and lorazepam) and propofol are GABA agonists that are often used for sedation in the ICU. Propofol has a fast onset and clearance, and is indicated for short-term sedation. Side effects of propofol are hypotension, respiratory depression, hypertriglyceridemia, pancreatitis, and propofol infusion syndrome. Propofol is useful for patients with neurologic injury, as it decreases intracranial pressure, cerebral blood flow, and cerebral metabolism. Flumazenil would be an example of a GABA antagonist. Opioids have their effect on mu receptors. They are agonists for these receptors, resulting in decreased pain perception. An example of a mu receptor antagonist would be naloxone. Dexmedetomidine is an alpha-2 agonist. It is often utilized as a sedative for patients in the intensive care unit. Mirtazapine is an example of an alpha-2 antagonist, which is often used for its antidepressant effects.

Answer: C

Jacobi J, Fraser GL, Coursin DB, *et al.* (2002) Clinical practices guidelines for the sustained use of sedatives and analgesics in the critically ill adult. *Critical Care Medicine* **30** (1), 119–41.

Mehta, S, McCullagh, I, Burry, L (2009) Current sedation practices: Lessons learned from international surveys. *Critical Care Clinics* **25**, 471–88.

Riker, RR, Fraser, GL (2009) Altering intensive care sedation paradigms to improve patient outcomes. *Critical Care Clinics* **25**, 527–38.

Sakata, RK (2010) Analgesia and sedation in intensive care unit. *Revista Brasileira de Anestesiologia* **60** (6), 648–58.

Surgical Critical Care and Emergency Surgery: Clinical Questions and Answers, First Edition. Edited by Forrest O. Moore, Peter M. Rhee, Samuel A. Tisherman and Gerard J. Fulda.

Wallace, S, Mecklenburg, B, Hanling, S. (2009) Profound reduction in sedation and analgesic requirements using extended dexmedetomidine infusions in a patient with an open abdomen. Military Medicine **174**, 1228–30.

3. *What combination of analgesia and sedation has been found to reduce the time of duration of mechanical ventilation?*

A. Administration of analgesia alone

B. Administration of sedation alone

C. Administration of analgesia prior to sedation

D. Administration of sedation prior to analgesia

E. Administration of analgesia and sedation at the same time

In a technique dubbed "analgesia first," drugs used for sedation are administered after the use of analgesics. Studies have found that this technique has led to a reduction in amount of sedatives required, as well as a decrease in the duration of mechanical ventilation. Administration of analgesia alone would not allow for adequate comfort for the patient. Administration of sedation alone would not relieve the patients' pain.

Answer: C

Riker RR, Fraser GL (2009) Altering intensive care sedation paradigms to improve patient outcomes. *Critical Care Clinics* **25**, 527–38.

Sakata, RK (2010) Analgesia and sedation in intensive care unit. *Revista Brasileira de Anestesiologia* **60** (6), 648–58.

4. *A 25-year-old man is involved in a car accident. Examination after being admitted to the hospital reveals an intracranial injury, fractured left humerus, two fractured ribs without pulmonary contusions, and multiple skin abrasions. Which medication would be contraindicated for pain control in this patient?*

A. Codeine

B. Fentanyl

C. Meperidine

D. Morphine

E. Remifentanil

Normeperidine is a metabolite of meperidine. Normeperidine is associated with an increase risk of having seizures. Patients with head injuries have a lower seizure threshold, and are more likely to have seizures. Using meperidine in a patient who has suffered a head injury would be ill advised. Codeine is a less potent pain medication. It would less likely be sufficient for pain control in the immediate post-injury period. However, its use would not be contraindicated. Fentanyl and morphine would be good choices for pain control in this patient. Remifentanil is a short-acting opioid. Its use would not be contraindicated but it effects would be short acting, making it an unlikely choice of analgesic.

Answer: C

Bodenham A, Shelly MP, Park GR (1988) The altered pharmacokinetics and pharmacodynamics of drugs commonly used in critically ill patients. *Clinical Pharmacokinetics* **14**, 347–373.

Power, BM, Forbes, AM, van Heerden, PV, *et al.* (1998) Pharmacokinetics of drugs in critically ill adults. *Clinical Pharmacokinetics* **34**, 25–56.

Sakata, RK (2010) Analgesia and sedation in intensive care unit. Revista Brasileira de Anestesiologia **60** (6), 648–58.

5. *Which of the following local anesthetics is classified as an amide?*

A. Benzocaine

B. Bupivacaine

C. Chloroprocaine

D. Cocaine

E. Tetracaine

Amides have an amide linkage between a benzene ring and a hydrocarbon chain, which is attached to a tertiary amine. The benzene ring confers lipid solubility for penetration of cell membranes. The tertiary amine attached to the hydrocarbon chain makes the anesthetic water soluble. The other choices are examples of esters. The important difference between amides and esters is that, in general, amides are metabolized in the liver, whereas esters are metabolized by plasma cholinesterases. Also, esters tend to have metabolites with higher allergenic potential.

Answer: B

Dorian, RS (2005) Anesthesia of the surgical patient. In: Brunicardi, FC (ed.) Schwartz's Principles of Surgery, McGraw-Hill, New York, pp. 1851–73.

6. *The first symptom of toxicity from a local anesthetic is:*

A. *Restlessness*

B. *Seizures*

C. *Slurred speech*

D. *Tinnitus*

E. *Unconsciousness*

Toxicity of a local anesthetic results from the absorption into the bloodstream. It first manifests in the central nervous system, and then the cardiovascular system. The symptoms progress from restlessness to tinnitus, slurred speech, seizures, and then unconsciousness. If the toxicity has progressed to seizure activity, administering a benzodiazepine or thiopental can treat it.

Answer: A

Dorian RS (2005) Anesthesia of the surgical patient. In: Brunicardi, FC (ed.) *Schwartz's Principles of Surgery*, McGraw-Hill, New York, pp. 1851–73.

7. *The target level of sedation for a patient not expected to require mechanical ventilation for greater than 48 hours is:*

A. *RASS +2 (agitated)*

B. *RASS +1 (restless)*

C. *RASS –1 (drowsy)*

D. *RASS –3 (moderate sedation)*

E. *RASS –4 (deep sedation)*

Unless contraindicated, the optimal level of sedation is where the patient is alert, not agitated, and able to maintain brief contact, and follow simple instructions. This correlates to RASS 0 to –2. RASS +1 or +2 would not provide enough sedation for the patient to be comfortable. This could lead to patient behavior that would be detrimental to their care, such as removing medical devices or thrashing in their bed. RASS –3 or –4 would be deeper sedation. This may be preferred if long-term sedation is expected. However, evaluating the mental status of patients with this level of sedation would be more difficult, as they would have a hard time participating.

Answer: C

Barr, J, Donner A (1995) Optimal intravenous dosing strategies for sedatives and analgesics in the intensive care unit. *Critical Care Clinics* **11**, 827–47.

Sessler CN, Gosnell M, Grap MJ, *et al.* (2002) The Richmond Agitation-Sedation Scale: Validity and reliability in adult intensive care patients. *American Journal of Respiratory and Critical Care Medicine* **166**, 1338–44.

Shapiro MB, West MA, Nathens AB, *et al.* (2007) Guidelines for sedation and analgesia during mechanical ventilation general overview. *The Journal of Trauma: Injury, Infection, and Critical Care* **63** (4), 945–50.

8. *The toxic dose of bupivacaine is:*

A. *3 mg/kg*

B. *5 mg/kg*

C. *7 mg/kg*

D. *9 mg/kg*

E. *11 mg/kg*

Bupivacaine is more cardiotoxic than other local anesthetics. It has a direct effect on ventricular muscle, and binds to sodium channels. Patients who receive a high dose of bupivacaine can experience hypotension, ventricular tachycardia, ventricular fibrillation, or complete atrioventricular heart block. These effects can be refractory to medical treatment. The toxic dose of bupivacaine is approximately 3 mg/kg. Using epinephrine as an additive to bupivacaine would allow for a greater amount of the drug to be used. Epinephrine is a vasoconstrictor that, when added to a local anesthetic, reduces bleeding, hastens the nerve blockade, lengthens its duration, and improves the quality of the nerve blockade. Higher amount of local anesthetic can be administered when epinephrine is added. Epinephrine containing injections should not be used where there are end arteries, as they can lead to distal ischemia.

Answer: A

Dorian, RS (2005) Anesthesia of the surgical patient. In: Brunicardi, FC (ed.) *Schwartz's Principles of Surgery*, McGraw-Hill, New York, pp. 1851–73.

9. *A 25-year-old woman is undergoing preoperative preparation for a planned Cesarean section. After injection of a local anesthetic into her dura sac, she complains of sensory and motor loss of her legs. Additionally, she reports that she is unable to control her urine continence. The effect of the local anesthetic is:*

A. Brown–Sequard syndrome

B. Cauda equina syndrome

C. Central cord syndrome

D. Guillian–Barre syndrome

E. Sheehan's syndrome

Cauda equina syndrome is the result of injury to the nerves emanating distal to the spinal cord. It results in bowel and bladder dysfunction. Additionally, there is an association of lower extremity sensory and motor loss. It is seen in cases where there is an indwelling spinal catheter and high concentrations of lidocaine. Brown–Sequard syndrome is the result of incomplete cord transection. It is associated with a penetrating injury, resulting in ipsilateral motor loss and contralateral loss of pain and temperature sensation. Central cord syndrome is a result of hyperflexion of the cervical spine. It results in the bilateral loss of motor function, pain, and temperature sensation in the upper extremities. The lower extremities are spared. Guillian–Barre syndrome is an acute inflammatory demyelinating polyradiculopathy. It often occurs after a viral infection, surgery, inoculation, or mycoplasma infection. Patients present with weakness ascending from the legs to the body, arms, and to cranial nerves, which progress over 2–4 weeks. Sheehan's syndrome is the resultant pituitary insufficiency of a mother after childbirth. It is caused by hypovolemia or shock following childbirth. This leads to ischemia of the pituitary, mostly affecting the anterior pituitary.

Answer: B

Dorian RS (2005) Anesthesia of the surgical patient. In: Brunicardi, FC (ed.) *Schwartz's Principles of Surgery*, McGraw-Hill, New York, pp. 1851–73.

10. *A patient is about to undergo a major abdominal operation. The anesthesiologist wants to use an induction agent that also has analgesic properties. Which of the following should he/she select?*

A. Thiopental

B. Diazepam

C. Etomidate

D. Ketamine

E. Midazolam

Ketamine differs from the other agents. It produces analgesia as well as amnesia, and is classified as a dissociative anesthetic. The other agents listed only have amnesic properties, and provide no analgesia. The use of a benzodiazepine, in addition to ketamine, has been shown to decrease the side effects of delirium and hallucinations, which are associated with ketamine.

Answer: D

Dorian RS (2005) Anesthesia of the surgical patient. In: Brunicardi, FC (ed.) *Schwartz's Principles of Surgery*, McGraw-Hill, New York, pp. 1851–73.

11. *Which of the following opioids undergoes rapid hydrolysis that is not effected by age, renal function, hepatic function, or weight?*

A. *Alfentanil*

B. *Meperidine*

C. *Morphine*

D. *Remifentanil*

E. *Sufentanil*

Remifentanil is an analog of fentanyl. It is a synthetic opioid that differs from nonsynthetic opioids in lipid solubility, tissue binding, and elimination profiles. This leads to differing potencies and durations of action. Remifentanil undergoes rapid hydrolysis and is unaffected by age, sex, weight, renal dysfunction, or hepatic dysfunction. Due to its rapid hydrolysis, it has little post-operative analgesia.

Answer: D

Dorian RS (2005) Anesthesia of the surgical patient. In Brunicardi FC (ed.) *Schwartz's Principles of Surgery*, McGraw-Hill, New York, pp. 1851–73.

12. *Succinylcholine is hydrolyzed by what mechanism?*

A. *Hofmann elimination*

B. *Plasma cholinesterase*

C. *Kidney metabolism only*

D. *Liver metabolism only*

E. *Kidney and liver metabolism*

Succinylcholine is a depolarizing neuromuscular blocker, which binds to the post-synaptic acetylcholine receptor. It has a rapid onset and offset. It should be avoided in patients who have suffered burns or tissue injury, as it can result in a significant rise in serum potassium. It is quickly hydrolyzed by plasma cholinesterase (pseudocholinesterase). Patients with low pseudocholinesterase levels have a delay in return of motor function. Cis-atracurium is an example of a drug that is metabolized by Hofmann elimination. Hofmann elimination is a temperature and plasma pH dependent process. An increase in pH favors the elimination process, whereas a decrease in pH slows down the process. Thus, cis-atracurium undergoes an organ independent metabolism. Pancuronium is an example of a medication that is eliminated almost completely unchanged by the kidney. Vecuronium and rocuronium are examples of medications that are metabolized by both the liver and kidneys.

Answer: B

Dorian RS (2005) Anesthesia of the surgical patient. In Brunicardi FC (ed.) *Schwartz's Principles of Surgery*, McGraw-Hill, New York, pp. 1851–73.

13. *A 59-year-old man is undergoing a ventral hernia repair. The man has a past medical history of coronary artery disease, diabetes mellitus, hypertension, and hyperlipidemia. Which muscle relaxant should be used in order to decrease the risk of myocardial ischemia perioperatively?*

A. *Cis-atracurium*

B. *Mivacurium*

C. *Pancuronium*

D. *Rocuronium*

E. *Succinylcholine*

Muscle relaxants with minimal or no effects on heart rate and blood pressure should be used in patients with high risk of myocardial ischemia. Rocuronium and vecuronium would be the most ideal choices for neuromuscular blockade in such conditions. The other neuromuscular blockers have a greater effect on the cardiovascular system, making them a less ideal choice.

Answer: D

Dorian RS (2005) Anesthesia of the surgical patient. In Brunicardi FC (ed.) *Schwartz's Principles of Surgery*, McGraw-Hill, New York, pp. 1851–73.

14. *A 55-year-old man with hepatic cirrhosis is undergoing an intra-abdominal operation. Which neuromuscular blocking agent should be avoided in this patient?*

A. Cis-atracurium

B. Mivacurium

C. Pancuronium

D. Rocuronium

E. Vecuronium

Mivacurium is the only non-depolarizing neuromuscular blocking agent that is metabolized by plasma cholinesterase, similar to succinylcholine. Patients with cirrhosis are more likely to have decreased levels of plasma cholinesterase, resulting in a hypersensitivity to mivacurium. Of the choices, mivacurium should be avoided in a patient with significant liver disease. Cis-atracurium is eliminated by Hofmann degradation and would not be affected by liver disease. Pancuronium is eliminated almost unchanged by the kidneys, and would be unaffected by liver disease. Both the liver and kidney metabolize rocuronium and vecuronium. While their elimination may be decreased in liver disease, this decrease would not be as significant as a drug exclusively reliant upon liver function.

Answer: B

Dorian RS (2005) Anesthesia of the surgical patient. In Brunicardi FC (ed.) *Schwartz's Principles of Surgery*, McGraw-Hill, New York, pp. 1851–73.

15. *Which of the following patients would be the best choice for using inhalation induction during the intubation sequence?*

A. A 9-year-old boy undergoing a laparoscopic appendectomy

B. A 45-year-old man undergoing an inguinal hernia repair

C. A 37-year-old woman undergoing a laparoscopic cholecystectomy

D. A 70-year-old man undergoing a colon resection

E. A 72-year-old woman undergoing a mastectomy

Patients who undergo an inhalation induction progress through three stages: 1. awake, 2. excitement, and 3. surgical level anesthesia. Adult patients are not good candidates for this type of induction for a number of reasons. First, the smell of the induction agent is unpleasant. Second, the excitement stage may last for several minutes. This could lead to hypertension, tachycardia, laryngospasm, vomiting, or aspiration. Children would be better candidates for this type of induction because they progress through the second stage quickly. The type of surgery (open versus. laparoscopic) would not be a rationale for the use of inhalational over intravenous induction.

Answer: A

Dorian RS (2005) Anesthesia of the surgical patient. In Brunicardi FC (ed.) *Schwartz's Principles of Surgery*, McGraw-Hill, New York, pp. 1851–73.

16. *Utilizing the Mallampati scale in a patient with a Class 3 airway, the practitioner would be able to visualize*

A. All the oral structures

B. The hard palate, soft palate, and uvula

C. The hard palate and soft palate

D. The hard palate

E. None of the above

Airway assessment should be conducted and is easily performed utilizing the Mallampati scale. Patients are placed in a comfortable sitting position and asked to open their mouth and protrude their tongue. The examiner then assesses the airway, noting the ability to visualize the faucial pillars, soft palate, and uvula. The patient with a Class 1 airway has all these structures visible. The pillars are masked by the tongue in a patient with a Class 2 airway. A patient with a Class 3 airway has only the hard and soft palate visualized in this position. A patient for whom only the hard palate is visible has a Class 4 airway. The Mallampati scale allows the examiner to recognize which patients may be at risk for difficult airway management, including difficult intubations. It has also been noted that obesity may contribute to airway difficulties. In addition to visualization of the airway, neck circumference and body mass index should also be assessed preoperatively and considered in the overall airway assessment.

Answer: C

Gonzalez H, Minville V, Delanoue K, *et al.* (2008) The importance of increased neck circumference to intubation difficulties in obese patients. *Anesthesia and Analgesia* **106** (4), 1132–6.

Mallampati SR, Gatt SP, Gugino LD, *et al.* (1985) A clinical sign to predict difficult tracheal intubation: a prospective study. *Canadian Anaesthetists Society Journal* **32** (4), 429–434.

17. *According to the American Society of Anesthesiologists Physical Status Classification, which of the following patients would be a good candidate for moderate sedation in most settings?*

A. *A declared brain-dead patient*

B. *Patient with mild-to-moderate systemic disease*

C. *Patient with severe systemic disease that is incapacitating and life-threatening*

D. *Patient with severe systemic disease with functional limitation that is not incapacitating*

E. *A moribund patient not expected to survive without surgical intervention*

The American Society of Anesthesiologists (ASA) has developed a physical status classification system to determine risk for complications among patients undergoing anesthesia (Table 11.1). This scale is frequently utilized in the moderate sedation setting and is easily performed on all patients in all settings. Patients in Class 1 and 2 are considered good candidates for moderate sedation procedures; those in Class 3 and Class 4 carry higher risks. Physicians providing sedation must recognize that Class 3 and 4 patients may benefit from sedation and should not be excluded based upon their ASA score. Additionally, sedation is frequently provided to intensive care unit (ICU) patients, most of whom are in Class 3 or 4, and these patients greatly benefit from the effects of the sedation.

Answer: B

American Society of Anesthesiologists Physical Status Classification

Class	Definition
P1	Normal healthy patient with no systemic disease
P2	A patient with mild-to-moderate systemic disease
P3	A patient with severe systemic disease with functional limitation that is nonincapacitating
P4	A patient with severe systemic disease that is incapacitating and life-threatening
P5	A moribund patient not expected to survive without surgical intervention
P6	A declared brain-dead patient whose organs are being removed for donor purposes

18. *End-tidal carbon dioxide monitoring allows early detection of*

A. *Hypoventilation*

B. *Airway obstruction*

C. *Malignant hyperthermia*

D. *Rising of* CO_2

E. *All of the above*

End-tidal carbon dioxide (CO_2) monitoring measures expired carbon dioxide and provides information on the patient's ventilation. This type of monitoring is most commonly utilized with deep sedation and general anesthesia but is becoming commonplace in monitoring patients undergoing moderate sedation. The advantage of this type of monitoring is that it allows early detection of developing hypoventilation and possible airway obstruction. Additionally, if the patient is developing the early stages of malignant hyperthermia, this can be recognized by rising CO_2 levels.

Two techniques are utilized for measuring expired carbon dioxide. The first utilizes a photodetector that calculates the CO_2 value as it passes through a transducer. The second method actually obtains a sample of expired air and diverts it to a machine (capnograph) that directly measures the carbon dioxide level. Both techniques are easily accomplished on intubated patients. Measurement of end-tidal CO_2 levels in nonintubated patients is also possible. Utilizing microstream technology, a nasal cannula-type device can be applied to the patient's nares to allow for end-tidal CO_2 measurements. These devices are comfortable for patients and provide the practitioner with additional information regarding the patient's ventilatory status.

Because pulse oximetry does not measure ventilation, its detection of oxygen desaturation occurs after a period of respiratory compromise. A randomized, controlled trial published in 2006 assessed the addition of microstream capnography to pulse oximetry in the monitoring of patients undergoing moderate sedation. The researchers found that capnography allowed early detection of arterial oxygen desaturation, before the development of oxygen desaturation, and resulted in improved patient outcomes. Other studies have supported the use of microstream capnography as a means to improve patient care during moderate sedation.

Answer: E

Lightdale JR, Goldmann DA, Feldman HA, *et al.* (2006) Microstream capnography improved patient monitoring during moderate sedation: a randomized, controlled trial. *Pediatrics* **117** (6), e1170–e1178.

McQuillen KK, Steele DW (2000) Capnography during sedation/analgesia in the pediatric emergency department. *Pediatric Emergency Care* **16** (6), 401–4.

Srinivasa V, Kodali BS (2004) Capnography in the spontaneously breathing patient. *Current Opinion in Anaesthesiology* **17** (6), 517–20.

19. *A patient who receives a score of 0 on the bispectral index is*

A. *An alert adult*

B. *An alert child*

C. *Moderately sedated*

D. *Displaying an isoelectric EEG pattern*

E. *Brain dead*

The bispectral index (BIS) has been developed as a method of objectively determining sedation status via electroencephalogram (EEG) recordings. Based on the index, sedation level can be determined mathematically based on the patient's EEG pattern. An alert adult would receive a score of 100, while a score of 0 is characterized by an isoelectric EEG pattern. The BIS score is a relatively new tool in addition to nursing evaluation, and research has indicated that it is a valid measure of depth of sedation. However, some studies have found its use to be questionable among some populations, such as pediatric patients. As BIS is used as a determinant of level of consciousness/sedation, it cannot be used as a measure of brain death.

Answer: D

Arbour R (2004) Using bispectral index monitoring to detect potential breakthrough awareness and limit duration of neuromuscular blockade. *American Journal of Critical Care* **13**, 66–73.

Brown McDermott N, VanSickle T, *et al.* (2003) Validation of bispectral index monitor during conscious and deep sedation. *Anesthesia and Analgesia* **97**, 39–43.

DeWitt JM (2008) Bispectral index monitoring for nurse-administered propofol sedation during upper endoscopic ultrasound: a prospective, randomized controlled trial. 2008; Epub ahead of print, www.springerlink.com /content/6713u8746l555073/ (accessed May 19, 2008).

Gill M, Green SM, Krauss B (2003) A study of the bispectral index monitor during procedural sedation and analgesia in the emergency department. *Annals of Emergency Medicine* **41**, 234–41.

Mason KP, Michna E, Zurakowski D, *et al.* (2006) Value of bispectral index monitor in differentiating between moderate and deep Ramsay Sedation Scores in children. *Paediatric Anaesthesiology* **16** (12), 1226–31.

Olson DM, Gambrell M (2005) Balancing sedation with bispectral index monitoring. *Nursing* **35** (5), 32.

20. *The development of hypovolemia and hemorrhage during moderate sedation requires*

A. *Vasodilating drugs*

B. *Vasopressors*

C. *Aggressive volume and blood replacement*

D. *Diligent monitoring to ensure that sedation is maintained*

E. *All of the above*

Hemodynamic instability is the most common cardiovascular complication occurring during moderate sedation. The direct cardiodepressant effect of many of the sedating drugs causes hypotension in the patient. The patient with a pre-existing compromised circulatory volume is at greatest risk for this complication. Hypovolemia and hemorrhage require aggressive volume and blood replacement to prevent dangerously low circulating pressures. In acute cases, vasoactive drugs may be required to supplement hemodynamic status. Recognition of the patient at risk for hypotension will allow the practitioner to supplement the patient's volume status prior to sedation, thereby circumventing this problem.

Other causes of hypotension include pain and the histamine release that occurs with a number of depressant agents. It is imperative that the cause of the hypotension be identified so that proper therapy can be instituted to reverse the cause and correct the problem.

Answer: C

Watson D. (1998) *Conscious Sedation/Analgesia,* CV Mosby Co., St. Louis, MO.

Chapter 12 Delirium, Alcohol Withdrawal, and Psychiatric Disorders

Meghan Edwards, MD and Ali Salim, MD, FACS

1. *Which of the following statements regarding delirium in the ICU is true?*

A. *Delirium is an independent predictor of higher six-month mortality*

B. *Delirium is a benign condition which occurs almost exclusively in elderly patients at night*

C. *Delirium is most often associated with multiple medical co morbidities and is therefore uncommon in postoperative patients*

D. *The diagnosis of delirium requires a formal psychiatric consultation*

E. *Delirium is synonymous with dementia*

A 2004 prospective cohort study of 275 mechanically ventilated critically ill patients identified delirium as an independent predictor of higher six-month mortality. Increased mortality associated with ICU delirium has been reported in many studies since that time. The mean age of patients experiencing delirium in Ely's study was 56 years, with a standard deviation of 17 years, demonstrating that delirium does not occur exclusively in elderly patients. Other publications have also described delirium in critically ill pediatric populations.

Though delirium may often occur in patients with multiple medical co morbidities, it is certainly common in postoperative patients. A 2009 prospective study of 134 postoperative patients demonstrated a delirium rate of 63%, and delirium was an independent predictor of longer ICU and hospital stays.

The diagnosis of delirium does not require a formal psychiatric consultation. There are screening tools available that have been shown to effectively and consistently identify delirium when implemented by nursing staff. Any clinician familiar with the DSM-IV criteria can make the diagnosis of delirium (please see question 5 below).

Delirium and dementia are not synonymous. Delirium is an acute change in condition; while dementia is a disease insidious in onset, which is diagnosed by history or serial mental status examination. According to the DSM-IV, dementia cannot be diagnosed during an episode of delirium.

Answer: A

Ely EW, Margolin R, Francis J, *et al.* (2001) Evaluation of delirium in critically ill patients: validation of the Confusion Assessment Method for the Intensive Care Unit (CAM-ICU). *Critical Care Medicine* **29** (7), 1370–9.

Ely EW, Shintani A, Truman B, *et al.* (2004) Delirium as a predictor of mortality in mechanically ventilated patients in the intensive care unit. *Journal of the American Medical Association*. **291** (14), 1753–62.

Lat I, McMillian W, Taylor S, *et al.* (2009) The impact of delirium on clinical outcomes in mechanically ventilated surgical and trauma patients. *Critical Care Medicine* **37** (6), 1898–905.

Smith HA, Boyd J, Fuchs DC, *et al.* (2011) Diagnosing delirium in critically ill children: Validity and reliability of the Pediatric Confusion Assessment Method for the Intensive Care Unit. *Critical Care Medicine* **39** (1), 150–7.

2. *A 68-year-old man, postoperative day 6 status post femoral-popliteal bypass surgery, is being monitored in the ICU after recent extubation. He has been afebrile and has not required pain medication in the past 24 hours. His heart rate is 115 beats/minute, blood pressure is 168/88 mm Hg, and oxygen saturations are 98% on 2L nasal cannula. The nursing staff attempts to move him to bed from his chair for the evening, but he becomes combative: waving his arms wildly and kicking the staff.*

Surgical Critical Care and Emergency Surgery: Clinical Questions and Answers, First Edition. Edited by Forrest O. Moore, Peter M. Rhee, Samuel A. Tisherman and Gerard J. Fulda.

He begins shouting, "Help! Someone is trying to kill me!" Which of the following medications should be used to treat delirium in this scenario?

A. *Lorazepam*

B. *Haloperidol*

C. *Diphenhydramine*

D. *Morphine*

E. *Midazolam*

Haloperidol is a traditional antipsychotic. Its mechanism of action is blocking dopamine receptors in the CNS. Side-effects of administration of haloperidol include extrapyramidal reactions, neuroleptic malignant syndrome, and QT interval prolongation/torsades de pointes. Currently, it is the recommended medical therapy for delirium.

Risperidone, olanzapine, and ziprasidone are newer antipsychotics. These are also approved for treatment of delirium and also cause QT interval prolongation. The MIND trial is a randomized, placebo-controlled trial that is currently underway to demonstrate the efficacy of antipsychotics for the treatment of ICU delirium.

Benzodiazepines, such as lorazepam and midazolam, are not recommended for acute treatment of delirium, because they can paradoxically exacerbate the episode. The amnestic properties of benzodiazepines can also confuse the scenario.

Diphenhydramine is an antihistamine. It is FDA approved as an antiparkinsonian agent as well as to treat allergies or motion sickness. Some of the adverse reactions associated with diphenhydramine include confusion, restlessness, and sedation. It is not a recommended treatment for delirium.

If a patient has pain, it is reasonable to consider treating with an analgesic, such as Morphine first. However, this patient has had adequate pain control without pain medications for the past 24 hours, so pain is less likely to be the cause of his delirium.

Answer: B

Fink MP, Abraham E, Jean-Louis V, Kochanek P (2005) *Textbook of Critical Care*, 4th edn, Elsevier, Philadelphia, PA.

Girard TD, Pandharipande PP, Carson SS, *et al.* (2010) Feasibility, efficacy, and safety of antipsychotics for intensive care unit delirium: the MIND randomized, placebo-controlled trial. *Critical Care Medicine* **38** (2), 428–37.

3. *All of the following are factors known to contribute to the development of delirium in the ICU except:*

A. *Sleep deprivation*

B. *Medications*

C. *Sepsis*

D. *Head CT scans*

E. *Advanced age*

Delirium can be caused by a variety of factors in hospitalized patients, particularly those in the ICU. Sleep deprivation, medications, and sepsis have all been well documented as contributors. Retrospective studies have also demonstrated increased delirium associated with advanced age. Head CT scans are frequently used to evaluate an acute change in mental status, but have not been shown to contribute to delirium. Two mnemonics which can be useful for remembering causes/contributors to delirium include:

Infection

Withdrawal
Acute metabolic
Trauma/pain
Central nervous system pathology
Hypoxia

Deficiencies (Vitamin B12, thiamine)
Endocrinopathies (thyroid, adrenal)
Acute vascular (hypertension, shock)
Toxins/drugs
Heavy metals

Or

Drugs
Electrolyte and physiologic abnormalities
Lack of drugs (withdrawal)
Infection
Reduced sensory input (blindness, deafness)
Intracranial problems (CVA, meningitis, seizure)

Urinary retention and fecal impaction
Myocardial problems (MI, arrhythmia, CHF)

Answer: D

Fink MP, Abraham E, Jean-Louis V, Kochanek P (2005) *Textbook of Critical Care*, 4th edn, Elsevier, Philadelphia, PA.

Mangnall LT, Gallagher R, Stein-Parbury J (2011) Post-operative delirium after colorectal surgery in older patients. *American Journal of Critical Care* **20** (1), 45–55.

4. *Which of the following assessment tools has been validated as an accurate tool for the measurement of delirium in the ICU?*

A. RASS scale

B. Riker scale

C. CAM-ICU scale

D. Glasgow coma scale

E. All of the above

In 2001, Ely and colleagues designed and tested a modified version of the Confusion Assessment Method for use in intensive care unit patients and named it the CAM-ICU. It includes an assessment of the timing and course of altered mentation, presence of inattention, and presence of disorganized thinking (consistent with the DSM-IV criteria). The CAM-ICU demonstrated both reliability and validity when used by nurses and physicians to identify delirium in the intensive care unit. Multiple studies have repeatedly demonstrated its usefulness as a measurement tool since that time. A major advantage of the CAM-ICU over previous assessment scales is that it can be used to assess delirium in patients who are mechanically ventilated, despite the barrier to communication.

The Ramsay, Riker (SAS), Motor Activity Assessment (MAAS), and Richmond Agitation Sedation (RASS) are tools that can be used to rate the level of a patient's sedation and/or agitation; however, they cannot measure delirium. Tables 1–4 depict these sedation scales.

The Glasgow Coma Scale is a neurologic scale used to rapidly assess a patient's state of consciousness. It is a 15-point score calculated by assessment of a patients' eye opening, verbal response, and movement. It does not measure delirium.

Answer: C

Devlin JW, Boleski G, Mlynarek M, *et al.* (1999) Motor Activity Assessment Scale: a valid and reliable sedation scale for use with mechanically ventilated patients in a adult surgical intensive care unit. *Critical Care Medicine* **27**, 1271–5.

Ely EW, Margolin R, Francis J, *et al.* (2001) Evaluation of delirium in critically ill patients: validation of the Confusion Assessment Method for the Intensive Care Unit (CAM-ICU). *Critical Care Medicine* **29** (7), 1370–9.

Fraser GL, Riker R (2001) Monitoring sedation, agitation, analgesia, and delirium in critically ill adult patients. *Critical Care Clinics* **17**, 1–21.

Mirski MA, LeDroux SN, Lewin JJ 3rd, *et al.* (2010) Validity and reliability of an intuitive conscious sedation scoring tool: the nursing instrument for the communication of sedation. *Critical Care Medicine* **38** (8), 1674–84.

Ramsay M, Savege T, Simpson BRJ, *et al.* (1974) Controlled sedation with alphaxalone/alphadolone. *British Medical Journal* **2**, 656–9.

Sessler CN, Gosnell MS, Grap MJ, *et al.* (2002) The Richmond Agitation-Sedation Scale: validity and reliability in adult intensive care unit patients. *American Journal of Respiratory and Critical Care Medicine* **166**, 1338–44.

Table 12.1 Ramsay Scale

Score	Response
1	Awake and anxious, agitated, or restless
2	Awake, cooperative, accepting ventilation, oriented, tranquil
3	Awake; responds only to commands
4	Asleep; brisk response to light glabellar tap or loud noise
5	Asleep; sluggish response to light glabellar tap or loud noise stimulus but does not respond to painful stimulus
6	Asleep; no response to light glabellar tap or loud noise

Source: Data from Ramsay M, Savege T, Simpson BRJ, *et al.* (1974) Controlled sedation with alphaxalone/alphadolone. *British Medical Journal* 1974; 2, 656–9.

Table 12.2 The Riker Sedation–Agitation Scale

Score	Response
7	Dangerous agitation. Pulls at endotracheal tube, tries to remove catheters, climbs over bed rail, strikes at staff, thrashes side-to-side
6	Very agitated. Does not calm, despite frequent verbal reminders; requires verbal reminding of limits, physical restraints; bites endotracheal tube
5	Agitated. Anxious or mildly agitated, attempts to sit up, calms down to verbal instructions
4	Calm and cooperative. Calm, awakens easily, follows commands
3	Sedated. Difficult to arouse, awakens to verbal stimuli or gentle shaking but drifts off again, follows simple commands
2	Very sedated. Arouses to physical stimuli but does not communicate or follow commands, may move spontaneously
1	Unarousable. Minimal or no response to noxious stimuli, does not communicate or follow commands

Source: Data from Fraser GL, Riker R (2001) Monitoring sedation, agitation, analgesia, and delirium in critically ill adult patients. *Critical Care Clinics* **17**, 1–21.

Table 12.3 MAAS (Motor Activity Assessment Scale)

Score	Response
0	Unresponsive. Does not move with noxious stimuli
1	Responsive only to noxious stimuli. Opens eyes or raises eyebrows or turns head toward stimulus or moves limbs with noxious stimuli
2	Responsive to touch or name. Opens eyes or raises eyebrows or turns head toward stimulus or moves limbs when touched or name is loudly spoken
3	Calm and cooperative. No external stimulus is required to elicit movement and patient adjusts sheets or clothes purposefully and follows commands
4	Restless and cooperative. No external stimulus is required to elicit movement and patient picks at sheets or tubes or uncovers self and follows commands
5	Agitated. No external stimulus is required to elicit movement and attempts to sit up or moves limbs out of bed and does not consistently follow commands (for example, lies down when asked but soon reverts back to attempts to sit up or move limbs out of bed)
6	Dangerously agitated, uncooperative. No external stimulus is required to elicit movement and patient pulls at tubes or catheters or thrashes side to side or strikes at staff or tries to climb out of bed and does not calm down when asked

Source: Data from Devlin JW, Boleski G, Mlynarek M, *et al.* (1999) Motor Activity Assessment Scale: a valid and reliable sedation scale for use with mechanically ventilated patients in a adult surgical intensive care unit. *Critical Care Medicine* **27**, 1271–5.

Table 12.4 Richmond Agitation Sedation Score (RASS)

Score	Response
+4	Combative. Overtly combative or violent, immediate danger to staff
+3	Very agitated. Pulls on or removes tubes or catheters or has aggressive behavior toward staff
+2	Agitated. Frequent nonpurposeful movement or patient ventilator dyssynchrony
+1	Restless. Anxious or apprehensive but movements not aggressive or vigorous
0	Alert and calm
−1	Drowsy. Not fully alert, but has sustained (more than 10 seconds) awakening, with eye contact/eye opening to voice
−2	Light sedation. Briefly (less than 10 seconds) awakens with eye contact to voice
−3	Moderate sedation. Any movement (but no eye contact) to voice
−4	Deep sedation. No response to voice, but any movement to physical stimulation
−5	Unarousable. No response to voice or physical stimulation

Source: Data from Sessler CN, Gosnell MS, Grap MJ, *et al.* (2002) The Richmond Agitation–Sedation Scale: validity and reliability in adult intensive care unit patients. *American Journal of Respiratory Critical Care Medicine* **166**, 1338–44

5. *According to DSM-IV, the diagnosis of delirium involves which of the following elements?*

A. *Fluctuating course*

B. *Inattention*

C. *Acute change in cognition*

D. *Caused by the direct physiological consequences of a general medical condition*

E. *All of the above*

Delirium is an acute, fluctuating change in mental status, with inattention and altered level of consciousness.

The DSM-IV criteria for diagnosis of delirium are as follows:

Disturbance of consciousness (i.e. reduced clarity of awareness of the environment) with reduced ability to focus, sustain, or shift attention (inattention).

Change in cognition (e.g. memory deficit, disorientation, language disturbance and perceptual disturbance) that is not better accounted for by a pre-existing, established, or evolving dementia.

Development over a short period of time (usually hours to days) and disturbance tends to fluctuate during the course of the day.

There is evidence from the history, physical examination, or laboratory findings that the disturbance is caused by the direct physiological consequences of a general medical condition.

Answer: E

American Psychiatric Association (2000) *Diagnostic and Statistical Manual of Mental Disorders*, 4th edn, American Psychiatric Association, Washington DC.

Fink MP, Abraham E, Jean-Louis V, Kochanek P (2005) *Textbook of Critical Care*, 4th edn, Elsevier, Philadelphia, PA.

6. *In a randomized, multicenter trial of dexmedetomidine versus midazolam by the SEDCOM study group, dexmedetomidine was shown to have which potential advantage as a sedative agent?*

A. *Associated with lower incidence of delirium*

B. *Not associated with cardiovascular adverse effects*

C. *Associated with shorter time to extubation*

D. *Both A and C*

E. *Associated with a statistically significant decrease in ICU length of stay*

Dexmedetomidine is a selective alpha-2 adrenergic agonist used for short-term sedation in the ICU. It exerts sedative effects via postsynaptic activation of alpha-2 receptors in the central nervous system, and analgesic action by inhibiting norepinephrine release presynaptically. It also inhibits sympathetic activity, including decreasing blood pressure and heart rate. Its advantages include easy dose titration due to rapid distribution and short half-life, as well as lack of respiratory depressive effect. It is used in the ICU as an adjunct or alternative to benzodiazepines, such as midazolam.

The SEDCOM study group published the results of their two-year, 68-center trial in *JAMA* in 2009. Results demonstrated no difference in percentage of time within the target RASS range for patients treated with dexmedetomidine versus those treated with midazolam (their primary endpoint). However, there were differences in secondary outcomes. The prevalence of delirium during treatment was 54% in dexmedetomidine-treated patients versus 76.6% in patients treated with midazolam ($P < 0.001$). Median time to extubation was 1.9 days shorter in dexmedetomidine-treated patients ($P = 0.01$). There was a trend toward decreased ICU length of stay in dexmedetomidine-treated patients (5.9 days compared to 7.6 days); however this was not statistically significant. Dexmedetomidine-treated patients were more likely to develop bradycardia, but had a lower likelihood of tachycardia or hypertension requiring treatment ($P = 0.02$). Answer B is false, because bradycardia was the most notable adverse effect associated with dexmedetomidine.

Answer: D

Fink MP, Abraham E, Jean-Louis V, Kochanek P (2005) *Textbook of Critical Care*, 4th edn, Elsevier: Philadelphia, PA.

Riker RR, Shehabi Y, Bokesch PM *et al.* (2009) Dexmedetomidine versus midazolam for sedation of critically ill patients: a randomized trial. *Journal of the American Medical Association* **301** (5), 489–99.

7. *A 67-year-old woman, postoperative day three status-post Hartmann's colostomy for perforated diverticulitis, is reported to be disoriented on morning rounds. Which of the following medications that she was given is least likely to contribute to her development of delirium?*

A. *Morphine*

B. *Lorazepam*

C. *Diphenhydramine*

D. *Albuterol*

E. *Nortriptyline*

Medications are the most common reversible cause of delirium. Elderly patients are at particularly increased risk for drug-induced delirium due to altered pharmacokinetics and pharmacodynamics. Contributing factors are the increase in total body fat, decrease in lean body mass and water, decrease in albumin, and decrease in glomerular filtration rate associated with aging.

Medical co-morbidities can increase the risk for medication-induced delirium. This is often due to decreased metabolism or decreased elimination resulting from organ dysfunction. Creatinine clearance should be measured regularly, and medication dosages should be renally adjusted as indicated.

Patients taking multiple medications are also at increased risk for interactions between medications, which consequently increases the risk for delirium.

Narcotics (morphine), benzodiazepines (lorazepam), antidepressants (Nortriptyline) and antihistamines (diphenhydramine) are all well documented contributors to delirium in hospitalized patients. Many other classes of medications have been frequently implicated in the development of delirium, including gastrointestinal agents, antiemetics, antibiotics, and cardiac medications. Several herbal and alternative medications can contribute as well. Some pulmonary medications, such as steroids and theophylline, have been associated with the development of delirium. However, there is currently no evidence to suggest albuterol-induced delirium.

Answer: D

Alagiakrishnan K, Wiens CA (2004) An approach to drug induced delirium in the elderly. *Postgraduate Medical Journal* **80** (945), 388–93.

Fink MP, Abraham E, Jean-Louis V, Kochanek P (2005) *Textbook of Critical Care*, 4th edn, Elsevier: Philadelphia, PA.

8. *A 52-year-old man is admitted to the ICU after diagnostic laparotomy with modified Graham patch for a perforated duodenal ulcer. Mechanical ventilation is continued postoperatively due to his hemodynamic instability requiring vasopressor support, as well as his persistent metabolic acidosis. The ICU nurse suggests you write for sedation per the unit protocol. Which of the following is true regarding sedation protocols?*

A. *Sedation protocols have been associated with increased ICU mortality due to over sedation of patients*

B. *Implementation of sedation protocols has been shown to prevent the development of ICU delirium*

C. *Sedation protocols have been associated with increased medication costs in the ICU*

D. *Sedation protocols have been associated with fewer ventilator days*

E. *Sedation protocols require monitoring patients with a bispectral index (BIS) monitor*

The optimal level of sedation for a mechanically ventilated patient varies with medical condition and treatment needs. Oversedation and undersedation have clinical and economic consequences. In 2010, a systematic review was published to examine the impact of sedation protocols for optimizing level of sedation in mechanically ventilated patients. Implementation of sedation guidelines and protocols, which includes daily interruption of sedation (sedation holidays), was uniformly associated with improvement in outcomes. Examples of measured improvements include ICU and hospital length of stay, duration of mechanical ventilation, and hospital costs. At least 15 studies reported a reduction in average duration of mechanical ventilation associated with the introduction of a sedation protocol. Mortality rates reported were decreased or statistically insignificant when analyzed after implementation of sedation protocols.

The incidence of nosocomial infections was also reduced in some studies. At least seven studies reported the impact of sedation protocols on the costs of sedative agents used. Results demonstrated a reduction in costs with protocolized sedation. Though sedation protocols may in theory help decrease delirium rates, they have not been demonstrated to be completely preventative. Few studies have specifically evaluated the impact of sedation protocols on the incidence of delirium; however, a few randomized controlled trials reported no statistically significant difference in incidence of delirium from protocolized sedation.

Sedation protocols can involve titration to clinical parameters, such as vital signs and clinical exam (see sedation scales, Tables 12.1 to 12.4). An alternative is to titrate to BIS value. The BIS monitor obtains EEG information from a sensor on the forehead, and quantifies the patient's level of consciousness with a number 0–100 (0 indicates no brain activity, while 100 indicates fully awake). BIS values have been shown to correlate with the above referenced commonly used sedation scales.

Answer: D

Feliciano DV, Mattox KL, Moore EE (2008) *Trauma*, 6th edn. McGraw Hill, New York.

Jackson DL, Proudfoot CW, Cann KF, Walsh T (2010) A systematic review of the impact of sedation practice in the ICU on resource use, costs and patient safety. *Critical Care*. **14** (2), R59. Epub 2010 Apr 9.

9. *The incidence of post-traumatic stress disorder (PTSD) in patients after discharge from the ICU has been reported to be approximately:*

A. 1–2%

B. <10%

C. 30%

D. 80%

E. Almost 100%

In the largest follow-up study to date in terms of the number of ICU survivors, Myhren *et al.* found a high prevalence (27%) of patients above case level for posttraumatic stress one year after ICU treatment. In this prospective cohort study, posttraumatic stress was evaluated by patient questionnaires weeks after discharge from the ICU. In addition to the high prevalence of patients found to have posttraumatic stress, half of the patients had PTSD-related symptoms that were judged "may be of clinical significance," even though they did not meet full criteria for the disorder. Post-traumatic stress disorder risk during the first year following ICU discharge did not differ between medical, surgical and trauma patients.

Post-traumatic stress disorder occurs after an individual experiences or witnesses a traumatic event involving actual or threatened death or serious injury. The event itself elicits a reaction of intense fear, helplessness, and horror, and subsequently symptoms of intrusion, avoidance, and arousal. Classic ongoing symptoms include dissociation, re-experiencing, and avoidance. The diagnosis is generally not considered until symptoms have been present for at least four weeks, and it is a chronic condition that is difficult to treat.

According to DSM-IV, the gold standard for diagnosis is the structured clinical interview to predefined criteria. This makes it a difficult diagnosis, and an even more difficult subject for large-scale studies. Clinical interviews are not always feasible but many studies like Myhren's have found high numbers of ICU patients to have symptoms consistent with PTSD using questionnaires. Pain, lack of control, and inability to express needs while in the ICU are factors suspected to contribute to the high incidence of PTSD after an ICU admission.

Answer: C

American Psychiatric Association (2000) *Diagnostic and Statistical Manual of Mental Disorders*, 4th edn, American Psychiatric Association, Washington DC.

Feliciano DV, Mattox KL, Moore EE (2008) *Trauma*, 6th edn. McGraw Hill, New York.

Griffiths J, Fortune G, Barber V, Young JD (2007) The prevalence of post traumatic stress disorder in survivors of ICU treatment: a systematic review. *Intensive Care Medical* **33**, 1506–18.

Myhren H, Ekeberg O, Tøien K, *et al.* (2010) Posttraumatic stress, anxiety and depression symptoms in patients during the first year post intensive care unit discharge. *Critical Care*. **14** (1), R14. Epub 2010 Feb 8.

10. *A 46-year-old man is admitted to the ICU with acute alcoholic pancreatitis. He has a history of drinking 12 to 14 cans of beer/day. Which of the following is false regarding an IV ethanol protocol compared to IV diazepam protocol for alcohol withdrawal?*

A. *Both have been advocated and used successfully for acute alcohol withdrawal in the ICU*

B. *Acute hepatic failure is more likely to be precipitated by diazepam than ethanol*

C. *Ethanol has a short duration of action and narrow margin of safety, which can make titration more difficult*

D. *A 2008 randomized controlled trial demonstrated a better agitation control profile with diazepam compared to ethanol*

E. *None of the above*

Heavy alcohol consumption prior to surgery is a known risk factor contributing to morbidity and mortality, and is also known to worsen ICU outcomes. Symptoms of withdrawal from alcohol may become evident within 24 hours of cessation. Benzodiazepines have been the recommended first-line therapy for prevention and management of alcohol withdrawal, although intravenous ethanol has been advocated and reported as a successful alternative in several case series. Ethanol has a short duration of action, a narrow margin of safety, and is associated with gastric irritation (even when administered intravenously). In addition, ethanol has the potential to precipitate acute hepatic failure and lowers the seizure threshold. Convulsions may occur in alcohol dependent patients despite having alcohol in their bloodstream. IV ethanol is also toxic to the tissues in the event of extravasation.

In 2008, the *Journal of Trauma* published a randomized controlled trial of 52 trauma patients admitted to the ICU with a history of daily alcohol intake greater than or equal to five drinks per day. In the study, patients were treated prophylactically for four days with either IV ethanol or IV diazepam. The results demonstrated that a scheduled-dose diazepam regimen had a superior sedation/agitation profile compared with intravenous ethanol.

Answer B

Feliciano DV, Mattox KL, Moore EE (2008) *Trauma*, 6th edn, McGraw Hill, New York.

Weinberg JA, Magnotti LJ, Fischer PE, *et al.* (2008) Comparison of intravenous ethanol versus diazepam for alcohol withdrawal prophylaxis in the trauma ICU: results of a randomized trial. *Journal of Trauma* **64** (1), 99–104.

11. *On the above patient's fourth day of hospitalization, his abdominal pain and nausea have resolved and his vital signs are all within normal limits. He is being transferred to the ward, and the intern inquires whether his lorazepam should be scheduled or given on an as needed basis. Which of the following is true of a symptom-driven lorazepam protocol for alcohol withdrawal?*

A. *May be as effective as fixed-dose therapy while reducing the amount of medication administered*

B. *Requires frequent assessments by a clinician with a validated monitoring scale*

C. *Can be instituted effectively without specific training*

D. *Decreases the incidence of withdrawal associated seizures*

E. *A and B*

The important aspects of alcohol withdrawal management include:

- ABCs;
- adequate IV access;
- CU monitoring if withdrawal symptoms are more than mild, seizures occur, the possibility of respiratory/airway compromise exists, or if there is hypotension, dysrhythmias, electrolyte disorders, advanced age, or co morbid conditions;
- exclude other conditions;
- correct electrolyte abnormalities (hypokalemia, hypomagnesemia, hypophosphatemia).

It has been demonstrated that symptom-triggered therapy may be as effective as fixed-dose therapy for alcohol withdrawal syndrome prophylaxis while reducing the amount of medication administered. A 2007 study compared patients on a fixed continuous benzodiazepine infusion with those on a symptom driven protocol. Patients in the symptom-triggered protocol group received intermittent doses of IV benzodiazepine, and were ultimately escalated to continuous on the protocol if needed. The symptom-triggered protocol resulted in a shorter time to control symptoms, lower cumulative benzodiazepine dose, shorter time receiving benzodiazepine continuous infusion, shorter ICU length of stay, and shorter hospital stay (though the last two outcomes did not reach statistical significance). With symptom-triggered therapy, some patients may require no medication at all.

Symptom-triggered therapy requires frequent assessments with a monitoring instrument such as the Clinical Institute Withdrawal Assessment-Alcohol (CIWA-A), and treatment is titrated to maintain symptoms in the mild range. Such assessment requires training and experience, and such resources are not always readily available. Symptom-triggered therapy has not been demonstrated to reduce the incidence of withdrawal associated seizures.

Answer: E

DeCarolis DD, Rice KL, Ho L, *et al.* (2007) Symptom-driven lorazepam protocol for treatment of severe alcohol withdrawal delirium in the intensive care unit. *Pharmacotherapy* **27** (4), 510–18.

Feliciano DV, Mattox KL, Moore EE (2008) *Trauma*, 6th edn, McGraw Hill, New York.

12. *Which of the following is FALSE regarding ICU patients with alcohol dependence compared to those without?*

A. *Patients with alcohol dependence have higher rates of sepsis*

B. *Patients with alcohol dependence have higher hospital mortality*

C. *Patients with alcohol dependence have higher rates of organ failure*

D. *Patients with alcohol dependence spend less time in the hospital*

E. *Patients with alcohol dependence who have sepsis or liver failure have more than twice the risk for hospital mortality*

A 2007 study published in *Critical Care Medicine* demonstrated that ICU patients with alcohol dependence had higher rates of sepsis (12.9% versus 7.6%, $p < 0.001$), organ failure (67.3% versus 45.8%, $p < 0.001$), septic shock (3.6% versus 2.1%, $p = 0.001$), and hospital mortality (9.4% versus 7.5%, $p = 0.022$), with fewer hospital-free days. Also, among patients with sepsis and liver failure, alcohol dependence increased the likelihood for hospital mortality by more than twofold. Patients with alcohol dependence may have a predilection to infection due to abnormalities in their immune systems (many such abnormalities have been demonstrated in animal models). In addition, patients with chronic excessive use of alcohol have complicating medical conditions resulting from the substance abuse, such as cardiomyopathy, dysrhythmias, and cirrhosis. Alcoholic patients are also at increased risk due to the possibility for alcohol withdrawal and the associated pathophysiologic process (such as tachycardia, hypertension, seizures, etc.).

Answer: D

Feliciano DV, Mattox KL, Moore EE (2008) *Trauma*, 6th edn, McGraw Hill, New York.

O'Brien JM Jr, Lu B, Ali NA, *et al.* (2007) Alcohol dependence is independently associated with sepsis, septic shock, and hospital mortality among adult intensive care unit patients. *Critical Care Medicine* **35** (2), 345–50.

13. *The incidence of depression in ICU survivors*

A. *Is as high as 30% in the year after ICU care*

B. *Is significantly greater in males*

C. *Increases with patient age*

D. *Has no impact on patient quality of life*

E. *All of the above*

In 2009, *Intensive Care Medicine* published a systematic review of ICU survivors conducted using

Medline, EMBASE, Cochrane Library, CINAHL, PsycINFO, and a hand-search of 13 journals. Fourteen studies were eligible for the study. Results demonstrated that the prevalence of substantial depressive symptoms is quite high in the year after ICU care (clinician-diagnosed depressive disorder was prevalent in 33%). Sex, age, and severity of illness at ICU admission were not consistent risk factors. Post-ICU depressive symptoms appeared to have substantial associations with both physical and mental health aspects of quality of life.

Answer: A

Davydow DS, Gifford JM, *et al.* (2009) Depression in general intensive care unit survivors: a systematic review. *Intensive Care Medicine* **35** (5), 796–809.

14. *A nurse calls you requesting an "as needed" lorazepam order for her patient, who was shouting at the medical assistant and removed his own foley catheter. Which of the following is true of this patient?*

A. *He is displaying signs of hyperactive delirium, which has a worse prognosis than hypoactive delirium*

B. *He is displaying signs of hyperactive delirium, which has a better prognosis than hypoactive delirium*

C. *He is displaying signs of hypoactive delirium, which has a worse prognosis than hyperactive delirium*

D. *He is displaying signs of hypoactive delirium, which has a better prognosis than hyperactive delirium*

E. *He is displaying signs of hyperactive delirium. Hyperactive and hypoactive delirium have a similar prognosis*

Signs of hyperactive delirium include agitation and combativeness. Patients may be extremely agitated, yell, call out for help, wander the hallways, or enter other patient's rooms. Patients with hyperactive delirium are at risk for self-extubation, harm to self by removal of catheters, and patient-ventilator asynchrony. Hypoactive delirium, conversely, is marked by calm, inattentiveness. Patients will often appear sluggish and lethargic, to the point of stupor. Like hyperactive delirium, the onset is sudden, and there is the distinguishing feature of fluctuating level of consciousness. The patient may sometimes be perceived to be depressed. Hypoactive is the less recognized form of delirium, and accordingly has a higher mortality rate.

Answer: B

Fink MP, Abraham E, Jean-Louis V, Kochanek P (2005) *Textbook of Critical Care*, 4th edn, Elsevier, Philadelphia, PA.

Guenther U, Popp J, Koecher L, *et al.* (2010) Validity and reliability of the CAM-ICU Flowsheet to diagnose delirium in surgical ICU patients. *Journal of Critical Care.* **25** (1), 144–51.

Chapter 13 Acid-Base, Fluid and Electrolytes

Charles Kung Chao Hu, MD, MBA, FACS, FCCP, Andre Nguyen, MD, and Nicholas Thiessen, MD

1. *Following the infusion of isotonic fluids in a normal, healthy subject, what mediators best regulate sodium level in the extracellular space?*

A. *Hypothalamic receptors*

B. *Antidiuretic hormone*

C. *Renin-angiotensin-aldosterone system*

D. *Thirst*

As the fluid is isotonic, plasma sodium concentration does not change. It is confined to the extracellular space. The extracellular system primarily regulates urinary sodium excretion. It is true that the amount of sodium in the extracellular space can vary depending on dietary sodium intake, but in homeostasis, the sodium concentration in the extracellular space remains constant due to physiological controls that regulate water intake and excretion. More sodium in the extracellular space means extracellular fluid expansion. Less sodium in the extracellular space results in contraction. Sodium balance is affected by numerous receptors. The renin-angiotensin-aldosterone system is the best known mediator of sodium regulation. In addition, atrial natriuetic peptide, baroreceptors, and the sympathetic nervous system are all important components of sodium regulation. The body has redundancy in sodium regulation.

Answer: C

Kraft MD, Btaiche IF, Sacks GS, Kudsk KA (2005) Treatment of electrolyte disorders in adult patients in the intensive care unit. *American Journal of Health-System Pharmacy* **62** (16), 1663–82.

Surgical Critical Care and Emergency Surgery: Clinical Questions and Answers, First Edition. Edited by Forrest O. Moore, Peter M. Rhee, Samuel A. Tisherman and Gerard J. Fulda.

Lindeman RD, Papper S (1975) Therapy of fluid and electrolyte disorders. *Annals of Internal Medicine* **82** (1), 64–70.

Weiner M, Epstein FH (1970) Signs and symptoms of electrolyte disorders. *Yale Journal of Biological Medicine* **43** (2), 76–109.

2. *Following infusion of electrolyte-free water in a normal, healthy subject, which of the following mediators best regulate plasma sodium concentration?*

A. *Arginine vasopressin*

B. *Hypothalamic receptors*

C. *Renin-angiogensen-aldosterone system*

D. *Thirst*

Electrolyte-free water is distributed throughout all fluid compartments, extracellular and intracellular space. Since one-third of body water is extracellular, electrolyte-free water only has one-third effect on extracellular space that isotonic saline has. Water balance and cell volume are regulate by arginine vasopressin secreted by the neurohypophysis. It activates V2 receptor in the renal collecting duct, which in turn activates aquaporins. Vasopressin is extremely low when plasma sodium concentration is below 135 meq/L. Above 135 meq/L, vasopressin level increases linearly in relationship to plasma sodium concentration. Intake of water, vasopressin secretion, and renal electrolyte-free water excretion respond to changes of plasma sodium concentration.

Answer: A

Kraft MD, Btaiche IF, Sacks GS, Kudsk KA (2005) Treatment of electrolyte disorders in adult patients in the intensive care unit. *American Journal of Health-System Pharmacy* **62** (16), 1663–82.

Lindeman RD, Papper S (1975) Therapy of fluid and electrolyte disorders. *Annals of Internal Medicine* **82** (1), 64–70.

Weiner M, Epstein FH (1970) Signs and symptoms of electrolyte disorders. *Yale Journal of Biological Medicine* **43** (2), 76–109.

3. *Your patient is post-operative day 1 from a pancreaticoduodenectomy for a tumor in the head of the pancreas. His serum sodium is 133 meq/L. Currently the patient is receiving an intravenous infusion of normal saline at 150 ml/hr. The urine output has been about 55 ml/hr. The patient appears warm, with mild edema in the lower extremities. What would you do next?*

A. *Increase normal saline rate to 175 ml/hr*

B. *Change IV fluids to D5 $^1/_2$ NS at 100 mL/hr*

C. *Change IV fluids to lactated Ringers at 150 mL/hr*

D. *Maintain current IV fluid and decrease rate to 100 mL/hr*

E. *Maintain current IV fluid and rate*

Hypotonic hyponatremia results from either massive water intake, exceeding the capacity to excrete free water, or impaired water excretion. There are multiple causes of acute hyponatremia such as the syndrome of inappropriate antidiuretic hormone release, psychogenic self-induced water intoxication, excessive sweating, or use of cyclophosphamide, ecstasy (MDMA), or oxytocin. Nonhypotonic causes of hyponatremia include IgG therapy, irrigant absorption in prostatectomy or intrauterine surgery, hyperglycemia, hyperlipidemia. In the above scenario, postoperative hyponatremia is caused by vasopressin secretion in response to surgical stress. Vasopressin could be secreted for two or more days postoperatively. Free water is retained. Sodium and potassium are excreted in the urine at high concentrations. As a result, isotonic fluids are "desalinated" and can lower the plasma sodium concentration. The treatment in this case is to avoid hypotonic fluid and excessive volume of isotonic fluids (NS, LR) after surgery. If symptoms of hyponatremia occurs, hypertonic saline and diuretics can be used.

Answer: D

Gowrishankar M, Lin SH, Mallie JP, *et al.* (1998) Acute hyponatremia in the perioperative period: insights into its pathophysiology and recommendations for management. *Clinical Nephrology* **50**, 352, 1998.

Steele A, Gowrishankar M, Abrahamson S, *et al.* (1997) Postoperative hyponatremia despite near-isotonic saline infusion: a phenomenon of desalination. *Annals of Internal Medicine* **126**, 20.

4. *A 58-year-old man is now post-operative day 4 after a colon resection for cancer. On examination, he has mild edema in his lower extremities. His chest x-ray shows mild congestive heart failure. He is receiving normal saline at 125 ml/hr and his serum sodium level is 132 meq/L. His urine output is 40–50 ml/hr. The patient states he takes diuretics at home on occasion when he develops edema in his legs. How would you treat his serum sodium?*

A. *Increase IV fluids to 150 ml/hr*

B. *Decrease IV fluids to 75 ml/hr*

C. *Treat with thiazide diuretics*

D. *Change his IV fluids to hypertonic saline*

E. *Treat with loop diuretics and ACE inhibitors*

One liter of normal saline will increase plasma sodium concentration by 1 mEq/L. Thus treating hyponatremia in edematous patients with saline will only exacerbate the problem. Thiazide diuretics are contraindicated since they block reabsorption of sodium and chloride in the distal tubules and prevent the generation of maximally dilute urine. Loop diuretics are the mainstay of treatment in this case. They improve free water excretion. With the addition of ACE inhibitors, it is effective in congestive heart failure and also reduces vasopressin secretion.

Answer: E

Adrogue HJ, Madias NE (2000) Hyponatremia. *New England Journal of Medicine* **342**, 1581.

Sonnenblick M, Friedlander Y, Rosin AJ (1993) Diuretic-induced severe hyponatremia: review and analysis of 129 reported patients. *Chest* **103**, 601.

Sterns RH, Silver SM, Spital A (2000) *Hyponatremia. The Kidney: Physiology and Pathophysiology*. Lippincott Williams &Wilkins, Philadelphia, PA.

5. *What is the free water deficit in a patient with a serum sodium of 140 meq/L?*

A. 0 liter

B. 1 liter

C. 2 liters

D. 3 liters

E. 4 liters

$$\text{Water deficit} = \text{normal body water} * (1 - (\text{Serum Na}/140))$$

The calculated water deficit is the amount of water that will return sodium concentration to normal. Common causes of hypernatremia are: insensible losses, neurogenic/nephrogenic diabetic insipidus, lithium, demeclocycline, gastric fluid losses, ingestion of excessive salt.

Answer: A

Androgue HJ, Madias NE (2000) Hypernatremia. *New England Journal of Medicine* **342**,1493.

Kraft MD, Btaiche IF, Sacks GS, Kudsk KA (2005) Treatment of electrolyte disorders in adult patients in the intensive care unit. *American Journal of Health-System Pharmacy* **62** (16), 1663–82.

6. *A 47-year-old man presents with lower extremity numbness and tingling sensation that has been going on for about 2 weeks. Recently, he states that he has developed some weakness in his muscles. His past medical history is unremarkable except for kidney stones. His metabolic panel reveals a potassium level of 6.8 mEq/dl, BUN 35 mg/dL, and Cr 1.5 mg/dL. Other values are within normal limits. A 12-lead EKG reveals elevated T waves, and slight widening of QRS complexes. You diagnosed him with hyperkalemia from Type 1 renal tubular acidosis (RTA). What is your next plan of action?*

A. Calcium chloride, glucose infusion with insulin, cation exchange resins

B. Glucose infusion with insulin then cation exchange resins

C. Glucose infusion with insulin, sodium bicarbonate, then lasix

D. Thiazide diuretics, glucose infusion with insulin, then cation exchange resin

E. Calcium chloride then dialysis

Multiple disorders are associated with impairment of renal potassium elimination. Most common etiologies are renal failure (impaired distal nephron excretion), severe dehydration, metabolic acidosis (loss of bicarbonate, diarrhea), rhabdomyolysis, RTA (Type 4, Hyperkalemic type 1), increased dietary intake, or medication induced (succinylcholine, Beta$_2$-adrenergic blockade, insulin deficiency).

Aggressive treatment to lower serum potassium and to stabilize the cell membrane should be started for high levels of potassium especially when EKG changes are present. Infusion of calcium raises the threshold excitability potential. Bicarbonate, glucose with insulin, and beta$_2$-adrenergic receptor stimulation lowers serum potassium by promoting potassium movement intracellularly. These measures are temporary, however. For severe or refractory cases, dialysis is warranted.

Answer: A

Allon M (1995) Hyperkalemia in end-stage renal disease: mechanisms and management. *Journal of the American Society of Nephrology* **6**, 1134.

Perazella MA (2000) Drug-induced hyperkalemia: old culprits and new offenders. *American Journal of Medicine* **109**, 307.

7. *Approximately how much potassium replacement is needed if serum level is at 2.0 mEq/L?*

A. 250 mEq

B. 500 mEq

C. 750 mEq

D. 1000 mEq

Hypokalemia can be caused by a multitude of etiologies. The most common include low dietary intake, movement across cell membranes (metabolic alkalosis, beta-$_2$-adrenergic stimulation, insulin administration, increased cell proliferation), body losses (use of diuretics, diarrhea, vomiting, profuse sweating, burns, RTA Type 1). Clinical manifestations are muscle weakness, cramps, EKG changes such as T wave depression and appearance of U waves.

Treatment involves normalization of the potassium levels in the plasma. For each 1 mEq/L fall in plasma potassium, the amount of storage falls by 200–400 mEq. At potassium level of 2.0 mEq/L, the total deficit can be greater than 1000 mEq.

Answer: D

Gennari FJ (1998) Hypokalemia. *New England Journal of Medicine* **339**, 451.

Kraft MD, Btaiche IF, Sacks GS, Kudsk KA (2005) Treatment of electrolyte disorders in adult patients in the intensive care unit. *American Journal of Health-System Pharmacy* **62** (16), 1663–82.

8. *A trauma patient is on the ventilator for four days and has failed to wean. Tube feedings had been started on the second hospital day and rapidly increased to her goal. Physical exam reveals a thin 19-year-old woman, weighing 48 kg and 177 cm height. Lungs have coarse breath sounds. She has 2+ pitting edema and hyperreflexia. Which of the following should be done next?*

A. *Give furosemide*

B. *Discontinue maintenance IV fluids*

C. *Give thiamine*

D. *Discontinue tube feeds*

E. *Stat CT of the head*

The patient has a BMI of 15.3 kg/m^2 and chilblains (tender red or purple bumps that occur as a reaction to cold), which suggest that the patient suffers from anorexia nervosa. Feeding the patient a carbohydrate diet of tube feeds has caused a refeeding syndrome (RFS). The body shifts back to carbohydrate metabolism from protein and fat catabolism, and glucose becomes the primary source of energy once again. The increased glucose causes an increase in the release of insulin, which shifts the following intracellular; glucose, potassium, magnesium, and phosphate. This shift causes hypokalemia, hypomagnesemia, and hypophosphatemia. The hypophosphatemia can have a profound effect on adenosine triphosphate and 2-3-diphosphoglycerate levels. Insulin exhibits a natriuretic effect on the kidneys. Sodium is retained in this instance. This can cause fluid retention and expansion of the extracellular fluid volume, leading to fluid overload, pulmonary edema, and congestive heart failure. The hypomagnesemia is characterized by hyperreflexia in this patient. The first step in managing RFS is to stop the influx of carbohydrates/tube feeds.

Answer: D

Attia E, Walsh BT (2009) Behavioral management for anorexia nervosa. *New England Journal of Medicine* **360** (5), 500–6.

Fuentebella J, Kerner JA (2009) Refeeding syndrome. *Pediatric Clinics of North America* **56** (5), 1201–10.

White KP, Rothe MJ, Milanese A, Grant-Kels JM (1994) Perniosis in association with anorexia nervosa. *Pediatric Dermatology* **11** (1), 1–5.

9. *A 70-year-old man was involved in an auto versus pedestrian accident three days ago. He suffered a traumatic brain injury and has been complaining of headaches and hallucinations. Laboratory data: Na 120 mEq/L, K 4.0 mEq/L, Cl 96 mEq/L, bicarbonate 25 mEq/L, BUN 30 mg/dl, Cr 1.8 mg/dl, glucose 160 mg/dl. Urine osmolality 475 mOsm/kg, urine sodium 196 mEq/L. CVP 4 mm Hg. Physical exam: cervical collar in place, spinal precautions, arousable but disoriented, lungs clear bilaterally with respiratory rate of 8 breaths/minute, heart rate 50 beats/minute. What would be the appropriate next step in his management?*

A. *Initiation of intravenous normal saline at 150 mL/hr*

B. *Demeclocycline 600 mg × 1 now and twice daily*

C. *Conivaptan 40 mg IV × 1 now and daily for 3 days*

D. *150 mL/hour of 3% saline infusion × 2 hours*

E. *Fluid restriction and furosemide 20 mg IV × 1 now*

The patient is exhibiting symptoms of acute hyponatremia. The laboratory and clinical findings suggest a possible cerebral salt wasting syndrome (CSW), with hypovolemia and high urinary sodium. From a metabolic stand point, 3% saline infusion is administered for hyponatremia to increase serum sodium by 2 mEq/L/hr but not more than 12 mEq/L in the first 24 hours to avoid central pontine myelinolysis. Central pontine and extrapontine myelinolysis, begins with lethargy and affective changes (generally after initial improvement of neurologic symptoms with treatment), followed by mutism or dysarthria, spastic quadriparesis, and pseudobulbar palsy. Once 3% saline infusion has begun, the symptoms should improve.

Answer: D

Ellison DH, Berl T (2007) The syndrome of inappropriate antidiuresis. *New England Journal of Medicine* **356** (20), 2064–72.

Rivkees SA (2008) Differentiating appropriate antidiuretic hormone secretion, inappropriate antidiuretic hormone secretion and cerebral salt wasting: the common, uncommon, and misnamed. *Current Opinion in Pediatrics* **20** (4), 448–52.

Sterns RH, Silver SM (2008) Cerebral salt wasting versus SIADH: what difference? *Journal of the American Society of Nephrology* **19** (2), 194–6.

10. *A 60-year-old woman underwent an upper endoscopy for GI bleeding, which was readily controlled. The patient was given benzocaine prior to the procedure to anesthetize the posterior oropharynx. Post procedure, the patient's oxygen saturation is 75% on 2 L nasal cannula. Blood gas reveals pH 7.40. $PaCO_2$ 40 mm Hg. PaO_2 115 mm Hg. HCO_3 24 mEq/l. Base excess 0.6 mmol/L. Her Hgb is 8 g/dl. Electrolytes are normal. Her temperature is 37.0 °C. Vital signs are heart rate 120 beats/minute. RR 22 breaths/minute. BP 100/80 mm Hg. The patient is dizzy and confused. What is the most appropriate next step in management?*

A. *Place the patient on facemask 10 L/min O_2*

B. *Give flumazenil 0.2 mg IV q1min × 1-5 doses prn*

C. *Obtain stat CT chest with pulmonary embolism protocol*

D. *Give naloxone 0.4 mg IV q2min prn*

E. *Give methylene blue, 1 mg/kg IV × 1*

The clinical scenario is methemoglobinemia, given the discrepancy in the PaO_2 and SaO_2, and the use of an oxidizing agent benzocaine. Methemoglobinemia is a condition caused by oxidation of iron within the hemoglobin molecule from the ferrous (Fe_2+) to the ferric (Fe_3+) state. This oxidation significantly diminishes the oxygen-carrying capacity of hemoglobin and can lead to central and peripheral cyanosis, metabolic acidosis due to inability of the cells to carry out aerobic metabolism, and eventually coma and death if left untreated. The enzyme, NADH-methemoglobin reductase maintains methemoglobin at very low levels. The leading cause of methemoglobinemia is drug toxicity caused by an oxidizing toxin. The agents most frequently associated with methemoglobinemia are aniline, benzocaine, dapsone, pyridium, nitrites, nitrates, and naphthalene. When these drugs are metabolized by the cytochrome P-450 system in the liver, oxygen radicals are produced which can lead to oxidation of the hemoglobin iron.

Answer: E

Kane GC, Hoehn SM, *et al.* (2007) Benzocaine-induced methemoglobinemia based on the Mayo Clinic experience from 28,478 transesophageal echocardiograms: incidence, outcomes, and predisposing factors. *Archives of Internal Medicine* **167** (18), 1977–82.

Moore TJ, Walsh CS, *et al.* (2004) Reported adverse event cases of methemoglobinemia associated with benzocaine products. *Archives of Internal Medicine* **164** (11), 1192–6.

11. *A 62-year-old woman was in a motor vehicle collision seven days ago. She is currently in the SICU and is oliguric and on vasopressor for septic shock. Her recent laboratory findings are: pH 7.32, $PaCO_2$ 28 mm Hg, PaO_2 120 mm Hg, HCO_3 10 mEq/l, Base Excess −7.5 mmol/L, SaO_2 100%, FiO_2 60%, Na 132 mmol/L, K 3.7 mmol/L, Cl 118 mmol/L, bicarbonate 10 mmol/L, BUN 45 mg/dl, Cr 4.8 mg/dl, albumin 1.3 g/dl, INR 2.5, total bilirubin 7.0 mg/dL. Which buffer should be added to the replacement fluid for continuous venovenous hemodiafiltration?*

A. *Acetate*

B. *Citrate*

C. *Lactate*

D. *Bicarbonate*

E. *Free water*

The patient has metabolic acidosis in the setting of acute renal failure. Hypoalbuminemia lowers the anion gap and masks the presence of acidifying anions. The patient also has liver failure. When oxidizing anions are used in the replacement fluids, the anion (acetate, lactate, and citrate) must be completely oxidized to carbon dioxide and water in order to generate bicarbonate. If the metabolic conversion of non-bicarbonate anions proceeds without accumulation, then their buffering capacity is equal to that of bicarbonate. However, when the metabolic conversion is impaired by liver dysfunction, the increased blood concentration of the anions leads to an increased anion with lactate or unmeasured anions with acetate and citrate, which can worsen the metabolic acidosis.

Answer: D

Brivet F, Kleinknecht D, Loirat P (1996) Acute renal failure in intensive care units—causes, outcome, and prognostic factors: a prospective, multicenter study. *Critical Care Medicine* **24**, 192–8.

Naka T, Bellomo R (2004) Bench-to-bedside review: treating acid-base abnormalities in the intensive care unit–the role of renal replacement therapy. *Critical Care* **8** (2), 108–14.

Palsson R, Laliberte KA, Niles JL (2006) Choice of replacement solution and anticoagulant in continuous venovenous hemofiltration. *Clinical Nephrology* **65** (1), 34–42.

12. (parts 1 and 2). *A 45-year-old woman who has had multiple previous abdominal operations was admitted with a small bowel obstruction presumably from adhesions. A nasogastric tube (NGT) was inserted. Over the past 4 days, NGT output has been greater than 5 L of bilious green output.*

Her vital signs are unremarkable except for a heart rate of 110 beats/minute. Her oral mucosa is dry. Her urine is dark amber brown.

Part 1. *Which of the following is most likely to be true?*

A. *Metabolic alkalosis; hypokalemia; aciduria*

B. *Metabolic alkalosis; hyperkalemia; alkaline urine ph*

C. *Metabolic acidosis; hypokalemia; aciduria*

D. *Metabolic acidosis; hyperkalemia; alkaline urine ph*

High volume NGT output from bowel obstruction will induce a metabolic alkalosis, hypokalemia, and a paradoxical aciduria.

Answer: A

Part 2. *What is the BEST intravenous fluid regimen to correct her acid-base derangement?*

A. *0.45% saline at 100 mL/hr*

B. *D5 0.45% saline at 100 mL/hr*

C. *0.9% saline and 30 mEq/L of KCl at 150 mL/hr*

D. *Lactated ringers at 150 mL/hr*

E. *0.45% saline with 20 mEq/L of KCl at 50 mL/hr*

Answer: C

The patient has a contraction metabolic alkalosis. High NG output, or excessive vomiting is a common cause of metabolic alkalosis. During volume contraction, bicarbonate is reabsorbed with sodium because there is insufficient chloride to maintain electrical neutrality. The distal convoluted tubules will exchange H+ and K+ for Na+, which produced inappropriate aciduria. Metabolic alkalosis associated with volume depletion will respond to volume, chloride, and potassium replacements. Common causes of metabolic alkalosis are vomiting (NG tube suctioning), mineralocorticoid excess (such as Cushing's, hyperaldosteronism, steroid administration), milk alkali syndrome, and hypokalemia. Clinical manifestations are rare but paresthesias, carpopedal spasms, ventricular irritability ($pH > 7.55$).

Answer D would be inadequate resuscitation. Answer A is not acceptable because the low rate, the hypotonicity and the absence of optimal potassium replacement are not good choices. Answer B is not acceptable because the low rate, the absence of optimal potassium replacement and hyperglycemic load on a poorly-controlled diabetic are not good choices. Answer C is a better choice of fluid.

Reilly RF, Perazella MA (2007) *Acid-base, Fluid Electrolytes.* McGraw-Hill, New York.

Sterns RH, Silver SM, Spital A (2000) *Hyponatremia. The Kidney: Physiology and Pathophysiology,* Lippincott Williams & Wilkins, Philadelphia, PA.

13. *A 55-year-old man was admitted with a ruptured cerebral aneurysm four days ago and he remains on mechanical ventilation. Past medical history is significant for hypertension and chronic kidney injury stage 3 (CKI-3). He is morbidly obese (132 kg; 5 feet-8 inch; BMI > 40). The aneurysm has been controlled via endovascular coiling. He has been receiving boluses of normal saline to maintain normal volume status and mild hypertension. He has been agitated intermittently.*

His spontaneous respiratory rate is 32 breaths/minute. An ABG reveals pH 7.28, pCO_2 25 mm Hg, PO_2 133 mm Hg, bicarbonate 18 mEq/L, base excess −9.2 mmol/L. His serum sodium is 155 mEq/L, potassium 3.8 mEq/L, chloride 128 mmol/L, HCO_3 17 mmol/L. BUN is 44 mg/dL, creatinine 2.5 mg/dL. Which of the following is the most likely acid-base disturbance?

A. *Metabolic acidosis with a base deficit of at least 300 mEq*

B. *Respiratory alkalosis and a nonanion gap metabolic acidosis*

C. *Metabolic acidosis with a hyperchloremic normal anion gap from a renal tubular acidosis*

D. *Metabolic acidosis with a hyperchloremic normal anion gap from mannitol diuresis and NS*

Patient has a primary metabolic acidosis and a primary respiratory alkalosis. Appropriate compensation can be estimated using Winters' formula [$pCO_2 = (1.5 \times HCO_3) + 8 \pm 2$]. His pCO_2 is too low for simple compensation for the metabolic acidosis.

He has a hyperchloremic nongap metabolic acidosis. The base deficit is (0.5) (weight)[(desired-observed HCO_3)]. Thus, (0.5)(132 kg)[(24 – 18)] = 396. Patient has a baseline chronic kidney injury stage 3 (CKI) given in his history. CKI is not renal tubular acidosis. Prolonged used of mannitol will increased water loss relative to serum sodium. Prolonged resuscitation with NS will induce a hyperchloremic normal anion gap metabolic acidosis.

Metabolic acidosis occurs due to increased in H+ production, decrease in H+ excretion, or loss of bicarbonate. Anion gap is the difference between measured cations (Na+) and anions (HCO_3- + Cl–). The difference represents the amount unmeasured anions typically proteins, phosphates, other salts. Normal anion gap is 3 to 11 mM/l. Besides excessive saline infusion, GI losses, diarrhea, fistulas, and renal tubular acidosis are also causes of metabolic acidosis.

Answer: B

DuBose TD, Finkel KW (2002) *Acid-Base and Electrolyte Disorders*, WB. Saunders & Co., Philadelphia, PA, Chapter 4.

Rose BD, Post TW (2001) *Clinical Physiology of Acid-Base and Electrolyte Disorders*. McGraw-Hill, New York, Chapter 17.

14. (parts 1 and 2). *A 54-year-old man was a pedestrian struck by a car at an estimated speed of 40 mph. His injuries included bilateral rib fractures, pelvic fractures, splenic and liver injuries. He underwent splenectomy, hepatorrhaphy and damage control laparotomy, plus on-table pelvic angiographic embolization. Upon arrived in the SICU, his ABG revealed: pH 7.21, pCO_2 38 mm Hg, pO_2 66 mm Hg, HCO_3 17 mEq/L.*

Part 1. *Which of the following best describes his acid base status?*

A. *Primary metabolic acidosis with compensatory respiratory alkalosis*

B. *Primary metabolic acidosis with superimposed respiratory acidosis*

C. *Primary respiratory acidosis with compensated metabolic alkalosis*

D. *Primary respiratory acidosis with superimposed metabolic acidosis*

Answer: B

The diagnosis of primary metabolic acidosis is present with a low pH and low plasma [HCO_3-]. Anion gap can be determined to help find an etiology. The respiratory compensation can be estimated by the Winters' formula:

$$\text{Expected } pCO_2 = (1.5 \times HCO_3-) + 8 \pm 2$$

The respiratory compensation is inadequate or a superimposed respiratory acidosis is present if the measured pCO_2 is higher than the expected value. The respiratory compensation is excessive or a superimposed respiratory alkalosis is present when pCO_2 is lower than expected value. In this scenario, the expected pCO_2 is calculated to be 33.5 ± 2 mm Hg. The measured pCO_2 is 38 mm Hg, making the respiratory compensation inadequate: superimposed respiratory acidosis.

Winters SD, Pearson R, Gabow PA, *et al.* (1990) The fall of the serum anion gap. *Archives of Internal Medicine* **150**, 311.

The patient developed worsening hypoxic respiratory failure over the next 48 hours, requiring high-frequency oscillation ventilation and inhaled nitric oxide. He also developed acute kidney injury. His labs include: Na-153 mEq/L; K-5.0 mEq/L; Cl-116 mEq/L; HCO_3-18 mEq/L; BUN-100 mEq/L; Cr-4.5 mEq/L; glucose 119 mg/dL; albumin-1.1 g/dL. The ABG revealed: pH 7.08, pCO_2 72 mm Hg, pO_2 85 mm Hg, HCO_3 21 mEq/L, BE-8 mmol/L

Part 2. *Which of the following best describes his current acid-base status?*

A. *Primary metabolic acidosis with compensatory respiratory alkalosis*

B. *Primary metabolic acidosis with superimposed respiratory acidosis*

C. *Primary respiratory acidosis with compensated metabolic alkalosis*

D. *Primary respiratory acidosis with superimposed metabolic acidosis*

Answer: D

The diagnosis of respiratory acidosis is low pH and elevated pCO_2. In general, an increase in 10 mm Hg pCO_2 is accompanied by 0.08 decrease in pH. Here the pH is less than is expected from this estimate. The patient also has a base deficit, suggesting a primary metabolic acidosis.

Reilly RF, Perazella MA (2007) *Acid-base, Fluid Electrolytes.* McGraw-Hill, New York.

Rose, BD, Post, TW (2001) *Clinical Physiology of Acid-Base and Electrolyte Disorders.* McGraw-Hill, New York, Chapter 17.

15. *After damage-control laparotomy for a gunshot wound to the abdomen, a patient developed a small bowel high-output enterocutaneous fistula. Which acid-base disturbance would be expected?*

A. *Metabolic acidosis. Hyperchloremia. Wide anion gap.*

B. *Metabolic acidosis. Hyperchloremia. Normal anion gap.*

C. *Metabolic acidosis. Hypochloremia. Normal anion gap.*

D. *Metabolic alkalosis. Hyperkalemia.*

E. *Metabolic alkalosis. Hypokalemia.*

High output from the gastrointestinal tract causes loss of bicarbonate. Non-anion gap metabolic acidosis can be expected from such a course. The treatment in this setting would be to replace fluids and electrolytes.

Answer: B

DuBose TD, Finkel KW (2002) *Acid-Base and Electrolyte Disorders,* WB. Saunders & Co., Philadelphia, PA, Chapter 4.

Rose BD, Post TW (2001) *Clinical Physiology of Acid-Base and Electrolyte Disorders.* McGraw-Hill, New York, Chapter 17.

16. *A 58-year-old, institutionalized woman has become vitamin D deficient and hypocalcemic. What is her expected physiological response?*

A. *Increased parathyroid hormone (PTH) release*

B. *Enhanced renal reabsorption of calcium and excretion of phosphate*

C. *Initial increase in calcitriol formation*

D. *Increased renal absorption of calcium and phosphate*

E. *A, B and C*

The physiologic effects of vitamin D and the regulation of calcium homeostasis involves the gastrointestinal tract, bone, and kidney. Hypocalcemia induces an increase in parathyroid hormone (PTH), controls the calcium absorption in those systems. The effects of PTH include osteoclastic bone resorption, increased reabsorption of calcium by the kidneys and increased excretion of phosphate. Initially, PTH can increase calcitriol levels, until substrate for its production are depleted. The majority of the calcium is stored in the bone (98%). Plasma calcium exists in ionic form (50%), protein bound (40%), and rest in complex forms (10%). Ionic calcium is the form that controls most cellular functions. True calcium concentration is based on the following formula:

$$[Ca_2+] = \text{measured}[Ca_2+] + 0.8 * (4 - [\text{albumin}])$$

Answer: E

Kapoor M, Chan GZ (2001) Fluid and electrolytes abnormalities. *Critical Care Clinics* **17** (3), 503–29.

Goldfarb S (2008) *Disorders of Calcium Balance: Hypercalcemia and Hypocalcemia*, McGraw Hill, New York, Chapter 6.

17. *A 55-year-old man comes into the emergency room with complaints of nausea, constipation, and fatigue. He has a history of kidney stones. His serum calcium level is 12 mg/dl. What is the most appropriate initial treatment for his current condition?*

A. Hydration with normal saline

B. Administration of bisphosphonates

C. Infusion of calcitonin

D. Dialysis

E. Administration of steroids

Hypercalcemia is defined as $[Ca_2+] > 10.4$ mg/dl. The most common cause is hyperparathyroidism. Other causes are malignancy, renal failure, or the use of thiazide diuretics. Symptoms of hypercalcemia are fatigue, depression, mental status changes, nausea and vomiting. Signs are typically nephrolithiasis and arrhythmias (short QT interval). Patients are frequently hypovolemic. Restoring normal volume status can help with renal excretion of calcium. Forcing a diuresis with a loop diuretic may be the next step. Using hydration for hypercalcemia, the onset is typically hours to maintain adequate urine output. For bisphosphonates and calcitonin, the effect takes a day or two. Dialysis can be effective but it is very rarely needed.

Answer: A

Kapoor M, Chan GZ (2001) Fluid and electrolytes abnormalities. *Critical Care Clinics* **17** (3), 503–29.

Reilly RF, Perazella MA (2007) *Acid-base, Fluid Electrolytes*, McGraw-Hill, New York.

18. *A 48-year-old woman has developed an enterocutaneous fistula after a bowel resection at another hospital for bowel obstruction. The fistula has been present for about 3 months and the output is around 400–500 ml/day. She is currently on parenteral nutrition but states that she has been noncompliant with it during the day since it restricts her activities. She is lethargic and a little bit confused. On examination, she develops carpopedal spasm with inflation of a sphygmomanometer and contraction of the ipsilateral facial muscles to tapping the facial nerve. What are the most likely electrolyte abnormalities?*

A. Hypomagnesemia and hypocalcemia

B. Hypermagnesemia and hypercalcemia

C. Hypercalcemia

D. Hypomagnesemia and hypercalcemia

Hypomagnesemia is due to insufficient intake or enhanced loss from GI tract. Increased renal excretion can be from diuretics. Other causes are endocrine (hypoparathyroid, hypothyroidism) or chronic alcoholism. Symptoms of hypomagnesemia are nausea, vomiting, lethargy, confusion. Signs can be Trousseau's and Chvostek's signs, tetany, convulsions, or torsades de pointes. Many findings are similar with hypocalcemia.

Answer: A

Reilly RF, Perazella MA (2007) *Acid-base, Fluid Electrolytes*, McGraw Hill, New York.

Riggs JE (2002) Neurological manifestations of electrolyte disturbances. *Neurological Clinics* **20**, 227–39.

Chapter 14 Metabolic Illness and Endocrinopathies

Therese M. Duane, MD, FACS and Andrew Young, MD

1. *A 67-year-old woman is admitted to the intensive care unit following a four-node parathyroidectomy with reimplantation for secondary hyperparathyroidism due to renal failure. She has a calcium level of 7.2 mg/dL 12 hours postoperatively. She is asymptomatic, but an ECG is obtained which shows a QT interval of 560 ms. Which of the following is the best treatment option for this patient?*

A. *Proceed urgently to the operating room for removal of the implanted parathyroid*

B. *Give 2 gm intravenous calcium gluconate*

C. *Electively re-explore the patient in the morning for a missed parathyroid gland*

D. *Double her calcitriol dose from 0.25 μg to 0.5 μg twice daily*

E. *Continue observation with no intervention at this time*

While several studies have tried to identify which factors predispose a patient to hypocalcemia after a parathyroidectomy, it is important to remember that all patients undergoing a parathroidectomy need frequent calcium level checks post operatively as there is a high incidence of hypocalcemia. Patients undergoing subtotal parathyroidectomy may only require oral calcium and vitamin D supplementation, while those patients undergoing total parathyroidectomy with/without reimplantation usually require more aggressive calcium replacement therapy intravenously. Patients with hypocalcemia are found to have peri-oral paresthesias, Trousseau sign, Chvostek's sign, hyper-reflexia and ECG changes including prolonged QT interval. Intravenous calcium should be initiated if a patient exhibits any of these signs or symptoms and if serum calcium levels are below the normal range.

Answer: B

Mittendorf EA, Merlino JI, McHenry CR (2004) Post-parathyroidectomy hypocalcemia: incidence, risk factors, and management. *The American Journal of Surgery* **70** (2), 114–19; discussion 119–20.

Torer N, Torun D, Torer N, *et al.* (2009) Predictors of early postoperative hypocalcemia in hemodialysis patients with secondary hyperparathyroidism. *Transplantation Proceedings* **41** (9), 3642–6.

2. *A 32-year-old man was admitted to the intensive care unit following a motor vehicle crash in which he suffered several small intracranial hemorrhages. A ventriculostomy catheter was placed to monitor his intracranial pressures. The patient has been receiving iso-osmotic intravenous fluids. On post trauma day 5, his plasma mOsm is now >320 mOsm. His urine mOsm is 130 mOsm. What is the best course of action?*

A. *Increase the amount of free water administration via his nasogastric feeding tube*

B. *Change his parenteral fluids to normal saline*

C. *Check placement of the venticulostomy tube to ensure the patient's intracranial pressures are not rising despite the improved readings*

D. *Begin low dose, twice daily dexamethasone*

This patient has diabetes insipidus (or a deficiency of antidiuretic hormone), which can be seen in traumatic brain injury patients. There are two types of diabetes insipidus—central (associated with traumatic brain injury) and nephrogenic. Exogenous ADH differentiates between the two. If the patient responds to the exogenous ADH then

Surgical Critical Care and Emergency Surgery: Clinical Questions and Answers, First Edition. Edited by Forrest O. Moore, Peter M. Rhee, Samuel A. Tisherman and Gerard J. Fulda.

the cause is central but if there is no response then the cause is nephrogenic. Diabetes insipidus is characterized by high plasma osmolarity with a paradoxical low urine osmolarity. Initial treatment consists of increasing free water to try and correct hyperosmolarity. Patients with more severe DI will require desmopressin (DDAVP) injection.

Answer: A

Agha A, Sherlock M, Phillips J, *et al.* (2005) The natural history of post-traumatic neurohypophysial dysfunction. *European Journal of Endocrinology* **152** (3), 371–7.

Kronenberg HM (2003) Diabetes Insipidus. In: Larsen PR (ed.) *Williams Textbook of Endocrinology*, 11th edn, Philadelphia, PA: WB Saunders, Philadelphia, PA. 2003.

3. *A 52-year-old man is developing sepsis in the ICU following a trans-thoracic esophagectomy. He requires early goal-directed therapy, including fluid resuscitation and high-dose vasopressor support. In addition to the fluid and vasopressor therapy, the Surviving Sepsis Campaign recommends which of the following?*

A. *Empirically adding double coverage of anaerobes*

B. *High dose steroids (>300 mg hydrocortisone per day)*

C. *Waiting until speciation of cultures before beginning antibiotics so as not to increase the likelihood of resistance*

D. *Low-dose steroids (200–300 mg hydrocortisone per day)*

The Surviving Sepsis Campaign recommends that low-dose steroids be given (200–300 mg per day) for seven days for patients who are in septic shock requiring vasopressor support and who have had adequate intravenous fluid. Additional studies have stated that there may be no difference in morbidity and mortality among those patients who did receive low dose steroids and those that did not. The study for which the Surviving Sepsis Campaign was based used patients who had a systolic blood pressure of less than 90 for at least an hour as an inclusion criteria, while later studies broadened this to any patient in sepsis. It is important to keep this distinction in mind and patients should be chosen carefully.

Answer: D

Dellinger RP, Carlet JM, Masur H, *et al.* (2004) Surviving Sepsis Campaign guidelines for management of severe sepsis and septic shock. *Intensive Care Medicine* **30** (4), 536–55.

Sprung CL, Annane D, Keh D, *et al.* (2008) CORTICUS Study Group. Hydrocortisone therapy for patients with septic shock. *New England Journal of Medicine* **358** (2), 111–24.

4. *A 19-year-old man has been in the intensive care unit for the last two days following an all-terrain vehicle crash in which he sustained multiple orthopedic injuries and a T2 spinal cord injury. In the last 24 hours his blood glucose has started to increase, and the last two readings were 190 mg/dL and 210 mg/dL respectively. You decide to begin a sliding scale insulin regimen. What is the best target blood glucose range for this patient?*

A. *70–90 mg/dL*

B. *81–110 mg/dL*

C. *<150 mg/dL*

D. *<180 mg/dL*

This is a trauma patient with a spinal cord injury and several orthopedic injuries who will require tight blood glucose control with intravenously administered insulin. While this patient may not have been diabetic prior to his injuries, there will be changes in metabolism throughout the body that will contribute to higher blood sugar levels. Trauma patients were found to be in a subgroup of critically ill patients that benefited from tight glucose control with a range of 81 to 108 mg/dL. It is important to note that in the same study that overall mortality *increased* when looking at the entire study group with this target range, while the group with a goal of less than 180 mg/dL had lower mortality. Therefore, this does not apply to nontrauma patients.

Answer: B

NICE-SUGAR Study Investigators, Finfer S, Chittock DR, Su SY, *et al.* (2009) Intensive versus conventional glucose control in critically ill patients. *New England Journal of Medicine* **360** (13), 1283–97.

Ziegler TR (2001) Fuel metabolism and nutrient delivery in critical illness. In: Becker K (ed.) *Principles and Practice of Endocrinology and Metabolism,* 3rd edn, Lippincott Williams & Wilkins, Philadelphia PA, pp. 2102–8.

5. *A 32-year-old woman is admitted to the ICU following a right laparoscopic adrenalectomy for an adrenal adenoma. The tumor was an active glucocorticoid secreting tumor. She will require postoperative steroids. What constellation of signs and/or symptoms would suggest that the patient is having acute adrenal dysfunction?*

A. *Hypertension, emesis, hypokalemia, paresthesias*

B. *Hypertension, nausea without emesis, hyperkalemia, hypocalcemia*

C. *Hypotension, emesis, hyperkalemia, hypercalcemia, hypoglycemia, confusion*

D. *Hypotension, low fibrin split products, bleeding from the incision and venipuncture sites*

An Addisonian crisis, or hypocortisolism, consists of hypotension, vomiting and diarrhea, hyperkalemia, hypercalcemia, hypoglycemia, fever, syncope, lethargy and possible abdominal pain. This can be due to the removal of a glucocorticoid producing adrenal adenoma. The over-production of glucocorticoids by the adenoma causes Cushing's Syndrome with the subsequent atrophy of the contralateral adrenal gland. Patients should be placed on replacement therapy prior to adrenalectomy and continue with therapy afterwards to prevent hypocortisolism.

Answer: C

Brunt L.M, Moley J (2004) The pituitary and adrenal glands. In: Townsend CM (ed.) *Sabiston Textbook of Surgery,* 17th edn, Elsevier, Philadelphia, PA, 1042–4.

6. *A 52-year-old man has been admitted to the ICU following emergent operation for a strangulated inguinal hernia. He is hypertensive despite adequate pain control. He has a history of hypertension and took lisinopril at home. What is the mechanism of lisinopril?*

A. *Breaks down bradykinin*

B. *Prevents conversion of angiotensinogen to angiotensin I*

C. *Prevents conversion of angiotensin I to angiotensin II*

D. *Blocks renin synthesis in the juxtaglomerular complex*

The renin angiotensin aldosterone system begins with renin production in the juxtaglomerular complex when decreased blood pressure is sensed. Renin cleaves angiotensinogen to angiotensin I. Angiotensin I is then cleaved by angiotensin converting enzyme (ACE) to create angiotensin II. Angiotensin converting enzyme also breaks down bradykinin into its inactive form. Angiotensin II has multiple effects across a range of tissues, but most importantly for the critically ill patient. Angiotensin II supports the circulatory system by causing release of aldosterone, stimulating thirst, increasing sympathetic tone, and causing release of antidiuretic hormone. Aldosterone is a mineralocorticoid secreted by the adrenal glands which causes increased sodium absorption and potassium secretion in the kidney.

Lisinopril inhibits ACE, which prevents the body's natural mechanism for volume retention. This is an important point especially in this particular case since the patient has just had a significant operation and his volume status is labile. While it is important to restart home medications in patients admitted to the hospital, the clinical situation should be considered. For this particular patient, a shorter acting anti-hypertensive medication from a different class should be chosen.

Answer: C

Corry DB, Tuck ML (2001) Renin-angiotensin system and aldosterone. In: Becker K (ed.) *Principles and Practice of Endocrinology and Metabolism,* 3rd edn, Lippincott Williams & Wilkins, Philadelphia, PA, pp. 764–72.

Haas CE, LeBlanc JM (2004) Acute postoperative hypertension: a review of therapeutic options. *American Journal of Health-System Pharmacy* **61** (16), 1661–73; quiz 1674–5.

7. *A 47-year-old woman underwent left adrenalectomy for a pheochromocytoma. In the ICU, she has been requiring low dose vasopressor support to maintain an adequate blood pressure. The proper order of medications* *that she should have received preoperatively for control of her hypertension is:*

A. *Metoprolol, phenoxybenzamine*

B. *Prazosin, phenoxybenzamine*

C. *Prazosin, metoprolol*

D. *Metoprolol, potassium chloride*

Pheochromocytomas produce excess catecholamines causing hypertension, headaches, sweats and sometimes a feeling of impending doom. It is also useful to remember the *rule of tens*: 10% are bilateral, 10% occur in children, 10% are extra-adrenal, and 10% are familial. Patients must be treated preoperatively to prevent hypertensive crisis due to tumor manipulation as well as circulatory collapse perioperatively. Preoperative treatment includes alpha blockade (with phenoxybenzamine or prazosin) followed by beta blockade. In addition patients must be given adequate volume in order to tolerate the sudden cessation of high amounts of circulating catecholamines once the tumor has been removed. Patients may require vasopressor or inotropic support postoperatively.

Answer: C

Allen CTB, Imrie D (1977) Hypoglycaemia as a complication of removal of a phaeochromocytoma. *Canadian Medical Association Journal* **116**, 363.

Williams DT, Dann S, Wheeler MH (2003) Phaeochromocytoma—views on current management. *European Journal of Surgery and Oncology* **29** (6), 483–90.

8. *A 35-year-old woman underwent an uncomplicated celiotomy for a tubo-ovarian abscess. Three hours after the operation she began to have chest pain, confusion, and hypertension that has been difficult to control. She had cardiac enzymes sent. Her ECG shows sinus tachycardia, and her chest x-ray appears normal. She has a past medical history of Graves' disease for which she takes methimazole although she had not been able to tolerate anything by mouth prior to her presentation. The most appropriate medication to give first is:*

A. *Methimazole 25 mg PO*

B. *Potassium iodide 5 drops PO*

C. *Aspirin 325 mg PO*

D. *Hydrocortisone 100 mg IV*

This patient is experiencing thyroid storm given her history of Graves' disease and operative stress. While three of the above answers may be correct, it is important to give them in the proper order as follows: stop new thyroid gland synthesis with antithyroid medication (methimazole or propylthiouracil), then treatment with iodine therapy to stop thyroid hormone release (potassium iodide or Lugol's solution), followed by treatment of adrenergic symptoms (hydrocortisone and/or beta-blockers). Giving iodine therapy prior to antithyroid therapy may exacerbate a thyroid storm. Furthermore, there should be a delay of 30 to 60 minutes prior to giving iodine therapy. She had been taking methimazole for her Graves' disease, but she may have missed doses secondary to her disease process or perhaps her maintenance dose is not enough given this new stress. The safe course of action is to give the methimazole first, then wait 30 to 60 minutes to give the potassium iodide.

Patients with Graves' disease can be treated with either propylthiouracil or methimazole, although the FDA recently issued a warning against propylthiouracil as it may cause hepatotoxicity. The cardiovascular affects of thyrotoxicosis can be severe and are treated with a beta blocker. Propanolol is preferred as it also blocks T4 to T3 conversion at higher doses. Thyroid storm, while rare, can occur in patients with clinical or subclinical hyperthyroid disease who experience a precipitating event (for example, infection, trauma, etc.). Mortality from thyroid storm ranges from 20 to 30%.

Answer: A

Klein I, Ojamaa K (2001) Thyroid hormone and the cardiovascular system. *New England Journal of Medicine* **344** (7), 501–9.

Nayak B, Burman K (2006) Thyrotoxicosis and thyroid storm. *Endocrinology Metabolism Clinics of North America* **35** (4), 663–86.

9. *A 28-year-old man suffered a severe traumatic brain injury from a motorcycle crash. There is concern for diffuse axonal injury. His current Glasgow Coma Scale is 6. He requires vasopressors to maintain an adequate* *cerebral perfusion pressure. A morning cortisol level is drawn and is 10 μg/dL. This patient most likely has:*

A. *Sheehan's syndrome*

B. *A normal ACTH*

C. *A normal cortisol level*

D. *Secondary adrenal insufficiency*

This patient has adrenal insufficiency secondary to traumatic brain injury. He is most likely suffering from hypopituitarism which, according to some studies, may be underdiagnosed in the TBI population. It is important to note the low level of cortisol in this patient and stress dose glucocorticoids should be considered given this patient's vasopressor requirement.

Answer: D

Blair JC (2010) Prevalence, natural history and consequences of posttraumatic hypopituitarism: a case for endocrine surveillance. *British Journal of Neurosurgery* **24** (1), 10–17.

Cohan P, Wang C, McArthur DL, *et al.* (2005) Acute secondary adrenal insufficiency after traumatic brain injury: a prospective study. *Critical Care Medicine* **33** (10), 2358–66.

10. *A 19-year-old man has been in the intensive care unit for the last 14 days following an assault in which he sustained a right occipital skull fracture and associated subarachnoid hemorrhage. Over the past 5 days he has become progressively more hyponatremic despite free water restriction. Today his serum sodium level is 118 mmol/L, his plasma osmolarity is 241 mOsm/kg, his urine osmolarity is 500 mOsm/kg water. What key test(s) need to be done before making the diagnosis of the syndrome of inappropriate antidiuretic hormone (SIADH)?*

A. *Demeclocycline challenge*

B. *Thyroid and Adrenal function tests*

C. *Urine creatinine*

D. *DDAVP challenge*

This patient most likely has SIADH, however there are certain criteria that must be met prior to diagnosis: plasma osmolarity <275 mOsm/kg, urine osmolarity >100 mOsm/kg water, normal renal function, clinical euvolemia, elevated urinary sodium excretion, and absence of other potential causes—namely hypothyroidism, hypocortisolism or recent diuretic use. Syndrome of inappropriate antidiuretic hormone is essentially a diagnosis of exclusion. Treatment begins with free water restriction, but can include salt tablets and/or hypertonic saline administration coupled with loop diruretics. Neurological effects are usually seen when plasma sodium decreases below 120 mmol/L. It is important to begin correction at a relatively slow rate if that patient has been experiencing hyponatremia for >48 hours to prevent central pontine myelinolysis .

Answer: B

Adrogué HJ, Madias NE (2000) Hyponatremia. *New England Journal of Medicine* **342** (21), 1581–9.

Moro N, Katayama Y, Igarashi T, *et al.* (2007) Hyponatremia in patients with traumatic brain injury: incidence, mechanism, and response to sodium supplementation or retention therapy with hydrocortisone. *Surgical Neurology* **68** (4), 387–93.

11. *A 65-year-old man has been in the ICU for two days following a motor vehicle crash for which he sustained four rib fractures and a left femur fracture, which have been repaired. He has a history of Crohn's disease and was on steroids for a recent flare-up prior to his accident. Stress-dose steroids were given shortly after arrival, and he had been doing well until today. Now he is not able to tolerate his diet and he has vomited twice. Plain films of the chest and abdomen show free air. What is the most likely cause of the free air?*

A. *Crohn's exacerbation with subsequent perforation following stress response to injury*

B. *Injury to bowel from initial crash, not identified secondary to steroid use*

C. *Bowel perforation secondary to ischemia from blood loss during femur repair*

D. *Beginning diet too soon after injury prior to subsequent femur operation*

E. *Gastric perforation from stress ulceration*

This patient most likely had occult bowel injury on presentation secondary to his steroid use. Even a CT of the abdomen may not show early bowel injury if there is no free air or there is no oral contrast that has reached the perforation. Given his steroid use, he may not develop peritonitis. A much higher index of suspicion for occult injury is required for patients who have been taking steroids chronically as their inflammatory response will be blunted.

Answer: B

Martin RF, Rossi RL (1997) The acute abdomen. An overview and algorithms. *Surgical Clinics of North America* **77** (6), 1227–43.

ReMine SG, McIlrath DC (1980) Bowel perforation in steroid-treated patients. Annals of Surgery **192** (4), 581–6.

12. *A 32-year-old woman has been transferred to the ICU following a celiotomy and right hemicolectomy for a Crohn's flare-up that resulted in perforation. She had been taking 10 mg of prednisone daily prior to her presentation and was started on stress dose steroids. To improve this patient's wound healing, what is one approach that may be of benefit?*

A. Prolong the taper of steroids to decrease the inflammatory response.

B. Topical vitamin E

C. Topical vitamin A

D. Topical mitomycin C

Glucocorticoids have anti-inflammatory effects. Because inflammatory effects are important for proper wound healing to occur. Patients who are on steroids therefore have impaired wound healing. Vitamin A is known to reverse many of the deleterious effects of steroids in wound healing, including the appearance of inflammatory cells, fibroblasts, deposition of ground substance, regeneration of capillaries, and epithelial migration. It should be noted that while steroids decrease wound contracture, vitamin A does not reverse this effect. While there are many animal models that demonstrate these effects of vitamin A, there is a lack of good randomized controlled trials to support the animal models.

Answer: C

Haws M, Brown RE, Suchy H, *et al.* (1994) A-soaked gelfoam sponges and wound healing in steroid-treated animals. *Annals of Plastic Surgery* **32** (4), 418–22.

Wicke C, Halliday B, Allen D, *et al.* (2000) Effects of steroids and retinoids on wound healing. *Archives of Surgery* **135** (11), 1265–70.

Chapter 15 Hypothermia and Hyperthermia

Raquel M. Forsythe, MD, FACS

1. *In a healthy 25-year-old man at rest in a neutral environment (28 °C), the majority of heat exchange occurs as heat loss via*

A. Convection

B. Radiation

C. Conduction

D. Transference

E. Evaporation

Radiation exchange is the transfer of energy between objects with no direct contact. It accounts for 50% to 70% of heat lost by humans at rest in a neutral environment. Conduction involves the direct exchange of heat between the body and an object in direct contact with the body. The speed of heat exchange is related to the thermal conductivity of the object. Water has much greater thermal conductivity than the body, which accounts for the rapid heat exchange that occurs when the body is submerged in water. Convection involves the exchange of heat with the warmer or cooler air molecules passing over the skin. The amount of heat exchange by convection depends on the speed of airflow around the body. Evaporative heat loss in humans is primarily through perspiration. Unlike the other mechanisms of heat exchange, evaporation can exchange heat even in a warmer environment than the body. It is therefore the major means that the body utilizes to prevent hyperthermia in a warm thermal environment. Transference is not a mechanism by which heat is exchanged by the body.

Surgical Critical Care and Emergency Surgery: Clinical Questions and Answers, First Edition. Edited by Forrest O. Moore, Peter M. Rhee, Samuel A. Tisherman and Gerard J. Fulda.

Answer: B

Irwin R, Rippe J (2008) *Irwin and Rippe's Intensive Care Medicine*, 6th edn, Lippincott Wiliams & Wilkins, Philadelphia, PA.

2. *Comparing a healthy 25-year-old and a healthy 75-year-old*

A. The younger patient has a lower basal metabolic rate

B. The younger patient has a higher heat conductance

C. The younger patient generates more heat by shivering

D. The older patient has a lower risk of hypothermia

E. The older patient has a lower sweat threshold

Older patients have deterioration of the ability to regulate temperature, putting them at higher risk for both hypothermia and hyperthermia. Older persons require a greater change in temperature to notice ambient changes. In some cases, they may need a change in temperature of >2 °C to notice a change. The sweat volume decreases and the threshold to produce sweat increases as we age. This significantly decreases evaporative cooling. Older people have lower basal metabolic rates than do younger individuals. A decline in body mass in older patients leads to a higher heat conductance as well as less heat generated by shivering. Some elderly patients lose the ability to shiver. Older people may also experience a loss of the ability to vasoconstrict cutaneous vessels in response to cold.

Answer: C

Irwin R, Rippe J (2008) *Irwin and Rippe's Intensive Care Medicine*, 6th edn, Lippincott Wiliams & Wilkins, Philadelphia, PA.

Questions 3 and 4 *A man becomes lost on a hiking trip in winter. He is found after 36 hours and brought to the emergency department. His skin is cool to the touch. He is lethargic with sluggish pupils. His EKG shows a heart rate of 52 beats/minute with J waves (Osborn waves) noted.*

3. *His expected core body temperature would be:*

A. *37 °C*

B. *35 °C*

C. *31 °C*

D. *26 °C*

E. *20 °C*

This patient demonstrates signs and symptoms consistent with moderate hypothermia. Mild hypothermia is classified based on core body temperature of 35 °C to 32.2 °C. One would expect to see confusion, slurred speech, impaired judgment and tachycardia. This patient exhibits moderate hypothermia, defined as core body temperature of <32.2 °C to 28 °C. Besides the symptoms noted above, a patient would also exhibit hypoventilation, decreased oxygen consumption and CO_2 production. The bradycardia that patients with moderate hypothermia exhibit is resistant to atropine. Severe hypothermia is defined as core temperature below 28 °C. At this temperature, patients may experience spontaneous ventricular fibrillation or asystole. Severe hypothermia causes a decline in blood pressure (BP) and cardiac output as well as a loss of cerebrovascular regulation. EEG activity is diminished in severe hypothermia.

Answer: C

Hanania NA, Zimmerman JL, Hypothermia. In: Hall JB, Schmidt GA, Wood LDH. *Principles of Critical Care*, 3rd edn: www.accesssurgery.com/content.aspx?aID=2282615 (accessed November 14, 2011).

4. *After removing the man's wet clothing and confirming core body temperature with a low-reading rectal thermometer, normal saline warmed to 42 °C is administered via short IV tubing. The next most appropriate step in this patient's management is:*

A. *Endotracheal intubation*

B. *Transcutaneous pacing*

C. *Placement of nasogastric tube with warm saline gastric lavage*

D. *Immersion in a 40 °C water bath*

E. *Placement of a forced air blanket over the body*

Although some controversy exists with regard to the optimal method and rate of rewarming, with moderate hypothermia (temperature <32.2 °C to 28 °C), active rewarming is indicated. There are no controlled studies that compare rewarming protocols, so there is no level 1 evidence to guide rewarming. After removing any wet clothing or other factors that may contribute to ongoing heat loss, the patient should be placed in a controlled, warm environment. Passive external rewarming, consisting of covering the patient with an insulating material to prevent any additional heat loss can increase body temperature by 0.5 °C to 2 °C per hour. This should be performed in patients with mild or moderate hypothermia and may be sufficient treatment in patients with mild hypothermia. For patients with moderate to severe hypothermia, any cardiovascular instability, or inadequate rewarming by passive methods, more aggressive rewarming is indicated. Active external rewarming methods include forced air rewarming (Bair Hugger-type blanket), heating pads, radiant heat and submersion in a 40 °C water bath. Active external rewarming may cause vasodilatation of the extremities, facilitating transport of colder peripheral blood to the warmer core and transiently lowering core body temperature. Peripheral vasodilatation may also worsen hypotension. There are technical challenges associated with immersion in a water bath with regards to monitoring and active resuscitation. Successful use of forced air blankets, which are readily available, as the primary rewarming method has been reported, even in cases with cardiopulmonary arrest. Active core warming may be needed if active external rewarming fails. Techniques include gastric lavage with warm saline, the delivery of heated oxygen via an endotracheal tube, pleural cavity lavage through chest tubes and peritoneal lavage. Rewarming rates average 1 °C to 3 °C per hour. In cases of severe hypothermia, cardiopulmonary bypass can provide circulatory support and raise core temperatures much more quickly, up to 1 °C to 2 °C every three to five minutes, though this takes time to initiate, may require systemic anticoagulation, and may not be readily available.

Answer: E

Hanania NA, Zimmerman JL, Hypothermia. In: Hall JB, Schmidt GA, Wood LDH. *Principles of Critical Care*, 3rd edn: www.accesssurgery.com/content.aspx?aID=2282615 (accessed November 14, 2011).

Koller R, Schnider TW, Neidhart P (1997) Deep accidental hypothermia and cardiac arrest—rewarming with forced air. *Acta Anaesthesiologica Scandinavica* **31**, 1359.

5. *A 22-year-old military recruit collapses at basic training. He is brought to the emergency department for treatment. Which of the following would differentiate heat exhaustion from heat stroke in this patient?*

A. *Lactic acidosis*

B. *Heart rate of 127 beats/minute*

C. *Orthostatic hypotension*

D. *Temperature of 39.8 °C*

E. *Sweating*

The spectrum of heat injury encompasses heat cramps, heat exhaustion and heat stroke. Treatment of heat exhaustion does not generally require intensive care management but it is important to differentiate it from heat stroke. There are two syndromes of heat stroke: classic heat stroke typically occurs in older individuals with underlying medical problems, while exertional heat stroke predominantly occurs in younger individuals who participate in vigorous activity in a hot environment. Both syndromes can present with tachycardia and orthostatic hypotension. Sweating is present in 50% of individuals presenting with heat stroke, so this is not a useful discriminating factor between heat stroke and heat exhaustion. Heat stroke most often presents with a history of exposure to heat, severe CNS dysfunction and temperature >40 °C. However, temperature alone does not rule out heat stroke, since frequently attempts at cooling the patient have been initiated in the prehospital setting. Heat stroke involves a systemic inflammatory response that leads to organ dysfunction, predominantly encephalopathy. Lactic acidosis would not be expected in heat exhaustion but may be seen as severe in heat stroke. In classic heat stroke, it is generally the result of hypoperfusion, while in exertional heat stroke it is usually caused by anaerobic muscle metabolism.

Answer: A

Zimmerman JL, Hanania NA. Hyperthermia. In: Hall JB, Schmidt GA, Wood LDH: *Principles of Critical Care*, 3rd edn, www.accesssurgery.com/content.aspx?aID=2282701, accessed November 14, 2011.

6. *In a patient who remains comatose after resuscitation from cardiac arrest, which of the following would be a contraindication to therapeutic hypothermia?*

A. *Initial rhythm of asystole*

B. *An elapsed time of six hours since the arrest*

C. *Need for norepinephrine at 0.1 μg/kg/min*

D. *Cardiac arrest as a result of a motor vehicle crash with a pelvic fracture*

E. *Glasgow coma motor score of 4 on exam*

At experienced centers, there are multiple indications for therapeutic hypothermia. The most common is cardiac arrest with coma (unable to follow commands) after return of spontaneous circulation (ROSC). Other indications include severe cerebral edema from acute liver failure (while awaiting transplantation) and refractory intracranial hypertension. In survivors of cardiac arrest, it is standard to induce therapeutic hypothermia regardless of the initial presenting rhythm. If more than 8 hours have elapsed since the return of spontaneous circulation, hypothermia may have limited value. Other contraindications include imminent cardiopulmonary collapse despite hemodynamic support or mechanical hemodynamic support, or the presence of any underlying existing terminal condition. Therapy with pressors would not, in and of itself, be a contraindication for hypothermia, unless the patient remains unstable despite aggressive support. In addition, hypothermia should be avoided in patients with life-threatening bleeding or infection. For this reason, hypothermia should not be induced in trauma patients with cardiac arrest unless bleeding can be effectively ruled out. In the case of a traumatic cardiac arrest, only if the trauma workup reveals no source of hemorrhage would hypothermia be appropriate.

Answer: D

Seder DB, Van der Kloot TE (2009) Methods of cooling: practical aspects of therapeutic temperature management. *Critical Care Medicine* **37** (7): S211–S222.

7. *In patients undergoing operative procedures, a body temperature of 35 °C in the recovery room is associated with:*

A. *Stimulation of the immune response to surgery*

B. *Improved wound healing*

C. *Increased risk of surgical site infection*

D. *Decreased hospital length of stay*

E. *Increased systemic vasodilation*

Perioperative hypothermia is defined as a temperature of <36 °C at any point in the perioperative period. There is significant evidence that it is associated with significant morbidity. The two main areas of increased morbidity are surgical site infection and cardiac complications. Perioperative hypothermia has a significant effect on the immune system including leukocyte migration, neutrophil phagocytosis and cytokine antibody production. These immune changes result in a decreased resistance to surgical site infections (SSI). Surgical site infections have been associated with an increased risk of death, increased length of hospital stay, and an increase in hospital costs. Perioperative hypothermia can also cause an increase in circulating catecholamine levels, systemic vasoconstriction, and systemic blood pressure. These effects increase cardiac demands and lead to an increased risk of cardiac morbidity. Perioperative hypothermia, however, remains common. Recent guidelines recommend that active measures be taken to the prevention of perioperative hypothermia in an effort to reduce the risk of SSIs and morbid cardiac events. These active measures include esophageal or oral thermometry, the use of IV fluid warmers for abdominal procedures of greater than one hour duration and the use of warm forced air devices for procedures that are expected to last greater than 30 minutes.

Answer: C

Forbes SS, Eskicioglu C, Nathens AB, *et al.* (2009) Evidence-based guidelines for prevention of perioperative hypothermia. *Journal of the American College of Surgeons* **209**, 492–503.

Melling AC, Ali B, Scott EM, *et al.* (2001) Effects of preoperative warming on the incidence of wound infection after clean surgery: a randomized controlled trial. *Lancet* **358**, 876–80.

8. *The cardiovascular and hemodynamic effect of mild hypothermia (33 °C) in a healthy euvolemic patient includes:*

A. *Increased heart rate*

B. *Decreased myocardial contractility*

C. *Increased cardiac output*

D. *Increased systolic function*

E. *No change in vascular resistance*

The effect of hypothermia on the myocardium and cardiovascular physiology are complex and depend on the patient's volume status and sedation level. It also depends on the depth of hypothermia. With mild hypothermia in an otherwise healthy, euvolemic patient, heart rate would decrease with an increase in myocardial contractility. Systolic function will improve while a mild degree of diastolic dysfunction may occur. With the decrease in heart rate, a decrease in cardiac output may be seen. Given that the metabolic rate decreases with hypothermia, the balance between oxygen supply and demand for tissues is generally stable or improved. In contrast to mild hypothermia, deep hypothermia (less than 30 °C) does decrease myocardial contractility and may also cause hypovolemia by inducing a cold diuresis and capillary leak.

Answer: D

Polderman KH (2009) Mechanisms of action, physiological effects and complications of hypothermia. *Critical Care Medicine* **37**, S186–S202.

9. *In the brain injured patient:*

A. *Fever occurs in approximately 30% of all patients with subarachnoid hemorrhage (SAH)*

B. *Fever in traumatic brain injury is associated with poor long-term outcomes*

C. *Fever has no impact on the outcome after ischemic stroke*

D. *An infectious cause for fever is rarely found after spinal cord injury*

E. *There is no relationship between fever and cerebral vasospasm in SAH*

Fever occurs in approximately 70% of all neurologically injured patients. Only half the febrile episodes can be attributed to infection, with pneumonia the most common source of infection in these patients. Early temperature elevation after brain injury is most commonly attributed to an acute phase response. Blood within the cerebrospinal fluid spaces, particularly the intraventricular spaces, may lead to fever. Patients with subarachnoid hemorrhage (SAH) have a high rate of fever—up to 70%—and this has been implicated in the development of cerebrovascular spasm. Fever in the acute phase of SAH has been independently associated with morbidity and mortality. Fever after traumatic brain injury (TBI) is associated with increased intracranial pressure, neurologic impairment and long-term poor outcome. Spinal-cord injured patients may have difficulty maintaining normothermia. Therefore, they will most commonly have an infection causing fever, generally pneumonia or a urinary tract infection; although fever of unknown origin can also occur. In ischemic stroke patients, early fever is associated with worse stroke severity and outcomes.

Answer: B

Badjatia N (2009) Hyperthermia and fever control in brain injury. *Critical Care Medicine* **37**, S250–S257.

Chapter 16 Acute Kidney Injury

Terence O'Keeffe, MB, ChB, MSPH, FACS

1. *Which of the following items is not part of the grading system for acute kidney injury (AKI), using the RIFLE criteria?*

A. *An increase in serum creatinine of more than or equal to 0.3 mg/dL, or increase to more than or equal to 150% to 200% from baseline*

B. *Anuria for eight hours*

C. *An increase in serum creatinine to more than 200% to 300% from baseline*

D. *Urine output of less than 0.5 ml/kg for more than six hours*

E. *A serum creatinine more than or equal to 4.0 mg/dL*

Acute renal failure (ARF) is a common complication in critically ill patients, associated with significant mortality as well as morbidity. However, not only the diagnosis but also the treatment of this condition has remained controversial and confusing for many years. There has therefore been an impetus in recent years to develop consensus regarding the classification of this clinical entity. Acute renal failure has been reclassified as acute kidney injury (AKI). The definition of acute kidney injury was originally proposed from a consensus conference in 2004 where a grading system was introduced with the acronym **RIFLE**, which stands for **R**isk, **I**njury, **F**ailure, **L**oss and **E**nd-stage kidney disease. The vast majority of critical care and nephrology organizations have accepted this definition. Table 16.1 sets out the Acute Kidney Injury Network criteria for the different stages of acute kidney injury. This is modified from the original RIFLE criteria, but stages 1, 2, and 3 correspond to "R", "I", and "F". Anuria of more than 12 hours was part of the original definition, but is no longer used; the diagnosis of AKI being based on increases in serum creatinine or decreases in urine output.

Table 16.1 Modified RIFLE criteria for staging acute kidney injury

Stage	Serum creatinine criteria	Urine output criteria
1	Increase in serum creatinine of more than or equal to 0.3 mg/dl or increase to more than or equal to 150% to 200% (1.5- to 2-fold) from baseline	Less than 0.5 ml/kg per hour for more than 6 hours
2	Increase in serum creatinine to more than 200% to 300% (>2- to 3-fold) from baseline	Less than 0.5 ml/kg per hour for more than 12 hours
3	Increase in serum creatinine to more than 300% (>3-fold) from baseline (or serum creatinine of more than or equal to 4.0 mg/dl with an acute increase of at least 0.5 mg/dl	Less than 0.3 ml/kg per hour for 24 hours or anuria for 12 hours

Only one criterion has to be fulfilled for qualify for a stage. Patients who undergo dialysis of any type are considered to have met the criteria for stage 3 irrespective of the stage they are in at the time of dialysis.

Answer: B

Bellomo R, Ronco C, Kellum JA, *et al.* (2004) Acute renal failure—definition, outcome measures, animal models, fluid therapy and information technology needs: the Second International Consensus Conference of the Acute Dialysis Quality Initiative (ADQI) Group. *Critical Care* **8**, R204–R212.

Surgical Critical Care and Emergency Surgery: Clinical Questions and Answers, First Edition. Edited by Forrest O. Moore, Peter M. Rhee, Samuel A. Tisherman and Gerard J. Fulda.

Mehta RL, Kellum JA, Shah SV, *et al.* (2007) Acute Kidney Injury Network: report of an initiative to improve outcomes in acute kidney injury. *Critical Care.* **11** (2), R31.

2. *Which of the following is not consistent with acute tubular necrosis in a patient with oliguria?*

A. *Fractional excretion of sodium (FENA) of 3%*

B. *Urine Osmolality of 260 mOsm/liter.*

C. *Urinary sodium of 12 mEq/L*

D. *Urine/plasma creatinine ratio of 16*

E. *The presence of granular casts on urine microscopy*

Acute tubular necrosis is one of many causes of oliguric renal failure, but can usually be distinguished from pre-renal azotemia by a low urine osmolality (<350 mOsm/L), a high urinary sodium (>40mEq/L), an elevated FENa (usually >2%), a low urine/plasma creatinine ratio of <20, and the presence of granular casts and renal tubular epithelial cells on microscopy. Urinary sodiums of less than 20 mEq/L are more typically found in patients with pre-renal azotemia. The FENa is the most discriminatory single test.

Answer: C

Fauci A, Braunwald E, Kasper DL, *et al.* (2008) Acute renal failure. In: *Harrison's Principles of Internal Medicine,* 17th edn, McGraw-Hill, New York, pp. 1752–61.

Lerma EV, Kelly B. Acute Tubular Necrosis, http://emedicine.medscape.com/article/238064-overview, accessed November 14, 2011.

3. *Which of the following would not be part of an appropriate initial workup for a post-operative surgical patient with oliguria, a BUN of 45 mg/dL and a creatinine of 2.2 mg/dL?*

A. *Sending urinary electrolytes and creatinine to calculate a fractional excretion of sodium (FENa)*

B. *Renal arteriography to assess for renal artery stenosis*

C. *Assessment of intravascular volume by invasive monitoring*

D. *Placement of a Foley catheter to assess hourly urine volume*

E. *Calculation of the BUN/Cr ratio*

The initial investigation of acute kidney injury should include urinary electrolytes, a plasma chemistry panel, a complete blood count, bladder scanning and/or placement of a Foley catheter as well as an assessment of intravascular fluid volume status. Urine microscopy and urinary tract ultrasound may also form part of these initial investigations. In the patient presented, a renal angiogram would not be indicated as one of the first line investigations, and in fact may exacerbate the situation by increasing the kidney injury due to the intravenous contrast required. A careful history together with a full physical examination may in fact provide more information regarding the likely source of the acute kidney injury than renal angiography, which is rarely indicated in the acute phase. The goal is to identify whether the patient is in AKI due to a prerenal, renal or post renal cause, as this will guide the management of the patient and help to identify what further testing may be necessary.

Answer: B

Parrillo JE, Dellinger RP (2007) Acute renal failure. In: *Critical Care Medicine. Principles of Diagnosis and Management in the Adult.* 3rd edn, Mosby, Philadelphia, PA.

4. *Workup for obstructive uropathy might include all of the following except*

A. *Rectal exam*

B. *Placement of a foley catheter*

C. *Ultrasonography of the urinary tract*

D. *Abdominal CT scan*

E. *Renal arteriography*

The history and physical exam, in addition to additional laboratory tests will help to guide the appropriate investigation. Rectal exam will give information regarding the size and character of the prostate, while foley catheterization may relieve the cause of the obstruction as well as enabling a clear quantification of the amount of urine produced. Ultrasonography of the urogenital tract is the preferred screening modality if obstruction is suspected, because it is highly sensitive for hydronephrosis, and is low cost as well as safe and repeatable. CT scanning is becoming more and more useful for evaluation of the upper urinary tract, particularly with the recent improvements in image quality from helical CT. Renal arteriography has no place in the management of obstructive renal failure, although it may be important to investigate renal hypertension and other renovascular disorders.

Answer: E

Frøkiaer J, Zeidel M (2007) Urinary tract obstruction. In: Brenner BM, ed. *Brenner and Rector's The Kidney*, 8th edn, WB Saunders, Philadelphia, PA, pp. 1239–48

5. *Regarding the use of fenoldopam in patients with acute kidney injury, which of the following is correct?*

A. *The use of fenoldopam is associated with a decrease in mean arterial pressure*

B. *Low-dose fenoldopam (<0.05 μg/kg/min) is as effective as high dose (0.07–0.1)*

C. *Fenoldopam is an effective therapy for reducing contrast-induced nephropathy*

D. *Therapy with fenoldopam is as effective as low-dose dopamine in preventing the need for dialysis in patients with acute renal failure*

E. *Fenoldopam is recommended in postcardiac surgery patients at high risk for acute tubular necrosis*

Fenoldopam was once heralded as a more attractive alternative to the use of low-dose dopamine for the prevention and/or treatment of acute kidney injury. Although controversial due to the lack of good scientific evidence, it has become clear that it is *not* an effective therapy for the prevention of contrast nephropathy. Neither is it particularly useful in the high-risk cardiac surgical group, if for no other reason than the significant risk of hypotension associated with use of this drug. High-dose therapy in one study demonstrated a significant decrease in serum creatinine levels compared to low-dose therapy. Neither dopamine nor fenoldopam are currently recommended as treatment for acute kidney injury or to prevent or treat contrast-induced nephropathy.

Answer: A

Kellum JA, Leblanc M, Venkataraman R (2008) Acute renal failure. *Clinical Evidence* (Online) **11**, September 3, pii 2001.

Samuels J, Finkel K, Gubert M, *et al.* (2005) Effect of fenoldopam mesylate in critically ill patients at risk for acute renal failure is dose dependent. *Renal Failure* **27** (1), 101–5.

6. *In patients with acute kidney injury from traumatic rhabdomyolysis, which of the following is true?*

A. *Treatment should be instituted when the creatine kinase (CK) levels rise to above 3000 U/L*

B. *Mannitol is strongly recommended as first line therapy in the treatment of this condition*

C. *Alkalinization of the urine using intravenous sodium bicarbonate, targeting a pH of greater than 6.0, can prevent renal failure in patients with rhabdomyolysis*

D. *Early aggressive fluid replacement with saline is the mainstay of treatment*

E. *Serum myoglobin levels remain elevated longer than serum CK levels*

Rhabdomyolysis is most commonly caused by trauma but may also be due to medications, exercise, toxins, infections, muscle enzyme deficiencies or endocrinopathies. It is associated with elevated levels of creatine kinase. Levels above 5000 U/L are associated with acute kidney injury; and treatment is recommended above this level. Neither mannitol nor urinary alkalinization with sodium bicarbonate have been convincingly shown to reduce the need for dialysis or mortality from this condition. The half-life of serum CK is 1.5 days, compared to 2–3 hours for serum myoglobin. The only effective treatment seems to be aggressive intravenous fluid replacement early in the course of the disease. This may require invasive monitoring with either a central line or a pulmonary artery catheter to prevent fluid overload.

Answer: D

Brown CV, Rhee P, Chan L, *et al.* Preventing renal failure in patients with rhabdomyolysis: do bicarbonate and mannitol make a difference? *Journal of Trauma* **56** (6), 1191–6.

Huerta-Alardín AL, Varon J, Marik PE (2005) Bench-to-bedside review: Rhabdomyolysis—an overview for clinicians. *Critical Care* **9** (2), 158–69.

7. *Which of the following would not be considered an indication for acute dialysis?*

A. *A pericardial friction rub in a patient with a BUN of 85 mg/dL*

B. *A patient with a prolonged international normalized ratio due to warfarin overdose*

C. *A central venous pressure of 20 mm Hg in a patient with AKI and acute pulmonary edema*

D. *A pH of 7.15, unresponsive to bicarbonate fluid therapy*

E. *A patient with primary hyperparathyroidism, with a serum calcium of 12 mg/dL, unresponsive to hydration and calcitonin*

The easily remembered mnemonic of AEIOU (Acid-base, Electrolytes, Intoxications, Overload, Uremic symptoms) still provides a good working guide for the indications for dialysis in the acute setting. Excessive uremia can lead to confusion as well as platelet dysfunction and generally dialysis is instituted with a BUN of greater than 100 mg/dL. Dialysis may be indicated for the removal of certain metabolic poisons and/or medications, however warfarin does not cross the dialysis membrane and so an overdose of this drug cannot be treated in this way. It will require reversal with vitamin K, prothrombin complex concentrate and/or fresh frozen plasma. Fluid overload, especially when symptomatic as demonstrated by pulmonary edema in a patient who will not respond to diuretics, is an appropriate indication for dialysis. Patients with severe metabolic acidosis that is unresponsive to more conservative therapy are also good candidates for acute dialysis. Finally dialysis can remove electrolyte abnormalities such as hypercalcemia, hyperkalemia and hyperphosphatemia. It should be noted that hypocalcemia is more common in acute kidney injury, with hypercalcemia being much more rare, usually associated with the diuretic phase of rhabdomyolysis associated AKI.

Answer: B

Clarkson MR, Friedewald JJ, Eusatace JA, Rabb H (2007) Acute kidney injury. In: Brenner BM, ed. *Brenner and Rector's The Kidney*, 8th edn, WB Saunders, Philadelphia, PA, pp. 943–86.

Palevksy P (n.d.) Renal replacement therapy (dialysis) in acute kidney injury (acute renal failure): indications, timing, and dialysis dose, www.uptodate.com/contents/renal-replacement-therapy-dialysis-in-acute-kidney-injury-acute-renal-failure-indications-timing-and-dialysis-dose (accessed March, 2011).

8. *Which of the following is recommended for the prevention of contrast-induced nephropathy?*

A. *500 mg of intravenous vitamin C before administration of contrast, followed by three doses every eight hours*

B. *An infusion containing sodium bicarbonate started prior to administration and continued for six hours post administration of IV contrast*

C. *Treatment with N-acetylcysteine both pre-and post administration of IV contrast*

D. *Administration of an intravenous fenoldapam infusion before the contrast administration*

E. *The use of low osmolality contrast media for contrast administration*

The data for beneficial effects from therapies for contrast nephropathy is both contradictory and of poor quality. A randomized controlled trial in 2007 on the use of vitamin C (given PO) for the prevention of contrast nephropathy found no significant benefit versus placebo. However, randomized controlled trials have shown benefit with the administration of sodium bicarbonate, N-acetylcysteine, and pre-procedure intravenous hydration with normal saline, prior to invasive procedures or CT scanning requiring the use of IV contrast. The use of low osmolality contrast media has also been shown to be beneficial. Current recommendations are for preprocedure hydration using 0.9% normal saline rather than other therapies due to the poor quality of the data surrounding the use of N-acetylcysteine and sodium bicarbonate.

Answer: E

Boschieri A, Weinbrenner C, Botzek B, *et al.* (2007) Failure of ascorbic acid to prevent contrast-media induced nephropathy in patients with renal dysfunction. *Clinical Nephrology* **68** (5), 279–86.

Kellum JA, Leblanc M, Venkataraman R. (2006) Acute renal failure. *Clin Evid* **15**, 1191–212.

9. *In a patient with Acute Kidney Injury Network grade 2 acute kidney injury ("I" in the RIFLE criteria), which one of the following medications requires adjustment for renal dosing?*

A. Unfractionated subcutaneous heparin, 5000 units subcutaneous three times daily

B. Low molecular weight heparin, 30 mg subcutaneous twice daily

C. Nafcillin 1 gm IV every 4 hours

D. Linezolid 600 mg IV every twelve hours

E. Phenytoin 100 mg PO three times daily

Of all the drugs listed above, only low molecular weight heparin (Lovenox) requires renal adjustment. Without this adjustment levels of low molecular weight heparin will build up in the bloodstream and can cause significant bleeding diatheses. Although the manufacturers package insert claims that adjustment can be performed to take into account the degree of acute injury kidney injury, this author strongly recommends that patients who develop AKI while on Lovenox are switched to unfractionated subcutaneous heparin at the earliest opportunity.

Answer: B

Dowling TC, Matzke GR, Murphy JE, Burckart GJ (2010) Evaluation of renal drug dosing: prescribing information and clinical pharmacist approaches. *Pharmacotherapy* **30** (8), 776–86.

Matzke GR, Frye RF (1997) Drug administration in patients with renal insufficiency. Minimising renal and extrarenal toxicity. *Drug Safety* **16** (3), 205–31.

10. *Which of the following signs and/or symptoms is unlikely to be observed in a patient with hyperkalemia due to grade 3 AKI?*

A. Peaked T waves on the EKG

B. Generalized fatigue

C. Left bundle branch block with a potassium level of 7.2 mEq/L

D. Widened QRS complex in a patient with a potassium level of 5.5 mEq/L

E. Ventricular fibrillation if untreated

Early changes on the EKG consist of peaked T waves, a shortened QT interval, and ST segment depression. These are followed by bundle branch blocks and widening of the QRS complex. Without treatment the QRS morphology will eventually widen to resemble a sine wave, with ventricular fibrillation or asystole following. The EKG changes are generally related to the serum potassium level, therefore a widened QRS complex would be unlikely in a patient with a potassium level of only 5.5 mEq/L. Patients may be asymptomatic or can report generalized fatigue, weakness, paresthesias, palpitations, or even paralysis.

Answer: D

Garth D (n.d.) Hyperkalemia in Emergency Medicine, http://emedicine.medscape.com/article/766479-overview (accessed February, 2011)

Nyirenda MJ, Tang JI, Padfield PL, Seckl PL (2009) Hyperkalaemia *British Medical Journal* **339**, b4114.

11. *In a patient with severe hyperkalemia (Potassium >6.5 mEq/L) and widened QRS complexes, which of the following treatments should be administered first to prevent malignant ventricular arrhythmias?*

A. Intravenous calcium gluconate

B. Dialysis

C. Intravenous insulin and glucose

D. *Intravenous furosemide*

E. *Intravenous sodium bicarbonate*

All the above treatment choices listed above can be used to treat hyperkalemia, however. calcium gluconate will have the most rapid effect by stabilizing the myocardium, decreasing the risk of arrhythmias. It is usually only indicated when EKG changes are present. Intravenous insulin will drive potassium back into the cells and the effects occur within 30 minutes of administration. Albuterol has a similar effect and onset of action. Kayexalate will bind potassium and can be given orally or rectally. Sodium bicarbonate raise pH, which results in potassium shifts into the intracellular space. Calcitonin is used in hypercalcemia, NOT hyperkalemia. Furosemide can be effective by inducing potassium loss through the kidney if the patient can still make urine, but the onset of action is slower, and large doses may be needed in AKI.

Answer: A

Garth D. Hyperkalemia in Emergency Medicine, http://emedicine.medscape.com/article/766479-overview (accessed February, 2011).

Nyirenda MJ, Tang JI, Padfield PL, Seckl, PL (2009) Hyperkalaemia. *British Medical Journal* **339**, b4114.

12. *Which of the following statements is correct regarding the use of furosemide in acute kidney injury (AKI)?*

A. *Furosemide will decrease the percentage of patients with AKI who will require renal replacement therapy*

B. *The use of high-dose furosemide for AKI is not associated with significant side effects*

C. *Administration of furosemide for AKI is associated with increased mortality*

D. *Furosemide can convert patients from an oliguric to non-oliguric state, which is associated with a decreased hospital length of stay*

E. *Furosemide will induce a diuresis in some patients with acute kidney injury*

Although furosemide may produce a diuresis in some patients with acute kidney injury, it has not been conclusively shown that this has an effect on the eventual need for renal replacement therapy, in-hospital mortality, or the number of dialysis sessions required until the recovery of renal function. Neither is there a significant effect on hospital length of stay. The high doses of furosemide required to induce a diuresis in this patient group carry a significant risk of ototoxicity, however data regarding an increase in mortality due to furosemide administration is questionable. In the absence of significant benefits the use of furosemide in acute kidney injury is to be discouraged.

Answer: E

Bagshaw SM, Delaney A, Haase M, *et al.* (2007) Loop diuretics in the management of acute renal failure: a systematic review and meta-analysis. *Critical Care and Resuscitation* **9** (1), 60–8.

Ho KM, Sheridan DJ (2006) Meta-analysis of frusemide to prevent or treat acute renal failure. *British Medical Journal* **333** (7565), 420.

13. *Dopamine, when used in the treatment of acute kidney injury, has all of the following effects except?*

A. *An increase in the glomerular filtration rate*

B. *A significant rise in the urine output in the majority of patients*

C. *Is often associated with tachycardia and other arrhythmias*

D. *Has been shown to effectively reduce the need for renal replacement therapy*

E. *Administration of low-dose dopamine at 5 μg/kg/min is as effective as 3 μg/kg/min in preventing the need for renal replacement therapy*

Treatment with low-dose dopamine for acute kidney injury was considered beneficial in the past. However, the largest meta-analysis performed in 2005 showed no beneficial effects of low-dose dopamine on mortality, the need for real replacement therapy, or adverse events. Therapy with low-dose dopamine will however increase the glomerular filtration rate by improving renal blood flow, subsequently causing an increase in urine output in the majority of patients. This may be associated with an improvement in the serum creatinine level, and measured creatinine clearance. There is no compelling data that 5 μg/kg/min is more effective than 3 μg/kg/min, other than increasing the risk of side effects. Unwanted effects from dopamine therapy included tachycardia and arrhythmias, which can limit the use of this medication. As stated previously, current recommendations are that dopamine should not be used for acute kidney injury.

Answer: D

Friedrich JO, Adhikari N, Herridge MS, Beyene J (2005) Meta-analysis: low-dose dopamine increases urine output but does not prevent renal dysfunction or death. *Annals of Internal Medicine* **142** (7), 510–24.

Marik PE (2002) Low-dose dopamine: a systematic review. *Intensive Care Medicine* **28** (7), 877–83.

14. *Which of the following medications would be the LEAST likely cause of acute kidney injury in a woman patient with a new rash, white blood cells in the urine, a normal white blood cell count and eosinophilia on urine microscopy?*

A. Amoxicillin

B. Phenytoin

C. Pantoprazole

D. Ketorolac

E. Heparin

This patient presents with findings consistent with acute interstitial nephritis. This typically begins abruptly, manifesting as acute kidney injury. In most instances, the nephritis occurs within days of exposure to the offending drug. However, in some instances (particularly with non-steroidal anti-inflammatory drugs), acute interstitial nephritis begins after several months of exposure. The analgesic nephropathy is 5–6 times more common in women, which is generally attributed to women taking more analgesics than men. However, a greater sensitivity to the toxic effects of analgesics or differences in analgesic metabolism in women cannot be ruled out. The most commonly associated drugs are: antibiotics (e.g., penicillins, fluoroquinolones, and sulfa drugs), rifampin, phenytoin, proton pump inhibitors, non-steroidal anti-inflammatory medications, diuretics (e.g., thiazides, furosemide), and allopurinol. Although any drug can theoretically cause acute interstitial nephritis, acute reactions to heparin are more likely to be generalized hypersensitivity or even anaphylactic. Additionally, thrombocytopenia occurs in up to 30% of patients, which can occur in a severe form as heparin-induced thrombocytopenia.

Answer: E

Alper, AB. Nephritis, Interstitial, http://emedicine.medscape.com/article/243597-overview (accessed February, 2011).

Remuzzi G, Perico N, De Broe ME (2007) Tubulointerstitial Diseases. In: Brenner BM, ed. *Brenner and Rector's The Kidney,* 8th edn, WB Saunders, Philadelphia, PA, pp. 1174–1202.

15. *Which of the following is not an advantage of continuous renal replacement therapy over intermittent dialysis?*

A. It can be used in hemodynamically unstable patients

B. Less expensive

C. Useful to remove fluid in smaller volumes

D. More effective in lowering intracranial pressure

E. Better removal of proinflammatory mediators

Although the type of renal placement therapy, as well as the dosing of the dialysis remains controversial, there are some circumstances in which continuous renal replacement therapy such as continuous venovenous hemodiafiltration offers advantages over intermittent hemodialysis. It is a much better tolerated process for the patient who is critically ill—for example in septic shock requiring vasopressor support—as there are fewer hemodynamic fluxes during dialysis. It can be available 24 hours a day, depending on the training of the nursing personnel and the equipment available in the intensive care unit. It can also remove small volumes of fluid at a time therefore allowing finer adjustments to be made regarding the amount of fluid removed. It may have benefit in septic shock by removing pro-inflammatory mediators, although this remains controversial. It also has fewer deleterious side effects on intracranial pressure, which may be important in those patients also suffering from traumatic brain injury. However, it is clear that it is not cheaper than other forms of hemodialysis, and may in fact be more expensive than other currently available therapies.

Answer: B

Pannu N, Klarenbach S, Wiebe N, *et al.* (2008) Renal replacement therapy in patients with acute renal failure: a systematic review. *Journal of the American Medical Association* **299**, 793–805.

Parrillo JE, Dellinger RP (2007) Acute renal failure. In: *Critical Care Medicine. Principles of Diagnosis and Management in the Adult.* 3rd edn, Mosby, Philadelphia, PA.

16. *Regarding nutrition for a patient with acute kidney injury requiring dialysis, which of the considerations below is correct?*

A. *Enteral formulas do not need to be low nitrogen*

B. *Caloric needs are not increased due to the acute kidney injury*

C. *Fat-soluble vitamin supplementation is important*

D. *Total caloric intake should be in the order of 35–40 kcal/kg/day*

E. *Parenteral nutrition is the preferred route while the patient is on continuous renal replacement therapy*

Nutritional management in patients with acute kidney injury requires close collaboration between the physicians, nurses and dietitians. Patients with AKI, particularly following surgery or trauma, and patients with multiorgan failure can frequently have protein catabolic rates above 1.5 g/kg/day. The objective of nutrition in AKI is to provide sufficient calories and protein to preserve lean body mass, avoid starvation ketoacidosis and promote healing, while minimizing production of nitrogenous waste. If the patient is not catabolic then protein intake should be restricted to below 0.8 g/kg/day. Catabolic patients, especially those on continuous renal replacement therapy, should receive at least 1.4 g/kg/day. Water-soluble vitamins should be provided with the exception of vitamin C, which, in high doses, promotes urinary oxalate excretion and store information. Total caloric intake should normally be in the range of 25 to 30 kcal/kg/day, and should not exceed 35 kcal/kg/day. Although vigorous parenteral nutrition has been claimed to improve prognosis in AKI, the enteral route is preferred because it avoids the morbidity and costs associated with parenteral nutrition.

Answer: A

Clarkson MR, Friedewald JJ, Eustace JA, Rabb H (2007) Acute kidney injury. In: Brenner BM, ed. *Brenner and Rector's The Kidney*, 8th edn, WB Saunders, Philadelphia, PA, pp. 943–76.

Brown RO, Compher C (2010) ASPEN clinical guidelines: nutrition support in adult acute and chronic renal failure. *Journal of Parenteral and Enteral Nutrition* **34** (4), 366–77.

17. *Which of the following is an appropriate indication for the use of sodium bicarbonate?*

A. *A trauma patient post-splenectomy with a pH of 7.15 and a hemoglobin of 7.0 mg/dL*

B. *Severe nongap metabolic acidosis (pH<7.0)*

C. *Post-cardiac arrest in a hospitalized patient who was cardioverted for ventricular fibrillation*

D. *A patient with gram-negative sepsis undergoing CRRT, with a pH of 7.3*

E. *A torsade de pointes ventricular arrythymia*

The use of intravenous sodium bicarbonate to treat metabolic acidosis, although practiced for over 50 years, remains contentious. The treatment for a trauma patient who has just undergone splenectomy and remains anemic should be to transfuse with packed red blood cells and or clotting factors as necessary. Treating this patient with sodium bicarbonate will only serve to mask the underlying hypovolemia. Sodium bicarbonate therapy has a definite role in the treatment of severe metabolic acidosis that is unresponsive to conventional fluid resuscitation, particularly in the face of any acute kidney injury. The primary treatment for ventricular fibrillation is cardioversion, and if this is performed rapidly after arrest then there is no need for the routine administration of sodium bicarbonate. Patients with mild acidosis, particularly those who undergo reorientation therapy, could have this adjusted using the buffers in the dialysis solution rather than the administration of intravenous sodium bicarbonate. Finally, the treatment for torsade de pointes is magnesium.

Answer: B

DuBose TD (2007) Disorders of Acid-Base Balance. In: Brenner BM, ed. *Brenner and Rector's The Kidney*, 8th edn, WB Saunders, Philadelphia, PA, pp. 943–76.

Vukmir RB, Katz L (2006) Sodium bicarbonate improves outcome in prolonged prehospital cardiac arrest. *American Journal of Emergency Medicine* **24** (2), 156–61.

Chapter 17 Liver Failure

Bellal Joseph, MD

1. *A 58-year-old man presents to the emergency department with an incarcerated umbilical hernia with leaking ascites. He is a known alcoholic and has been previously diagnosed with cirrhosis. Which of the following scoring systems is the most accurate predictor of increased risk for morbidity and mortality in a cirrhotic patient after an abdominal operation?*

A. *APACHE II*

B. *APACHE III*

C. *Childs Class*

D. *MELD (model for end-stage liver disease) score*

E. *Child–Turcotte–Pugh score (CTP)*

Prognostic models are useful in estimating disease severity and survival and are used to make decisions regarding specific medical interventions. Several prognostic models are currently used in healthcare settings. Some focus on generalized health status, such as the Acute Physiology and Chronic Health Evaluation System (APACHE III). Cirrhosis of the liver is associated with increased morbidity and mortality when a patient must undergo exploration. Two models that are used commonly in the care of patients with chronic liver disease are the Child–Turcotte–Pugh (CTP) score and the more recently described Model for End-stage Liver Disease (MELD).

The MELD is a prospectively developed and validated chronic liver disease severity scoring system that uses a patient's laboratory values for serum bilirubin, serum creatinine, and the international normalized ratio for prothrombin time (INR) to predict survival. The CTP score was found to be better than the APACHE II and APACHE III scores in predicting short-term mortality of cirrhotic patients. The MELD score is the most precise tool to assess operative risk in the same patient population. The MELD score has been confirmed to be more precise in categorizing risks of cirrhotic patients for both hepatic and other abdominal operations and to be superior to the CTP score. The revised model is currently used by the United Network for Organ Sharing (UNOS) in prioritizing allocation of deceased donor organs for liver transplantation.

Answer: D

Chatzicostas C, Roussomoustakaki M, Notas G, *et al.* (2003) A comparison of Child-Pugh, APACHE II and APACHE III scoring systems in predicting hospital mortality of patients with liver cirrhosis. *BMC Gastroenterology* **3**, 7.

Farnsworth N, Fagan SP, Berger DH, *et al.* (2004) Child-Turcotte-Pugh versus MELD score as a predictor of outcome after elective and emergent surgery in cirrhotic patients. *American Journal of Surgery* **188**, 580–3.

2. *A 65-year-old woman with a history of severe alcohol abuse is brought to the emergency department after her first episode of hematemesis. After initial resuscitation with four units of packed RBC's the patient's vital signs are stable and the bleeding has subsided. The patient undergoes upper endoscopy and esophageal varices are noted. All of the following statements concerning initial management are correct except:*

A. *Transjugular intrahepatic portosystemic shunt (TIPS) is indicated if endoscopic varix ablation is unsuccessful*

B. *Liver transplantation is considered in the acute situation for the management of variceal bleeding*

C. *Activated Factor VII is used in exceptional circumstances to control coagulopathic bleeding*

D. *Ablative therapy to eliminate varices is appropriate for hemorrhage secondary to esophageal varices*

Surgical Critical Care and Emergency Surgery: Clinical Questions and Answers, First Edition. Edited by Forrest O. Moore, Peter M. Rhee, Samuel A. Tisherman and Gerard J. Fulda.

E. *Band ligation of varices is preferred over sclerotherapy because it is associated with fewer complications such as perforations and strictures*

In patients with presumed cirrhosis and upper gastrointestinal bleeding, the source of the bleeding must be identified. After initial patient stabilization, upper endoscopy is indicated to search for the etiology. Transjugular intrahepatic portosystemic shunt (TIPS) and operative portosystemic shunting are options if endoscopic ablation is unsuccessful. Liver transplantation is never considered in the acute situation. Patients with a history of severe alcohol abuse would not meet transplant criteria. Activated factor VII is used in rare circumstances to control coagulopathic bleeding, but is never indicated in a patient for whom standard measures have been successful. Finally, ablative therapy to eliminate the varices is appropriate for hemorrhage secondary to esophageal varices. This is considered first-line therapy. Methods for ablating varices without open operation include endoscopic sclerotherapy and endoscopic band ligation. Band ligation is usually chosen because it is associated with fewer complications such as perforation and stricture.

Answer: B

Brunicardi F, Andersen D, Billiar T (2010) *Schwartz's Principles of Surgery*. 9th edn, McGraw-Hill, New York.

Rosemurgy AS, Zervos EE (2003) Management of variceal hemorrhage. *Current Problems in Surgery* **40**, 263–343.

3. *A 65-year-old alcoholic man with ascities undergoes emergent colectomy for a lower gastrointestinal bleed. During his postoperative recovery the urine output is consistently low. The patient has a presumed diagnosis of hepatorenal syndrome. All of the following findings are consistent with hepatorenal syndrome except:*

A. *Absence of proteinuria*

B. *Oliguria (<500 ml per day)*

C. *High sodium concentration in the urine*

D. *Increased urine-plasma osmolality ratio (U:P >1.0)*

E. *Azotemia*

Hepatorenal syndrome is quite common in the cirrhotic population and is found in approximately 10% of individuals admitted to the hospital with ascites. It is characterized by azotemia, oliguria (<500 mL per day), low urinary sodium excretion (<10 mEq per liter), and increased urine-plasma osmolality ratio (U:P > 1.0) in the absence of urinary sedimentation. Histology of renal tissue from patients with hepatorenal syndrome is normal. Hepatorenal syndrome occurs in patients with pre-existing parenchymal liver disease after a precipitating event such as surgery or a hypotensive episode (e.g., GI bleed, dialysis, sepsis). The etiology of hepatorenal syndrome is not completely understood but appears to involve vasodilation, decreased effective arterial volume, and further reduction of glomerular filtration by the renin-angiotensin-aldosterone system. Hepatorenal syndrome progress over days to weeks after the precipitating event. While initially partly responsive to volume expansion, it is ultimately refractory to all interventions except liver transplantation.

Answer: C

Arroyo, V, Guevara M, Ginès P, *et al.* (2002) Hepatorenal syndrome in cirrhosis: pathogenesis and treatment. *Gastroenterology* **122** (6), 1658–76.

Mulholland MW, Lillemoe KD, Doherty G *et al.* (2010) *Greenfield's Surgery: Scientific Principles and Practice*, Lippincott Williams & Wilkins, Philadelphia, PA.

4. *The stent placed during transjugular intrahepatic portosystemic shunt (TIPS)*

A. *Should be followed with computed tomography scan every six months after placement*

B. *Is not covered*

C. *Is associated with postprocedure encephalopathy rates of 80%*

D. *Has a stenosis rate of greater than 50%*

E. *Is dilated until a gradient of less than 20 mm Hg is obtained*

Transjugular intrahepatic portosystemic shunts (TIPS) involve creation of a low-resistance channel between the hepatic vein and the intrahepatic portion of the portal vein using angiographic techniques. The indications for TIPS include bleeding refractory to endoscopic and medical management, refractory ascities, Budd–Chiari syndrome, and hepatorenal syndromes. The stent is expanded to a diameter that reduces the portosytemic gradient to less than 12 mm Hg. TIPS is associated with postprocedure encephalopathy rates of approximately 25%, and patients with renal insufficiency are at risk for worsened renal function. The long-term problem with TIPS is stenosis of the shunt, which is reported in as many as two-thirds of patients. Most centers advocate an aggressive Doppler ultrasound monitoring program with prompt balloon dilation for identified stenosis of the stent.

Answers: D

Boyer TD, Haskal ZJ, American Association for the Study of Liver Diseases (2010) The role of transjugular intrahepatic portosystemp shunt (TIPS) in the management of portal hypertension: update 2009. *Hepatology* **51**, 306.

Mulholland MW, Lillemoe KD, Doherty G *et al.* (2010) *Greenfield's Surgery: Scientific Principles and Practice*, Lippincott Williams & Wilkins, Philadelphia, PA.

5. *Appropriate treatments in a patient with hepatic encephalopathy include all of the following except?*

A. *Limiting dietary protein*

B. *Construction of a side-to-side portocaval shunt*

C. *Addition of glucose to the diet*

D. *Administration of lactulose*

E. *Control of any active bleeding*

Hepatic encephalopathy has been related to hyperammonemia with ammonia intoxication. Ammonia is produced when intestinal bacteria break down blood in the gastrointestinal tract. Active bleeding should be controlled and dietary protein should be limited to reduce protein load to the liver. Prolonged restriction of protein intake should be considered with caution because of protein-calorie malnutrition that is common in these patients. There may be benefit to administering relatively higher levels of branch-chain amino acids with minimized aromatic amino acids. Glucose in the diet inhibits ammonia production by bacteria. Lactulose acts as a mild cathartic, and its breakdown products acidify the luminal contents in the colon and thereby decrease production of ammonia by intestinal bacteria and interfere with transfer of ammonia across the colonic mucosa. Portosystemic shunts interfere with ammonia metabolism in the liver. Side-to-side shunts are indicated when the patient has hepatic venous outflow obstruction.

Answer: B

Cameron, J (2008) *Current Surgical Therapy*, 9th edn, Mosby, New York.

Mulholland MW, Lillemoe KD, Doherty G *et al.* (2010) *Greenfield's Surgery: Scientific Principles and Practice*, Lippincott Williams & Wilkins, Philadelphia, PA.

6. *Which of the following statements is true regarding spontaneous bacterial peritonitis?*

A. *Infection is most commonly polymicrobial*

B. *Diagnosis can be made clinically without paracentesis*

C. *Antibiotic therapy is reserved for patients with positive ascitic fluid cultures*

D. *Gram-negative enteric bacteria are often present.*

E. *Diagnosis is established by elevated ascitic fluid absolute polymorphonuclear leukocyte count (PMN) > 100 cells/mm*^{3}

The diagnosis of spontaneous bacterial peritonitis is established by a positive ascitic fluid bacterial culture and an elevated ascitic fluid absolute polymorphonuclear leukocyte (PMN) count ($\geq$250 cells/mm^3). Spontaneous bacterial peritonitis is a lethal complication of ascites that affects about 10% of patients with cirrhotic ascities. Fever and abdominal pain are common manifestations. Antibiotic therapy should be instituted promptly based on elevated ascitic fluid PMN count or on symptoms even if the PMN count is lower. The infection is usually from one organism and most commonly *Escherichia coli,* or Klebsiella. Initial therapy is usually a third-generation cephalosporin. Secondary bacterial peritonitis is usually a polymicrobial infection that rarely responds to antibiotics without an operative or radiologic intervention.

Answer: D

Brunicardi F, Andersen D, Billiar T (2010) *Schwartz's Principles of Surgery*. 9th edn, McGraw-Hill, New York.

Runyon BA, AASLD Practice Guidelines Committee (2009) Management of adult patients with ascites due to cirrhosis: an update. *Hepatology* **49**, 2087.

7. *Which of the following is appropriate for prevention of variceal hemorrhage in a patient with varices that have never bled?*

A. Endoscopic sclerosis

B. TIPS

C. Surgical selective shunt

D. Propranolol

E. Inhaled vasopressin

Of the currently available therapies most studies show some decrease in the incidence of bleeding with prophylactic propranolol. Endoscopic sclerotherapy as prohpholaxis has not yielded consistent benefit and may be detrimental to some patients. Surgical therapy in the form of portacaval shunts as prophylaxis showed a decreased risk of bleeding in operated patients but an increased risk of hepatic failure and encephalopathy and decreased survival.

Answer: D

Cameron, J (2008) *Current Surgical Therapy,* 9th edn, Mosby, New York.

D'Amico G, Criscuoli V, Fili D, Mocciaro F, Pagliaro L (2002) Meta-analysis of trials for variceal bleeding. *Hepatology* **36**, 1023.

8. *A 65-year-old man with a model for end-stage liver disease (MELD) score of 15 has intractable ascites and esophageal varices. Which of the following is the best treatment for the ascites?*

A. Surgical side- to-side portacaval shunt

B. Surgical end-to-side portacaval shunt

C. Transjugular intrahepatic portosystemic shunt (TIPS)

D. Peritoneovenous shunt

E. Distal splenorenal shunt

Medically intractable ascites occurs in 10% of patients with cirrhosis and ascites. The only definitive therapeutic option is liver transplantation. TIPS is effectively a side-to-side portacaval shunt placed through the right internal jugular vein under local anesthesia. TIPS has been shown to lead to an increase in urine output and a marked or complete reduction in ascites. A peritoneovenous shunt that drains into the internal jugular vein, reinfuses ascites into the vascular space. However, this procedure has been virtually abandoned due to an excessive rate of complications. Surgical shunts are not indicated for the treatment of ascites alone in a patient who has not had bleeding varices. Surgical shunts for ascites require a nonselective, side-to-side arrangement; therefore an end-to-side portacaval or distal splenorenal shunt are contraindicated. Shunt surgery has been associated with a high morbidity and mortality.

Answer: C

Cameron, J (2008) *Current Surgical Therapy,* 9th edn, Mosby, New York.

Ochs A, Rössle M, Haag K, *et al.* (1995) The transjugular intrahepatic portosystemic stent-shunt procedure for refractory ascites. *New England Journal of Medicine* **332**, 1192.

9. *A 60-year-old man with liver cirrhosis secondary to alcohol abuse presents to the emergency room with hematemesis and lightheadedness. The patient still drinks alcohol and appears cachectic and pale. On examination the patient has significant ascites and large collateral veins on the abdominal wall. Stool is guaiac positive. The patient has two large-bore IVs placed and aggressive hydration is started. He is also treated with IV famotidine and an IV octreotide drip. The patient continues to* *have hematemesis and is intubated for airway protection. Which of the following statements is most correct regarding management of this patient?*

A. *If emergent endoscopy is not immediately available, esophageal balloon tamponade is indicated*

B. *Immediate angiogram with possible embolization needs to be performed*

C. *Sclerotherapy and esophageal balloon tamponade have comparable efficacy in controlling esophageal bleeding*

D. *Transfusion of fresh frozen plasma is indicated prior to procedural interventions*

E. *Patient should be aggressively resuscitated with crystalloids and blood transfusions, pending an endoscopy and anatomic diagnosis of bleeding*

The patient should be resuscitated with aggressive crystalloid resuscitation and the transfusion of blood products as needed. Once this is accomplished, or if the patient has persistent bleeding, emergent endoscopy should be performed in order to establish a diagnosis and attempt hemostasis of bleeding lesion. An esophageal balloon tamponade with a Sengstaken–Blakemore or Minnesota tube is indicated in cases of confirmed esophageal variceal hemorrhage in which endoscopy therapy is unavailable, technically not feasible or unsuccessful. Placement of an esophageal balloon should not be performed without anatomical diagnosis. Although the patient in this case is at high risk for esophageal variceal hemorrhage, severe gastrointestinal bleeding in patients with signs of chronic liver disease can result from other causes in up to 35% of cases. Endoscopic therapy with sclerotherapy or banding has been demonstrated to be more effective than an esophageal balloon tamponade in treating acute esophageal variceal hemorrhage. Without documentation of coagulopathy, there is no reason to transfuse fresh frozen plasma in this patient.

Answer: E

Cameron, J (2008) *Current Surgical Therapy*, 9th edn, Mosby, New York.

D'Amico G, Criscuoli V, Fili D *et al.* (2002) Meta-analysis of trials for variceal bleeding. *Hepatology* **36**, 1023.

10. *A 25-year-old woman is brought to the hospital by family members after being found unresponsive. The patient has no significant past medical history, however the family reports that she has been depressed. The patient is lethargic, and has mild diffuse abdominal tenderness, with no guarding and decreased bowel sounds. Laboratory data are significant for: alanine amino transferase 3800 U/L, aspartate aminotransferase 4300 U/L, total bilirubin 7.5 mg/dL, and INR of 2.5. Which of the following is the most likely to result in mortality in this patient?*

A. *Uncontrolled bleeding*

B. *Septic shock*

C. *Brain edema*

D. *Respiratory failure*

E. *Acute myocardial infarction*

The patient presents with a clinical picture that is consistent with fulminant liver failure (FLF). Acute liver failure (ALF) is defined as a rapid deterioration of hepatic function, manifested by an increase in prothrombin time (PT) and a decrease of factor V, without evidence of hepatic encephalopathy. Fulminant hepatic failure involves severe, acute liver dysfunction complicated by hepatic encephalopathy in a patient with no previous liver disease. Usually one of the first findings of liver failure is jaundice. The onset of hepatic encephalopathy is less than two weeks. The most common cause of ALF and FHF in the USA is acetaminophen toxicity. Complications related to ALF and FHF include coagulopathy, cerebral edema and intracranial hypertension, acute portal hypertension, renal failure, infections, and multiple organ failure. The most common cause of death in patients with FHF is cerebral edema leading to increased intracranial pressure and herniation. The care for patients with FHF and ACF is supportive along with management of the underlying cause, if possible. It is important to identify patients at higher risk of death for rapid referral to transplant centers, since, in most patients, liver transplant is the only curative therapeutic modality.

Answer: C

Kulkarni S, Cronin DC (2005) Fulminant hepatic failure. In: Hall JB, Schmidt GA, Wood LDH (eds) *Principles of Critical Care*, 3rd edn, McGraw-Hill Co., New York.

11. *All of the following regarding acetominophen toxicity are true except:*

A. *Toxicty in adults is likely to occur with single ingestion greater than 250 mg/kg or 12 g over a 24-hour period*

B. *Doses greater than 350 mg/kg cause severe liver toxicity*

C. *Acute alcohol ingestion is an additional risk factor for hepatotoxicity*

D. *The initial manifestations of acetominophen poisoning are often mild and nonspecific*

E. *A serum acetaminophen level must be obtained in every patient suspected of overdose*

Acute alcohol ingestion is not a risk factor for hepatotoxicity and may even be protective by competing with acetaminophen for metabolism of the cytochrome p450 enzymes, reducing the amount of toxic metabolite produced (N-acetyl-p-benzoquinoneimine (NAPQI)). Toxicity is likely to occur with single ingestions greater than 250 mg/kg or those greater than 12 g over a 24-hour period for adults. Virtually all patients who ingest doses in excess of 350 mg/kg develop severe liver toxicity (defined as peak aspartate aminotransferase (AST) or alanine aminotransferase (ALT) levels greater than 1000 IU/L) unless appropriately treated. Acetaminophen is rapidly and completely absorbed from the gastrointestinal tract. Serum concentrations peak between one-half and two hours after an oral therapeutic dose. All patients with a clear history of acetaminophen overdose should undergo measurement of serum acetaminophen concentration. If any doubt exists about the time of ingestion, a serum concentration should be obtained immediately at the time of presentation. A serum concentration should also be obtained four hours following the time of acute ingestion or presentation.

Answer: C

Lee WM (2003) Drug-induced hepatotoxicity. *New England Journal of Medicine* **349**, 474.

12. *Which of the following is true regarding the clinical manifestations of acute acetaminophen intoxication?*

A. *Laboratory studies are typically elevated within 8 hours of ingestion of acetaminophen*

B. *Liver function abnormalities peak from 24 to 36 hours*

C. *Patients who develop hepatic injury usually demonstrate elevation of aminotransferase*

D. *Acute renal failure rarely occurs as a result of acetaminophen toxicity*

E. *Chronic hepatic dysfunction is a common sequel of acetaminophen poisoning*

The clinical course of acetaminophen poisoning is often divided into four sequential stages. Stage I: In the first 24 hours after overdose, patients often manifest nausea, vomiting, diaphoresis, pallor, lethargy, and malaise. Some patients remain asymptomatic. Laboratory studies are typically normal. Stage II: from 24 to 72 hours after ingestion, the clinical and laboratory evidence of hepatotoxicity and, occasionally, nephrotoxicity become evident. Of patients that develop hepatic injury, over one half will demonstrate aminotransferase elevation within 24 hours and all have elevations by 36 hours. Stage III: liver function abnormalities peak from 72 to 96 hours after ingestion. The systemic symptoms of stage I reappear in conjunction with jaundice, confusion (hepatic encephalopathy), a marked elevation in hepatic enzymes, hyperammonemia, and a bleeding diathesis. Acute renal failure occurs in 25% of patients with significant hepatotoxicity and in more than 50% of those with frank hepatic failure. Stage IV patients who survive stage III enter a recovery phase that usually begins by day 4 and is complete by 7 days after overdose. It is notable that chronic hepatic dysfunction is not typically a sequel in survivors of acetaminophen poisoning.

Acetylcysteine is the accepted treatment for acetaminophen poisoning and is given to all patients at significant risk for hepatotoxicity. Some recommend administering acetylcysteine for all patients with fulminant hepatic failure, even if not caused by acetaminophen toxicity.

Answer: C

Rowden AK, Norvell J, Eldridge DL, Kirk MA (2005) Updates on acetaminophen toxicity. *Medical Clinics of North America* **89**, 1145–59.

Chapter 18 Nutrition

Rifat Latifi, MD, FACS

1. *Which of the following is true?*

A. *The stress response is divided into the ebb, catabolic flow, and anabolic flow phases*

B. *The ebb phase is dominated by catabolism, typically lasts 3 to 10 days*

C. *The catabolic flow phase is dominated by circulatory changes that require resuscitation over 8 to 24 hours*

D. *The acute phase should be treated with blood and blood products*

E. *In the catabolic phase metabolism shifts to synthetic activities and reparative processes*

The response to stress and injury consist of three phases: the ebb phase, the catabolic flow phase, and the anabolic flow phase. Each of these phases has distinct changes that require specific interventions in order to eliminate or minimize the consequences of illness and/or injury. The ebb phase is dominated by circulatory changes that require resuscitation (with fluid, blood, and blood products) over a period of 8 to 24 hours. The catabolic flow phase, dominated by catabolism, typically lasts 3 to 10 days but may last longer. The anabolic flow phase emerges as the patient's metabolism shifts to synthetic activities and reparative processes. The catabolic flow phase is driven by cytokine mediators released from lymphocytes and macrophages in the cellular immune reaction, dominated by interleukin-6 (IL-6). The release of these mediators is proportional to the intensity of the injury but the release of cytokines themselves is upregulated by hormonal and humoral events. The early nonspecific response to systemic tissue injury that is responsible for the reprioritization of protein synthesis in the liver is termed the acute phase response (APR). Depending on the magnitude and the severity of the injury, APR is characterized by an exponential increase in positive acute phase proteins and a decrease in negative acute phase proteins. The regulation of APR, a complex process, depends on many factors. Tissue injury or infection leads to a local inflammatory response, which in turn leads to the release of many cytokines at the site of inflammation; the cytokines are eventually carried to the liver, where they act on the hepatocytes. Crystalloids, blood and blood products may be required for the initial resuscitation based on the severity and the magnitude of the injury.

Answer: A

Azimuddin, K, Latifi R, Ivatury R (2003) Acute Phase Proteins in Critically Ill Patients. In: Latifi R., Dudrick SJ (eds) *The Biology and Practice of Current Nutritional Support*, 2nd edn, Landes Bioscience, Austin TX.

Hill AG, Hill GL (1998) Metabolic response to severe injury. *British Journal of Surgery* **85**, 884–90.

2. *Which of the following is true?*

A. *IL-1, IL-6, and TNF are all implicated in the production of acute phase proteins*

B. *IL-1 and IL-6 effect the gastrointestinal tract and have no effect on APP*

C. *IL-12 has no effect on Th1-mediated inflammatory responses*

D. *IL-1 is not implicated in the production of acute phase proteins*

E. *IL-6 effects APP but do not affect the gastrointestinal tract*

The catabolic flow phase is driven by cytokine mediators released by lymphocytes and macrophages in the cellular immune reaction, dominated by interleukin-6 (IL-6). The release of these mediators is proportionate to the amount

Surgical Critical Care and Emergency Surgery: Clinical Questions and Answers, First Edition. Edited by Forrest O. Moore, Peter M. Rhee, Samuel A. Tisherman and Gerard J. Fulda.

of the injury. The release of cytokines is linked to upregulation of hormonal and humoral events. The hormonal events include the release of glucagon and catecholamines, thyroid hormone, growth hormone, and cortisol, and their effects—hyperglycemia, metabolic rate, release of free fatty acids and associated ketosis, insulin growth factor 1 (IGF1), and negative nitrogen balance from gluconeogenesis. A variety of cytokines have been implicated in the production of acute phase proteins from the liver, including interleukin 1 and 6 (IL-1, IL-6) and tumor necrosis factor-alpha (TNF). Interleukin-12 is a key cytokine that initiates Th1-mediated inflammatory responses. This pattern is predictable and reproducible. First, the serum concentration decreases for most of the acute phase proteins, both for positive and for negative reactants. Later, the hepatic synthesis of negative acute phase proteins decreases, and the concentration of serum albumin remains depressed for days to weeks after the injury. Albumin reaches the lowest point by the 5th post-injury day. Whether nutritional support in the immediate post-injury phase can alter or blunt the acute phase response has not been adequately answered.

Answer: A

Ingenbleek Y, Bernstein L (1999) The stressful condition as a nutritionally dependent adaptive dichotomy. *Nutrition* **15**, 305–20.

Issihiki H, Akira S, Sugita T, *et al.* (1991)Reciprocal expression of NF-IL6 and C/EBP in hepatocytes: possible involvement of NF-IL6 in acute phase protein gene expression. *New Biologist* **3** (1), 63–70.

3. *Glutamine is:*

A. *An essential amino acid which cannot be synthesized in sufficient quantities during periods of stress*

B. *Involved in immune functions, but not the production of heat shock proteins*

C. *Associated with a decrease in gram-negative bacteremia with parental administration*

D. *Contraindicated in critically ill patients*

E. *Classified as a branch-chain-amino acids and should be given to patients with liver failure*

Glutamine is an amino acid that serves as the primary fuel for small bowel enterocytes and other rapidly proliferating cells, such as cells in wounds. It is classified as a nonessential amino acid because the human body can synthesize it in sufficient quantities. Yet, during periods of stress, the body's requirements may exceed its capacity to synthesize glutamine. Glutamine is involved in many immune functions, including the production of heat shock proteins. Studies have shown that supplementation with glutamine may lead to a decrease in nosocomial infections in patients with systemic inflammatory response and a decrease in pneumonia, sepsis, and bacteremia in trauma patients. Parenterally administered glutamine has been associated with a decrease in gram-negative bacteremia. Thus, the addition of glutamine to enteral nutrition has been recommended for burn, trauma, and other intensive care unit (ICU) patients.

Answer: C

McClave SA, Martindale RG, Vanek VW, *et al.* (2009) Guidelines for the Provision and Assessment of Nutrition Support Therapy in the Adult Critically Ill Patient: Society of Critical Care Medicine (SCCM) and American Society for Parenteral and Enteral Nutrition (A.S.P.E.N.). *Journal of Parenteral and Enteral Nutrition* **33** (3), 277–316.

Ziegler TR, Ogden LG, Singleton KD, *et al.* (2005) Parenteral glutamine increases serum heat shock protein 70 in critically ill patients. *Intensive Care Medicine* **31** (8), 1079–86.

4. *Which of the following is true regarding prealbumin, retinol-binding protein, and transferrin?*

A. *They are all negative acute phase proteins*

B. *They are all positive acute phase proteins*

C. *Prealbumin and transferrin and are negative acute phase protein, but retinol-binding protein is a positive acute phase protein*

D. *Negative acute phase proteins increase with stress or injury*

E. *Prealbumin and retinol binding protein are positive acute phase protein, while transferrin is negative acute phase protein*

Positive acute-phase proteins seem to be a protective response to tissue injury. They have diverse functions as antioxidants, proteolytic inhibitors, and mediators of coagulation. The negative acute phase proteins are albumin, prealbumin, retinol-binding protein, and transferrin. Their serum concentrations fall immediately after the injury, in proportion to its severity. They are used to monitor the nutritional status of acutely ill patients. Continued and prolonged production of acute phase proteins in critically ill patients may be an indicator of ongoing sepsis and tissue damage and is associated with higher mortality rates. Perhaps some of the changes at this stage are responsible for what is defined as compensatory anti-inflammatory response syndrome (CARS).

Answer: A

Ward NS, Casserly B, Ayala A (2008) The Compensatory Anti-inflammatory Response Syndrome (CARS) in critically ill patients. *Clinical Chest Medicine* **29** (4), 617–27.

5. *Significant muscle losses, negative nitrogen balance, increased nutriment requirements and redistribution of amino acids from peripheral tissue to splanchnic organs is noted:*

A. *During daily hemodialysis*

B. *In critically ill patients*

C. *Only after liver transplantation*

D. *Only in severe burns*

E. *Only in bowel ischemia*

Severely injured and critically ill patients characteristically demonstrate significant muscle losses, negative nitrogen balance, increased requirements two to three times, and redistribution of amino acids from peripheral tissues to splanchnic organs. Metabolic response to injury is the striking increase in protein catabolism. Skeletal muscle and nitrogen losses following injury occur as well. The process of increased nitrogen losses is complex and correlates with increased metabolic rate, which peaks several days after injury and gradually returns towards normal over several weeks. This phenomenon occurs consistently following major surgery, blunt injury, burns, sepsis and various other major injuries. This results in mobilization and increased utilization of nutrient substrates such as fatty acids, amino acids and glucose. An increased muscle protein catabolism following injury has been demonstrated. Although plasma amino acid levels have been measured in critically ill and injured patients in an effort to identify specific changes related to the catabolic response, the results have been inconsistent. Nonetheless, the adverse consequences for the critically ill patient are a rapid loss of muscle mass and subsequent marked debility. All amino acids are required for optimal protein synthesis; however, alanine and glutamine are the major carriers of nitrogen from muscle, constituting as much as 70% of the amino acids released from skeletal muscle following injury.

Answer: B

Essen P, McNurlan MA, Gamrin L, *et al.* (1998) Tissue protein synthesis rates in critically ill patients. *Critical Care Medicine* **26**, 92–100.

Latifi R, Dudrick SJ (eds) (1995) *Surgical Nutrition: Strategies in Critically Ill,* Springer-Verlag/RG Landes, Austin TX.

6. *Protein synthesis:*

A. *Occurs on the surface of ribosome, or multiprotein, multi-RNA complexes that provides the enzyme, peptidyl-transferase*

B. *Has four steps: initiation, elongation, rotation, and termination.*

C. *Ribosomes moves from the 3′-end to the 5′-end of the mRNA that is being translated*

D. *Final step occurs in response to termination signals, after the final amino acid residue is placed at the amino terminal of the newly synthesized protein*

E. *Is called transcription*

Protein synthesis occurs on the surface of ribosome, or multiprotein, multi-RNA complexes that provide the enzyme, peptidyl-transferase. Peptidyl-transferase is one of many proteins of the larger ribosomal subunit and is imbedded in the surface of the subunit. It catalyzes peptide bond formation and covalent linkage of one amino acid residue to another. The process of protein synthesis itself is called "translation," because the "language" of the nucleotide sequence on the mRNA is translated into the language of an amino acid sequence. The mRNA is translated from its 5′-end to its 3′-end producing a protein synthesized from its amino-terminal end to its carboxyl-terminal end. The direction of translation is precisely defined, with the amino terminal of the evolving protein being synthesized first and the carboxyl terminal synthesized last. The polypeptide chains produced by translation may be modified further after translation. Protein synthesis has *three* steps: initiation, elongation, and termination. Initiation involves assembly of the components of the translational system before the peptide bonds are formed. The termination, as the final step of protein synthesis, occurs in response to termination signals, after the final amino acid residue is placed at the carboxyl terminal of the newly synthesized protein.

Answer: A

Latifi, R, Dudrick SJ (1993) Amino Acids in Critically Ill and Cancer Patients, RG Landes, Austin TX.

7. *Arginine:*

A. *Levels are increased in trauma and critical care patients*

B. *Is found in TPN*

C. *And glutamine are present only in immune-modulating enteral diets*

D. *And glutamine are present in only immune-enhancing diets*

E. *None of the above are true*

Arginine is a semi or conditionally essential amino acid, and its requirements are increased during sepsis and tissue injury. Through its role in the urea cycle, arginine takes part in the synthesis of other amino acids, urea and nitric oxide. Arginine is important for cell mediated immunity. It is required for the growth and function of T lymphocytes in cultures. *In vivo,* arginine retards thymic involution by encouraging production of thymic hormones and thymocyte proliferation. Arginine also promotes leukocyte-mediated cytotoxicity. Growth hormone receptors are widely distributed in the immune system, and by releasing growth hormone, arginine may increase the cytotoxic activity of macrophages, neutrophils, NK cells and cytotoxic T cells. Furthermore, nitric oxide, a product of arginine metabolism, has important tumoricidal, antimicrobial and inflammatory activities.

Glutamine is the most abundant amino acid in blood and in the body's free amino acid pool. Lymphocytes and macrophages use glutamine as a source of energy. After entering the cell, glutamine is converted to glutamate and ammonia by the action of glutaminase in the inner mitochondrial membrane. Further processing results in production of aspartate and oxidation of about 25% of glutamine to carbon dioxide. This "glutaminolysis" pathway works in conjunction with the glycolytic pathway to allow the combined use of glucose and glutamine as an energy source for macrophages and lymphocytes. Thus, a relative deficiency of glutamine stores that occurs during critical illness is likely to lead to poor immune responses. Both arginine and glutamine are present in large quantities in immune-modulating formulas (example Oxepa) and immune-enhancing formulas (Impact and others). Neither of them is part of current TPN formulas.

Answer: E

Latifi R, Dudrick SJ (eds) (1995) *Surgical Nutrition: Strategies in Critically Ill,* Springer-Verlag/RG Landes, Austin TX.

8. *TPN is indicated in which of the following clinical scenario:*

A. *All critically ill patients with open abdomen admitted to the intensive critical care unit*

B. *Only those patients who cannot eat within ten days of hospitalization*

C. *High output eneterocutaneous fistulas*

D. *Patients with acute pancreatitis*

E. *First phase of management of short gut syndrome*

The general indications for the use of TPN are: 1. provision of adequate nutrition for as long as necessary intravenously when use of the gastrointestinal tract is impractical, inadequate, ill-advised, or impossible; 2. reduction of mechanical and secretory activity of the alimentary tract to basal levels in order to achieve a state of "bowel rest"; provision of specially tailored formulas to improve nutritional status in patients with kidney or liver failure; and 4. reduction of the urgency for surgical intervention in patients who might eventually require operation, but in whom prolonged, progressive malnutrition will greatly increase the risk of operation and postoperative complications. TPN efficacy has been demonstrated clearly in many pathophysiologic conditions including short-gut syndrome, fistulas, severe inflammatory bowel disease, severe acute hemorrhagic pancreatitis, chemotherapy and radiation induced enteritis, transplant patients and severely malnourished cancer patients in their perioperative management, when provision of nutrition enterally is not possible. Other conditions in which TPN is indicated but in which its efficacy has not been clearly demonstrated in the literature include acute exacerbations of chronic pancreatitis, anorexia nervosa, cardiac cachexia, hyperemesis gravidarum, chronic protein losses and cancer patients with mild malnutrition. In general, when GI tract cannot be used for more than five days in patients in a catabolic state with or without evidence of malnutrition, or when patients cannot be fed for more than 4–5 days after major surgery, parenteral nutrition should be started. Areas of intense clinical investigation in which TPN may eventually be shown to be of great value are cancer patients in general, sepsis and trauma, and general perioperative support to prevent or correct malnutrition. Answer A is incorrect, as it has been clearly demonstrated that patients with open abdomen can be fed enterally successfully. Patients who cannot eat, should not eat, or cannot eat for more than 3–5 days should be started on TPN or peripheral parenteral nutrition. One should not wait 7 to 10 days to start TPN. Patients with acute pancreatitis may be fed enterally. TPN should be reserved for only those patients who have severe hemorrhagic acute pancreatitis complicated with severe ileus and potentially fistulas. Short-gut syndrome patients should be supported with TPN. The length of TPN depends on the patient's condition; however, most patients eventually will be able to eat. If they cannot meet caloric requirements, than TPN is given to support oral intake, usually at night.

Answer: C

Dudrick SJ, Latifi R (1992) Total parenteral nutrition: current status. *Contemporary Surgery* **41**, 41–8.

Joseph, B, Kulvatunyou, K, Tang, A, *et al.* (2011) Total parenteral nutrition in critically ill and injured patients. European Surgery **43** (1), 19–23.

9. *Which of the following statement about TPN are true?*

A. Dr Stanley Dudrick described the growth of intravenously fed mice that experienced normal weight gain and normal growth, as compared with their orally fed counterparts.

B. Early nutritional support via TPN has the potential to reduce disease severity, diminish complications, and decrease the intensive care unit (ICU) length of stay.

C. TPN cannot give clinicians the ability to parenterally fulfill patients' ongoing requirement for calories, protein, electrolytes, vitamins, minerals, trace elements, and fluids.

D. The rate of TPN use in the critical care setting has increased in recent years.

E. TPN is imperative in all critically ill patients.

In 1967 Dudrick *et al.* described the growth of intravenously fed beagle puppies that experienced normal weight gain and normal growth, as compared with their orally fed counterparts. Early nutritional support via TPN has the potential to reduce disease severity, diminish complications, and decrease the length of stay in the intensive care unit (ICU). When enteral nutrition is not possible, TPN gives clinicians the ability to fulfill patients' ongoing requirement for calories, protein, electrolytes, vitamins, minerals, trace elements, and fluids parenterally. TPN use has been studied in patients with a wide array of clinical conditions, such as trauma, cancer, inflammatory bowel disease, short gut syndrome, radiation enteritis, poor wound healing, and gastrointestinal (GI) fistula. Yet few well-designed, randomized, controlled trials of the efficacy of TPN in critically ill and injured patients have been conducted. It is well known that 20% to 40% of critically ill and injured patients exhibit some form of malnutrition. Of that subgroup, 85% to 90% can be treated with enteral nutrition. In the remaining 10% to 15%, enteral nutrition is contraindicated; TPN, delivered intravenously, provides the only support. Many interacting biologic and clinical factors are responsible for the development of malnutrition in critically ill and injured hospitalized patients, including a history of pre-injury or disease-specific causes, the hypercatabolic states associated with trauma, sepsis, cancer, and surgical interventions. Although a recent Review by Rhee *et al.* showed that the rate of TPN use in the critical care setting has declined, intensivists continue to encounter many cases where enteral feeding fails and TPN is imperative.

Answer: B

Heyland DK, Dhaliwal R, Drover JW, *et al.* (2003) Canadian clinical practice guidelines for nutrition support in mechanically ventilated critically ill adult patients. *Journal of Parenteral and Enteral Nutrition* **27**, 355.

Ziegler, T (2009) Parenteral nutrition in the critically ill patient. *New England Journal of Medicine* **361**, 1088–97.

10. *Which of the following is true regarding lipid use in critically ill patients?*

A. *Lipid emulsions should be avoided in critically ill patients in the first week of ICU stay*

B. *Essential fatty acid deficiency occurs when patients do not receive lipids in the first seven days*

C. *Omega-3 and not omega-6 fatty acid are currently used in TPN formulas*

D. *There is no reliable biochemical test to diagnose fatty acid deficiency*

E. *None of the above is true*

The nature of the lipids that should be administered is currently the focus of much debate; so is the question of whether or not such innovations as structured lipids and triglycerides of varying chain lengths are of any benefit. A study by Dudrick *et al.* proved that the fear of essential fatty acid deficiency, if fatty emulsions are not given to critically ill and injured patients, is unfounded. In that study, designed to arrest and eliminate atherosclerotic plaque formation in patients with severe heart disease, TPN was administered, with no lipids, for 3 months. None of the patients on TPN without lipids developed fatty acid deficiency, as measured by the triene: tetraene ratio and by clinical examinations. A subsequent study found that trauma patients on TPN with no lipids had better clinical outcomes than patients on TPN with lipids. The latest guidelines of the American Society for Parenteral and Enteral Nutrition call for no fat in the first week in the ICU. Until intravenous omega-3 fatty acids become available everywhere, we should be very cautious when using fat emulsions in critically ill and injured patients because the effect may actually be detrimental.

Answer: A

McClave SA, Martindale RG, Vanek VW, *et al.* (2009) Guidelines for the Provision and Assessment of Nutrition Support Therapy in the Adult Critically Ill Patient: Society of Critical Care Medicine (SCCM) and American Society for Parenteral and Enteral Nutrition (ASPEN). *Journal of Parenter and Enteral Nutrition* **33** (3), 277–316.

Schneider P (2006) Nutrition support teams: an evidence-based practice. *Nutrition in Clinical Practice* **21**, 62.

11. *Branched-chain amino acids:*

A. *Are contraindicated in liver failure*

B. *Should not be used in critically ill patients*

C. *Are contraindicated in sepsis*

D. *Should be used in 3% concentration*

E. *Are not recommended in sepsis*

After injury and sepsis, an energy deficit that may develop in skeletal muscle is met by increased oxidation of branched-chain amino acids (BCAAs). Evidence indicates that skeletal muscle is the major site of BCAA degradation. A recent study demonstrated that critically ill patients who were unable to be fed enterally but who were given total parenteral nutrition (TPN) fortified with BCAAs at high concentration (at either 23% or 45%) had significantly lower morbidity and mortality, as compared with patients on standard TPN (1.5 g/kg/day of protein). The decrease in mortality correlated with higher doses of BCAAs (at 0.5 g/kg/day or higher). Furthermore, BCAA-rich parenteral nutrition formulas have been shown to correct the plasma amino acid imbalance that consistently exists in critically ill patients. Such formulas also improve plasma concentrations of prealbumin and retinol- binding protein in septic patients. In a series of trauma patients, BCAA supplementation improved nitrogen retention, transferrin levels, and lymphocyte counts. Since the concentration of BCAAs is low in septic patients, probably as a result of overuse of BCAAs, supplementation with BCAAs may be beneficial. Despite few studies showing benefit in sepsis, there are no recommendations for use of BCAA in sepsis.

Answer: E

Calder PC (2006) Branched-chain amino acids and immunity. *Journal of Nutrition* **136** (1 Suppl), 288S–293S.

García-de-Lorenzo A, Ortíz-Leyba C, Planas M *et al.* (1997) Parenteral administration of different amounts of branch-chain amino acids in septic patients: clinical and metabolic aspects. Critical Care Medicine **25** (3), 418–24.

12. *Critically ill patients who fulfill all ARDS criteria should:*

A. *Not be fed enterally due to the risk of aspiration*

B. *Be placed on TPN until extubated*

C. *Be kept NPO as long as they are on high PEEP*

D. *Be given immune-enhancing formulas*

E. *Be given immune-modulating formulas*

Immunonutrition has gained wider use in the care of critically ill and injured patients. This trend follows an increasing body of literature supporting the idea that different substrates will enhance a depressed immune system (immune-enhancing formulas) or modulate an over-reactive one (immune-modulating formulas). Although the biologic properties of immune-enhancing nutritional substrates have been well studied, their role in routine clinical care is still controversial. Multiple meta-analyses have shown that immune-modulating formulations are associated with a reduction in ventilator days, in infectious morbidity, and in hospital length of stay, as compared with standard nutritional regimens.

For example, studies have shown that nutritional formulas containing medium-chain triglycerides (MCTs)—when given in a 1:1 LCT: MCT ratio—may be beneficial to septic patients with ARDS, as evidenced by changes in the venous admixture (Qva/Qt), in the mean pulmonary artery pressure (MPAP), and in the P/F ratio. Not only does a high-fat, low-carbohydrate nutritional regimen appear to be beneficial for patients in acute respiratory failure requiring ventilatory support, but the type of fatty acids provided may also have an effect on recovery. A prospective, multicenter, double-blinded, randomized, controlled trial involving 146 patients with ARDS first showed a benefit of the eicosapentaenoic acid, gamma-linolenic acid (EPA + GLA) + antioxidants diet on pulmonary neutrophils recruitment, gas exchange, mechanical ventilation requirements, length of ICU stay, and new organ failures. In that trial, patients in the two randomization arms received, for at least 4 to 7 days, either (1) an enteral compound with EPA + GLA or (2) an is nitrogenous is caloric standard diet. Subsequent studies by the same authors also showed a decrease in inflammatory mediators from bronchoalveolar lavage fluids (BALFs), namely, a decrease in IL-8 and in LTB_4, as well as an associated decrease in BALF neutrophils and protein permeability, suggesting a possible mechanism for the observed benefit. A subsequent single-center, prospective, randomized, controlled, unlabeled study expanded the criteria to include patients with ALI in addition to ARDS; oxygenation and lung compliance improved. Subsequently, another prospective, multicenter, double-blinded, randomized, controlled trial involving 165 patients showed a significant decrease in the 28-day mortality rate in patients with sepsis or septic shock requiring mechanical ventilation who received the EPA + GLA + antioxidants diet, as compared with the control group. Moreover, in patients on that diet vs. the control group, the number of ventilator-free days (13.4 versus 5.8 days) and ICU-free days

(10.8 versus 4.6 days) also increased, and new organ dysfunction significantly decreased.

Answer: E

Pontes-Arruda A, Aragao AM, Albuquerque JD (2006) Effects of enteral feeding with eicosapentaenoic acid, gamma-linolenic acid, and antioxidants in mechanically ventilated patients with severe sepsis and septic shock. *Critical Care Medicine* **34** (9), 2325–33.

Singer P, Theilla M, Fisher H, *et al.* (2006) Benefit of an enteral diet enriched with eicosapentaenoic acid and gamma-linolenic acid in ventilated patients with acute lung injury. *Critical Care Medicine* **34** (4), 1033–8.

13. *Immune-enhancing formulas are:*

A. *Contraindicated in trauma patients*

B. *Contraindicated in sepsis*

C. *Contraindicated in cancer*

D. *Expensive and not cost effective*

E. *Responsible for reduction in morbidity and septic and infectious complications*

Although it is difficult to isolate the precise impact of nutritional support, enteral formulas fortified with immune-enhancing substrates have been associated with a significant reduction in the risk of infectious complications and a reduction in overall hospital stay. It has been demonstrated that certain nutrients can modulate inflammatory, metabolic, and immune processes, while other can enhance the immune system. Amino acids such as arginine and glutamine improve body defenses and tumor cell metabolism, increase wound healing; and reduce nitrogen loss. RNA and omega-3 fatty acids also modulate the immune function. Immune-enhancing formulas have improved the immune response in burn, trauma, and surgical patients and have reduced infections, total complications, and length of stay. One prospective, blinded study found that an immune-enhancing enteral diet containing glutamine reduced septic complications in patients with severe trauma. Of 390 critically ill surgical and medical patients, 101 received early enteral nutrition (within 72 hours). Of those 101 patients, 50 received immune-enhancing diets and had significantly reduced requirements for mechanical ventilation and a shorter hospital stay, as compared with control patients. A recent prospective, double-blind, randomized trial of patients with major burns (>50% body surface) demonstrated that supplemental intravenous glutamine, infused continuously over 24 hours, was significantly better than just isonitrogenous amino acid solutions. According to a meta-analysis of 11 randomized controlled clinical trials of enteral nutrition with an immune-enhancing formula that included 1009 patients, nutritional support supplemented with key nutrients (arginine, glutamine, branched-chain amino acids, nucleotides, and omega-3 fatty acids) significantly reduced the risk of developing infectious complications and reduced the overall hospital stay in critically ill patients and in patients with GI cancer. A consensus panel from a recent conference on immune-enhancing enteral therapy recommended the use of immune-enhancing diets in the following 2 groups of patients: (1) severely malnourished patients (albumin <3.5 g/dL) undergoing upper GI surgery and patients with albumin <2.8 g/dL undergoing lower GI surgery and (2) patients with blunt or penetrating torso trauma with an injury severity score (ISS) >18 or an abdominal trauma index >20.

Answer: E

Fukuda T, Seto Y, Ymada K, *et al.* (2008) Can immune-enhancing nutrients reduce postoperative complications in patients undergoing esophageal surgery? Diseases of the Esophagus **21**, 708–11.

Giger U, Buchler M, Farhadi J, *et al.* (2007) Preoperative immunonutrition suppresses perioperative inflammatory response in patients with major abdominal surgery—a randomized controlled pilot study. *Annals of Surgical Oncology* **14** (10), 2798–806.

14. *Which statement is true about nucleotides in critically ill patients?*

A. *Are part of the standard TPN formula*

B. *Can be synthesized by T lymphocytes when stressed*

C. *Supplementation significantly decreases infections*

D. *Should be given only in combination with glutamine*

E. *Are present only in speciality TPN formulas*

Nucleotides are perhaps best known for their role in the synthesis of deoxyribonucleic acid (DNA) and ribonucleic acid (RNA) and, hence, for their role in genetic coding. However, nucleotides also play a role in adenosine triphosphate (ATP) metabolism; they are a part of many coenzymes involved in carbohydrate, protein, and lipid synthesis. Nucleotides may be synthesized by some cells. But it is believed that rapidly dividing cells, such as epithelial cells and T lymphocytes, are unable to produce nucleotides and that, during periods of stress, a relative deficit of nucleotides develops. Nucleotides have been implicated in the modulation of immune function. Exogenous nucleotides have been found to be needed for the helper/inducer T-cell response. In the clinical setting, IED containing nucleotides have been shown to significantly reduce infections, ventilator days, and length of hospital stay, for both critically ill and postsurgical patients. However, those studies have not addressed the isolated effects of nucleotides as a substrate, so further studies addressing them are needed. Nucleotides are not present in current TPN formulas.

Answer: C

Beale RJ, Bryg DJ, Bihari DJ (1999) Immunonutrition in the critically ill: a systematic review of clinical outcome. *Critical Care Medicine* **27** (12), 2799–805.

Grimble GK, Westwood OM (2001) Nucleotides as immunomodulators in clinical nutrition. *Current Opinion in Clinical Nutrition and Metabolic Care* **4** (1), 57–64.

Chapter 19 Neurocritical Care

Scott H. Norwood, MD, FACS and Herb A. Phelan, MD, FACS

1. *Intracranial hypertension immediately following blunt traumatic brain injury is most commonly a result of:*

A. *Epidural hematoma*

B. *Intracellular edema*

C. *Diffuse axonal injury*

D. *Vasogenic edema*

E. *Both intracellular edema and vasogenic edema*

The most common cause of intracranial hypertension following blunt traumatic brain injury is intracellular brain edema. Vasogenic edema, although occasionally present in the early stages, is not a common early cause, but may result in prolonged intracranial hypertension after about seven to ten days. Epidural hematomas and diffuse axonal injury by themselves are infrequent causes.

Answer: B

Marmarou A, Signoretti S, Fatourous P, *et al.* (2006) Predominance of cellular edema in traumatic brain swelling in patients with severe head injuries. *Journal of Neurosurgery* **104**, 720–30.

2. *Steroid therapy for blunt traumatic brain injury*

A. *Increases the chance of death from all causes*

B. *Reduces the mortality rate at two weeks post injury*

C. *Is associated with decreased infection rates*

D. *Must be started within 48 hours to be effective*

E. *Prevents late vasogenic edema if started within five days of injury*

Surgical Critical Care and Emergency Surgery: Clinical Questions and Answers, First Edition. Edited by Forrest O. Moore, Peter M. Rhee, Samuel A. Tisherman and Gerard J. Fulda.

A number of studies have consistently demonstrated no role for steroids in the management of acute traumatic brain injury. The MRC CRASH trial, published in 2004, was stopped after enrolling approximately 10 000 patients because of the clear increase in mortality from all causes in the group of patients receiving steroids. Higher infection rates were also reported. Steroids are still occasionally used to treat headaches that accompany concussion syndrome, but this is usually in the later stages of the injury and presumably reduces the mild vasogenic edema. The vasogenic edema associated with brain tumors are also treated with steroids on occasion with good symptomatic relief.

Answer: A

Bratton SL, Chestnut RM, Ghajar J, *et al.* (2007) XV. Steroids. Guidelines for the management of severe traumatic brain injury, 3rd edn. *Journal of Neurotrauma* **24**, S91–S95.

Edwards P, Arango M, Balica L, *et al.* (2005) Final results of MRC CRASH, a randomized placebo-controlled trial of intravenous corticosteroid in adults with head injury-outcomes at six months. *Lancet* **365**, 1957–9.

3. *The main objective of intracranial cerebral pressure monitoring following traumatic brain injury is to*

A. *Maintain cerebral perfusion pressure over >70 mm Hg*

B. *Maintain intracranial pressures <15 mm Hg*

C. *Maintain adequate cerebral perfusion and oxygenation to the non-injured brain tissue*

D. *Prevent secondary seizure development*

E. *Maintain cerebral perfusion pressure >55 mm Hg and intracranial pressure <10 mm Hg*

The primary objective of ICP monitoring is to maintain adequate brain tissue perfusion and oxygenation while simultaneously avoiding secondary brain injury while the injured portions of the brain are allowed to heal. Generally, treatment of the intracranial pressure should be initiated when the ICP increases >20 mm Hg. The ideal cerebral perfusion pressure currently is controversial, but lies somewhere between 50 to 70 mm Hg.

Answer: C

Bratton SL, Chestnut RM, Ghajar J, *et al.* (2007) VI. Indications for intracranial pressure monitoring. Guidelines for the management of severe traumatic brain injury, 3rd edn. *Journal of Neurotrauma* **24**, S37–S44.

Bratton SL, Chestnut RM, Ghajar J, *et al.* (2007) VII. Intracranial pressure thresholds. Guidelines for the Management of severe traumatic brain injury, 3rd edn. *Journal of Neurotrauma* **24**, S55–S59.

Bratton SL, Chestnut RM, Ghajar J, *et al.* (2007) IX. Cerebral perfusion thresholds. Guidelines for the management of severe traumatic brain injury, 3rd edn. *Journal of Neurotrauma* **24**, S59–S64.

4. *A 25-year-old man is admitted to the emergency department following a motor vehicle crash. He arrives comatose and intubated with a blood pressure of 140/85 mm Hg, heart rate of 100 beats per minute,* SpO_2 *of 100%, and breathing spontaneously at a rate of 14 breaths per minute. A CT scan of the brain confirms a right frontal intraparenchymal cerebral hematoma. Indications for immediate operative intervention include:*

A. *Midline shift of 3 mm on CT scan*

B. *A Glasgow Coma Scale Score of 12 (intubated) with the intracerebral hematoma volume measurement equal to 10 cm*^{3}

C. *A Glasgow Coma Scale Score of 7 (intubated) with a measured intracranial pressure of 8 mm Hg, a midline shift of 2 mm, and a mass lesion measuring 8 cm*^{3}

D. *A mass lesion on CT measuring over 50 cm*^{3}

E. *None of the above*

Patients with intraparenchymal hematomas are candidates for surgery if they develop signs of progressive neurological deterioration and the lesion is of sufficient size to warrant operative intervention. Patients with Glasgow Coma Scale Scores of 6 to 8 with frontal or temporal contusions greater than 20 cm^3 in volume with midline shift of at least 5 mm and/or cisternal compression on the CT scan, and patients with any lesion greater than 50 cm^3 in volume should generally be treated operatively. Patients with intraparenchymal mass lesions who do not show evidence of neurological compromise, have well controlled intracranial pressure, and no significant signs of mass effect on CT scan are generally managed nonoperatively with intensive monitoring and serial imaging.

Answer: D

Bullock MR, Chestnut R, Ghajar J, *et al.* (2006) Surgical management of traumatic parenchymal lesions. *Neurosurgery* **58**, S2 25–S2 46.

5. *A 37-year-old woman is admitted following a fall from a horse. Her initial Glasgow Coma Score prior to intubation is 8 and her vital signs are stable. A CT scan shows multiple small intraparenchymal hemorrhages in the frontal and temporal lobes with a small amount of subarachnoid hemorrhage in the right posterior parietal area. A ventriculostomy is inserted for intracranial pressure monitoring. Her initial intracranial pressure is 10 mm Hg. Approximately 30 hours following admission the patient's intracranial pressure increases to 25 mm Hg. There is no change in neurological examination. Initial management of the patient's change in intracranial pressure includes all of the following except:*

A. *Drainage of cerebral spinal fluid through the ventriculostomy*

B. *Immediate CT scan of the brain to rule out development of a mass lesion*

C. *Osmotic diuretics*

D. *Maintenance of normothermia*

E. *Hyperventilation to a* $PaCO_2$ *of 25 to 30 torr*

Initial management of an elevated intracranial pressure in a patient with a ventriculostomy should be drainage of cerebral spinal fluid. Additionally, an emergency CT scan should be obtained as soon as possible to rule out development of a mass lesion that might require operative intervention. Osmotic diuretics and maintenance of body temperature within normal limits are also appropriate. Hyperventilation is not usually recommended since it may result in ischemia to normal brain tissue. Generally, hyperventilation to this level is a last resort in patients who are showing obvious signs of impending cerebral herniation.

Answer: E

Valadka AB, Dannenbaum MJ (2008) pathophysiology, clinical diagnosis, and prehospital and emergency center care. Head and central nervous system injuries. In: Asensio J, Trunkey D (eds) *Current Therapy of Trauma and Surgical Critical Care,* Mosby Elsevier, Philadelphia, PA, pp. 147–52.

6. *Mannitol for osmotic therapy to reduce intracranial pressure*

A. *Should never be given prior to insertion of an intracranial pressure monitor*

B. *Is usually given at a dose of 0.1 g/kg*

C. *Should not be given if the serum osmolality is over 295 mosm/l*

D. *Works initially by creating osmotic gradients between blood plasma and brain cells, reducing cellular volume*

E. *Initially reduces intracranial pressure by expanding intravascular volume, reducing blood viscosity, and increasing cerebral blood flow*

Mannitol remains a standard therapy for reducing intracranial pressure. The initial dose of mannitol is 1 g/kg and can be given emergently without intracranial pressure monitoring as long as the patient is normotensive. Mannitol is particularly useful if the patient is showing any signs or symptoms of impending herniation. Subsequent dosing to a serum osmolality up to 320 mosm/l is usually recommended as needed. Dosing to higher levels has not been shown to improve outcome and increases the risk of acute renal failure. Mannitol reduces intracranial pressure through two mechanisms. The immediate mechanism is expansion of intravascular volume which reduces blood viscosity. This results in an increase in cerebral blood flow in the areas of the brain where cerebral autoregulation remains intact and ICP falls. The second mechanism, which occurs later, involves the establishment of osmotic gradients between the serum plasma and the brain cells. This ultimately decreases intracellular volume and reduces intracranial pressure. Since mannitol also functions as a diuretic there is always a risk of reducing blood pressure and therefore cerebral perfusion pressure if the patient is not adequately volume resuscitated. For this reason, hypertonic saline has gained favor as an osmotic agent for increased ICP since it is less likely to cause hypotension.

Answer: E

Muizelaar JP, Lutz HA, Becker DP (1984) Effect of mannitol in ICP and CBF and correlation with pressure autoregulation in severely head-injured patients. *Journal of Neurosurgery* **61**, 700.

Vialet R, Albanese J, Thomachot L, *et al.* (2003) Isovolume hypertonic solutes (sodium chloride or mannitol) in the treatment of refractory posttraumatic intracranial hypertension: 2 mL/kg 7.5% saline is more effective than 2 mL/kg 20% mannitol. *Critical Care Medicine* **31**, 1683.

7. *Clinical studies in both the prehospital and hospital setting following traumatic brain injury*

A. *Have definitely shown that correcting hypotension and hypoxia improves mortality rate*

B. *Have shown a correlation with increased mortality and systolic blood pressure <90 mm Hg*

C. *Have failed to show any relationship between avoidance of hypoxemia and improved mortality rates*

D. *Are inconsistent with current recommendations for treating hypotension and hypoxemia following traumatic brain injury*

E. *Suggest that systolic blood pressure is a better parameter than mean arterial pressure for monitoring patients with traumatic brain injury*

There is an abundance of Level II evidence to support the dictum of avoiding hypotension and hypoxemia in patients with traumatic brain injury. Secondary brain injury may occur from episodes of hypotension and hypoxemia. Chestnut *et al.*, in reviewing data from the Traumatic Coma Data Bank, showed a correlation between a single prehospital systolic blood pressure measurement <90 mm Hg and increased morbidity and mortality. Other studies support that repeated episodes of hypotension in the hospital setting may significantly and negatively affect mortality rates. Current Level II recommendations are that in patients with traumatic brain injury, systolic blood pressure <90 mm Hg, and PaO_2 <60 mm Hg (or SpO_2 <90%) should be avoided. For obvious ethical reasons, there are no definitive Level I studies to prove this Level II evidence. There is no evidence to suggest that systolic blood pressure is a better parameter to monitor compared to mean arterial pressure. There is no consistent relationship between systolic blood pressure and mean arterial pressure. Mean arterial pressure is used to calculate cerebral perfusion pressure, so it is reasonable to maintain mean arterial pressure at levels considerably higher than those represented by a systolic blood pressure of 90 mm Hg.

Answer: B

Bratton SL, Chestnut RM, Ghajar J, *et al.* (2007) I. Blood pressure and oxygenation. In Bullock MR, Povlishock JT (eds) *Guidelines for the Management of Severe Traumatic Brain Injury*, 3rd edn, Leibert, New York, NY, pp. S7–S13.

Chestnut RM, Marshal LF, Clauber MR, *et al.* (1993) The role of secondary brain injury in determining outcome from severe head injury. *Journal of Trauma* **34**, 216–22.

8. *A 30-year-old man is admitted to the intensive care unit following a gunshot wound to the head. He is hemodynamically stable with a systolic blood pressure of 140/100, a heart rate of 115 bpm, and a spontaneous respiratory rate of 22 breaths per minute. The best predictor of a poor outcome is*

A. *Bihemispheric injury*

B. *Bullet fragmentation*

C. *Pupillary changes*

D. *An admission Glasgow Coma score of <6*

E. *Presence of intraventricular blood*

A number of studies in the mid to late 1990s showed that patients arriving post gunshot wound to the brain and a Glasgow Coma Score of 3, 4 or 5 have extremely poor outcomes in terms of mortality or survival in a chronic vegetative state. The decision to subject these patients to aggressive resuscitation remains controversial. The presence of disseminated intravascular coagulopathy (DIC) is always associated with a poor outcome. Diffuse fragmentation, bihemispheric injury, intraventricular hemorrhage, and absence of pupillary response all predict a poor outcome, but a Glasgow Coma score of <6 is the most consistently reported negative predictor.

Answer: D

Levy ML (2000) Outcome prediction following penetrating craniocerebral injury in a civilian population; aggressive surgical management in patients with admission Glasgow Coma Scale scores of 6 to 15. *Neurosurgery* **8**, 1–6.

Levy ML, Masri LS, Lavine S, Apuzzo MLJ (1994) Outcome prediction after penetrating craniocerebral injury in a civilian population: Aggressive surgical management in patients with admission Glasgow Coma Scale scores of 3, 4, or 5. *Neurosurgery* **35**, 77–85.

9. *Subarachnoid hemorrhage secondary to a ruptured cerebral artery aneurysm*

A. *Can be excluded with a normal CT scan of the brain*

B. *Usually requires a lumbar puncture to make a definitive diagnosis*

C. *Is treated in the early preoperative stages with maintenance of blood pressure < 160/90 mm Hg with intravenous anti-hypertensive medications*

D. *Does not require anticonvulsant prophylaxis*

E. *Is not associated with xanthochromia or red blood cells in the cerebral spinal fluid*

A ruptured cerebral artery aneurysm usually presents with severe headache of sudden onset, lethargy and nuchal rigidity. Smaller bleeds may not present with severe symptoms. The initial diagnosis of subarachnoid hemorrhage is usually made by non-contrast CT scan of the brain.

However, about 10% of patients presenting with early subarachnoid hemorrhage related to a ruptured cerebral artery aneurysm will have a normal CT, and the diagnosis will need to be confirmed with lumbar puncture. Lumbar puncture will typically show xanthochromia or high red blood cell counts that do not clear across serial cerebral spinal fluid samples. In addition to assuring that airway and breathing are optimized, early treatment includes maintaining blood pressure <160/90 mm Hg. Prophylactic anticonvulsants are recommended for prevention of seizures in all cases.

Answer: C

Cowan Jr. JA, Thompson BG (2010) Neurosurgery. In: Doherty GM, Thompson NW (eds) *Current Diagnosis and Treatment Surgery*, 13th edn, McGraw-Hill, New York, pp. 858–9.

10. *Vasospasm following surgical or endovascular occlusion of a cerebral artery aneurysm*

A. *Is best managed with a combination of "permissive" hypertension, hemodilution, and hypervolemia*

B. *Is usually self-limited and requires no treatment*

C. *Is not typically treated with nimodipine*

D. *Is often heralded by the development of hypothermia*

E. *Is often treated with cerebral angioplasty for distal cerebral lesions*

Vasospasm following surgical or endovascular management of cerebral artery aneurysms is common and can lead to severe disability and death. Hyperthermia and mental status changes are early signs of vasospasm. Typical treatment includes "permissive" hypertension to maintain systolic blood pressure between 180–200 mm Hg (adding vasopressors if necessary), hemodilution with intravenous fluids to keep the hematocrit at approximately 30%, and hypervolemia with albumin and hypertonic saline to maintain a central venous pressure between 8–14 mm Hg. The peak time for occurrence is 4 to 14 days following the development of subarachnoid hemorrhage. Vasospasm should always be treated since approximately 30% of patients will develop permanent neurological deficits. Nimodipine is a commonly used drug following surgical or endovascular intervention to reduce vasospasm. Cerebral angioplasty is used for proximal vasospasm, but generally is not used for distal or diffuse vasospasm.

Answer: A

Cowan Jr. JA, Thompson BG (2010) Neurosurgery. In: Doherty GM, Thompson NW (eds) *Current Diagnosis and Treatment Surgery*, 13th edn, McGraw-Hill, New York, p. 860.

11. *The incidence of infection from external ventriculostomy catheters for cerebral spinal fluid drainage and intracranial pressure monitoring*

A. *Increases linearly over time*

B. *Is reduced by exchanging the catheters every five days*

C. *Is reduced with the use of antibiotic impregnated catheters*

D. *Is reduced by administering intravenous antibiotics for prophylaxis just prior to insertion*

E. *None of the above*

As with most medical devices used in the intensive care unit, ventriculostomy removal should occur as soon as possible when the perceived risk of complications outweighs the benefits of their use. Ventriculostomy catheters are used extensively for both elective and traumatic brain injury neurosurgical patients but there are very little controlled randomized data to definitively answer the question of true infection risk. Zambramski *et al.* performed a prospective randomized study on patients of all types requiring ventriculostomy. These investigators found a lower infection rate (1.3% versus 9.4%) in those patients randomized to receive a catheter impregnated with rifampin and minocycline. Park *et al.* showed a nonlinear relationship between infection risk and duration of catheter use. He found an extremely low infection rate that rose over the initial four days, but then remained constant even with prolonged catheter use for greater than 10 days. All patients in this retrospective study received antibiotics for prophylaxis, and no antibiotic impregnated catheters were used.

A positive cerebral spinal fluid culture was considered an infection. Multiple other studies have failed to demonstrate a benefit in using systemic antibiotics for prophylaxis with ventriculostomy catheter insertion. There is also no evidence to support the use of routine ventriculostomy exchange at a predetermined period to prevent infection. If ventriculostomies are placed carefully, under sterile conditions, and used with closed drainage systems, minimizing manipulations and flushing, then the risk of a device-related infection is very low. Further studies are needed to arrive at a definition for ventricular device related infection versus colonization so that the true incidence can be better defined.

Answer: C

Park P, Garton HJL, Kocan MJ, *et al.* (2004) Risk of infection with prolonged ventricular catheterization. *Neurosurgery* **55**, 594–601.

Wong GKC, Poon WS, Wai S, *et al.* (2002) Failure of regular external ventricular drain exchange to reduce cerebrospinal fluid infection: result of a randomized controlled trial. *Journal of Neurology, Neurosurgery and Psychiatry* **73**, 759–61.

Zambramski JM, Whiting D, Darouiche RO, *et al.* (2003) Efficacy of antimicrobial-impregnated external ventricular drain catheters: a prospective, randomized, controlled trial. *Neurosurgery* **98**, 725–30.

12. *An 80-year-old man with a Glasgow Coma Scale score of 15 is admitted to the intensive care unit three hours following a fall from ground level. Bilateral proximal humerus fractures have been splinted. CT scans of the brain and cervical spine show a 1 cm left frontal lobe intracerebral contusion and chronic degenerative changes to the cervical spine without acute fracture. Neurological assessment show good motor strength and reflexes in the lower extremities. Motor strength in the upper extremities is difficult to fully assess due to the fractures, but the patient appears to have bilateral loss of fine motor movement in the fingers and weakness with wrist flexion and extension. These findings are most consistent with:*

A. *Conus medullaris syndrome*

B. *The findings on the brain CT scan*

C. *Anterior spinal cord syndrome*

D. *Brown–Sequard syndrome*

E. *Central cord syndrome*

Central cord syndrome is commonly associated with falls in the elderly. The injury affects motor strength in the upper extremities more severely than the lower extremities. These patients frequently have spinal stenosis and the mechanism of injury is usually a hyperextension injury resulting in vascular compromise to the central portion of the cervical spinal cord. Since the cervical fibers controlling motor function to the upper extremities are located more medially than the lower motor fibers, the effects are more prominent in the upper extremity motor neurons. Sensory findings are variable and sphincter control may also be affected.

Answer: E

Cowan Jr. JA, Thompson BG (2010) Neurosurgery. In: Doherty GM, Thompson NW (eds) *Current Diagnosis and Treatment Surgery*, 13th edn, McGraw-Hill, New York, p. 829.

13. *A ventricular catheter connected to an external strain gauge transducer for intracranial pressure monitoring:*

A. *Provides measurements that are usually lower than parenchymal ICP transducer systems*

B. *Is more accurate than subarachnoid, subdural and epidural monitoring systems*

C. *Is associated with a 10% risk of significant intracerebral hematoma formation at the time of insertion*

D. *Is the most expensive method of monitoring intracranial pressure*

E. *Is much less accurate than parenchymal ICP transducer systems*

There are a number of devices currently used to measure intracranial pressure. The optimal device should be accurate, reliable, cost-effective, and associated with minimal patient morbidity during insertion and during the life of the device.

The two most accurate systems currently available are the ventriculostomy catheter and parenchymal catheter insertion systems. Published studies show similar results in terms of measurement accuracy. Systems using subarachnoid, subdural, and epidural catheters are less accurate. In the current state of technology, ventriculostomy is considered the most accurate, reliable, and cost effective method and remains the reference standard for comparison of all other systems. The risk of significant hematoma formation is less than 1% during insertion of a ventriculostomy. Ventriculostomy also allows therapeutic drainage of cerebral spinal fluid if the intracranial pressure is elevated, an advantage when compared to other monitoring systems.

Answer: B

Bratton SL, Chestnut RM, Ghajar J, *et al.* (2007) VII. Intracranial pressure monitoring technology. In Bullock MR, Povlishock JT (eds) *Guidelines for the Management of Severe Traumatic Brain Injury*, 3rd edn, Liebert, New York, NY, pp. S45–S54.

14. *Seizures following traumatic brain injury*

A. *Are higher following blunt traumatic brain injury compared to penetrating traumatic brain injury*

B. *Are best prevented in the late stages of injury (after 4 weeks) with early administration of phenytoin for prophylaxis*

C. *Are associated with increased mortality rates if they occur early (less than 2 weeks) following traumatic brain injury*

D. *Are reduced in the early stages of injury (less than 2 weeks) with phenytoin*

E. *Are not affected by administration of anti-seizure medications for prophylaxis*

Anticonvulsants are recommended to decrease the incidence of early post-traumatic seizures. Risk factors for developing seizures following trauma include penetrating brain injury (>50% of cases), Glasgow Coma Scale scores <10, depressed skull fractures, subdural and epidural hematomas, and intracerebral hematomas. Temkin *et al.* showed a significant reduction in early post-traumatic seizures with administration of phenytoin early after injury. No reduction in late post-traumatic seizures occurred and no difference in mortality rates was identified between those patients who developed seizures early following injury versus those without seizures. The current body of evidence indicates that anticonvulsants administered for prophylaxis prevent early post-traumatic seizures but do not significantly reduce the incidence of late post-traumatic seizures.

Answer: D

Temkin NR, Dikmen SS, Wilensky AJ, *et al.* (1990) A randomized, double-blind study of phenytoin for the prevention of post-traumatic seizures. *New England Journal of Medicine* **323**, 497–502.

Yablon SA (1993) Posttraumatic seizures. *Archives of Physical Medicine and Rehabilitation* **84**, 983–1001.

15. *Barbiturate therapy in the management of traumatic brain injury*

A. *May effectively reduce ICP in patients with intracranial hypertension refractory to other forms of therapy*

B. *Improves outcome when used as initial therapy in patients with diffuse brain injury*

C. *Has minimal effect on cardiac function and hemodynamic status*

D. *Is superior to standard forms of therapy for reducing ICP*

E. *Is best monitored for effective reduction in cerebral metabolism and cerebral blood flow by monitoring serum pentobarbital levels*

The use of barbiturates, specifically pentobarbital, to treat refractory intracranial hypertension following traumatic brain injury remains controversial. A number of randomized controlled studies were performed in the 1980s. Eisenberg *et al.* randomly allocated patients to receive pentobarbital versus continuing standard therapy in patients with Glasgow Coma Scale scores of 4 to 8. A large number of the control patients in this study crossed over to receive barbiturates, thus confusing the interpretation of the final results. In addition, all of these studies were performed at a time when prolonged hyperventilation, strict fluid restriction, and steroids were considered optimal conventional therapy. Therefore, the question of improving mortality and outcome with today's conventional therapy remains unanswered. This has led one group to conclude that there is no evidence that barbiturate therapy in patients with acute severe head injury improves outcome. It is well known that barbiturates can significantly reduce cardiac output and if this form of therapy is utilized, strict monitoring techniques to prevent reduction in cardiac output should be implemented. Barbiturate therapy will effectively reduce intracranial pressure. It is believed that this effect is due to a reduction in both cerebral metabolism and cerebral blood flow. Barbiturate therapy as an initial treatment is not indicated. One study actually showed increased mortality rates when barbiturates were used compared to mannitol as initial treatment. Standard forms of therapy should always be utilized initially since barbiturates have not been definitively shown to reduce ICP in the early stages following injury. If barbiturates are used in patients with intracranial hypertension refractory to standard forms of therapy, treatment is best monitored for effective reduction in cerebral metabolism and cerebral blood flow by monitoring the electroencephalogram pattern of burst suppression. Optimal reductions in cerebral metabolism and cerebral blood flow are believed to occur when burst suppression is induced. A goal of therapy remains achievement of serum pentobarbital levels in the range of 3-4 mg/dL. However, there is poor correlation among serum levels, systemic complications secondary to pentobarbital therapy, and ultimate therapeutic benefit.

Answer: A

Eisenberg HM, Frankowski RF, Contant CF, *et al.* (1988) High dose barbiturate control of elevated intracranial pressure in patients with severe head injury. *Journal of Neurosurgery* **69**, 15–23.

Schwartz M, Tator C, Rowed D, *et al.* (1984) The University of Toronto head injury treatment study: a prospective, randomized comparison of pentobarbital and mannitol. *Canadian Journal of Neurological Science* **11**, 434–40.

16. *The best order of initial management of a patient presenting with a blunt cervical spinal cord injury at the C3-C4 level is*

A. Airway management, high dose methylprednisolone, volume resuscitation, beta-agonist support, and alpha-agonist support

B. Airway management, volume resuscitation, beta-agonist support, alpha-agonist support, high-dose methylprednisolone

C. Volume resuscitation, vasopressor support, and high-dose methylprednisolone

D. Airway management, volume resuscitation, and vasopressor support

E. Airway management, volume resuscitation, beta-agonist support, alpha- agonist support, high-dose methylprednisolone

Patient with cervical spinal cord injuries are at high risk for acute respiratory failure from hypoventilation. While this may not be apparent initially, the risk may increase within the first 12 to 48 hours post-injury due to temporary ascending spinal cord edema. Therefore, airway concerns and close observation for signs of ventilatory failure should always be the first priority. Hypotension from neurogenic shock should be treated with prompt initiation of volume expansion. Decreased systolic blood pressure refractory to volume expansion is typically followed by a beta-agonist followed by an alpha-agonist if needed. A beta-agonist is initially preferred because of the possibility of bradycardia, which may be exacerbated by a pure alpha-agonist. High-dose methylprednisolone is still offered as an option for acute blunt spinal cord injury as a guideline by the AANS, but it is presented with the caveat that "evidence supporting harmful side effects is more consistent than any suggestion of clinical benefit." Generally, high-dose methylprednisolone is being used less and less due to the high risk of infectious complications.

Answer: D

Cowan Jr. JA, Thompson BG (2010) Neurosurgery. In: Doherty GM, Thompson NW (eds) *Current Diagnosis and Treatment Surgery,* 13th edn, McGraw-Hill, New York, p. 828.

Matsumoto T, Tamaki T, Kawakami M, *et al.* (2001) Early complications of high-dose methylprednisolone sodium succinate treatment in the follow-up of acute cervical spinal cord injury. *Spine* **26**, 426.

Robertson CS, Gopinath SP, Goodman JC, *et al.* (1995) SjvO2 monitoring in head-injured patient. *Journal of Neurotrauma* **12**, 891–6.

17. *All of the following statements concerning brain oxygenation monitoring techniques are true except:*

A. *Increased mortality rates are associated with just one episode of jugular venous oxygen desaturation (SjO_2)*

B. *SjO_2 levels > 75% are associated with poor neurologic outcomes*

C. *SjO_2 levels <60% are associated with poor neurologic outcomes*

D. *Brain tissue oxygenation tension ($P_{br}O_2$) <15 mm Hg is associated with a poor neurologic outcome.*

E. *A high SjO_2 level is associated with cerebral infarction*

A number of observational studies suggest a correlation between low brain oxygenation parameters and poor outcome following traumatic brain injury. Current thresholds to initiate therapy to improve brain tissue oxygenation, based on Level III evidence include an SjO_2 level less than 50% and a $P_{br}O_2$ level <15 mm Hg. A high SjO_2 (>75%) is associated with cerebral infarction as necrotic brain tissue does not extract oxygen. The question still remains whether goal directed therapy to restore SjO_2 and $P_{br}O_2$ to normal improves outcome. Technological deficiencies in SjO_2 monitoring and studies specifically addressing what area of the brain in which $P_{br}O_2$ measurements should be performed (most injured versus least injured hemisphere for example) need to be performed before these techniques in monitoring are uniformly adopted.

Answer: C

Bratton SL, Chestnut RM, Ghajar J, *et al.* (2007) X. Brain oxygen monitoring and thresholds. In Bullock MR, Povlishock JT (eds) *Guidelines for the Management of Severe Traumatic Brain Injury*, 3rd edn, Leibert, New York, NY, pp. S65–S70.

Cormio M. Valadka AB, Robertson CS (1999) Elevated jugular venous oxygen saturation after severe head injury. *Journal of Neurosurgery* **90**, 9–15.

18. *Progesterone for the treatment of traumatic brain injury*

A. *Has serious side effects that prevent its use*

B. *Has not been shown to reduce mortality following traumatic brain injury*

C. *Reduces mortality, but not morbidity following traumatic brain injury*

D. *Has neuroprotective effects that works primarily by mechanisms other than reducing cerebral edema*

E. *Has been shown to reduce both mortality and improve functional outcomes following traumatic brain injury*

Progesterone is a naturally occurring hormone and in most clinical studies has been shown to have a very high safety profile. Two Phase-II trials have been published and both have shown promising benefit in progesterone's neuroprotective effects and potential benefits in reducing both early and late mortality and improving functional outcomes following traumatic brain injury. A Phase III multicenter trial has been approved by the National Institutes of Health. A number of studies to determine the molecular mechanisms of this neuroprotective effect have been performed. These molecular effects include reduced inflammation and reduced lipid peroxidation, maintenance of blood-brain barrier, integrity and improved ionic stability. All of these molecular effects directly reduce cerebral edema following traumatic brain injury. Further studies are needed to determine whether progesterone becomes a standard therapy in the armamentarium of treatments following traumatic brain injury.

Answer: E

Phelan HA, Shafi S, Parks J, *et al.* (2007) Use of a pediatric cohort to examine gender differences in outcome after trauma. *Journal of Trauma* **63**, 1127–31.

Schumacher M, Guennoun R, Stein DG, De Nicola AF (2007) Progesterone: therapeutic opportunities for neuroprotection and myelin repair. *Pharmacology and Therapeutics* **116**, 77–106.

Wright DW, Kellerman AL, Hertzberg DS, *et al.* (2007) ProTECT: a randomized clinical trial of progesterone for acute traumatic brain injury. *Annals of Emergency Medicine* **49**, 391–402.

Xiao G, Wei J, Yan W *et al.* (2008) Improved outcomes from the administration of progesterone for patients with acute traumatic brain injury: a randomized controlled trial. *Critical Care* **12**, R61.

19. *The zone of normal cerebral autoregulation:*

A. *Is usually between 50 mm Hg and 150 mm Hg (cerebral perfusion pressure)*

B. *Is usually maintained following traumatic brain injury*

C. *Has no relationship to actual cerebral blood flow*

D. *Can be reproduced following traumatic brain injury by increasing cerebral perfusion pressure to >70 mm Hg*

E. *Results in maximum cerebral vasoconstriction as cerebral perfusion pressure decreases*

Under normal conditions cerebral blood flow is maintained relatively constant between cerebral perfusion pressures of 50–150 mm Hg. Cerebral autoregulation is disrupted following traumatic brain injury. In the mid to late 1990s it became popular to push cerebral perfusion pressure to >70 mm Hg or higher in order to enhance cerebral blood flow. This practice is generally no longer observed and in more recent years maintaining cerebral perfusion pressure to a value of approximately 60 mm Hg is recommended. The ultimate goal of managing both cerebral blood flow and the level of perfusion is to meet the metabolic demands of the brain. As cerebral perfusion pressure decreases maximal intracerebral vasodilatation occurs in order to maintain constant flow. As cerebral perfusion pressure increases the opposite occurs and cerebral vasoconstriction occurs to reduce flow and maintain normal perfusion.

Answer: A

Chestnut RM. (2006) Head trauma. In: MW Mulholand, KD Lillemoe, GM Doherty, *et al.* (eds) *Greenfield's Surgery Scientific Principles and Practice*, Lippincott Williams & Wilkins, Philadelphia, PA, pp. 374–5.

Lang EW, Chestnut RM (2000) A bedside method for investigating the integrity and critical thresholds of cerebral pressure autoregulation in severe traumatic brain injury patients. *British Journal of Neurosurgery* **14**, 117–26.

20. *Controlling elevated intracranial pressure is an important factor in pediatric patient survival following traumatic brain injury. Appropriate measures to maintain intracranial pressure <20 mm Hg include all of the following except:*

A. *3% normal saline by continuous infusion*

B. *Prophylactic hyperventilation to maintain $PaCO_2$ <35 mm Hg*

C. *Mannitol*

D. *Sedation and neuromuscular blockade*

E. *Ventriculostomy with cerebrospinal fluid drainage*

Prophylactic hyperventilation, as in adults, should be avoided in infants and children with traumatic brain injury since hyperventilation can compromise cerebral perfusion at a time when cerebral blood flow may be reduced. Aggressive hyperventilation ($PaCO_2$ <30 mm Hg) should be considered only as a second tier option when all other forms of therapy have failed. Even in this situation, either brain tissue oxygen monitoring or jugular venous oxygen saturation should be monitored to identify ischemic changes in the brain. All of the other options given above are acceptable first tier therapeutic responses for reducing intracranial pressure in infants and children.

Answer: B

Adelson PD, Bratton SL, Carney NA, *et al.* (2003) Guidelines for the acute medical management of severe traumatic brain injury in infants, children, and adolescents. Pediatric Critical Care Medicine **4**, S1–S75.

Jagannathan J, Okonkwo D, Yeoh H, *et al.* (2008) Long-term outcomes and prognostic factors in pediatric patients with severe traumatic brain injury and elevated intracranial pressure. *Journal of Neurosurgery Pediatrics* **2**, 240–9.

21. *A surgical colleague consults you on a 33-year-old man on whom he performed diagnostic laparoscopy for right lower quadrant pain 12 days previously. Intraoperatively, the appendix was found to be normal and turbid fluid was found in the pelvis which later grew out Campylobacter jejuni. The patient had an uneventful postoperative course, but came to his clinic check yesterday complaining of weakness, malaise, and shortness of breath. He was admitted, and a subsequent chest x-ray was normal as was a chest CT. Over the ensuing 48 hours, his extremity weakness has progressed while his work of breathing has increased to the point that his surgeon now wishes to place him in the ICU. Which of the following is an incorrect statement about this patient's likeliest diagnosis?*

A. *Guillain Barre Syndrome (GBS) typically presents 2-4 weeks after a relatively benign gastrointestinal or respiratory illness*

B. *Campylobacter seropositivity is found in 40–70% of patients*

C. *GBS has a low lethality, with an expected mortality rates of less than 3%*

D. *Plasmapheresis is no longer considered a mainstay of therapy for GBS*

E. *Corticosteroids are ineffective when used as monotherapy*

This patient has a fairly typical history and presenting picture for Guillain Barre Syndrome. This progressive demyelinating disorder is usually preceded by a bacterial or viral infection, with *C. jejuni* being a common etiology. Patients often initially complain of finger dysthesias and proximal lower extremity weakness which is progressive. A minority of patients will progress to needing mechanical ventilation. Both plasma exchange and intravenous immunoglobulin are effective treatments, but their concomitant use has not been shown to shorten symptoms. Steroids alone have not been shown to shorten symptoms or affect long term neurologic function, and they do cause higher rates of insulin requirement. While a minority of patients will exhibit permanent neurologic sequelae, a large review of 5000 GBS patients showed an overall mortality rate of 2.6%.

Answer: D

Alshekhlee A. Hussain Z. Sultan B, Katirji B (2008) Guillain-Barre syndrome: incidence and mortality rates in US hospitals. *Neurology* **70** (18), 1608–13.

Cortese I. Chaudhry V, So YT, *et al.* (2011) Evidence-based guideline update: Plasmapheresis in neurologic disorders: report of the Therapeutics and Technology Assessment Subcommittee of the American Academy of Neurology. *Neurology* **76** (3), 294–300.

Dalakas MC (2002) Mechanisms of action of IVIg and therapeutic considerations in the treatment of acute and chronic demyelinating neuropathies. *Neurology* **59** (12 Suppl. 6), S13–21.

Hughes RA, Swan AV, van Doorn PA (2010) Corticosteroids for Guillain-Barré syndrome. *Cochrane Database Systematic Reviews* **2**: CD001446.

Chapter 20 Venous Thromboembolism

Herb A. Phelan, MD, FACS and Scott H. Norwood, MD, FACS

1. *A 37-year-old man is admitted after suffering a grade II spleen injury in a motor vehicle collision. He is hemodynamically stable, and you undertake a course of nonoperative management. On postinjury day 3 he develops acute shortness of breath and a workup reveals a pulmonary embolism. What should be the next step in your management?*

A. *Placement of a permanent vena cava filter*

B. *Placement of a retrievable vena cava filter*

C. *Immediate initiation of systemic anticoagulation*

D. *Performance of splenectomy followed by systemic anticoagulation*

E. *An echocardiogram to assess for signs of right heart strain followed by initiation of systemic anticoagulation at 5 days post-injury if no heart strain is found*

Prophylactic and therapeutic anticoagulation in patients with nonoperatively managed solid organ injuries is a controversial topic with a paucity of data to support any opinion. Santaniello and colleagues examined a series of 20 patients with blunt aortic injuries and concomitant Grade I or II spleen or liver injuries, which were being managed nonoperatively. These patients all underwent systemic heparinization with bypass during the repair of their blunt aortic injuries at a mean of 1.5 days post-injury, and the authors reported no failures of splenic/liver nonoperative management. Further, others have shown that low molecular weight heparin can be used as prophylaxis at 48 hours post-injury without an increase in transfusion requirement or failure rates. While extrapolation of data should always be undertaken with caution, in the setting described above systemic anticoagulation would seem to be suitable management by post-injury day 3. Because "c" is a safe option, which is the least invasive and does not involve a delay in care, it represents the best answer.

Answer: C

Alejandro KV, Acosta JA, Rodriguez PA, *et al.* (2003) Bleeding manifestations after early use of low-molecular-weight heparins in blunt splenic injuries. *American Journal of Surgery* **69** (11), 1006–9.

Santaniello JM, Miller PR, Croce MA, *et al.* (2002) Blunt aortic injury with concomitant intra-abdominal solid organ injury: treatment priorities revisited. *Journal of Trauma* **53** (3), 442–5.

2. *Regarding intermittent pneumatic compression devices (IPCs) and graduated compression stockings (GCSs), which of the following statements is incorrect?*

A. *When IPCs were initially created, some systems used cuffs with large bladders and slow inflation rates, which weakens the value of older studies on the subject*

B. *Incorrect GCS sizing or application can lead to a reverse gradient of flow which creates greater pressure proximally and increases DVT risk*

C. *The complementary physiologic mechanisms of action for IPC and GCS account for studies that show an additive efficacy when used simultaneously*

D. *The 2008 ACCP recommendations do not discriminate between IPCs and GCS when making recommendations about mechanical DVT prophylaxis*

E. *If a DVT is diagnosed in a patient wearing IPCs, the device on that leg should be removed*

While many high-quality studies on the utility of IPCs are available, the various methods of application frequently make comparisons difficult, particularly in regard to older literature.

Surgical Critical Care and Emergency Surgery: Clinical Questions and Answers, First Edition. Edited by Forrest O. Moore, Peter M. Rhee, Samuel A. Tisherman and Gerard J. Fulda.

Other issues with the research in the field is that studies do not specify between foot, calf, and thigh-high devices, nor do they always describe the patient and nursing compliance with the device's application (a persistent clinical problem). GCS can come in up to 12 sizes, and the limb has to be measured accurately to prevent incorrect pressure gradients. This incorrect gradient can occur in up to 50% of applied GCS. GCS work by reducing venous diameter and increasing venous flow, while IPCs do the same by periodically emptying the deep venous system. It is therefore not recommended that they be used in tandem. The ACCP guidelines do not differentiate between the two in making mechanical prophylaxis recommendations, but weak data suggests that IPCs are superior for the prevention of DVT. If a DVT is found in a patient wearing IPCs, the IPC should be removed since their action may cause embolization.

Answer: C

Best AJ, Williams S, Crozier A, *et al.* (2000) Graded compression stockings in elective orthopaedic surgery: An assessment of the in vivo performance of commercially available stockings in patients having hip and knee arthroplasty. *Journal of Bone and Joint Surgery (British Volume)* **82**, 116 –18.

Geerts WH, Bergqvist D, Pineo GF, *et al.* (2008) Prevention of Venous Thromboembolism: American College of 2). Chest Physicians Evidence-Based Clinical Practice Guidelines, 8th edn. *Chest* **133**, 381S-453S.

Morris RJ, Woodcock JP (2010) Intermittent pneumatic compression or graduated compression stockings for deep vein thrombosis prophylaxis? A systematic review of direct clinical comparisons. *Annals of Surgery* **251**, 393–6.

3. *After a 12-foot fall, a 48-year-old woman suffers a pelvic fracture which requires anterior plating on post-injury day 2. On post-injury day 5 she develops a swollen left leg and an ultrasound confirms that she has a superficial femoral DVT for which she is started on therapeutic anticoagulation. When you see her in clinic on post-injury day 32 after her discharge from a rehabilitation facility, she is complaining of a painful, swollen, heavy leg. On exam, the leg has normal skin color with no breakdown and is swollen and mildly tender to palpation. As you begin to explain her condition to her, which of the following statements about post-thrombotic syndrome (PTS) would be incorrect?*

A. *Eighty percent of symptomatic DVTs are proximal to the knee; of these, the incidence of PTS 2 years post-DVT will be 50%.*

B. *Up to 10% of patients with PTS will manifest leg ulcerations.*

C. *Studies have shown that the quality of life of patients suffering from PTS is poorer than patients of similar age with arthritis, chronic lung disease, or diabetes.*

D. *For patients with DVT, no benefit has been shown for anticoagulation for 3 to 6 months and the use of graduated compression stockings for 2 years in reducing the incidence of PTS.*

E. *The societal costs of PTS are considerable as the mean age of affected patients is 56, and more than 50% of patients are of working age.*

Thrombosis damages the deep venous valves and frequently renders them incompetent. This results in venous reflux and venous hypertension. Venous hypertension in turn can affect segments of veins and valves not involved in the original area of thrombus. This is the fundamental pathophysiology of PTS, which is characterized by pain, heaviness, and edema of the involved extremity. When it occurs in the leg, these symptoms are exacerbated by standing and ambulating. As the disease becomes more severe, it can progress to subcutaneous atrophy, hyperpigmentation, and ulceration. This condition markedly diminishes quality of life, particularly given the fact that it often affects younger patients and affects their ability to earn a livelihood. Fortunately, good data exists, which suggests that a regimen of anticoagulation and graduated compression stockings can reduce its frequency.

Answer: D

Kahn SR, Shbaklo H, Lamping DL, *et al.* (2008) Determinants of health-related quality of life during the 2 years following deep vein thrombosis. *Journal of Thrombosis and Haemostasis* **6**, 1105–12.

Patterson BO, Hinchliffe R, Loftus IM, *et al.* (2010) Indications for Catheter-Directed Thrombolysis in the Management of Acute Proximal Deep Venous Thrombosis. *Arteriosclerosis, Thrombosis and Vascular Biology* **30**, 669–74.

Prandoni P, Lensing AW, Prins MH, *et al.* (2004) Below-knee elastic compression stockings to prevent the post-thrombotic syndrome: a randomized, controlled trial. *Annals of Internal Medicine* **141**, 249–56.

4. *A 27-year-old man remains intubated in your SICU on post-injury day 6 after a motor vehicle collision in which he suffered multiple left-sided rib fractures with a large pulmonary contusion and underwent laparotomy with splenectomy. After noting that his left lower extremity is swollen, an ultrasound is obtained which shows a superficial and common femoral DVT which appears to extend above the inguinal ligament. Therapeutic anticoagulation is initiated. The following day a CT scan of the abdomen is performed to assess for an abscess. No abscess is found but the CT scan demonstrates that the DVT extends proximally to just below the cava. In discussing this with his family, all of the following statements about catheter-directed thrombolytics (CDT) are correct except:*

A. *While systemic thrombolysis has been shown to be effective but associated with excessively high bleeding complications, CDT uses a more localized delivery of drug to achieve lysis with lower rates of systemic complications*

B. *Freshly formed thrombus responds better to CDT*

C. *A filter should be placed prior to performing CDT as the lysing clot has been shown to be at high risk for embolization*

D. *Venous stent placement in conjunction with thrombolysis may improve patency rates in select cases*

E. *Phlegmasia caerulea dolens is a well accepted indication for CDT*

Early studies examining the question of systemic thrombolytics for DVT lysis demonstrated that the technique achieved success but with unacceptably high rates of serious bleeding complications, particularly retroperitoneal and intracranial hemorrhage. By instilling the lytic agent locally, CDT appears to markedly reduce these risks. While CDT seems to be effective in achieving lysis, the indications for the procedure remain vague. The 2008 American College of Chest Physicians (ACCP) guidelines recommend that patients with a life expectancy greater than one year, good functional status, extensive ileofemoral thrombosis, and presentation within 14 days of symptom onset be considered candidates for CDT. Ongoing studies are evaluating whether this window can be pushed to 21 days. By successfully achieving recanalization, it is hoped that post-thrombotic syndrome (PTS) can be avoided by maintaining valvular competence and avoiding venous hypertension. Filters need not be used routinely as CDT has not been shown to increase the rate of embolization. Venous stents are occasionally indicated, particularly if abnormal venous anatomy is demonstrated. In the most common of these conditions, May–Thurner syndrome, the left common iliac vein is compressed by the overlying iliac artery causing not only an extrinsic compression but chronic low-grade venous trauma from the arterial pulse as well. Given the lack of an effective alternative and the high mortality if left untreated, phlegmasia is an accepted indication for CDT.

Answer: C

Comerota AJ (2010) The ATTRACT trial: rationale for early intervention for iliofemoral DVT. *Perspectives in Vascular Surgery and Endovascular Therapy* January 3, E-pub ahead of print.

Enden T, Sandvik L, Klow N, *et al.* (2007) Catheter-directed venous thrombolysis in acute iliofemoral vein thrombosis: the CaVenT study: rationale and design of a multicentre, randomized controlled, clinical trial (NCT00251771). *American Heart Journal* **154**, 808–14.

Geerts WH, Bergqvist D, Pineo GF, *et al.* (2008) Prevention of venous thromboembolism: American College of 2). Chest Physicians evidence-based clinical practice guidelines, 8th edn. *Chest* 133, 381S–453S.

Protack C, Bakken A, Patel N, *et al.* (2007) Long-term outcomes of catheter directed thrombolysis for lower extremity deep venous thrombosis without prophylactic inferior vena cava filter placement. *Journal of Vascular Surgery* **45**, 992–7.

5. *Which of the following statements about VTE in pregnancy is incorrect?*

A. *Pelvic vein thromboses account for 50% of all pregnancy-related VTE.*

B. *Normal pregnancy is accompanied by increased levels of fibrinogen, von-Willebrand factor, and factors VII, VIII, and X.*

C. *The risk of VTE in pregnancy is as high during the first trimester as it is during the third trimester.*

D. *About 33% of pregnancy-related DVT and 50% of pregnancy-related PE occur post-partum.*

E. *When DVT occurs in pregnancy it is more likely to be proximal and massive.*

The hypercoagulability of pregnancy is an evolutionary response to protect women from exsanguination during childbirth. Indeed, hemorrhage is still the leading cause of maternal death worldwide. In industrialized countries, however, it is VTE. Other factors that increase maternal risk for VTE are hormonally induced decreased venous capacitance, decreased venous outflow from the pelvis, and lower levels of mobility. Since the risk of VTE has been shown to be as high during the first trimester as the last, it suggests that the anatomic changes of pregnancy are less important than the hypercoagulable state that develops. Pelvic vein thromboses account for less than 1% of all DVTs, and about 10% of DVT in pregnancy. Not only are the DVTs of pregnancy more commonly proximal and massive, they are more frequently left-sided (likely due to the longer course of the left common iliac vein). Further, about one-third of pregnancy-related DVT and 50% of PE occur post-partum. Despite these risks, most women do not require anticoagulation as its complication rates are generally accepted to be higher than the risks of VTE. The exception is those women who have a history of thrombosis for whom anticoagulation can not only potentially decrease VTE risk but decrease the likelihood of spontaneous abortion as well.

Answer: A

Chang J, Elam-Evans LD, Berg CJ, *et al.* (2003) Pregnancy-related mortality surveillance–United States, 1991–1999. *MMWR Surveillance Summary* **52**, 1– 8.

Goldhaber SZ, Tapson VF (2004) A prospective registry of 5,451 patients with ultrasound-confirmed deep vein thrombosis. *American Journal of Cardiology* **93**, 259–62.

Gordon M (2002) Maternal physiology in pregnancy. In: Gabbe S, Niebyl J, Simpson J (eds) *Normal and Problem Pregnancies*, 4th edn, Churchill Livingstone, New York, pp. 63–92.

James AH, Tapson VF, Goldhaber SZ. (2005) Thrombosis during pregnancy and the postpartum period. *American Journal of Obstetrics and Gynecology* **193**, 216–9.

Macklon NS, Greer IA, Bowman AW (1997) An ultrasound study of gestational and postural changes in the deep venous system of the leg in pregnancy. *British Journal of Obstetrics and Gynaecology* **104**, 191–7.

Ray JG, Chan WS (1999) Deep vein thrombosis during pregnancy and the puerperium: a meta-analysis of the period of risk and the leg of presentation. *Obstetrical and Gynecological Survey* **54**, 265–71.

6. *Which of the following statements about echocardiography and its use in diagnosing PE is incorrect?*

A. *Transthoracic echo (TTE) is only able to visualize thrombus in right heart chambers approximately 15% of the time and thrombi in the pulmonary artery at an even lower frequency*

B. *A right ventricular size of 30 mm or greater in the precordial view is the most specific TTE finding for pulmonary embolism*

C. *Transesophageal echo (TEE) relies upon visualization of the embolus for the diagnosis of pulmonary embolism*

D. *The value of echocardiography is in identifying those patients with a higher mortality risk who may benefit from more aggressive management of their embolism*

E. *For central pulmonary embolism, TEE has a sensitivity of 95% and a specificity of 100%*

In general, TTE relies on detecting general signs of right ventricular strain as a surrogate for diagnosing pulmonary embolism, whereas TEE relies on direct visualization of thrombus to make the diagnosis. Given that another etiology of right ventricular enlargement and hypokinesis is the common condition of volume overload, it is not a very specific sign. TEE is highly sensitive and specific for central PE, but loses some of this accuracy for more peripheral emboli as the left mainstem bronchus interferes with the ultrasound beam. While TTE has much lower sensitivity for the detection of pulmonary embolism, it provides valuable information about hemodynamics, the status of the right ventricle, and the presence of pulmonary hypertension. Other TTE findings suggestive of pulmonary embolism are tricuspid regurgitation, abnormal motion of the interventricular septum, and lack of collapse of the inferior vena cava during inspiration. One of the values of echocardiography is that it can assist in risk stratification by identifying proximal emboli and giving information regarding cardiac function and compensation. Knowledge of these factors can inform decisions about thrombolytic therapy or surgical embolectomy.

Answer: B

Mookadam F, Jiamsripong P, Goel R, *et al.* (2010) Critical appraisal on the utility of echocardiography in the management of acute pulmonary embolism. *Cardiology Review* **18** (1), 29–37.

7. *Which of the following statements about the incidence and management of DVT and PE is incorrect?*

A. *Twenty to 30% of untreated calf thrombi propagate into the thigh where they pose a 40–50% chance of embolizing if they remain untreated.*

B. *The diagnostic properties of the history and physical exam have been shown to be of very low utility in screening for DVT in critically ill patients.*

C. *Neither antiembolic stockings nor pneumatic compression devices have been evaluated with randomized controlled trials in general medical-surgical ICU patients.*

D. *The new anticoagulant fondaparinux holds promise as an anticoagulant in critical care due to the fact that it has an antidote which provides easy reversibility.*

E. *Autopsy studies have shown that over 75% of PE found on post-mortem examination were clinically unsuspected prior to death.*

Not only are DVT common, but they are almost universally under-recognized as multiple studies in centers that utilize aggressive screening have shown incidences of 10–30%. Further, clinical screening techniques that are of utility in ambulatory patients have been shown to be of almost no worth in ICU populations due to the infrequency of unilateral limb swelling (due to being recumbent) and the frequency of intubation, sedation, and analgesia interfering with reports of leg pain. The dearth of literature comparing mechanical prophylaxis methods in general medical-surgical patients is striking. Fondaparinux is approved for pharmacologic prophylaxis in high-risk patients, but has not been widely embraced due to its long half life, renal mode of clearance, lack of an antidote, and a lack of data on its effects in general medical-surgical units. In a 25-year longitudinal study, 9% of patients were found to have PE at autopsy, and 84% of these were clinically unsuspected.

Answer: D

Crowther MA, Cook DJ, Griffith LE, *et al.* (2005) Deep vein thrombosis: Clinically silent in the ICU. *Journal of Critical Care* **20**, 334-40.

Kakkar VV, Howe CT, Flanc C, *et al.* (1969) Natural history of postoperative deep vein thrombosis. *Lancet* **2**, 230–2.

Karwinski B, Svendsen E (1989) Comparison of clinical and postmortem diagnosis of pulmonary embolism. *Journal of Clinical Pathology* **42**, 135–9.

Limpus A, Chaboyer W, McDonald E, *et al.* (2006) Mechanical thromboprophylaxis in critically ill patients: A systematic review and meta-analysis. *American Journal of Critical Care* **15**, 402–10.

8. *Which of the following statements regarding the use of low-molecular-weight heparins (LMWHs) is correct?*

A. *They have been shown to have equivalent rates of heparin-induced thrombocytopenia (HIT) to unfractionated heparin (UFH)*

B. *LMWHs have a shorter half-life than UFH*

C. *LMWHs are dependent on hepatic clearance*

D. *In patients with impaired clearance, therapeutic doses of LMWHs have been shown to bioaccumulate over time while prophylactic doses do not*

E. *Due to decreased binding of LMWHs to plasma proteins as compared to UFH, hypoalbuminemic patients have less predictable dose responses with LMWH*

LMWHs are glycosaminoglycans derived from UFH with a molecular weight of about 5 kDa. In comparison with UFH, they are known for having greater bioavailability, longer half-lives, more predictable dose-response curves, better safety profiles, lower rates of HIT, and no need for lab monitoring. LMWHs are also known for being renally cleared, however, and this has led to some trepidation on the part of clinicians in their use in patients with a creatinine clearance <30 mL/min. Cook and co-workers have done a considerable amount of work in this area and have published relatively strong data that suggests that bleeding is less of a concern at prophylactic doses. In fact, in their work they have shown that for the LMWH dalteparin, bleeding complications at prophylactic doses in the setting of renal impairment are related to the concomitant use of aspirin rather than the dalteparin itself.

Answer: D

Cook D, Douketis J, Meade M, *et al.* (2008) Venous thromboembolism and bleeding in critically ill patients with severe renal insufficiency receiving dalteparin thromboprophylaxis: prevalence, incidence and risk factors. *Critical Care* **12**, R32.

Lim W, Dentali F, Eikelboom JW, *et al.* (2006) Meta-analysis: Low-molecular-weight heparin and bleeding in patients with severe renal insufficiency. *Ann Intern Med* **144**, 673–84.

Rabbat CG, Cook DJ, Crowther MA, *et al.* (2005) Dalteparin thromboprophylaxis for critically ill medical-surgical patients with renal insufficiency. *J Crit Care* **20**, 357–63.

9. *All of the following statements about D-dimer and its utility in the diagnosis of DVT and PE are true except:*

A. *D-dimer is primarily stored in the alpha granules of platelets and endothelial cells where, after platelet or cell activation, it translocates to the surface and is released into the plasma in soluble form*

B. *In the setting of low to intermediate risk, a negative D-dimer value can rule out PE with a sensitivity of 95% and a negative predictive value of 99% and no further testing is necessary*

C. *In prospective cohort studies, an elevated D-dimer has been shown to be associated with a threefold increased risk for future first-time DVT or PE*

D. *For patients stopping anticoagulation after DVT or PE, D-dimer has been shown to be an accurate predictor of recurrence*

E. *D-dimers accuracy in predicting risk is even higher in patients with congenital thrombophilias*

D-dimer is a degradation product of cross-linked fibrin that is formed immediately after clots are degraded by plasmin. It reflects a systemic activation of clot promotion and degradation. P-selectin is a cell-adhesion molecule important in clot formation which is stored in platelets and endothelial cells in the manner described, and its use as a serum marker for DVT and PE diagnosis is currently under investigation. While the negative predictive value of a normal D-dimer is very good, its lack of specificity and elevation by general states of hypercoagulability has limited its use as a sole tool for the positive diagnosis of PE. Both observational and interventional studies have demonstrated that D-dimer is a useful predictor of recurrence of DVT and PE. To that end, a strong body of evidence suggests that if a D-dimer is still elevated after the discontinuation of anticoagulation after an event, it should be restarted.

Answer: A

Cushman M, Folsom AR, Wang L, *et al.* (2003) Fibrin fragment D-dimer and the risk of future venous thrombosis. *Blood* **101**, 1243–8.

Palareti G, Cosmi B, Legnani C, *et al.* (2006) D-dimer testing to determine the duration of anticoagulation therapy. *New England Journal of Medicine* **355**, 1780–9.

Verhovsek M, Douketis JD, Yi Q, *et al.* (2008) Systematic review: D-dimer to predict recurrent disease after stopping anticoagulant therapy for unprovoked venous thromboembolism. *Annals of Internal Medicine.* **149**, 481–90, W494.

10. *Given the difficulty of using clinical diagnosis to make the diagnosis of pulmonary embolism (PE), two major, validated scoring systems have been created which stratify clinical risk for PE (the Wells score and the revised Geneva score). Which of the following is NOT a variable to be factored into the calculation of the revised Geneva score?*

A. *Age greater than 65*

B. *Previous surgery requiring general anesthesia within 1 month*

C. *Hemoptysis*

D. *Heart rate of 75 to 94 beats per minute*

E. *Index of suspicion for PE*

While they are largely the same in many respects, the primary difference between the Wells score and the Geneva score is that the Wells score gives points for the degree of clinical suspicion for PE while the Geneva score is completely standardized. It is thought that this reliance on only objective findings as the basis for score generation makes the Geneva score of more utility for the less experienced practitioner. A criticism of the original Geneva score was that the arterial blood gas required in the scoring system had to be performed on room air, and 15% of patients were not able to tolerate this in the original study. Therefore, the revised Geneva Score dropped that component. Other variables to be taken into account besides those listed in the question are a previous history of DVT or PE, an active malignant condition, unilateral limb pain, a heart rate greater than 95 beats per minute (which gives more points than someone with a heart rate of 75 to 94 beats per minute), and pain on lower limb deep palpation. Scores are assigned based on these findings, and total scores stratify patients as being low-, moderate-, or high-risk for PE.

Answer: E

Le Gal G, Righini M, Roy PM, *et al.* (2006) Prediction of pulmonary embolism in emergency patients: the revised Geneva score. *Annals of Internal Medicine* **144**, 165–71.

Wells PS, Anderson DR, Rodger M, *et al.* (2000) Derivation of a simple clinical model to categorize patients' probability of pulmonary embolism: increasing the model's utility with the SimpliRed D-dimer. *Journal of Thrombosis and Haemostasis* **83**, 416–20.

11. *After admitting a 63-year-old man with a flail chest to the surgical intensive care unit, you consult the pain service to place an epidural catheter for pain control. The consultant asks for your plans regarding VTE prophylaxis, and you articulate a desire to initiate a low molecular weight heparin (LMWH) when the patient is a candidate for anticoagulation. Which of the following is not a recommendation of the 2002 Consensus Statement of the American Society of Regional Anesthesia and Pain Medicine (ASRA) on the topic of LMWHs and epidurals?*

A. *The monitoring of anti-Xa levels is not recommended while the catheter is in place*

B. *The presence of blood during needle and catheter placement requires that LMWH initiation be delayed for 24 hours post-procedure*

C. *After pulling the catheter, the practitioner should wait 12 hours before initiating LMWH*

D. *Catheter placement can be safely performed as soon as 12 hours after a prophylactic dose of LMWH*

E. *Catheter placement can be safely performed as soon as 24 hours after discontinuing a therapeutic dose of LMWH*

The ASRA drew on the extensive European experience with LMWHs and epidural analgesia to generate their recommendations in 2002. It should be noted, however, that many of the studies which served as the basis for these recommendations were done using once-daily LMWH dosing. Anti-Xa levels are not recommended to be followed as they have not been shown to be predictive of the risk of bleeding. The ASRA also states that while LMWH initiation should be delayed for 24 hours by a "bloody tap", this does not serve as a rationale for an automatic cancellation of an elective surgery. The ASRA states that LMWH can be initiated after a two hour delay from the completion of catheter removal. Given the predictable nature of LMWH bioavailability, catheter placement can be safely performed 12 hours after a prophylactic dose and 24 hours after a therapeutic dose.

Answer: C

Horlocker TT, Wedel DJ, Benzon H, *et al.* (2003) Regional anesthesia in the anticoagulated patient: defining the risks (the second ASRA Consensus Conference on Neuraxial Anesthesia and Anticoagulation). *Reg Anesth Pain Med.* **28**(3), 172–97.

12. *Which of the following statements about the 2008 Clinical Practice Guidelines on VTE prevention from the American College of Chest Physicians (ACCP) is correct?*

A. *Duplex ultrasound screening for DVT should be performed routinely after major trauma*

B. *Prophylactic vena cava filters should be placed after complete spinal cord injury*

C. *For trauma patients with impaired mobility who undergo inpatient rehabilitation, pharmacologic prophylaxis can be discontinued in favor of mechanical prophyalxis at the time of transfer*

D. *For major trauma patients in whom ongoing bleeding is not a concern, first-line pharmacologic VTE prophylaxis constitutes low-molecular-weight heparin*

E. *For incomplete spinal cord injury, unfractionated low dose heparin should be first-line therapy for VTE prophylaxis*

Routine screening with Duplex ultrasound has not been shown to be an effective strategy for the prevention of clinically significant VTE, and the cost is generally considered to be prohibitive. Selective screening may be of benefit, however, in those major trauma patients in whom the initiation of early prophylaxis was delayed. The ACCP guidelines do not recommend the use of prophylactic vena cava filters under any circumstances. Major trauma patients with impaired mobility should receive prophylaxis with a low-molecular-weight heparin or a vitamin K antagonist through their inpatient stay. Strong level I evidence exists which suggests that low-molecular-weight heparin is superior to low dose unfractionated heparin as VTE prophylaxis after major trauma. Similarly, low molecular weight heparin constitutes first line therapy after incomplete spinal cord as well.

Answer: D

Geerts WH, Bergqvist D, Pineo GF, *et al.* (2008) Prevention of venous thromboembolism: American College of Chest Physicians evidence-based clinical practice guidelines, 8th edn. *Chest* **133**, 381S–453S.

13. *Which of the following statements about the Factor V Leiden mutation is incorrect?*

A. *Five percent of Caucasians are heterozygous for the mutation*

B. *The mutation causes resistance to activated protein C*

C. *Long-term anticoagulation with a vitamin K antagonist is recommended for patients who are heterozygous for the mutation*

D. *Venous thromboses are more common than arterial thromboses in patients with Factor V Leiden mutation*

E. *Venous thrombosis after general surgical or orthopedic procedures does not appear to be increased in patients heterozygous for the Factor V Leiden mutation when they are managed with well-reasoned protocols for VTE prophylaxis*

Five percent of Caucasians are heterozygous for the mutation, making it the most common inherited hypercoagulable state, as approximately 1 person in 5000 is homozygous for the disorder among the general population. Platelets carry an endogenous protein C inhibitor, which makes arterial thrombosis less common. The preponderance of the literature suggests that for patients undergoing major general surgical or orthopedic procedures, the incremental risk carried by possession of the mutation is overwhelmed by well-reasoned prophylaxis measures. Therefore, there is no basis for altering their perioperative management based on a history of Factor V Leiden. The same cannot be said for arterial thrombosis after a vascular procedure, however. Asymptomatic heterozygosity for Factor V Leiden does not constitute an indication for intervention.

Answer: C

Donahue BS (2004) Factor V Leiden and perioperative risk. *Anesthesia and Analgesia* **98**, 1623–34.

Slusher KB (2010) Factor V Leiden: A case study and review. *Dimensions of Critical Care Nursing* **29** (1), 6–10.

14. *For a patient preparing to undergo a total knee or hip replacement who is deemed to be at baseline risk for both PE and bleeding, the American Academy of Orthopedic Surgery's (AAOS) 2009 guidelines recommend that all of the following are acceptable prophylaxis regimens except:*

A. *Aspirin 325 mg twice a day starting on the day of surgery and continuing for six weeks*

B. *Low molecular weight heparin starting 12 to 24 hours postoperatively for 7 to 12 days and dosed per package insert*

C. *Unfractionated heparin 5000 U every 12 hours starting 24 hours postoperatively and continuing for 14 days*

D. *A synthetic pentasaccharide starting 12 to 24 hours postoperatively for 7 to 12 days and dosed per package insert*

E. *Warfarin starting the night before surgery at a dose sufficient to obtain an INR < 2.0 for 2–6 weeks*

Patients deemed to be at a baseline risk for bleeding and PE represent the majority of patients undergoing total knee and hip replacement. Further, this referral to a "standard" PE risk is relative to other joint replacement patients and not general surgical or medical patients (who are at lower overall risk). The bleeding risk with these regimens is felt to be in the range of 3–5%. Much of the early work done in this area suggested that the time-frame for PE occurrence was six weeks, and the time frame for aspirin was created to conform to this interval. Several reports on the low molecular weight heparins suggest that the utility of their use is much shorter. Of note, unfractionated heparin is not felt by the AAOS to have a role in prophylaxis. The AAOS recommendations can be summarized as follows:

PE Risk	Bleeding Risk	Recommendation
Baseline	Baseline	Any of: ASA 325 bid starting the day of surgery and continuing for 6 weeks LMWH starting 12 to 24 h postop for 7 to 12 days, dosed per package insert A synthetic pentasaccharide starting 12 to 24 h postop for 7 to 12 days, dosed per package insert. Warfarin starting the night before surgery at a dose sufficient to obtain an INR <2.0 for 2 to 6 weeks.
Baseline	Increased	Any of: ASA 325 bid starting the day of surgery and continuing for 6 weeks Warfarin starting the night before surgery at a dose sufficient to obtain an INR <2.0 for 2 to 6 weeks No prophylaxis
Increased	Baseline	Any of: LMWH starting 12 to 24 h postop for 7 to 12 days, dosed per package insert. A synthetic pentasaccharide starting 12 to 24 hrs postop for 7 to 12 days, dosed per package insert. Warfarin starting the night before surgery at a dose sufficient to obtain an INR <2.0 for 2 to 6 weeks.
Increased	Increased	Any of: ASA 325 bid starting the day of surgery and continuing for 6 weeks Warfarin starting the night before surgery at a dose sufficient to obtain an INR <2.0 for 2 to 6 weeks No prophylaxis

Answer: C

Johanson NA, Lachiewicz, Lieberman JR, *et al.* (2009) Prevention of symptomatic pulmonary embolism in patients undergoing total hip or knee arthroplasty. *Journal of the American Academy of Orthopedic Surgeons* **135**, 513–20.

15. *According to the 2008 ACCP guidelines, which of the following statements about the management of acute PE is incorrect?*

A. *In selected highly compromised patients who are unable to receive thrombolytics because of bleeding risk, surgical embolectomy may be used*

B. *For a patient with PE and vena cava filter insertion due to a contraindication to anticoagulation, anticoagulation should be initiated if the contraindication resolves*

C. *For patients with acute PE and severe renal failure, unfractionated heparin is preferred over low molecular weight heparin for systemic anticoagulation*

D. *For patients with acute, central pulmonary embolism treated with low molecular weight heparin, anti-factor Xa levels should be followed*

E. *For patients with PE due to a transient, reversible risk factor, treatment should consist of three months of warfarin followed by discontinuation and no assessment of the risk/benefit ratio of long-term anticoagulation*

Surgical embolectomy should also be considered to rescue those patients in whom thrombolytic therapy has not been successful. Outcomes are better when patients are operated on prior to the onset of cardiogenic shock, and should optimally be performed on a warm beating heart without cross-clamping, cardioplegia, or fibrillatory arrest. While vena cava filters decrease pulmonary embolism, they also cause increased rates of DVT due to the endothelial damage caused by accessing and dilating the insertion site. Therefore, anticoagulation can decrease the short- and long-term local complications associated with this condition. The ACCP does not recommend that anti-factor Xa levels be followed, regardless of whether or not the embolism is central. Patients suffering an "unprovoked PE" in the parlance of the ACCP should undergo three months of anticoagulation followed by an assessment of their risk factors for recurrence as well as for bleeding in patients with persistent risk factors for VTE. If risk factors for bleeding are absent and monitoring of anticoagulation parameters is feasible, the ACCP recommends long-term anticoagulation. Of note, no time frame is specified beyond the three months. If the PE was felt to be due to a transient condition that has resolved at the three-month time point, anticoagulation can be discontinued and no further assessment or consideration given to anticoagulation is necessary.

Answer: D

Geerts WH, Bergqvist D, Pineo GF, *et al.* (2008) Prevention of Venous Thromboembolism: American College of Chest Physicians Evidence-Based Clinical Practice Guidelines, 8th edn. *Chest* **133**, 381S–453S.

16. *Which of the following statements about the antiphospholipid syndrome (APS) is incorrect?*

A. *Presence of the antiphospholipid antibody on a single determination constitutes a diagnosis of the syndrome*

B. *For patients diagnosed with APS, indefinite anticoagulation with warfarin is recommended*

C. *In APS, arterial thrombosis tends to recur on the arterial side and venous thrombosis tends to recur on the venous side*

D. *Management of anticoagulation in APS can be complicated by artifactual elevation of the INR, requiring alternate strategies for monitoring*

E. *The syndrome is referred to as "primary APS" when it occurs by itself and as "secondary APS" when it occurs in conjunction with another autoimmune condition*

Antiphospholipid antibodies can occur in 5–10% of healthy donors, but these titers normally disappear over time. The diagnostic criteria for APS involves a characteristic clinical picture of thrombosis and a persistent antiphospholipid antibody titer on two separate occasions at least 12 weeks apart. Patients diagnosed with APS have high rates of recurrent thrombosis after discontinuation of anticoagulation for a period of years. Therefore, the consensus treatment is to continue anticoagulation indefinitely. Beginning an anticoagulation regimen can be difficult as the syndrome is known for occasionally interfering with standard assays. This necessitates specific inquiries with your hematology lab as to whether INR-reagents resistant to this effect are being used, and potentially following functional factor II and X assays. For reasons that are unclear, recurrences of thrombosis in APS tend to occur on the same side of the circulation as the original event.

Answer: A

Dentali F, Crowther M (2010) Antiphospholipid antibodies in critical illness. *Critical Care Medicine* **38** (Suppl.), 51–6.

Chapter 21 Transplantation, Immunology, and Cell Biology

Leslie Kobayashi, MD

1. *Which of the following would be the most helpful in differentiating pre-renal azotemia from hepato-renal dysfunction in a patient with liver failure?*

A. *Fractional excretion of sodium that is less than 1% (FeNa <1%)*

B. *Urine sodium of less than 10 (U_{Na} <10)*

C. *Urine osmolality greater than 400 (U_{Osm} >400)*

D. *Lack of response to fluid resuscitation*

E. *BUN/Creatinine ratio greater than 20*

Hepato-renal dysfunction refers to acute kidney injury within the setting of severe liver failure. It may have an insidious onset or present acutely if precipitated by a stressor, such as infection, gastro-intestinal bleeding, or dehydration. It can affect up to 40% of patients with cirrhosis. The likely etiology is nitric oxide-induced splanchnic vasodilation with activation of the renin-angiotensin-aldosterone system resulting in renal vasoconstriction and reduction in glomerular filtration rate. It presents similarly to pre-renal azotemia, and is, in essence, a pre-renal disease with decreased renal blood flow. The FeNa will be <1%, urine sodium will be low, urine osmoles will be high, and urinary sediment will generally be benign. However, because of the low serum oncotic pressure, and the high output, low resistance state of cirrhotic patients, hepato-renal syndrome generally will not respond to fluid challenge. This is markedly different from pre-renal azotemia, which will generally respond to volume replacement within 24 to 72 hours. The best treatment for hepato-renal syndrome is liver transplantation. Treatment of exacerbating conditions such as gastro-intestinal bleeding or infection is also critical. Some promising treatments include intravenous clonidine, midodrine, octreotide, norepinephrine in patients with a low mean arterial pressure, and combination therapy with terlipressin and albumin.

Answer: D

Gines A, Escorsell A, Gines P, *et al*. (1993) Incidence, predictive factors, and treatment of the hepatorenal syndrome with ascites. *Gastroenterology* **105**, 229–36.

Uriz J, Gines P, Cardenas A, *et al*. (2000) Terlipressin plus albumin infusion: an effective and safe therapy of hepatorenal syndrome. *Journal of Hepatology*. **33**, 43–8.

Wong F, Pantea L, Sniderman K (2004) Midodrine octreotide, albumin, and TIPS in selected patients with cirrhosis and type 1 heptorenal syndrome. *Hepatology* **40**, 55–64.

2. *Increased tacrolimus levels can be seen with co-administration with which of the following drugs?*

A. *Ketoconazole*

B. *Phenobarbital*

C. *Phenytoin*

D. *Rifampin*

E. *Carbamazipine*

Tacrolimus binds to FK binding protein-12 and blocks proliferation of calcineurin, preventing interleukin-2 (IL-2) expression/production, thus preventing an immune response from lymphocytes. It is metabolized by cytochrome P450 3A4 (CYP3A4) in both the liver and small intestine, and clearance is primarily from biliary excretion and fecal elimination. Very little drug is cleared by the kidneys. Any medications that inhibit CYP3A4 will increase drug concentrations, and in contrast,

Surgical Critical Care and Emergency Surgery: Clinical Questions and Answers, First Edition. Edited by Forrest O. Moore, Peter M. Rhee, Samuel A. Tisherman and Gerard J. Fulda.

medications that induce CYP3A4 will decrease drug concentrations. Ketoconazole, an antifungal and an inhibitor of CYP3A4, will result in increased levels of tacrolimus. By contrast phenobarbital, phenytoin, rifampin, and carbamazipine are all CYP3A4 inducers and co-administration will result in decreased tacrolimus levels. See Tables 21.1 and 21.2.

Table 21.1 CYP3A4 inhibitors: increase tacrolimus levels

Class	Examples
Antifungal agents	Fluconazole, voriconazole, ketoconazole
Calcium channel blockers	Diltiazem, nifedipine, nicardipine, verapamil
Macrolide antibiotics	Erythromycin, clarithromycin
Promotility agents	Metoclopramide
Protease inhibitors	Indinavir, ritonavir, atazanavir
Misc.	Metronidazole, cimetidine, ciprofloxacin, amiodarone
Herbals	Echinacea
Foods	Grapefruit juice, star fruit

Table 21.2 CYP3A4 inducers: decrease tacrolimus levels

Class	Examples
Anticonvulsants	Carbamazepine, phenytoin, phenobarbital
Rifamycins	Rifampin, rifabutin
Misc.	Glucocorticoids, pioglitazone
Herbals	St. John's wort

Answer: A

Lake KD and Canafax DM (1995) Important interactions of drugs with immunosuppressive agents used in transplant recipients. *Journal of Antimicrobial Chemotherapy* **36** (supplement B), 11–22.

Page RL, Klem PM, Rogers C (2005) Potential elevation of tacrolimus trough concentrations with concomitant metronidazole therapy. *Annals of Pharmacotherapy* **39** (6), 1109–13.

Vicari-Christensen M, Repper S, Basile S, *et al.* (2009) Tacrolimus: review of pharmacokinetics, pharmacodynamics, and pharmacogenetics to facilitate practitioners' understanding and offer strategies for educating patients and promoting adherence. *Progress in Transplantation* **19** (3), 277–284.

3. *Regarding cyclosporine and tacrolimus and their use in liver transplant recipients, which of the following is true?*

A. *Cyclosporine has more nephrotoxicity than tacrolimus*

B. *Cyclosporine has less nephrotoxicity than tacrolimus*

C. *Cyclosporine has a similar nephrotoxicity to tacrolimus*

D. *Cyclosporine is more potent than tacrolimus*

E. *Cyclosporine results in improved graft survival compared to tacrolimus*

Tacrolimus has a mechanism of action similar to cyclosporine, but is 10 to 100 times more potent, although both have similar nephrotoxicity. They both cause vasoconstriction of the afferent glomerular arteriole and decrease glomerular filtration, additionally they may exert direct cellular stress on renal tubular cells. When administered together, tacrolimus and cyclosporine have a synergistic immunosuppressive affect and have an increased renal toxicity when compared to either agent given alone. Several studies have revealed that while the two agents have similar long-term mortality, tacrolimus is associated with significantly fewer episodes of rejection and increased graft survival.

Answer: C

Lake KD and Canafax DM (1995) Important interactions of drugs with immunosuppressive agents used in transplant recipients. *Journal of Antimicrobial Chemotherapy* **36** (supplement B), 11–22.

Mukherjee S and Mukherjee U (2009) A comprehensive review of immunosuppression used for liver transplantation. *Journal of Transplantation* 701464 Epub 2009 Jul 16.

Vicari-Christensen M, Repper S, Basile S, *et al.* (2009) Tacrolimus: review of pharmacokinetics, pharmacodynamics, and pharmacogenetics to facilitate practitioners' understanding and offer strategies for educating patients and promoting adherence. *Progress in Transplantation* **19** (3), 277–284.

4. *A patient with cirrhosis requires anticoagulation for a pulmonary embolus. A heparin bolus followed by infusion fails to increase the aPTT. What is the next step in management?*

A. Transfuse with fresh frozen plasma

B. Administer systemic tissue plasminogen activator (tPA)

C. Change to an argatroban infusion

D. Change to a lepirudin infusion

E. Increase the dose of heparin

Patients with liver failure have decreased synthetic liver function, and decreased levels of clotting factors result in elevations in prothrombin time (PT) and international normalized ratio (INR). However, the liver also synthesizes natural anticoagulants such as Protein C and S and antithrombin III (AT-III). Patients may suffer from microvasular consumption as well, causing further decreases in AT-III levels. As a result these patients may be hypercoagulable despite having an elevated PT/INR. They may also demonstrate heparin resistance due to diminished AT-III levels, similar to the resistance seen in patients undergoing cardiopulmonary bypass. It has been shown that decreases in AT-III levels to 70% and 50% of normal will result in a decrease in heparin activity to 65% and 20% of baseline. Resistance is unlikely to respond to increases in heparin dose. AT-III deficiency can be reversed by transfusion with fresh frozen plasma (FFP) which contains high concentrations of Protein C and S as well as AT-III. Alternatively concentrates of AT-III are also available and may aid in avoiding volume overload associated with transfusion of large amounts of FFP.

Answer: A

Carmassi F, Morale M, DeNegri F, *et al.* (1995) Modulation of hemostatic balance with antithrombin III replacement tehrapyin a case of liver cirrhosis associated with recurrent venous thrombosis. *Journal of Molecular Medocome* **73**, 89–93.

Garcia-Fuster MJ, Abdilla N, Fabia MJ, *et al.* (2008) Venous thromboembolism and liver cirrhosis. *Revista Española de enfermedades digestivas* **100** (5), 259–62.

Spiess BD (2008) Treating heparin resistance with antithrombin or fresh frozen plasma. *Annals of Thoracic Surgery* **85**, 2153–60.

5. *What is the treatment of choice for invasive fungal infection with Candida glabrata in a patient following renal transplant?*

A. Voriconazole

B. Amphotericin B

C. Fluconazole

D. Meropenem

E. Caspofungin

The risk of invasive fungal infection (IFI) is increased in patients after solid organ transplant and is associated with decreased survival. Candida and Aspergillus species are the most common organisms, with non-albicans species increasing in frequency. Historically amphotericin B was the antifungal of choice, but it is associated with significant liver and renal toxicity. Newer liposomal formulations have decreased these risks. However, because of their clinical efficacy, broad spectrum of activity, and favorable side effect profile, echinocandins are becoming the antifungal of choice in many patient populations. Echinocandins include caspogungin, micafungin and anidulafungin. Comparisons of caspofungin to amphotericin B have shown equivalent efficacy and a more favorable side effect profile. In solid organ transplant recipients, caspofungin was found to be effective as both a first and second line treatment, with success in 87% of Candidal and 74% of Aspergillus infections. *In vitro* studies have found efficacy against non-albicans species such as *C. glabrata, C. krusei, C. Parapsilosis,* and *C. tropicalis,* as well as fluconazole resistant albicans isolates. The echinocandins also have the benefit of fewer drug-drug interactions in transplant patients. Specifically, unlike the azoles, they are not inhibitors of cytochrome P450 and are unlikely to alter pharmacodynamics of the calcineurin inhibitors used for immunosuppression. In general guidelines for fungal treatment and prophylaxis recommend posiconazole for prophylaxis in bone marrow transplant patients, caspofungin in confirmed or suspected Candidal IFI in neutropenic and non-neutropenic patients and for febrile neutropenia, and voriconazole in invasive Aspergillosis. Amphotericin B in liposomal preparation should be considered a second line agent for IFI.

Answer: E

Gullo A (2009) Invasive fungal infections: the challenge continues. *Drugs* **69**(Suppl), 65–73.

Ruping MJ, Vehreschild JJ, Cornely OA (2008) Patients at high risk of invasive fungal infections: when and how to treat. *Drugs* **68** (14), 1941–62.

Winkler M, Pratschke J, Schulz U, *et al.* (2010) Caspofungin for post solid organ transplant invasive fungal disease: results of a retrospective observational study. *Transplant Infectious Diseases* **12**, 230–7.

6. *A patient with Childs C cirrhosis secondary to hepatitis B presents with fevers, watery diarrhea, and large violaceous, bullous skin lesions on the legs after consuming raw oysters at a seafood restaurant two nights ago. What is the next step in treatment?*

A. *Doxycycline*

B. *Piperacillin/tazobactam*

C. *Vancomycin*

D. *Colistin*

E. *Penicillin*

This patient is infected with *Vibrio vulnificus,* an invasive, gram-negative bacillus found in warm seawater. Greater than 90% of cases can be traced to ingestion of oysters within one to three days of clinical presentation. Cirrhosis is the most common risk factor for Vibrio infection; however, other immunosuppressed states have also been implicated. Infection can occur as a result of ingestion or from exposure of unhealed wounds to contaminated water. Fever, malaise, and diarrhea generally precede the appearance of the typical skin lesions, which present within 36–48 hours of initial symptoms. The characteristic findings are large violaceous bullae, especially on the lower extremities. Blood, stool, and wound cultures can confirm the diagnosis, but because the spread is rapid and lethal, a high index of clinical suspicion must be present and treatment should be instituted prior to confirmatory cultures. The mortality of patients with Vibrio septicemia can be as high as 50% and increases to greater than 90% if septic shock occurs, or necrotizing soft tissue infection is present. Treatment is with doxycycline and ceftazadime. Alternative regimens include cefotaxime or ciprofloxacin. Additionally, there should be aggressive local wound care with drainage of any fluid collections and wide debridement of necrotic tissue.

Answer: A

Bross MH, Soch K, Morales R, *et al.* (2007) Vibrio vulnificus infection: diagnosis and treatment. *American Family Physician* **76** (4), 539–544.

Jones MK and Oliver JD (2009) Vibrio vulnificus: disease and pathogenesis. *Infection and Immunity* **77** (5), 1723–33.

Lupi O, Madkan V, Tyring SK (2006) Tropical dermatology: bacterial tropical diseases. *Journal of the American Academy of Dermatology* **54** (4), 559–78.

7. *What is the most common cause of late deaths in patients following renal transplant?*

A. *Viral infection*

B. *Bacterial infection*

C. *Chronic rejection*

D. *Cardiovascular disease*

E. *Squamous cell cancer*

The survival following renal transplantation has improved to 95% at one year. The mortality of post-transplant patients is higher than the general population, but significantly better than patients with end-stage renal disease without transplantation. The three leading causes of late death are cardiovascular disease, malignancy and infections. Cardiovascular disease is the leading cause of mortality, implicated in 42–57% of deaths. Malignancy is increasing in frequency and is now the second most common cause, accounting for 9–27% of deaths. The increase in malignancy-related deaths is likely multi-factorial, due to increased potency of immunosuppressive medications, longer post-transplant survival, and malignancy inducing infections such as human papilloma virus and Epstein Barr virus. In general malignancy is more frequent in post-transplant patients than in the general population, the most common are squamous cell skin cancers. However, fatalities due to skin cancers are uncommon. Solid organ malignancies occur less frequently but result in higher mortality. In contrast to malignancy, infection, which accounts for 11–22% of deaths, has been decreasing in frequency, and deaths due to infection are most prevalent in the early time period.

Answer: D

Briggs DJ (2001) Causes of death after renal transplantation. *Nephrology Dialysis Transplantation* **16**, 1545–9.

Marcen R (2009) Immunosuppressive drugs in kidney transplantation: Impact on patient survival, and incidence of cardiovascular disease, malignancy and infection. *Drugs* **69** (16), 2227–37.

Porazko T, Boratynska M, Patrzalek D, *et al.* (2002) Causes of death among cadaver kidney graft recipients between 1983 and 2000. *Transplant Proc* **34**, 2066–7.

8. *Regarding hyperacute rejection which of the following statements is true?*

A. *Its incidence can be decreased by the use of ABO cross-matching*

B. *It is mediated by activated T cells*

C. *It occurs within the first three to seven days post-transplant*

D. *Biopsy reveals peri-vascular lymphocytic infiltrate*

E. *Treatment consists of pulsed steroids and OKT3*

Hyperacute rejection is seen within minutes to hours of reperfusion. It is most commonly seen in renal and cardiac transplants, although there have been case reports in pulmonary and hepatic transplants. It is caused by activation of complement by preformed antibodies to antigens present on the donor vascular endothelial cells. It is similar to an acute hemolytic transfusion reaction, and results in rapid agglutination, small vessel thrombosis and graft loss, additionally if the graft is not removed a severe systemic inflammatory response may occur. The graft itself will become soft, mottled and cyanotic in appearance. Biopsy will demonstrate vascular wall edema and capillary microthrombi. Hyperacute rejection can be prevented by performing a preoperative cytotoxic cross match, and not utilizing ABO incompatible organs. The only treatment is graft removal and emergent re-transplantation.

Answer: A

Della-Guardia B, Almeida SP, Meira-Filho MA, *et al.* (2008) Antibody-mediated rejection: Hyperacute rejection reality in liver transplantation? A case report. *Transplant Proceedings* **40**, 870–1.

Sureshkumar KK, Hussain SM, Carpenter BJ, *et al.* (2007) Antibody-mediated rejection following renal transplantation. *Expert Opinion in Pharmacotherapy* **8** (7), 913–21.

9. *Cardiac allograft vasculopathy (CAV) is an accelerated form of coronary artery disease (CAD) seen in post-cardiac transplant patients, and is one of the leading causes of death after the first post-transplant year. However, it differs from traditional CAD in many ways, regarding these differences, which of the following is true?*

A. *CAV affects proximal vessels whereas CAD is more prominent in distal and intramyocardial vessels*

B. *The plaque pattern of CAV is diffuse and concentric, compared to focal and eccentric in CAD*

C. *Calcium deposition is prominent in CAV, but is rarely seen in CAD*

D. *Disruption of the internal elastic lamina is common in CAV, but rare in CAD*

E. *Active inflammation and progressive intimal hyperplasia and fibrosis are prominent in CAV, but not CAD*

Following cardiac transplantation, median survival is approximately nine years, and increases to 12 years for those who survive the first year. However, long term success continues to be limited by CAV. Cardiac allograft vasculopathy can be seen in 7–8% of patients at one year, but increases to 45–47% at eight years post transplant. Cardiac allograft vasculopathy affects all cardiac vessels including intra-myocardial arteries and, in some cases, coronary veins, this is in contrast to CAD which tends to affect proximal coronary arteries. Cardiac allograft vasculopathy is a progressive inflammation of the intima resulting in fibrosis which is diffuse and concentric, calcium deposition and disruption of the internal elastic lamina are rare. The inflammatory process involves both immune and non-immune factors including; cytomegalovirus infection, dyslipidemia, hyperhomocysteinemia, diabetes, hypertension, and ischemia reperfusion injury. Cardiac allograft vasculopathy also appears to be more prominent among patients with repeated episodes of graft rejection.

Answer: E

Kass M and Haddad H (2006) Cardiac allograft vasculopathy: pathology, prevention and treatment. *Current Opinion in Cardiology* **21**, 132–7.

Ramzy D, Rao V, Brahm J, *et al*. (2005) Cardiac allograft vasculopathy: a review. *Canadian Journal of Surgery* **48** (4), 319–25.

Schmauss D, Weis M. Cardiac allograft vasculopathy: Recent developments. *Circulation* 2008; **117**, 2131–41.

10. *Which of the following medications has been shown to decrease cardiac allograft vasculopathy (CAV) in heart transplant patients?*

A. *Beta blockers*

B. *Cyclosporin*

C. *Steroids*

D. *Aspirin*

E. *Statins*

Cardiac allograft vasculopathy is a progressive inflammatory vasculopathy that is a significant cause of death after cardiac transplant. It is best diagnosed using intravascular ultrasound, as the sensitivity and specificity of angiography are much lower than with traditional CAD. However, as this is not always readily available and is invasive, the best screening test is dobutamine stress echocardiography, which has a sensitivity and specificity of 79% and 83% respectively. Prevention and treatment of CAV should be aimed at decreasing risk factors in post-transplant patients. Hyperlipidemia is common both pre and post-transplant and can be exacerbated by use of immunosuppressants like corticosteroids and cyclosporine. Treatment with statins, in particular pravastatin and simvastatin, has been associated with decreased rates of CAV, decreased allograft rejection, and improved mortality. Additionally, treatment with calcium channel blockers, such as diltiazem, especially in combination with ACE inhibitors has been shown to prevent development of CAV. Prevention and treatment of cytomegalovirus infection with ganciclovir has also been shown to reduce progression of CAV. Lastly immunosuppressive regimens based on tacrolimus and mycophenolate mofetil appear to have less CAV compared to cyclosporine and azathioprine regimens. Newer areas of research show promise with folic acid, everlimus, and L-arginine. Antiplatelet agents, including aspirin, though commonly used in this patient population, have not been shown to prevent CAV.

Answer: E

Kass M and Haddad H (2006) Cardiac allograft vasculopathy: pathology, prevention and treatment. *Current Opinion in Cardiology* **21**, 132–7.

Mehra MR, Raval NY (2004) Metaanalysis of statins and survival in de novo cardiac transplantation. *Transplantation Proceedings* **36**, 1539–41

Ramzy D, Rao V, Brahm J, *et al*. (2005) Cardiac allograft vasculopathy: a review. *Canadian Journal of Surgery* **48** (4), 319–25.

Schmauss D and Weis M (2008) Cardiac allograft vasculopathy: Recent developments. *Circulation* **117**, 2131–41.

11. *A patient develops sudden oliguria following renal transplant, what is the best method to diagnose renal artery thrombosis?*

A. *Ultrasound*

B. *Operative exploration*

C. *Angiography*

D. *Renal biopsy*

E. *CT scan*

Renal artery thrombosis is a rare but serious complication following renal transplant, affecting less than 1% of patients, but often resulting in graft loss. Thrombosis often presents with sudden onset of oliguria in the early post-operative period. Common causes include acute and hyperacute rejection, surgical trauma, kinking of the vessel and hypercoagulable state. Ultrasound is a useful diagnostic tool and has the benefit of being rapidly available, easily performed, noninvasive, and repeatable. Additionally, ultrasound can provide information about venous flow, flow in the renal parenchyma, and dilation of the collecting system. Lastly, while angiography is an excellent option for diagnosis and therapy, ultrasound has the benefit of avoiding contrast exposure. Ultrasound will reveal absence of flow in the artery distal to the thrombus, as well as the vein.

Answer: A

Friedewald SM, Molmenti EP, Friedewald JJ, *et al.* (2005) Vascular and nonvascular complications of renal transplants: sonographic evaluation and correlation with other imaging modalities, surgery, and pathology. *Journal of Clinical Ultrasound* **33** (3), 127–38.

Irshad A, Ackerman S, Sosnouski D, *et al.* (2008) A review of sonographic evaluation of renal transplant complications. *Current Problems in Diagnostic Radiology* **37**, 67–79.

Libicher M, Radeleff, Grenacher L, *et al.* (2006) Interventional therapy of vascular complications following renal transplantation. *Clinical Transplantation* **20** (Suppl 17), 55–9.

12. *Which of the following is a contraindication to liver transplantation?*

A. Hepatitis B

B. Hepatitis C

C. Extrahepatic malignancy

D. Hepatocellular carcinoma with a single 4 cm lesion

E. Hepatocellular carcinoma with three lesions, ranging in size from 1 to 3 cm

Indications for liver transplant include liver failure due to hepatitis B and C, cholestasis, metabolic disorders, alcohol abuse, autoimmune disorders, Budd–Chiari, polycystic liver disease, and primary biliary or hepatic malignancies. Hepatitis B currently has the highest survival rate following liver transplantation, and hepatitis C is the most common indication for liver transplant. Hepatocellular carcinoma (HCC) is now the firth most common cancer worldwide, and less than 15% of patients with HCC are candidates for resection. Additionally, HCC patients have better survival and lower rates of recurrence after liver transplant compared to resection when using the Milan criteria, or UCSF extension of the Milan criteria. The Milan criteria allow transplantation for a single HCC lesion up to 5 cm, and up to three lesions each 3 cm or less. With these criteria, four-year survival is 85%, and the recurrence rate is 8%. Extended criteria from UCSF allow a single lesion up to 6.5 cm or up to three lesions as large as 4.5 cm with a total tumor burden of 8 cm or less. Studies have revealed outcomes equivalent to the Milan criteria in experienced centers. Absolute contraindications to transplantation include extrahepatic malignancy, uncorrectable cardiac or pulmonary disease, irreversible neurologic impairment and uncontrolled sepsis.

Answer: C

Alsina A (2010) Liver transplantation for hepatocellular carcinoma. *Cancer Control* **17** (2), 83–6.

Hanto DW and Johnson S (2007) Liver transplantation. In: Fischer JE and Bland KI (eds) *Mastery of Surgery*, 5th edn, Lippincott Williams & Wilkins, Philadelphia, PA, pp. 1196–211.

13. *What is the mechanism of action of tacrolimus and cyclosporine?*

A. Prevention of activation of T-cells

B. De-activation of T-cells

C. Inhibition of antibody production

D. Prevent proliferation of T and B cells

E. Inhibit antigen recognition of T cells by binding CD3

Both tacrolimus and cyclosporine are calcineurin inhibitors that block interleukin-2 (IL-2) mediated T-cell activation. Tacrolimus binds to FK binding protein and cyclosporine binds to cyclophilin. The drug-protein complexes then bind to calcineurin and inhibit transcription of multiple cytokines including IL-2, IL-3, IL-4, granulocyte-macrophage colony stimulating factor (GM-CSF), interferon gamma, and TNF-alpha.

Answer: A

Mukherjee S and Mukherjee U (2009) A comprehensive review of immunosuppression used for liver transplantation. *Journal of Transplantation* 701464 Epub 2009 Jul 16.

US Multicenter FK506 Liver Study Group (1994) A comparison of tacrolimus (FK 506) and cyclosporine for immunosuppression in liver transplantation. *New England Journal of Medicine* **331** (17), 1110–15.

14. *Which of the following side effects associated with calcineurin inhibitors is known to be more prominent with tacrolimus when compared to cyclosporine?*

A. Hypertension

B. Diabetes

C. Hirsutism

D. Gingival hyperplasia

E. Dyslipidemia

Calcineurin inhibitors are associated with a myriad of side effects, including nephrotoxicity, hypertension, and dyslipidemia. Nephrotoxicity appears to be equivalent between the two drugs, while hypertension and dyslipidemia appear slightly more prominent with cyclosporine. Diabetes is significantly more common with tacrolimus, and gastroenterologic (nausea, diarrhea) and neurologic (headache, tremor, seizure) symptoms also appear to be more prominent. In contrast hirsutism and gingival hyperplasia are more frequently associated with cyclosporine.

Answer: B

Mukherjee S and Mukherjee U (2009) A comprehensive review of immunosuppression used for liver transplantation. *Journal of Transplantation* 701464 Epub Jul 16.

Vicari-Christensen M, Repper S, Basile S, *et al.* (2009) Tacrolimus: review of pharmacokinetics, pharmacodynamics, and pharmacogenetics to facilitate practitioners' understanding and offer strategies for educating patients and promoting adherence. *Progress in Transplantation* **19** (3), 277–284.

15. *A patient develops acute respiratory deterioration, with airspace disease on chest x-ray, worsening hypoxemia, and increased airway pressures, 14 hours after lung transplant. What is the most likely etiology?*

A. Cytomegalovirus pneumonia

B. Ischemia reperfusion injury

C. Pseudomonas aeruginosa pneumonia

D. Obliterative bronchiolitis

E. Pulmonary embolism

Early respiratory failure is a common occurrence after lung transplant, affecting between 20–55% of patients. The most common cause of early respiratory failure, accounting for greater than 50% of cases, is ischemia reperfusion lung injury (IRLI). This commonly occurs within the first 72 hours of surgery. It is characterized by rapid development of airspace disease, progressive hypoxemia with PaO_2/FiO_2 ratio less than 200, and increased pulmonary pressures. Risk factors for IRLI include preoperative pulmonary hypertension, right ventricular dysfunction, cardiopulmonary bypass, and prolonged cold ischemia times. Ischemia reperfusion lung injury, along with episodes of acute rejection, has been associated with increased risk of obliterative bronchiolitis (OB). Obliterative broncitis is most prominent in the late postoperative period with a median time to diagnosis of 16–20 months. Bacterial and fungal pneumonias are also common in the early postoperative period, but generally present later than IRLI with a median time to occurrence of 34 days. Bacterial pneumonia is the earliest and most common, followed in timing and frequency by fungal and viral pneumonias. Pseudomonas, Aspergillosis, and CMV are the most common bacterial, fungal, and viral etiologies respectively. Pulmonary embolus may be an under-diagnosed cause of post-lung transplant respiratory failure in the first month. However, it usually presents between 72 hours and 1 week, and generally does not result in infiltrate on chest x-ray.

Answer: B

Aguilar-Guisado M, Givalda J, Ussetti P, *et al.* (2007) Pneumonia after lung transplantation in the Resitra Cohort: A multicenter prospective study. *American Journal of Trasplantation* **7**, 1989–96.

Campos S, Caramori M, Teixeira R, *et al.* (2008) Bacterial and fungal pneumonias after lung transplantation. *Transplant Proc* **40** (3), 822–4.

Chatila W, Furukawa S, Gaughan JP, *et al.* (2003) Respiratory failure after lung transplantation. *Chest* **123**, 165–73.

Granton J (2006) Update of early respiratory failure in the lung transplant recipient. *Current Opinion in Critical Care* **12**, 19–24.

16. *In cases of severe or life threatening cytomegalovirus (CMV) enteritis what is the treatment of choice?*

A. *Oral ganciclovir*

B. *Oral valganciclovir*

C. *IV ganciclovir*

D. *IV valganciclovir*

E. *Acyclovir*

For CMV prophylaxis oral or IV ganciclovir, or valganciclovir can be used with similar efficacy. Both are superior to acyclovir. Prophylaxis is begun in the early post-transplant period and continued for 3–6 months. However, in cases of CMV infection the gold standard is IV ganciclovir. Studies have shown equivalent efficacy and similar outcomes using oral valganciclovir for nonlife-threatening infections in adult patients. However, IV ganciclovir remains the treatment of choice for pediatric patients and in those with severe life-threatening infections. Additionally, IV ganciclovir should be chosen for those patients in whom oral formulations would be poorly tolerated or unlikely to be absorbed, such as in enteritis. Consensus recommendations from the Infectious Diseases Section of The Transplantation Society recommend IV ganciclovir twice daily until viral eradication is seen on two consecutive titers, and for no fewer than two weeks.

Answer: C

Asberg A, Humar A, Rollag H, *et al.* (2007) Oral valganciclovier is noninferior to intravenous ganciclovir for the treatment of cytomegalovirus disease in solid organ transplant recipients. *American Journal of Transplantation* **7**, 2106–13.

Kotton CN, Kumar D, Caliendo AM, *et al.* (2010) International consensus guidelines on the management of cytomegalovirus in solid organ transplantation. *Transplantation* **89** (7), 779–95.

17. *During the second post-operative week after lung transplant a patient develops pneumonia. Which of the following is the most likely organism involved?*

A. *Pneumocystis jiroveci*

B. *Pseudomonas aeruginosa*

C. *Staphylococcus aureus*

D. *Aspergillus fumigates*

E. *Cytomegalovirus*

Pneumonia is a common complication following lung transplant. It is the second leading cause of postoperative respiratory failure in the early (less than 1 month) period. Gram negative rods (GNR) predominate, accounting for 83% of pneumonias, with the most common organisms being Pseudomonas, Acinetobacter and *E. coli.* Gram positive bacterial infections are most commonly due to *Staphylococcus aureus,* but are less common than GNR pneumonias and appear later in the post-transplant period. Aspergillus and cytomegalovirus (CMV) are less common causes of pneumonia and occur later than bacterial pneumonias, largely due to antimicrobial prophylaxis. Prophylaxis has also decreased the risk of pneumonia from atypical organisms, such as Pneumocystis from 10–12% to almost nil in most centers.

Answer: B

Aguilar-Guisado M, Givalda J, Ussetti P, *et al.* (2007) Pneumonia after lung transplantation in the Resitra Cohort: A multicenter prospective study. *American Journal of Trasplantation* **7**, 1989–96.

Campos S, Caramori M, Teixeira R, *et al.* (2008) Bacterial and fungal pneumonias after lung transplantation. *Transplantation Proceedings* **40** (3), 822–4.

Gavalda J, Roman A (2007) Infection in lung transplantation. *Enfermedades infecciosas y microbiología clínica* **25** (10), 639–49.

18. *A patient who recently underwent kidney transplant presents to clinic with swelling in the lower* *abdomen and drainage of milky fluid from his surgical wound. Creatinine levels of the fluid are low and ultrasound reveals an anechoic fluid collection and hydronephrosis of the allograft. What is the most likely diagnosis?*

A. *Urinoma*

B. *Surgical dehiscence*

C. *Abscess*

D. *Lymphocele*

E. *Hematoma*

Lymphocele occurs in 8–15% of renal transplants. They occur as a result of disruption of the lymphatics in the retroperitoneum during surgical dissection. They can exert a mass effect on the transplanted kidney, and generally appear as anechoic or minimally complex perinephric fluid collections. They are generally asymptomatic, but mass effect may result in hydronephrosis or ipsilateral lower extremity edema. Presentation usually occurs between the fourth and eighth postoperative weeks. Treatment consist of percutaneous drainage.

Answer: D

Atray NK, Moore F, Zaman F, *et al*. (2004) Post transplant lymphocele: A single center experience. *Clinical Transplantation* **18** (Suppl 12), 46–9.

Irshad A, Ackerman S, Sosnouski D, *et al*. (2008) A review of sonographic evaluation of renal transplant complications. *Current Problems in Diagnostic Radiology* **37**, 67–79.

19. *A patient is postoperative day 10 following a liver transplant. He has become progressively septic and complains of right upper quadrant pain. Labs reveal an increased white blood cell count and elevated liver function tests. CT scan reveals air in the biliary tree. What is the most likely diagnosis?*

A. *Ascending cholangitis*

B. *Portal vein thrombosis*

C. *Hepatic artery thrombosis*

D. *Hepatic abscess*

E. *Acute rejection*

Hepatic artery thrombosis (HAT) is a rare but serious complication of liver transplant. It occurs in 2.5–15% of cases, and is subdivided into early and late thrombosis. Early thrombosis generally occurs in the first days to weeks and is characterized by sepsis/SIRS syndrome, elevated liver function tests, and right upper quadrant pain; it can also result in fulminant liver failure. Late thrombosis occurs a few months to a year after transplant, and can present with intermittent recurrent sepsis, delayed bile leak or stricture, or asymptomatic elevation in liver function tests. Risk factors for HAT include obesity, hypercoagulable state, history of transarterial chemotherapy, surgical trauma, and technical error. Additionally, incidence of HAT is increased among pediatric and living donor liver transplants. The gold standard for diagnosis of HAT is angiography. Imaging can also include CT scan, which will show absence of opacification of the hepatic artery, liver abscess or necrosis, and stricture or necrosis of the biliary tree. Ultrasound can also be used to diagnose HAT, and has the benefit of ease of use, repeatability and independence from contrast. However, it has a lower sensitivity when compared to angiography, ranging from 50–60% compared to 80–90% in angiography. Treatment includes surgical revasularization, endovascular thrombolysis/ thrombectomy, and systemic heparinization. However, urgent/emergent re-transplantation is required in 50–90% of cases. Associated mortality is 50–55%, and is better with late compared to early thrombosis.

Answer: C

Duffy JP, Hong JC, Farmer DG, *et al*. (2009) Vascular complications of orthotopic liver transplantation: Experience in more than 4200 patients. *Journal of the American College of Surgeons* **208**, 896–905.

Goralczyk AD, Meir V, Ramadori G, *et al*. (2010) Acute paranoid psychosis as sole clinical presentation of hepatic artery thrombosis after living donor liver transplantation. *BMC Surgery* **10**, 7.

Proposito D, Segurola CL, Garcia, GI, *et al*. (2000) Diagnosis and treatment of hepatic artery thrombosis after liver transplantation. *Chirurgia italiana* **52**(5), 505–25.

20. *Successful pancreatic transplant will result in correction of insulin dependence in up to 80% of patients at* *one year. It can also reverse or stabilize all of the following complications of diabetes except?*

A. Retinopathy

B. Gastroparesis

C. Nephropathy

D. Macrovascular disease

E. Neuropathy

Pancreatic transplant has improved greatly in modern times. Survival is now greater than 95% at one year and 90% at three years. Graft survival is 85% in combined kidney/pancreas transplants and slightly less for solitary pancreas transplant. Insulin independence is achieved in 80% of patients at one year. Additionally, transplantation can stabilize diabetic retinopathy and can reverse neuropathy, gastroparesis, orthostatic hypotension, and nephropathy in the native kidneys. While there has been no evidence to suggest a benefit in macrovascular disease, there is some evidence that transplant can improve microvasculr microangiopathy. Lastly, transplant recipients nearly uniformly report immunosuppression management to be easier than management of labile diabetes.

Answer: D

Gruessner AC, Sutherland DE (2008) Pancreas transplant outcomes for the United States cases as reported to the United Network for Organ Sharing and the International Pancreas Transplant Registry. *Clinical Transplantation* 45–56.

Sutherland DE, Gruessner RWG, Gruessner AC (2001) Pancreas transplantation for treatment of diabetes mellitus. *World Journal of Surgery* **25** (4), 487–96.

Chapter 22 Obstetric Critical Care

Gerard J. Fulda, MD, FACS, FCCM, FCCP and Anthony Sciscione, MD

1. *A 28-year-old primigravid pregnant woman at 21 weeks gestation is admitted to the ICU following a motor vehicle collision and minor head injury. She was a belted driver. She was intoxicated with alcohol and cocaine. Her BP = 140/60 mm Hg, HR = 110 beats/minute, and the fetal heart rate is 120 beats/minute. The patient is now complaining of new-onset uterine contractions and is noted to have a moderate amount of vaginal bleeding. The most appropriate next step is to*

A. *Proceed with an emergency bedside Cesarean section for uterine rupture*

B. *Perform an emergency ultrasound looking for fetal injury*

C. *Administer 300 mg RhoGAM STAT for this Rh positive mother*

D. *Perform an emergency ultrasound looking for a hypoechoic collection between the placenta and myometrium*

E. *Obtain a STAT pelvic x-ray and determine the need for pelvic angiography with embolization*

This patient has a placental abruption and at this gestational age the fetus would be non-viable. The focus should be on keeping the mother stable. Major trauma is associated with placental abruption and may be as high as 1–5%. The greater the energy transfers the higher the incidence of abruption. Motor vehicle collisions are one of the leading causes of abruption as well as uterine rupture; the most likely mechanism is due to mechanical shearing forces of the placenta along with uterine stretching during deceleration. The diagnosis of abruption is usually made by emergency ultrasound. Early hemorrhage is typically hyperechoic or isoechoic, whereas resolving hematomas are hypoechoic within 1 week and sonolucent within 2 weeks of the abruption. Acute hemorrhage can be misinterpreted as uterine fibroids or a thickened placenta.

While an assessment of the bony pelvis is necessary, plain films alone would not dictate the need for embolization, especially in the face of stable vital signs. If the physical examination suggests a major pelvic fracture then a CT of the pelvis with contrast would be indicated. Extravasation of contrast with hemodynamic or fetal instability would be an indication for angio-embolization.

RhoGAM is administered to mothers with placental abruption when they are Rh negative only. As the fetus is not viable, an emergency Cesarean section is not an option and it is unlikely for a fetal ultrasound to lead to any useful predelivery interventions.

Answer: D

Harris CM (2004) Trauma and pregnancy. In: Foley MR, Strong Jr TH, Garite TJ (eds) *Obstetric Intensive Care Manual*, 2nd edn, McGraw-Hill, New York, p. 239.

Nyberg DA, Cyr DR, Mack LA, *et al.* (1987) Sonographic spectrum of placental abruption. *American Journal of Roentgenology* **148**, 161.

Nyberg DA, Mack LA, Benedetti TJ, *et al.* (1987) Placental abruption and placental hemorrhage: Correlation of sonographic findings with fetal outcome. *Radiology* **358**, 357.

2. *You are called to the delivery suite for a woman in protracted labor who has suddenly developed acute respiratory distress and has been intubated. She is now hypotensive and on vasopressors. You suspect she has had an amniotic fluid embolism and anticipate all of the following EXCEPT*

A. *Hemorrhage and accompanying disseminated intravascular coagulopathy (DIC)*

B. *Left ventricular dysfunction*

C. *Prolonged pulmonary vasoconstriction*

D. *Fetal distress and the need for immediate delivery*

Surgical Critical Care and Emergency Surgery: Clinical Questions and Answers, First Edition. Edited by Forrest O. Moore, Peter M. Rhee, Samuel A. Tisherman and Gerard J. Fulda.

E. *Fetal squamous cells in the pulmonary arterial circulation*

The diagnosis of amniotic fluid embolism is generally made on clinical grounds and after other common causes of sudden shock are potentially ruled out. Amniotic fluid embolism has an incidence of about 1 in 30 000 and is associated with protracted labor. There is a very high mortality rate if unrecognized. The underlying physiologic response to amniotic fluid embolism is vasomotor collapse due to vasodilation (not vasoconstriction) and left ventricular dysfunction. The patient presents with profound shock and hypoxia. If obtained, the chest x-ray will likely demonstrate bilateral interstitial and alveolar infiltrated. DIC can be the presenting symptom in amniotic fluid embolism and if present, increases the likelihood of the diagnosis. Fetal squamous cells have been recovered from maternal pulmonary artery blood in suspected cases.

Treatment is directed to the presenting symptoms which usually require aggressive volume resuscitation, inotropic support, mechanical ventilation, and blood component therapy. Rapid delivery of the fetus is definitely indicated for an amniotic fluid embolism in a viable fetus.

Answer: C

Clark SL, Pavlova Z, Greenspoon J (1986) Squamous cells in the maternal pulmonary circulation. *American Journal of Obstetrics and Gynecology* **154**, 104–6.

Gist RS, Stafford IP, Leibowitz AB, Beilin Y (2009) Amniotic fluid embolism. *Anesthesia and Analgesia* **108** (5), 1599.

3. *You are caring for a 21-year-old G1 P1 woman admitted to the ICU five days after a Cesarean delivery for arrest of descent. Her labor was complicated by prolonged rupture of the membranes. She was placed on piperacillin/tazobactam on the third postoperative day when the fever began. She is postoperative day 5 and she looks and feels well. She currently has a BP 105/75 mm Hg, HR = 115 beats/minute, T = 38.2, RR = 20 breaths/minute and WBC = 13.2 × 10^3/microL. Her wound appears to be healing well and a CT of the pelvis and blood cultures are all negative. The most appropriate next step is to:*

A. *Add fluconazole to her antimicrobial regime*

B. *Perform venography*

C. *Begin systemic anticoagulation with heparin*

D. *Recommend the patient undergo an urgent hysterectomy*

E. *Administer drotrecogin*

This patient has septic pelvic thrombophlebitis. While some patients can present several weeks post partum, most patients present 3–5 days post partum with a persistent fever *despite* antibiotics. The clinical exam may be relatively benign and the patient not appearing severely ill. Rick factors include Cesarean section, arrested decent and pelvic infections. Antibiotic administration along with systemic anticoagulation is the initial treatment of choice for this condition. Diagnosis can be difficult and requires a high index of suspicion. While most patients will have an elevated white blood cell count blood cultures are frequently negative. Still blood culture should be done because, if positive, it can assist in antibiotic selection. Without a positive culture antibiotics should be directed towards Gram positive cocci, and enteric organisms including anaerobes.

There is no single imaging study that can reliably diagnose septic pelvic thrombophlebitis, especially septic thrombophlebitis of the deep veins. While CT and MRI have a better sensitivity than ultrasound, a negative study does not rule out the presence of a septic pelvic thrombophlebitis. Venography will not visualize the uterine veins.

There is no evidence that the patient has a systemic fungal infection and with only two days of antibiotic therapy this is unlikely. Similarly, the patient does not have any signs or symptoms of severe sepsis or septic shock and as such drotrecogin is not indicated. Removal of the uterus is rarely indicated for septic pelvic thrombophlebitis and in this patient it is not a first choice for management.

Answer: C

Garcia J, Aboujaoude R, Apuzzio J, Alvarez JR (2006) Septic pelvic thrombophlebitis: diagnosis and management. *Infectious Diseases in Obstetrics and Gynecology* 15614.

Pastorek JG (1994) Septic pelvic-vein thrombophlebitis. In: Pastorek JG (ed.) *Obstetric and Gynecologic Infectious Disease,* Raven Press, New York, p. 165.

Twickler DM, Setiawan AT, Evans RS, *et al.* (1997) Imaging of puerperal septic thrombophlebitis: prospective comparison of MR imaging, CT, and sonography. *American Journal of Roentgenology* **169** (4), 1039.

4. *A previously healthy, 31-year-old G1 P1 woman at 39 weeks gestation is found to have a Hb of 11.6 mg/dL and a platelet count of 40 000 and Cr = 2.6 mg/dL. The rest of her lab values are normal. Her BP = 160/100 mm Hg, HR = 88 beats/minute, and RR 16 breaths/minute. Urinary output is decreased at <30 ml/hr for the last 3 hours. The most appropriate next step is to:*

A. Begin induction of labor with oxytocin

B. Perform a Cesarean delivery

C. Central Swan–Ganz monitoring

D. Plasmapheresis

E. Begin plasma expansion with colloid

This patient has anemia, thrombocytopenia, and renal insufficiency. This triad is associated with thrombotic thrombocytopenic purpura (TTP) and hemolytic uremic syndrome (HUS). The distinction between the two is that neurologic symptoms predominate in TTP and renal failure is the hallmark of HUS. This patients increasing Cr and decreasing urinary output suggest she has HUS. This condition has a very high maternal and fetal mortality and needs prompt action. The clinical presentation can be confused with severe sepsis and DIC, which are more common and should be ruled out as soon as possible. The placental vessels can thrombose so that a viable fetus should be delivered as soon as possible. Induction with oxytocin and a vaginal delivery would be preferable to performing a Cesarean section in this coagulopathic woman. There is some evidence that HUS can resolve with the delivery. Since there could be some confusion that this represents severe pre-eclampsia with or without HELLP syndrome, prompt delivery of the fetus would also be indicated. Failure to respond following delivery confirms the diagnosis of HUS over these other causes.

Further management of the patient who fails to improve following delivery is plasmapheresis. While consideration for plasmapheresis prior to delivery should be entertained induction of labor should begin as soon as the diagnosis is entertained. While the patient likely would benefit from volume expansion and invasive monitoring they are secondary considerations in the management scheme.

Answer: A

Fujimura Y, Matsumoto M, Kokame K, *et al.* (2009) Pregnancy-induced thrombocytopenia and TTP, and the risk of fetal death, in Upshaw–Schulman syndrome: a series of 15 pregnancies in 9 genotyped patients. *British Journal of Haematology* **144** (5), 742.

Natelson EA, White D (1985) Recurrent thrombotic thrombocytopenic purpura in early pregnancy: effect of uterine evacuation. *Obstet Gynecol.* **66** (3 Suppl), 54S.

Vesely SK, Li X, McMinn JR, *et al.* (2004) Pregnancy outcomes after recovery from thrombotic thrombocytopenic purpura-hemolytic uremic syndrome. *Transfusion* **44** (8), 1149.

5. *A woman in her 36th week of gestation presents with generalized malaise, headache right upper quadrant pain, and mild hypertension. Which clinical features favor the diagnosis of acute fatty liver of pregnancy (AFLP) versus HELLP syndrome?*

A. Fibrinogen is decreased in AFLP and normal or increased in HELLP

B. DIC is more common in HELLP

C. Both are likely to have decreased glucose levels

D. Increased bilirubin levels are diagnostic for HELLP

E. CT scanning is used to distinguish the two conditions

Acute fatty liver of pregnancy (AFLP) is a rare condition with a very high mortality rate. The condition is thought to be due to an inherited defect in lipid metabolism. A mutation, G1528C, results in a defect in a mitochondrial protein long-chain 3-hydroxyacyl CoA dehydrogenase (LCHAD). This leads to an accumulation of hepato-toxic long chain fatty acids. It is important to distinguish AFLP from HELLP syndrome. HELLP syndrome leads to areas of hepatic necrosis while the pathology of AFLP is due to fatty infiltration of the liver. The definitive diagnosis can be made with hepatic biopsy but is usually made clinically due to the risk and delay in performing the biopsy. Clinically, AFLP patients have a decrease in both fibrinogen and glucose, with severe hypoglycemia common. HELLP patients usually have normal levels of glucose and fibrinogen. Both conditions increase bilirubin and are associated with DIC but DIC is twice as common in AFLP (75% versus 20–40%). Diagnostic imaging with CT and ultrasound is not diagnostic but can be used to rule out other conditions leading to hepatic failure.

Treatment is directed to early delivery of the fetus. Most patients are in their trimester when AFLP develops and it usually resolves following delivery of the fetus. Intravenous glucose infusion and a combination of factor concentrates are usually required to correct the hypoglycemia and coagulopathy in preparation for delivery. When diagnosed and treated early there is a good chance for recovery, delays in management are often fatal.

Answer: A

Castro MA, Ouzounian JG, Colletti PM, *et al.* (1996) Radiologic studies in acute fatty liver of pregnancy. A review of the literature and 19 new cases. *Journal of Reproductive Medicine* **41** (11), 839.

Knight M, Nelson-Piercy C, Kurinczuk JJ, *et al.* (2008) A prospective national study of acute fatty liver of pregnancy in the UK. *UK Obstetric Surveillance System, Gut* **57** (7), 951.

Rajasri AG, Srestha R, Mitchell J (2007) Acute fatty liver of pregnancy (AFLP)—an overview, *Journal of Obstetrics and Gynaecology* **27** (3), 237.

6. *A 17-year-old G1 P1 is admitted to the ICU for the diagnosis of severe pre-eclampsia with a persistent BP of 165/112 mm Hg, 4+ proteinuria and decreased urinary output (< 30 ml/hr). Which is the best initial agent for controlling her hypertension?*

A. Nitroprusside

B. Captopril

C. Furosemide

D. Losartan

E. Labetalol

Critical care pharmacotherapy in the pregnant patient involves a comprehensive understanding of the risk and benefits to both the mother and fetus. This is best accomplished in a multiprofessional model of critical-care delivery including a pharmacist in the team. All antihypertensive agents can cross the placenta. Angiotensin receptor antagonist (losartan) and angiotensin converting enzyme inhibitors (captopril) are known to be harmful to the fetus and should not be used if possible. Nitroprusside has the potential to develop toxic metabolites over time and with high doses and should not be the initial agent selected unless treating a life-threatening malignant hypertensive crisis. Furosemide can be used for management of hypertension and is thought to be safe for the fetus. The risk in using a diuretic in a pregnant patient is volume depletion and for this reason they should be use with caution. Labetalol can be used in the pregnant patient and due to the fact that it has both alpha and beta blocking properties which may preserve placental blood flow better than other beta blockers. While not listed as a choice, calcium channel blockers such as nifedipine have also been used to manage hypertension in pregnancy.

Answer: E

Cooper WO, Hernandez-Diaz S, Arbogast PG, *et al.* (2006) Major congenital malformations after first-trimester exposure to ACE inhibitors. *New England Journal of Medicine* **354** (23), 2443.

Magee LA, Duley L (2003) Oral beta-blockers for mild to moderate hypertension during pregnancy. Cochrane Database Systematic Review.

7. *A 35-year-old African-American woman one month post-partum undergoes laparoscopic cholecystectomy due to symptomatic gallstones presenting during her pregnancy. She is transferred to the ICU post operatively for hypotension unresponsive to fluids during the surgery. On questioning, she has been short of breath, fatigued, and has developed a nonproductive cough, worse at night, which began during the last couple of weeks of her pregnancy. Management of this patient should include:*

A. Cardiac catheterization to evaluate the LAD

B. The administration of corticosteroids

C. The administration of immune globulin

D. A cardiac biopsy to rule out myocarditis

E. Standard heart failure care

This patient has developed peripartum cardiomyopathy, which should be managed in a similar way to other causes of congestive heart failure. This condition occurs late in pregnancy, within one month of delivery, and up to five months postpartum. The diagnosis is usually made clinically in a patient who develops heart failure (LV ejection fraction less than 40%) during this timeframe without a history of prior heart disease or other identifiable cause of heart failure. The etiology is unknown with immunologic and inflammatory hypothesis most often proposed. Risk factors for the development of postpartum cardiomyopathy have included older multiparous mothers, those with hypertension, drug abuse, and long-term tocolytic therapy. Since the diagnosis is made on a clinical basis, invasive diagnostic test are not indicated unless attempting to rule out other causes of heart failure which this patient does not have. While some authors have suggested a myocarditis as an explanation results of myocardial biopsy have not been uniform and do not alter the management. There is no proven benefit to immunosuppressive therapy or the administration of immunoglobulin.

The treatment is directed to the management of heart failure. The main caveat during pregnancy is to avoid drugs such as angiotensin receptor antagonist and angiotensin converting enzyme inhibitors, which are known to be harmful to the fetus. Selective beta blockers are safe and frequently used. Diuretics should be used with caution predelivery due to the potential for volume depletion. Digoxin can be safely added as a second-line agent, hydralazine and nitroglycerine are options for vasodilators,

The prognosis is guarded with a mortality rate of 10% and most women are left with some residual cardiac dysfunction.

Answer: E

Bozkurt B, Villaneuva FS, Holubkov R, *et al.* (1999) Intravenous immune globulin in the therapy of peripartum cardiomyopathy. *Journal of the American College of Cardiology* **34** (1), 177.

Mason JW, O'Connell JB, Herskowitz A, *et al.* (1995) A clinical trial of immunosuppressive therapy for myocarditis. *New England Journal of Medicine* **333** (5), 269.

Sliwa K, Fett J, Elkayam U (2006) Peripartum cardiomyopathy. *Lancet* **368** (9536), 687.

8. *A 21-year-old G1 P0 woman at 30 weeks gestation is admitted to the hospital with the diagnosis of preterm labor and is 3 cm dilated. She is admitted to Labor and Delivery and given 4 gm IV magnesium sulfate load followed by a 2 gm/h infusion. Soon after the loading dose of magnesium sulfate is infused she becomes lethargic, acutely short of breath and her SaO_2 decreases to 87%. The most appropriate next step is to:*

A. Administer 5000 units heparin IV and obtain a STAT spiral CT

B. Perform an emergency Cesarean section

C. Administer 10 ml of 10% Calcium chloride

D. Administer 20 μg/min terbutaline infusion

E. Administer 250 ml of 3% sodium chloride solution

This woman has tocolytic associated pulmonary edema. While volume overload is usually a contributing factor and patients present with signs and symptoms similar to other forms of pulmonary edema the initial management consist of discontinuing the offending tocolytic, in this case magnesium sulfate. It is important to rule out other causes of hypoxia, in this patient who had symptoms develop with the infusion of magnesium along with the accompanying lethargy suggest magnesium sulfate as the etiology. Without this association consideration to a sudden pulmonary embolism should be given and heparin and spiral CT scan would be a reasonable answer. The management tocolytic associated pulmonary endemia from magnesium includes administration of 10 ml of 10% Calcium chloride to counteract the effects of the magnesium. Other standard therapies such as oxygen and judicious diuresis should be given as well.

Unless there is evidence given of fetal distress Cesarean section and urgent delivery are not necessary. However, discontinuation of the tocolytic can result in a return of preterm labor. Resolution of the pulmonary edema usually occurs within

12–24 hours. Adding an additional tocolytic (terbutaline) or additional volume expansion (3% sodium chloride) will likely worsen the pulmonary edema and should not be chosen.

Answer: C

Samol JM, Lambers DS (2005) Magnesium sulfate tocolysis and pulmonary edema: the drug or the vehicle? *American Journal of Obstetrics and Gynecology* **192** (5), 1430.

Sciscione AC, Ivester T, Largoza M, *et al.* (2003) Acute pulmonary edema in pregnancy. *Obstetrics and Gynecology* **101** (3), 511.

9. *A 26-year-old G1 P1 woman at 32 weeks has had a normal prenatal course but has a long standing history of severe asthma which has been poorly controlled. She presents with acute shortness of breath and is admitted to the ICU for close monitoring. The asthma progresses and requires intubation. Intubation and ventilation should take into account the fact that normal physiologic changes of pregnancy lead to all of the following except?*

A. *An increased tidal volume of 40%*

B. *An increase in oxygen consumption of 30–40 mL/min*

C. *A decrease in functional residual capacity (FRC) by 25%*

D. *An increase in A-a gradient by 10–15%*

E. *An increase in $PaCO_2$ to 45 mm Hg*

The pregnant woman has an increased metabolic demand secondary to the needs of the fetus. This leads to several predictable physiologic alterations of the respiratory system. The most notable change is an increase in oxygen requirements of about 30–40 ml/min. The respiratory compensation is to increase the minute volume by increasing the tidal volume by about 40%, some of this is accomplished by a decrease in the FRC by 25%. There is a predictable increase in the A-a gradient, which improves the availability of oxygen to the mother. All of these compensations lead to a decrease in $PaCO_2$. The mother is able to maintain a relatively normal pH due to the gradual nature of these changes which allows the kidneys time to excrete excess bicarbonate.

Answer: E

Fundamental Critical Care Support Manual 3rd edition, Critical Care in Pregnancy, *Society of Critical Care Medicine*. Janice L. Zimmerman (ed.), pp. 14-1–14-12.

10. *Which of the following is characteristic of venous thromboembolism (VTE) in pregnancy?*

A. *Antepartum VTE is most common in the third trimester*

B. *Calf involvement occurs early in the process and spreads to the proximal veins*

C. *VTE occurs more frequently on the right side*

D. *Resistance to activated protein C occurs in the second and third trimester*

E. *D-dimer is a valuable invasive screening tool for VTE*

Venous thromboembolic disease occurs more frequently (10–50 times) in pregnant versus nonpregnant women. The increased risk appears to occur with the onset of pregnancy and results in VTE being equally distributed throughout all trimesters. One contributing factor is increased resistance to activated protein C in the last two trimesters and increases the hypercoagulable state of pregnancy.

Eighty percent to 90% of VTE in pregnancy occurs on the left side, presumably due to the pelvic venous anatomy. In many cases these VTE originate in the pelvis and are not the result of calf DVT, which extended proximally.

D-dimer is an ELISA assay that detects the products of fibrin degradation. Routinely used in the emergency department, a negative D-dimer makes the presence of VTE unlikely. A positive result is used to further evaluate the patient. However, in the pregnant patient D-dimer levels routinely increase in the second and third trimesters, with more than half of normal pregnant women having an elevated D-dimer level. Thus D-dimer is much less valuable as a screening tool in the pregnant patient than the nonpregnant.

Answer: D

Bourjeily G, Paidas M, Khalil H, *et al.* (2010) Pulmonary embolism in pregnancy. *Lancet* **375** (9713), 500.

Heit JA, Kobbervig CE, James AH, *et al.* (2005) Trends in the incidence of venous thromboembolism during pregnancy or postpartum: a 30-year population-based study. *Annals of Internal Medicine* **143** (10), 697.

Marik PE, Plante LA (2008) Venous thromboembolic disease and pregnancy. *New England Journal of Medicine* **359** (19), 2025.

Walker MC, Garner PR, Keely EJ, *et al.* (1997) Changes in activated protein C resistance during normal pregnancy. *American Journal of Obstetrics and Gynecology* **177** (1), 162.

11. *A 23-year-old woman in her second trimester is in the emergency department due to the sudden onset of shortness of breath while at home. She has no history of pulmonary disease and has had an uncomplicated pregnancy. She is anxious and diaphoretic. She has received one liter normal saline and is using her accessory muscles to breath. Her chest X-ray is unremarkable. Her current BP = 80/70 mm Hg, HR = 146 beats/minute, RR = 36 breaths/minute, SaO_2 = 82% on a 100% nonrebreathing mask.*

A. *TPA should be administered if she remains hypotensive*

B. *Fondaparinux administration in the first hour is associated with improved outcomes*

C. *D-Dimer levels can be used to determine if a spiral CT is justified*

D. *Heparin is contraindicated without a confirmatory test*

E. *Helical CT scan is associated with a significant fetal radiation exposure*

The risk of venous thromboembolic disease is significantly increased in pregnancy. A patient in her third trimester who presents with the sudden onset of hypoxia, hypotension, and a normal chest X-ray should be considered to have a pulmonary embolism until proven otherwise.

The use of thrombolytic agents in pregnancy associated pulmonary embolism has been used successfully. The key is to balance the risk and benefits based on the patient's condition. Compared to heparin, thrombolytics have an increased risk of causing bleeding. This patient is profoundly hypotensive and hypoxic and if uncorrected rapidly threatens both the mother and fetus. In this situation thrombolytics should be administered. The risk of bleeding is about 6% in these patients.

There is no demonstrated benefit directly associated with early fondaparinux administration in VTE. Due to a paucity of safety information fondaparinux is not recommended in pregnancy. While low molecular weight heparin is used in pregnancy, especially for long term treatment, this patient is hypotensive and heparinization via IV unfractionated heparin is effective immediately and can be reversed with protamine in the event of bleeding. Heparin should be administered when there is a strong clinical suspicion for a pulmonary embolism and before all diagnostic testing is complete.

D-dimer is an ELISA assay that detects the products of fibrin degradation. Routinely used in the emergency department, a negative D-dimer makes the presence of VTE unlikely. A positive result is used to further evaluate the patient. However, in the pregnant patient D-dimer levels routinely increase in the second and third trimesters, with more than half of normal pregnant women having an elevated D-dimer level. Thus D-dimer is much less valuable as a screening tool in the pregnant patient than the nonpregnant.

Spiral CT is the diagnostic study of choice for pulmonary embolism and should not be withheld due to a fear of radiation exposure to the fetus. While all ionizing radiation can lead to radiation damage, it is generally believed that the amount of radiation from a spiral CT scan is insufficient to cause fetal deformity.

Answer: A

Ahearn GS, Hadjiliadis D, Govert JA, Tapson VF (2002) Massive pulmonary embolism during pregnancy successfully treated with recombinant tissue plasminogen activator: a case report and review of treatment options. *Archives of Internal Medicines* **162** (11), 1221.

Bourjeily G, Paidas M, Khalil H, Rosene-Montella K, Rodger M (2010) Pulmonary embolism in pregnancy. *Lancet* **375** (9713), 500.

Turrentine MA, Braems G, Ramirez MM (1995) Use of thrombolytics for the treatment of thromboembolic disease during pregnancy. *Obstetrical and Gynecological Survey* **50** (7), 534.

Winer-Muram HT, Boone JM, Brown HL, *et al.* (2002) Pulmonary embolism in pregnant patients: fetal radiation dose with helical CT. *Radiology* **224** (2), 487.

12. *A woman in her first trimester is admitted to the ICU and requires mechanical ventilation and has associated renal insufficiency. Which of the following is most correct?*

A. *Lorazepam is preferred over midazolam for sedation*

B. *Cisatracurium is preferred over vecuronium as a paralytic agent*

C. *ACE inhibitors are preferred over digoxin in treating congestive failure*

D. *Fosphenytoin is preferred over levetiracetam as an anticonvulsant*

E. *Epinephrine is preferred over ephedrine for vasopressor support*

Critical care for the pregnant patient requires a broad understanding of the fetal risk of common ICU medications. Among benzodiazepines lorazepam has been shown to be teratogenic in animal studies, for this reason midazolam is theoretically a superior agent. Cisatracurium is classified as FDA category B in pregnancy versus C for Vecuronium. Cisatracurium has a very favorable metabolism occurring via plasma ester hydrolysis, Hoffman Degradation. Vecuronium is metabolized by the liver and not desirable in pregnant patients with hepatic dysfunction.

Digoxin is safe in pregnancy and can be used in the management of peripartum cardiomyopathy. However digoxin is secreted into the breast milk. ACE inhibitors have shown a definitive fetal risk and should not be generally used in pregnancy.

Fosphenytoin, which is metabolized to phenytoin, is a category D agent that can cause fetal hydantoin syndrome or fetal anticonvulsant syndrome and should generally not be used in pregnancy. While there are no controlled studies levetiracetam is listed as a pregnancy category C medication and would be preferred over fosphenytoin.

There is no preferred vasopressor in pregnancy. Ephedrine has been shown to increase both maternal blood pressure and fetal blood flow compared to epinephrine, which does not increase fetal blood flow due to vasoconstriction.

Answer: B

Lee A, Ngan Kee WD, Gin T (2002) A quantitative, systematic review of randomized controlled trials of ephedrine versus phenylephrine for the management of hypotension during spinal anesthesia for cesarean delivery. *Anesthesia and Analgesia* **94** (4), 920.

13. *A woman at 36 weeks gestation is admitted to the ICU with severe eclampsia. Antihypertensive therapy is initiated and her blood pressure is 180/110 mm Hg. The patient complains of headaches, visual disturbances and appears to be confused. Computed tomography (CT) demonstrates symmetric hypodensities that involve the occipitoparietal regions of the brain. An MRI of the brain demonstrates punctate and confluent hyperintense areas in the parieto-occipital lobes. With respect to this condition:*

A. *These radiographic findings are expected to resolve in 1–2 weeks with treatment*

B. *Frequently presents with status epilepticus resistant to magnesium sulfate*

C. *Rarely necessitates delivery of the fetus*

D. *Is generally limited to patients in their third trimester of pregnancy*

E. *Is associated with a high risk of intracerebral hemorrhage*

This patient has posterior reversible encephalopathy syndrome or PRES, also referred to as, reversible posterior cerebral edema syndrome or posterior leukoencephalopathy syndrome. Risk factors for PRES include hypertensive conditions, preeclampsia, and the immunosuppressants tacrolimus and cyclosporine. Clinically patients have headaches, mental status changes, confusion, and seizures. Diagnosis is confirmed with an MRI demonstrating vasogenic edema predominantly localized to the posterior cerebral hemispheres. With prompt treatment the patient improves rapidly and the MRI changes usually resolve in 1 to 2 weeks. In the pregnant patient with preeclampsia, magnesium sulfate is the drug of choice for PRES seizures. Prompt delivery of the fetus is usually therapeutic. PRES can occur any time in the peripartum period as well in non-pregnant patients. There is no increased risk of intracranial hemorrhage in the patients with PRES.

Answer: A

Finocchi V, Bozzao A, Bonamini M, *et al.* (2005) Magnetic resonance imaging in posterior reversible encephalopathy syndrome: report of three cases and review of literature. *Archives of Gynecology and Obstetrics* **271** (1), 79.

Lamy C, Oppenheim C, Méder JF, Mas JL (2004) Neuroimaging in posterior reversible encephalopathy syndrome. *Journal of Neuroimaging* **14** (2), 89.

14. *A woman presents to the emergency department one week after an emergency Cesarean section now complaining of lower abdominal tenderness and fever. Her temperature is 38.3 °C and the WBC count is 14.2 × 10^3/microL with two bands. The wound appears clean and is nontender. You are concerned she has postpartum endometritis. In this condition:*

A. *Early hysterectomy improves outcomes*

B. *The predominant organism is Streptococus*

C. *The diagnosis is confirmed by visualizing gas in the uterus on CT scan*

D. *Amikacin is the drug of choice*

E. *Can be reduced by a prophylactic dose of ampicillin*

Prophylactic antibiotics (ampicillin) can reduce the incidence of endometritis by two-thirds to three-quarters in women having a Cesarean section. The majority of cases are polymicrobial and involving both aerobes and anaerobes. For this reason recommended antimicrobial coverage needs to be broad spectrum. An agent like Amikacin has no anaerobic activity and would require an additional agent such as clindamycin.

Regimens with activity against penicillin resistant anaerobic bacteria are better than those without.

The diagnosis is usually made on the clinical basis of fever, foul lochia and uterine tenderness in a woman following Cesarean section. Imaging studies are used to rule out other diagnoses such as pelvic abscess. Most often the CT is nonspecific and does not rely on visualizing gas in the endometrium.

Once uncomplicated endometritis has clinically improved with intravenous therapy, oral therapy is not needed. Failure to respond in 48 hours should raise the possibility of another condition and investigated. The differential diagnosis should include septic pelvic thrombophlebitis and pelvic abscess as well as other common post operative infections.

Answer: E

French LM, Smaill FM (2004) Antibiotic regimens for endometritis after delivery. *Cochrane Database Systematic Reviews.*

Smaill F, Hofmeyr GJ (2002) Antibiotic prophylaxis for cesarean section. *Cochrane Database Systematic Review.*

Chapter 23 Envenomations, Poisonings and Toxicology

Michelle Strong, MD, PhD

1. *Whole-bowel irrigation (WBI) is a technique to prevent absorption of drugs. Large volumes of polyethylene glycol electrolyte (PEG) solution are administered until the rectal effluent is clear. Which of the following statements about WBI are incorrect?*

A. *A nasogastric tube may be necessary to administer the electrolyte solution*

B. *This technique has been suggested for enhancing elimination of substances not well absorbed by activated charcoal*

C. *It is contraindicated for patients with ileus, GI obstruction, or hemodynamic instability*

D. *It should not be used for sustained-release or enteric-coated medications*

E. *The head of the bed should be elevated to 45°*

Whole-bowel irrigation is a technique to prevent absorption of drugs by administering large volumes of polyethylene glycol solution until the rectal effluent is clear or toxin elimination is confirmed. A nasogastric tube is often necessary to effectively administer the electrolyte solution. The airway must be protected in patients with a depressed level of consciousness or respiratory depression. The head of the bed should be elevated to 45° to decrease the likelihood of aspiration. Whole-bowel irrigation is contraindicated in patients with ileus, GI obstruction or perforation, hemodynamic instability or intractable vomiting. This technique has been suggested to enhance elimination of substances that are not absorbed well by activated charcoal such as iron or lithium, potentially toxic ingestions of sustained-release or enteric coated medications, or in the situation of packaged illicit drug ingestion (body packing/stuffing). Currently, Whole-bowel irrigation has no other indications than those mentioned above.

Surgical Critical Care and Emergency Surgery: Clinical Questions and Answers, First Edition. Edited by Forrest O. Moore, Peter M. Rhee, Samuel A. Tisherman and Gerard J. Fulda.

Answer: D

Mokhlesi B, Leiken JB, Murray P, *et al.* (2003) Adult Toxicology in Critical Care: Part I: General approach to the intoxicated patient. *Chest* **123**, 577–92.

Zimmerman JL (2003) Poisonings and overdoses in the intensive care unit: General and specific management issues. *Critical Care Medicine* **31**, 2794–2801.

Zimmerman JL, Rudis M (2001) Poisonings. In: Parrillo JE, Dellinger RP (eds) *Critical Care Medicine*, 2nd edn. Mosby, St. Louis, pp. 1501–24.

2. *Antidepressant overdose is a significant source for patient mortality with the majority due to tricyclic antidepressants (TCA). The clinical presentation of TCA toxicity can be categorized as anticholinergic effects, cardiovascular effects, and seizures. Which agent used in the management of the cardiovascular toxicity of TCA overdose is correct:*

A. *Bretylium*

B. *Sodium bicarbonate*

C. *Physostigmine*

D. *Procainamide*

E. *Dobutamine*

The cardiovascular toxicity of tricyclic antidepressants (TCA) poisoning consists of sinus tachycardia with the prolongation of the QRS, QTc and PR intervals. Serum alkalinization remains the mainstay of therapy. Patients should receive sodium bicarbonate immediately when there is widening of the QRS interval and it should be continued until the QRS interval narrows or the pH >7.55. Therapy is based on studies that show that sodium bicarbonate narrows the QRS complex, improves systolic blood pressure and controls ventricular arrhythmias in TCA overdose. Lidocaine is the drug of choice in cyclic antidepressant overdose complicated by refractory ventricular arrhythmias. Bretylium can exacerbate hypotension. Procainamide and other class 1a antiarrhythmics can add to cardiac toxicity and should be avoided. Hypotension tends to be refractory to fluid resuscitation and many patients will require vasopressors. Direct acting alpha-adrenergic agonists (norepineprine, phenylephrine) are preferred because they counter act the alpha-adrenergic antagonist effects of TCAs. Dobutamine is not used because it will likely worsen hypotension and not counteract the alpha-adrenergic antagonistic effects although TCAs possess some anticholinergic effects, cardiotoxicity is prominent. Physostigmine may worsen cardiac function and is associated with cardiac arrest in the setting of TCA overdose.

Answer: B

Blackman K, Brown SG, Wilkes GJ (2001) Plasma alkalinization for tricyclic antidepressant toxicity: a systematic review. *Emergency Medicine (Fremantle)* **13**, 204–10.

Mokhlesi B, Leiken JB, Murray P, *et al.* (2003) Adult toxicology in critical care: Part II: specific poisonings. *Chest* **123**, 897–922.

Pentel P, Peterson CD (1980) Asystole complicating physostigmine treatment of tricyclic antidepressant overdose. *Annals of Emergency Medicine* **9**, 588–90.

Tran TP, Panacek EA, Foulke GE. (1997) Response to dopamine vs. norepinephrine in tricyclic antidepressant-induced hypotension. *Academic Emergency Medicine* **4**, 864–8.

Zimmerman JL (2003) Poisonings and overdoses in the intensive care unit: General and specific management issues. *Critical Care Medicine* **31**, 2794–801.

3. *Analgesics are the most common agents that result in toxicity necessitating hospitalization throughout the world. Acetaminophen accounts for the majority of toxicity. Which of the following statements about acetaminophen toxicity is incorrect?*

A. *Acetaminophen accounts for the highest number of deaths from poisonings in the USA*

B. *The Rumack–Matthew nomogram uses acetaminophen levels to determine the need for N-acetylcysteine administration in patients with repeated ingestions or extended release formulations of acetaminophen*

C. *N-acetylcysteine therapy is most effective when initiated in the first eight hours of ingestion*

D. *Concomitant use of activated charcoal and N-acetylcysteine therapy improves patient outcomes*

E. *King's College criteria for prognosis in acetaminophen-induced hepatotoxicity indicate that if serum creatinine is >3.4 mg/dL, INR >6.5, and grade III or worse encephalopathy occur within a 24-hour period the patient should be listed for transplantation*

Acetaminophen accounts for the majority of deaths from poisoning in the USA. N-acetylcysteine (NAC) is an antidote used in preventing acetaminophen-induced hepatotoxicity. The Rumack–Matthew nomogram uses acetaminophen levels to determine the need for NAC administration. The nomogram is useful *only* for single acute ingestions. N-acetylcysteine therapy is most effective when initiated in the first eight hours following ingestion but is recommended to be initiated as late as 24 hours after significant ingestion. The Rumack–Matthew nomogram should *not* be used for chronic ingestions and is inaccurate in sustained-release products. Activated charcoal adsorbs acetaminophen and many coingestants and should be administered to patients with concern for acetaminophen or multiple drug overdoses. The concomitant use of activated charcoal and NAC therapy improves patient outcomes. No NAC dose adjustment is necessary. Acetaminophen-induced hepatitis may progress to fulminant hepatic failure, and appropriate referral to liver transplantation may be necessary. King's College criteria for prognosis of acetaminophen-induced hepatotoxicity are often used and the patient should be listed for transplantation if the arterial pH <7.3 after adequate fluid or resuscitation or if all three of the following occur within a 24-hour period: serum creatinine is >3.4 mg/dL, INR > 6.5, and grade III or worse encephalopathy.

Answer: B

Alapat PM, Zimmerman JL (2008) Toxicology in the critical care unit. *Chest* **133**, 1006–13.

Rumack BH, Matthew H (1975) Acetaminophen poisoning and toxicity. *Pediatrics* **55** (6), 871–6.

Spiller HA, Sawyer TS (2007) Impact of activated charcoal after acute acetaminophen overdoses treated with N-acetylcysteine. *Journal of Emergency Medicine* **33**, 141–4.

Zimmerman JL (2003) Poisonings and overdoses in the intensive care unit: General and specific management issues. *Critical Care Medicine* **31**, 2794–801.

4. *Toxidromes are combinations of specific signs and symptoms that reflect effects of a drug class on particular neuroreceptors. Which signs, drug/toxin and drug treatments (listed in order of signs: drug/toxin:treatment) are incorrect:*

A. *Mydriasis, blurred vision, dry skin, ileus, urinary retention: atropine: benztropine*

B. *Salivation, lacrimation, urination, diarrhea, GI cramps, emesis: organophosphates: pralidoxime*

C. *Hypertension, tachycardia, mydriasis, diaphoresis: cocaine: benzodiazepines*

D. *Confusion, stupor, slurred speech, apnea: benzodiazepines: flumazenil*

E. *Altered mental status, slow shallow breaths, miosis: opiates: naloxone*

Management strategies are often geared toward the syndrome and not a specific agent. The anticholinergic toxidrome is manifested by mydriasis, blurred vision, tachycardia, dry skin, hypoactive bowel sounds, and urinary retention. It is caused by antihistamines, atropine, tricyclic antidepressants (TCA), benztropine, and phenothiazines. It is treated by physostigmine, except in life threatening TCA overdose because of worsening of conduction disturbances. Benztropine causes this syndrome; it does *not* treat it. Cholinergic toxidrome includes salivation, lacrimation, urination, diarrhea, GI cramps, emesis (SLUDGE). It is caused by organophosphates and is treated by pralidoxime. Signs of sympathomimetic toxidrome are hypertension, tachycardia, mydriasis, and diaphoresis. It is caused by cocaine, amphetamines, and phencyclidine (PCP) and treated by benzodiazepines. Sedative/hypnotic toxidrome is reflected by confusion, stupor, slurred speech, and apnea. It is caused by anticonvulsants, antipsychotics, benzodiazepines, and ethanol. Flumazenil is an antidote for benzodiazepine overdose. The narcotic toxidrome consists of altered mental status, slow shallow breaths, and miosis. It is caused by opiates and treated by the antidote naloxone.

Answer: A

Mokhlesi B, Leiken JB, Murray P, *et al.* (2003) Adult Toxicology in Critical Care: Part I: General approach to the intoxicated patient. *Chest* **123**, 577–92.

Weier A, Kleinschmidt K (2010) How are patients who are admitted to the intensive care unit after common poisonings diagnosed and managed? In: Deutschman CS, Neligan PJ (eds) *Evidence-based Practice of Critical Care*, Saunders, Philadelphia, PA, pp. 632–6.

5. *A 25-year-old woman ingested 10 tablets of carisoprodol 350 mg, 30 tablets of ibuprofen 200 mg and 10 tablets of cephalexin 500 mg 2 hours ago. On presentation to the emergency department (ED), she is lethargic but arouses to voice.*

Which of the following is the most appropriate method of gastric decontamination?

A. *Syrup of Ipecac*

B. *Whole-bowel irrigation*

C. *Sorbitol cathartic*

D. *Activated charcoal*

E. *Gastric lavage*

There is little evidence that any method of gastric decontamination is of benefit in overdose patients, however, activated charcoal is the best response. Activated charcoal adsorbs most ingested drugs and is generally effective and well tolerated. It is especially effective if given early. Ipecac syrup should not be used routinely in the management of poisoned patients. There is no evidence that ipecac improves outcomes and insufficient data to support administration soon after ingestion. Whole-bowel irrigation may be used in intoxications where activated charcoal is ineffective. It is considered for drugs such iron, lithium, sustained-release agents and illicit drug packets. Cathartics have been used to decrease the transit time through the GI tract and thus, decrease absorption. No evidence exists to support this theory and, thus, they generally are not recommended. Gastric lavage should not be used in the management of poisoned patients because of complications including hypoxia, laryngospasm, gastrointestinal perforation and aspiration pneumonia. There is also no clear benefit to its clinical outcome.

Answer: D

Chyka PA, Seger D, Krenzelok EP, *et al.* (2005) Position paper: single-dose activated charcoal. *Clinical Toxicology* **43**, 61–87.

Krenzelok EP, McGuigan M, Lheureux P, *et al.* (2004) Position paper: Ipecac syrup. *Journal of Toxicology and Clinical Toxicology* **42**, 133–43.

Tenenbein M, Lheureux P (2004) Position paper: whole-bowel irrigation. *Journal of Toxicology and Clinical Toxicology* **42**, 843–54.

Vale JA, Krenzelok EP, Barceloux GD (1999) Position statement and practice guidelines on the use of multi-dose activated charcoal in the treatment of acute poisoning. *Clinical Toxicology* **37**, 731–51.

Vale JA, Kulig K (2004) Position paper: gastric lavage. *Journal of Toxicology and Clinical Toxicology* **42**, 933–43.

6. *Salicylates poisonings is very common and sometimes fatal. Which one of the following features of salicylate toxicity or treatment of salicylate toxicity is incorrect:*

A. *The toxidrome for salicylates includes nausea, vomiting, dyspnea, diaphoresis, dizziness, and tinnitus*

B. *Significant ingestions of salicylates result in respiratory acidosis or mixed metabolic alkalosis and respiratory acidosis*

C. *Administration of sodium bicarbonate to raise the plasma pH to 7.45 to 7.50 induces urinary alkalinization that in turn increases renal clearance of salicylates*

D. *Hemodialysis is indicated for salicylate levels >100 mg/dL, significant metabolic derangements that do not rapidly clear with resuscitation, or renal insufficiency*

E. *Activated charcoal is useful for acute salicylate ingestions, but not in cases of toxicity from chronic exposure*

The salicylate toxidrome includes nausea, vomiting, dyspnea, diaphoresis, dizziness, and hearing changes. Poisoned patients suffer from respiratory alkalosis or mixed anion-gap metabolic acidosis and respiratory alkalosis. At toxic levels, salicylates are metabolic poisons that affect multiple organ systems by uncoupling oxidative phosphorylation. This leads to accumulation of organic acids, such as lactic acid and ketoacids, and metabolic acidosis with an elevated anion gap. Respiratory alkalosis occurs through direct central stimulation. Sodium bicarbonate is administered to raise the plasma pH to between 7.45 and 7.5 to induce renal clearance. Raising the urinary pH from 6.1 to 8.1 results in a >18-fold increase in renal clearance by trapping the salicylate ion in the renal tubules. Hemodialysis is indicated for salicylate levels >100 mg/dL, significant metabolic derangements that do not rapidly clear with resuscitation, or renal insufficiency. Activated charcoal is only useful in acute salicylate ingestions. Multidose activated charcoal to enhance elimination is controversial.

Answer: B

Mokhlesi B, Leiken JB, Murray P, *et al.* (2003) Adult toxicology in critical care: Part II: specific poisonings. *Chest* **123**, 897–922.

O'Malley GF (2007) Emergency department management of the salicylate-poisoned patient (abstract). *Emergency Medicine Clinics of North America* **25**, 333–46.

Prescott LF, Balali-Mood M, Critchley JA, *et al.* (1982) Diuresis or urinary alkalinisation for salicylate poisoning? *British Medical Journal (Clinical Research Edition)* **285**, 1383–6.

Temple AR (1981) Acute and chronic effects of aspirin toxicity and their treatment. *Archives of Internal Medicine* **141**, 364–9.

7. *Carbon monoxide (CO) is a nonirritating, colorless, odorless gas that is a common cause of morbidity and mortality. Which statement about CO poisoning is correct?*

A. *CO gas is formed by the complete combustion (oxidation) of carbon-containing materials*

B. *Pulse oximetry accurately reflects oxygen saturation because it can distinguish carboxyhemoglobin from oxyhemoglobin*

C. *CO binds to hemoglobin more readily than oxygen and decreases oxyhemoglobin and blood oxygen-carrying capacity*

D. *The severity of CO poisoning is independent of concentration and duration of exposure*

E. *Delayed neuropsychiatric sequelae from CO poisoning are directly correlated to the clinical severity of the toxin*

CO is an insidious gas that is formed by the *incomplete* combustion of carbon-containing materials. Complete oxidation of these materials produces carbon dioxide. CO poisoning occurs from smoke inhalation, automobile exhaust, and poorly ventilated charcoal or gas stoves. CO binds to hemoglobin with an affinity 240 times greater than oxygen and decreases oxyhemoglobin saturation and oxygen-carrying capacity. CO toxicity results in impaired transport and release of oxygen causing cellular hypoxia and cyctochrome oxidase blockade causing direct inhibition of cellular respiration. The severity of CO poisoning is dependent on the concentration of CO, duration of exposure and the minute ventilation. Mild exposure (carboxyhemoglobin 5–10%) may result in headache and mild dyspnea. Higher carboxyhemoglobin concentrations (10–30%) cause headache, dizziness, dyspnea, irritability, nausea, and vomiting. Concentrations >50% lead to coma, seizures, cardiovascular collapse and death. However, the delayed neuropsychiatric sequelae (DNS) *do not* correlate with the clinical severity of CO poisoning. Delayed neuropsychiatric sequelae may occur over a long period of time (three to 240 days) and there is no accurate way of predicting which patients will acquire DNS. At one year, 50 to 75% of patients with DNS will have a full recovery. Administration of 100% supplemental oxygen decreases the half-life of carboxyhemoglobin from 5–6 hours to 45–90 min. Hyperbaric oxygen decreases the half-life to 15–30 minutes. Hyperbaric oxygen treatment at 6–12 hour intervals within a 24 hour period of exposure has been shown to decrease significantly DNS at both 6 weeks and 12 months.

Answer: C

Mokhlesi B, Leiken JB, Murray P, *et al.* (2003) Adult toxicology in critical care: Part II: specific poisonings. *Chest* **123**, 897–922.

Weaver LK, Hopkins RO, Chan KJ, *et al.* (2002) Hyperbaric oxygen for acute carbon monoxide poisoning. *New England Journal of Medicine* **347**, 1057–67.

Zimmerman JL (2003) Poisonings and overdoses in the intensive care unit: general and specific management issues. *Critical Care Medicine* **31**, 2794–801.

8. *An obtunded, hemodynamically stable patient with bipolar disorder is admitted to the ICU. She is chronically treated with lithium but had an ingestion of a large number of sustained-release lithium approximately 4 hours prior to admission. The patient's lithium level upon admission is 3.7 mEq/L (therapeutic range 0.5 to 1.25 mEq/L).*

Which one of the following is the most appropriate intervention at this time?

A. *Normal saline solution diuresis*

B. *Hemodialysis*

C. *Administer activated charcoal*

D. *Close observation and repeat lithium level in 6–8 hours*

E. *Administer sodium polystyrene sulphonate (Kayexalate®)*

Lithium is a monovalent cation used for the treatment of bipolar disorders. It is rapidly absorbed via the GI tract and eliminated by glomerular filtration with 80% being reabsorbed in the renal tubules. The greatest risk of lithium ingestion is central nervous system toxicity including delirium, tremor, ataxia, hyperreflexia, seizures and coma. Toxicity is more likely to occur in individuals who chronically ingest lithium. In this patient, hemodialysis should be instituted. Lithium is a prototypical dialyzable agent because of its low molecular weight, lack of protein binding and prolonged half-life (18 hours). Hemodialysis is indicated for serum levels > 3.5 mEq/L in acute indigestion, 2.5 mEq/L in chronic ingestion, symptomatic patients or patients with renal insufficiency. The level will be decreased effectively by hemodialysis; however, repeat levels must be obtained after dialysis to assess for rebound increase as lithium shifts from the intracellular to extracellular space. Close observation and repeat levels are necessary after initial hemodialysis. Saline diuresis is not effective in enhancing the elimination of lithium. Volume replacement is appropriate in these patients because lithium causes a nephrogenic diabetes insipidus. Sodium polystyrene sulfonate

(Kayexalate®) does bind lithium and may decrease absorption, it will also cause hypokalemia and is thus, not recommended. Activated charcoal is ineffective since lithium is not adsorbed to it.

Answer: B

Markowitz GS, Radhakrishnan J, Kiambham N, *et al.* (2000) Lithium nephrotoxicity: a progressive combined glomerular and tubulointerstitial nephropathy. *Journal of the American Society of Nephrology* **11**, 1439–48.

Mokhlesi B, Leiken JB, Murray P, *et al.* (2003) Adult toxicology in critical care: Part II: specific poisonings. *Chest* 123, 897–922.

Scharman EJ (1997) Methods used to decrease lithium adsorption or enhance elimination. *Journal of Toxicology and Clinical Toxicology* **35**, 601–8.

Timmer RT, Sands JM (1999) Lithium intoxication. *Journal of the American Society of Nephrology* 666–74.

9. *Toxicity due to nonethanol alcohols is encountered in the ICU. Which of the following statements about nonethanol alcohols is correct?*

A. *Ethylene glycol is metabolized by alcohol dehydrogenase to formaldehyde and then to formic acid*

B. *Accumulation and precipitation of oxalic acid to calcium oxalate in the renal tubules produces crystals and contribute to the development of renal tubular necrosis after methanol ingestion*

C. *Propylene glycol toxicity in the ICU is usually associated with prolonged, high dose infusions of midazolam*

D. *The treatment of choice for ethylene glycol and methanol poisoning is to enhance elimination of metabolites by administering fomepizole or ethanol which induces the alcohol dehydrogenase enzyme*

E. *The classic characterization of ethylene glycol and methanol ingestions is an anion gap metabolic acidosis and/or an osmolar gap*

Toxicity due to nonethanol alcohols is encountered in the ICU. These ingestions are infrequent but can result in significant morbidity and mortality. Ethylene glycol is metabolized by alcohol dehydrogenase to glycoaldehyde and glycolic acid and then eventually to glyoxylic acid and oxalic acid. Methanol is metabolized by alcohol dehydrogenase to formaldehyde, which is then converted to formic acid. Accumulation and precipitation of calcium oxalate crystals in the renal tubules that leads to the development of acute tubular necrosis occurs after *ethylene glycol* ingestion. Fomepizole and ethanol are *inhibitors* of alcohol dehygrogenase (not inducers) and thus, inhibit the formation of toxic metabolites of both substances. Fomepizole is the preferred agent because it does not exacerbate the inebriated state. Metabolic acidosis with an elevated anion gap and an elevated osmolar gap are classic features of nonethanol intoxication. Late presentations may not manifest an osmolar gap if the alcohol has already been metabolized to acid metabolites, but an anion gap acidosis will be obvious.

Answer: E

Ammar KA, Heckerling PS (1996) Ethylene glycol poisoning with a normal anion gap caused by concurrent ethanol ingestion: Importance of the osmolar gap. *American Journal of Kidney Disorders* **27**, 130–3.

Kruse JA (1992) Methanol poisoning. *Intensive Care Medicine* **18**, 391–7.

Mokhlesi B, Leiken JB, Murray P, *et al.* (2003) Adult toxicology in critical care: Part II: specific poisonings. *Chest* **123**, 897–922.

Zimmerman JL (2003) Poisonings and overdoses in the intensive care unit: general and specific management issues. *Critical Care Medicine* **31**, 2794–801.

10. *The American Academy of Clinical toxicology and the European Associations of Poison Centres and Clinical Toxicologists (AACT/EAPCCT) have published position papers on the management of poisoned patients. Which one of the following statements from these guidelines is incorrect?*

A. *Gastric lavage should not be used routinely in the management of poisoned patients because of complications including hypoxia, laryngospasm, gastrointestinal perforation and aspiration pneumonia*

B. *Ipecac syrup should not be used routinely in the management of poisoned patients due to insufficient evidence that it improves outcomes*

C. *Single dose activated charcoal should not be used routinely in the management of poisoned patients. It should be considered if the toxin is known to be adsorbed by charcoal and has been ingested within 1 hour*

D. *Urine alkalinization is not considered a first line treatment for patients with severe salicylate poisoning who do not meet criteria for hemodialysis*

E. *Administration of multi-dose activated charcoal should be considered for patients that have ingested life-threatening amounts of carbamazepine, dapsone, phenobarbital, quinine, or theophylline*

The American Academy of Clinical Toxicology and the European Associations of Poison Centres and Clinical Toxicologists (AACT/EAPCCT) have published position papers on the management of poisoned patients. These papers function as clinical practice guidelines for elimination strategies for poisoned patients. Gastric lavage should not be used routinely in the management of poisoned patients because of complications including hypoxia, laryngospasm, gastrointestinal perforation and aspiration pneumonia. In addition, there is no clear benefit to clinical outcome. Ipecac syrup should not be used routinely in the management of poisoned patients. There is no evidence that ipecac improves outcomes and insufficient data to support administration soon after ingestion. Single-dose activated charcoal should not be used routinely in the management of poisoned patients. However, it should be considered if the toxin is known to be adsorbed by charcoal and has been ingested within 1 hour. Studies reveal the effectiveness decreases after the first hour. Administration of multidose activated charcoal should be considered for patients that have ingested life-threatening amounts of carbamazepine, dapsone, phenobarbital, quinine, or theophylline. Studies have shown enhanced elimination of these drugs. None have demonstrated clinical benefit. Urine alkalinization is a *recommended* first-line treatment for patients with severe salicylate poisoning who do not meet criteria for hemodialysis.

Answer: D

Chyka PA, Seger D, Krenzelok EP, *et al.* (2005) Position paper: single-dose activated charcoal. *Clinical Toxicology* **43**, 61–87.

Krenzelok EP, McGuigan M, Lheureux P, *et al.* (2004) Position paper: Ipecac syrup. *Journal of Toxicology and Clinical Toxicology* **42**, 133–43.

Proudfoot AT, Krenzelok EP, Vale JA (2004) Position paper on urine alkalinization. *Journal of Toxicology and Clinical Toxicology* **42**, 1–26.

Vale JA, Krenzelok EP, Barceloux GD (1999) Position statement and practice guidelines on the use of multi-dose activated charcoal in the treatment of acute poisoning. *Clinical Toxicology* **37**, 731–51.

Vale JA, Kulig K. (2004) Position paper: gastric lavage. *Journal of Toxicology and Clinical Toxicology* **42**, 933–43.

Weier A, Kleinschmidt K. (2010) How are patients who are admitted to the intensive care unit after common poisonings diagnosed and managed? In: Deutschman CS and Neligan PJ (eds) *Evidence-based Practice of Critical Care*, WB Saunders, Philadelphia, PA, pp. 632–36.

11. *A 66-year-old obese man who was recently discharged from the inpatient medical service is found down by his wife with a small hematoma on his scalp. His finger stick glucose by paramedics was 24 mg/dL. He is given 1 ampule of 50% dextrose and arouses. He is brought in as trauma activation to the ED. He is initially alert and answering questions with the following vital signs: BP 150/88 mm Hg, HR 84 beats/min, RR 13 breaths/min, temperature 37.1 °C. His physical exam is unremarkable except for the small cephalohematoma and his trauma workup is negative. The patient's wife states that he is a diabetic and takes an oral medication. During a recent admission he had renal failure that resolved. During this evaluation, the patient becomes confused, lethargic and diaphoretic. His repeat finger stick glucose is 33 mg/dL. He again responds to 50% dextrose, but becomes unresponsive 30 minutes later. The patient is intubated for airway protection and admitted to the ICU. He is started on an IV infusion of 10% dextrose, but still requires several boluses of 50% dextrose for hypoglycemia.*

Which one of the following treatments is most likely to benefit this patient?

A. *Administration of 50% dextrose via nasogastric tube*

B. *Administration of subcutaneous octreotide*

C. *Administration of intravenous thiamine 100 mg*

D. *Administration of intramuscular glucagon*

E. *Administration of 20% dextrose via peripheral IV*

This patient's presentation is suggestive of possible overdose with a hypoglycemic agent. Severe, prolonged hypoglycemia is characteristic of ingestion of large doses of sulfonylureas. Sulfonylurea agents stimulate insulin release from the pancreas, resulting in hypoglycemia. Risk factors for hypoglycemia from therapeutic use include: age $>$ 65 years, multiple medications, frequent hospitalizations, use of agents with longer durations of action (e.g., chlorpropamide and glyburide), and impaired drug clearance; renal insufficiency can increase the risk of hypoglycemia four-fold. Patients with a sulfonylurea overdose and symptomatic hypoglycemia are immediately treated with IV dextrose. However, IV dextrose should not be used as monotherapy because it may cause hyperglycemia that triggers increased insulin release, leading to recurrent episodes of hypoglycemia. Octreotide is a somatostatin analogue that inhibits release of insulin from the pancreas and has been found to be effective in treating hypoglycemia and shortening the period of hypoglycemia. The most important mechanism of action is G-protein-mediated decrease in calcium influx through voltage-gated channels in pancreatic beta islet cells, which diminishes calcium-mediated insulin release. The dose of octreotide is 50 to 150 μg administered by intramuscular, or subcutaneous, injection every six hours. If thiamine deficiency (from alcoholism or other forms of malnutrition) is suspected, IV thiamine 100 mg is given in conjunction with glucose, but will not treat symptomatic hypoglycemia. Glucagon given IM stimulates hepatic glycogenolysis and raises serum glucose levels slightly. The efficacy of glucagon is dependent upon hepatic glycogen stores, which may be depleted in the setting of prolonged hypoglycemia. The short duration of action of glucagon further limits its effectiveness. Central venous access is required for administering concentrated glucose solutions due to hyperosmolarity that can cause endothelial damage. Oral administration of dextrose in a severely ill patient is unreliable.

Answer: B

Carr R, Zed PJ (2002) Octreotide for sulfonylurea-induced hypoglycemia following overdose. *Annals of Pharmacotherapy* **36**, 1727–32.

Fasano CJ, O'Malley G, Dominici P, *et al.* (2008) Comparison of octreotide and standard therapy versus standard therapy alone for the treatment of sulfonylurea-induced hypoglycemia. *Annals of Emergency Medicine* **51**, 400–6.

Green RS, Palatnik W. (2003) Effectiveness of octreotide in a case of refractory sulfonylurea-induced hypoglycemia. *Journal of Emergency Medicine* **25**, 283–7.

Shorr RI, Ray WA, Daugherty JR, *et al.* (1997) Incidence and risk factors for serious hypoglycemia in older persons using insulin or sulfonylureas. *Archives of Internal Medicine* **157**, 1681–6.

12. *A lethargic 35-year-old man is admitted to the ICU. The patient had been brought to the emergency department for evaluation by some friends after hiking. Upon admission, his vitals are BP 105/62 mm Hg, HR 125 beats per minute, RR 28 breaths per minute, temperature 36.5 °C. His physical examination is remarkable for bleeding gums and an ecchymotic, edematous left lower extremity from foot to knee with a small wound near the ankle. A surgical consult was obtained and compartment pressures are 21 mm Hg. He has a Foley catheter in place with brownish red urine. His laboratory studies are remarkable for platelets 92 × 10^3/μL, PTT 43 and INR 1.8; BUN 35 mg/dL, serum creatinine 1.6 mg/dL and CK 5416 U/L.*

Which one of the following interventions would be most beneficial to this patient?

A. *Placement of tourniquet to the thigh of the left lower extremity*

B. *Administration of piperacillin/tazobactam 3.375 gm IV every 6 hours*

C. *Transfusion of platelets and fresh frozen plasma*

D. *Administration of Crotalinae (pit viper) antivenom (Polyvalent Crotalidae ovine immune Fab)*

E. *Fasciotomy of the left lower extremity*

The physical findings in this patient are concerning for compartment syndrome. However, the wound on the lower leg and history are concerning for a snakebite. FabAV consists of the purified Fab fragments of sheep immunoglobulin (IgG) raised against the antivenom of four snakes. These Fab fragments bind venom in the intravascular space and are renally excreted. The half-life of FabAV is shorter than Crotalinae venom substances. Thus, recurrent toxicity is possible despite initial control of local and systemic effects and may necessitate repeated FabAV administration. FabAV appears most effective when given within six hours of envenomation. Methods, such as tourniquets, incision and oral suction, mechanical suction devices, cryotherapy, surgery, and electric shock therapy, have been advocated in the past, but are *no longer recommended*. Tourniquets can damage nerves, tendons, and blood vessels, and oral suction can lead to infection. Although snake bites may result in the inoculation of bacteria, infections are rare. Antibiotics should *not* be administered unless there is established infection or heavily contaminated wounds. Transfused platelets and coagulation factors in fresh frozen plasma are inactivated by Crotalinae venom and should be avoided in patients with Crotalinae-induced coagulopathy unless the patient has significant bleeding that is uncontrolled by high-dose antivenom administration. Increased compartment pressures result from this extrinsic pressure and can be reduced with the administration of adequate amounts of antivenom and elevation. Elevation, which is usually avoided in true compartment syndrome, results in the drainage of subcutaneous edema and contributes to the reduction of the source of increased tissue pressure. If there is a concern for clinically significant, increased tissue, or compartment pressures, direct measurement with an appropriate device should be performed to guide additional management with antivenom and elevation. The indications for fasciotomy in this context are unclear. An animal model of direct compartmental injection of venom demonstrated improved outcomes with antivenom alone versus antivenom plus fasciotomy. However, in this model, fasciotomy was performed immediately after venom injection. Thus, surgical intervention for elevated compartment pressures following Crotalinae snake bite is controversial and should be guided by a medical toxicologist and surgeon with extensive experience caring for victims with snake bite. In this patient, compartment pressures are still below the recommended value for performing extremity fasciotomy (30 mm Hg).

Answer: D

Gold BS, Barish RA, Dart RC (2004) North American snake envenomation: diagnosis, treatment and management. *Emergency Medical Clinics of North America* **22**, 423–43.

Gold BS, Dart RC, Barish RA, *et al.* (2003) Resolution of compartment syndrome after rattlesnake envenomation utilizing non-invasive measures. *Journal of Emergency Medicine* **24**, 285–8.

Gold BS, Dart RC, Barish RA (2002) Bites of venomous snakes. *New England Journal of Medicine* **347**, 347–56.

Lovecchio F, Klemens J, Welch S, *et al.* (2002) Antibiotics after rattlesnake envenomation. *Journal if Emergency Medicine* **23**, 327–8.

McKinney PE (2001) Out-of-hospital and interhospital management of crotaline snakebite. *Annals of Emergency Medicine* **37**, 168–74.

Seifert SA, Boyer LV, Benson BE, *et al.* (2009) AAPCC database characterization of native US venomous snake exposures, 2001–2005. *Clinical Toxicology* **47**, 327–35.

Tanen DA, Danish DC, Grice GA, *et al.* (2004) Fasciotomy worsens the amount of myonecrosis in a porcine model of crotaline envenomation. *Annals of Emergency Medicine* **44**, 99–104.

13. *All of the following statements are true regarding valproic acid overdose except:*

A. *Hypernatremia has been associated with high drug levels.*

B. *Administration of L-carnitine is recommended for patients with hyperammonemia, lethargy, coma, and hepatic dysfunction.*

C. *Cerebral edema may occur 24–72 hours after ingestion.*

D. *There is no concern for toxicity if there are therapeutic drug levels and no CNS depression 2 hours after ingestion.*

E. *Hemodialysis or combined hemodialysis and hemoperfusion methods have been effective in severe toxicity.*

Increased use of valproic acid (VPA) for bipolar disorder, seizures, migraine headaches, and neuropathic pain has led to increased overdose. Central nervous system depression is the most common symptom of acute overdose or toxicity ranging in severity from mild drowsiness to coma or fatal cerebral edema. The onset and progression of CNS depression is usually rapid but may be delayed as long as 72 hours with ingestion of delayed release preparations. Valporic acid serum levels often peak several hours after ingestion. Thus, levels should be assessed every two to four hours until a decline in level is noted indicating that a peak level has been reached. If peak levels have not yet been achieved, there is concern for rebound levels that could lead to increased CNS depression. Supportive care is the principal treatment for VPA intoxication and results in good outcomes in the vast majority of patients. Because VPA-induced hyperammonemia and hepatotoxicity may be mediated in part by carnitine deficiency, the administration of L-carnitine (50 mg/kg/day) is recommended for patients with hyperammonemia, lethargy, coma, and hepatic dysfunction. Although experience is limited, hemodialysis and hemodialysis-hemoperfusion modalities have been reported be to be effective in severe toxicity. Recent reports show that early intervention may correlate with rapid clinical improvement.

Answer: D

Licari E, Calzavacc P, Warrillow SJ, *et al.* (2009) Life-threatening sodium valproate overdose: A comparison of two approaches to treatment. *Critical Care Medicine* **37**, 3161–4.

Ohtani Y, Endo F, Matsuda I. (1982) Carnitine deficiency and hyperammonemia associated with valproic acid therapy. *Journal of Pediatrics* **101**, 782–5.

Szthankrycer MD (2002) Valproic acid toxicity. *Journal of Toxicology and Clinical Toxicology* **40**, 789–801.

14. *A 25-year-old man with known drug abuse history is brought to the ED for evaluation after fleeing police and then collapsing clutching his chest. On arrival to the hospital, EMS reports that he had a witnessed generalized tonic-clonic seizure enroute. His current vitals are BP 180/93 mm Hg, HR 125 beats/min, RR 20 breaths/min, temperature 38.7 °C. He is agitated, diaphoretic, and mumbling.*

Which one of the following should NOT be administered to this patient?

A. *Nitroglycerin*

B. *Metoprolol*

C. *Lorazepam*

D. *Oxygen*

E. *Phentolamine*

This patient presents with sympathomimetic syndrome consistent with cocaine or amphetamine intoxication. Clinical symptoms include tachycardia, hypertension, hyperthermia, agitation, mydriasis and psychosis. Cocaine-associated chest pain (CACP) accounts for approximately 40% of all cocaine-related visits to the emergency department and evaluation of these patients includes an ECG, chest radiograph, and biochemical markers to exclude myocardial infarction. Early management of patients with CACP includes administration of oxygen and reduction of sympathetic outflow using benzodiazepines given intravenously. Benzodiazepines should be given to patients who are anxious, agitated, hypertensive, or tachycardic; nitroglycerin should be given in addition to patients with hypertension. Beta blockers are **contraindicated** in patients who have recently used cocaine (<24 hours), and in patients with CACP. Beta blockers may lead to unopposed alpha-adrenergic stimulation which can cause coronary arterial vasoconstriction, ischemia, and infarction. Phentolamine, an alpha-adrenergic antagonist, can be used to reduce cocaine-induced coronary artery vasoconstriction when managing CACP or hypertension that is unresponsive to benzodiazepines.

Answer: B

Hollander JE (1995) The management of cocaine-associated myocardial ischemia. *New England Journal of Medicine* **333**, 1267–72.

Lange RA, Cigarroa RG, Yancy CW Jr, *et al.* (1989) Cocaine-induced coronary-artery vasoconstriction. *New England Journal of Medicine* 321, 1557–62.

Lange RA, Hillis LD (2001) Cardiovascular complications of cocaine use. *New England Journal of Medicine* **345**, 351–8.

15. *A 20-year-old woman is brought to the hospital after being found down next to a bottle of sustained-release metoprolol. By history from family, the patient was last seen awake three hours prior to arrival. Initial vital signs revealed a temperatire pf 37.0 °C, BP 102/40 mm Hg, HR 122 beats per minute, respirations 20 breaths/min. The patient was given activated charcoal. Approximately 90 minutes later, the patient has decreased mental status, BP 73/30 mm Hg and HR 55 beats per minute.*

Which one of the following would be the appropriate sequence of interventions most appropriate to stabilize this patient assuming the preceding intervention is unsuccessful?

A. *Calcium chloride IV, transcutaneous pacing, then transvenous pacing*

B. *Atropine 1 mg IV, then transcutaneous pacing*

C. *Glucagon IV, calcium chloride IV, then transcutaneous pacing*

D. *Transcutaneous pacing then transvenous pacing*

E. *Calcium chloride IV, glucagon IV, then transvenous pacing*

β-Adenergic blockers produce adverse effects primarily through bradycardia and hypotension. Central nervous system depression may occur with lipid-soluble agents such as propranolol, timolol, metoprolol, and acebutolol. Hypotension often results from negative inotropic effects rather than bradycardia. Glucagon is considered the *initial drug of choice*, because it produces chronotropic and inotropic effects and does not require β-receptors for activity. The goal of treatment is improvement in blood pressure and perfusion rather than increase in heart rate. Calcium chloride 10% may be effective in reversing hypotension. Transcutaneous pacing and transvenous pacing may be considered in refractory cases. Additional drugs that had variable efficacy include atropine, epinephrine, isoproterenol, and dopamine. Milrinone (phosphodiesterase inhibitors), intra-aortic balloon pump, or cardiopulmonary bypass may be considered if there is no response to other interventions.

Answer: C

Alapat PM, Zimmerman JL (2008) Toxicology in the critical care unit. *Chest* **133**, 1006–13.

Bailey B (2003) Glucagon in β-blocker and calcium channel blocker overdoses: a systemic review. *Journal of Toxicology and Clinical Toxicology* **41**, 595–602.

Mokhlesi B, Leiken JB, Murray P, *et al.* (2003) Adult toxicology in critical care: Part II: specific poisonings. *Chest* **123**, 897–922.

16. *A 56-year-old woman with chronic renal failure is status post a left carotid endarterectomy. She is admitted to the ICU with severe hypertension. The surgeon would like the systolic blood pressure <140 mm Hg. After 24 hours of treatment with nitroprusside, the patient develops confusion and metabolic acidosis. Her symptoms are best prevented/treated with administration of which one of the following agents?*

A. *Cyanocobalamin*

B. *Thiosulfate*

C. *Glucagon*

D. *Sodium bicarbonate*

E. *Calcium chloride*

This patient is developing signs and symptoms consistent with cyanide toxicity from nitroprusside. Nitroprusside has been shown to cause toxicity through the release of cyanide and accumulation of thiocyanate. Cyanide toxicity presents with unexplained cardiac arrest and changes in mental status, including convulsions, encephalopathy, and coma. Metabolic acidosis may also be present as a late finding. Risk of cyanide toxicity can be decreased by utilizing recommended doses of nitroprusside for short periods of time. An infusion of thiocynate is used to prevent and treat the symptoms of cyanide toxicity. Hydroxocobalamin is safe and effective in preventing and treating cyanide toxicity associated with the use of nitroprusside. However, cyanocobalamin is not effective as an antidote or able to prevent cyanide toxicity. Glucagon and calcium chloride are used to counteract the effects of β-blockers and calcium channel blockers, respectively. Sodium bicarbonate is used to treat tricyclic antidepressant toxicity.

Answer: B

Curry, SC (2005) Sodium nitroprusside. In: Brent J, Wallace K, Burkhart K *et al.* (2005) *Critical Care Toxicology*, Mosby Philadelphia, PA.

Schulz V, Gross R, Pasch T, *et al.* (1982) Cyanide toxicity of sodium nitroprusside in therapeutic use with and without sodium thiosulfate. *Klinische Wochenschrift* **60**, 1393–400.

Varon J, Marik PE (2000) The diagnosis and management of hypertensive crises. *Chest* **118**, 214–27.

Chapter 24 Common Procedures in the ICU

Adam D. Fox, DPM, DO and Daniel N. Holena, MD

1. *When preparing to place a central venous catheter (CVC) in a hemodynamically stable patient, all of the following have been shown to help reduce the risk of catheter-related blood stream infection (CRBSI) except:*

A. *Antisepsis of the skin with povidone-iodine solution rather than chlorhexadine*

B. *Maximal sterile barrier precautions*

C. *Antibiotic-coated catheters*

D. *Preferentially placing the CVC in the subclavian vein*

E. *Preprocedural hand washing*

Catheter-related blood stream infections remain a significant problem in the intensive care unit (ICU) setting. Prevention of these infections begins with the appropriate preparation. Standard hand washing prior to insertion should apply in all cases. Current recommendations call for antiseptic cleansing of the skin insertion site with 2% aqueous chlorhexadine gluconate solution. Studies have shown a significantly reduced infection rate with this preparation as compared to povidone-iodine or alcohol. When deciding on location for the CVC, placement in the subclavian vein has been shown to have the lowest rate of infection as compared to the internal jugular and femoral approaches. The choice of catheter may also play a role in reducing infection. Using an antimicrobial or antiseptic-impregnated CVC is recommended for patients in whom it is expected that the catheter will remain in place for >5 days. Once the site and catheter has been selected, it is imperative that maximal barrier protection be utilized. This includes cap, mask, sterile gown, sterile gloves, and a large sterile sheet. Additional methods that have been recommended include limiting the number of ports/lumens to those essential the management of the patient, avoidance of routine CVC changes, and replacing the dressing if it becomes dampened, loosened, or soiled.

Surgical Critical Care and Emergency Surgery: Clinical Questions and Answers, First Edition. Edited by Forrest O. Moore, Peter M. Rhee, Samuel A. Tisherman and Gerard J. Fulda.

Answer: A

Goetz AM, Wagener MM, Miller JM, *et al.* (1998) Risk of infection due to central venous catheters: effect of site of placement and catheter type. *Infection Control and Hospital Epidemiology* **19**, 842–5.

Guidelines for the Prevention of intravascular Catheter-Related Infections. MMWR. August 9, 2002/51(RR10); 1–26.

Maki DG, Ringer M, Alvarado CJ (1991) Prospective randomized trial of povidone-iodine, alcohol, and chlorhexadine for prevention of infection associated with central venous and arterial catheters. *Lancet* **338**, 339–43.

Maki DG, Stolz SM, Wheeler S, *et al.* (1997) Prevention of central venous catheter-related bloodstream infection by use of an antiseptic-impregnated catheter: a randomized, controlled trial. *Annals of Internal Medicine* **127**, 257–66.

Merrer J, De Jonghe B, Golliot F, *et al.* (2001) Complications of femoral and subclavian venous catheterization in critically ill patients: a randomized controlled trial. *Journal of the American Medical Association* **286**, 700–7.

Raad II, Hohn DC, Gilbreath BJ, *et al.* (1994) Prevention of central venous catheter-related infections by using maximal sterile barrier precautions during insertion. *Infection Control and Hospital Epidemiology* **15**, 231–8.

Veenstra DL, Saint S, Saha S, *et al.* (1999) Efficacy of antiseptic-impregnated central venous catheters in preventing catheter-related blood stream infections: a meta-analysis. *Journal of the American Medical Association* **281**, 261–7.

2. *Regarding the use of ultrasound guidance versus the landmark technique for the routine placement of a CVC, all of the following statements are true except:*

A. *Ultrasound reduces the number of passes necessary to achieve cannulation of the internal jugular as compared to the landmark technique*

B. *The landmark technique has a higher incidence of carotid puncture*

C. *Ultrasound use results in faster venous cannulation times*

D. *The benefits of ultrasonic localization can be applied to all access sites*

E. *Fewer failed procedures*

Anatomic landmarks have traditionally been used to guide CVC placement, but .with increasing use of portable ultrasound (US) in the ICU, there have been multiple studies evaluating its use in the placement of central venous catheters. In general, these studies have supported the use of two-dimensional US for placement of CVCs. Findings include: reduction in the number of passes to cannulation, lower incidence of carotid artery puncture/hematoma complications, and higher overall success rate. There are several caveats to these findings. First, the majority of studies examining the use of US have been conducted using the internal jugular vein as the access site, and therefore may not be generalizable to femoral and subclavian access sites. In addition, no study has compared the efficacy of US guided vs. landmark technique in patients needing emergent central venous access. However, given the overall data, the Agency for Healthcare Research and Quality recommends that real-time ultrasound guidance be utilized for CVC insertion as a way to improve patient care.

Answer: D

Denys BG, Uretsky BF, Reddy PS (1993) Ultrasound-assisted cannulation of the internal jugular vein: a prospective comparison to the external landmark-guided technique. *Circulation* **87**, 1557–62.

Hayashi H, Amano M (2002) Does ultrasound imaging before puncture facilitate internal jugular vein cannulation? Prospective randomized comparison with landmark-guided puncture in ventilated patients. *Journal of Cardiothoracic Vascular Anesthesiology* **16**, 572–5.

University of California at San Francisco (UCSF)-Stanford University Evidence-based Practice Center (2001) *Making Health Care Safer: A Critical Analysis of Patient Safety Practices.* Agency for Healthcare Research and Quality, Rockville, MD.

Slama M, Novara A, Safavian A, *et al.* (1997) Improvement in internal jugular vein cannulation using an ultrasound-guided technique. *Intensive Care Medicine* **23**, 916–19.

3. *All the following are true regarding arterial catheterization except:*

A. *The need for frequent arterial blood gasses (3 or more in a 24 hour time period) is an indication for arterial catheterization*

B. *Carpal tunnel syndrome is a relative contraindication*

C. *The Allen test should be performed prior to radial artery catheterization to ensure adequate ulnar collateral flow*

D. *End arteries such as the brachial artery should be avoided except when more preferable sites are not available*

E. *The risk of permanent ischemic complications in radial artery cannulation is rare*

As with any procedure, understanding the indications for and complications of arterial catheterization is crucial. Indications for indwelling arterial catheter placement include hemodynamic monitoring, frequent arterial blood gas sampling (three or more per 24 hours), and arterial administration of medications.. Complications include bleeding, infection, arteriovenous fistula formation, and distal ischemia secondary to thrombosis or embolization. Radial artery cannulation is a relatively safe procedure that has an incidence of permanent ischemic complications of 0.09% Multiple sites can be utilized for cannulation, but to minimize complications, sites with limited collateral circulation (such as the brachial artery) should be avoided. The Allen test attempts to assess ulnar arterial flow to the hand prior to radial arterial line placement. While theoretically pleasing, the clinical utility of this test is dubious. As such, many practitioners have abandoned this as a precursor to radial artery cannulation. Relative contraindications to arterial cannulation include trauma or burns to the ipsilateral extremity, carpal tunnel syndrome, damaged or infected skin at the access site, coagulopathy, and Raynaud's disease.

Answer: C

Brzezinski M, Luisetti T, London MJ (2009) Radial artery cannulation: A comprehensive review of recent anatomic and physiologic investigations. *Anesthesia and Analgesia* **109** (6), 1763–81.

Gabrielli A, Layon AJ, Yu Mihae (eds) (2009) *Civetta, Taylor, and Kirby's Critical Care*, Lippincott Williams & Wilkins. Philadelphia, PA, pp. 409–28.

Glavine RJ, Jones HM (1989) Assessing collateral circulation in the hand-four methods compared. Anesthesia **44**, 594.

Irwin RS, Ripe JM (eds) (2008) Intensive Care Medicine. Lippincott Williams & Wilkins, Philadelphia, PA, Table 3-1, pp. 38–47.

4. *When placing a percutaneous endoscopic gastrostomy (PEG), all the following have been utilized to reduce complications except:*

A. *Preprocedural antibiotic*

B. *Transillumination*

C. *1:1 ballottement*

D. *Placing the patient in the reverse trendelenburg position*

E. *Visualizing simultaneous air return while aspirating a syringe at the same time as endoscopic visualization of an intragastric needle*

PEG tube placement has become the preferred method for enteral access in the patient who will require long-term feeding access. It is less invasive than an open gastrostomy tube and can be performed in a variety of locations, including the ICU. Considerations prior to placement should include previous abdominal surgery and known anatomic variation of the gastrointestinal tract. PEG tubes are associated with ~1% mortality rate, ~3% major complication rate, and a 13% minor complication rate. Prior to beginning the procedure, prophylactic antibiotics (i.e. a first generation cephalosporin) should be given to reduce infection rate. Because PEG placement requires the blind passage of a needle, wire, and ultimately gastrostomy tube between the skin and gastric lumen, techniques have been developed to minimize the risk of injuring intervening structures (e.g. colon). After adequate endoscopic insufflation of the stomach, digital indentation of the skin should be visualized as directly translated to the gastric wall (a phenomenon known as 1:1 ballottement). In addition, light from the endoscope should be visualized passing through the abdominal wall (transillumination). Lastly, there are several papers that describe using a "finder" needle and fluid filled syringe to appropriately locate the stomach. Advancing the needle while simultaneously aspirating should show air return when in the lumen. If this air return is noted prior to gastric visualization of the needle, the assumption is that there is an interposed loop of bowel between the stomach and abdominal wall. There is no evidence that positioning the patient in Trendelenburg position can help reduce complication rates.

Answer: D

Larson DE, Burton DD, Schroeder KW, DiMagno EP (1987). Percutaneous endoscopic gastrostomy. Indications, success, complications, and mortality in 314 consecutive patients. *Gastroenterology* **93** (1), 48–52.

Lin HS, Ibrahim HZ, Kheng JW, *et al.* (2001) Percutaneous endoscopic gastrostomy: strategies for prevention and management of complications. *Laryngoscope* **111** (10), 1847–52.

Lipp A, Lusardi G (2006) Systemic antimicrobial prophylaxis for percutaneous endoscopic gastrostomy. *Cochrane Database of Systematic Review.* Issue 4 Art. No.: CD005571.

Sherwin PS, Sharma R, Jaik N (2007) complications related to percutaneous endoscopic gastrostomy (PEG) tubes. A comprehensive review. *Journal of Gastrointestinal Liver Disorders* **16** (4), 407–18.

5. *Regarding percutaneous dilatational tracheostomy (PDT), which of the following statements is correct?*

A. *Can only safely be performed in the operating room*

B. *Cannot safely be performed in patients undergoing cervical spine immobilization*

C. Is safe in patients who have previously undergone open tracheostomy

D. Has superior outcomes compared to open tracheostomy

E. Is absolutely contraindicated in the thrombocytopenic patient

PDT was first introduced in the mid-1980s and has since become a standard technique in the ICU due to multiple reports of its safety, cost savings, and ease of performance. There are no outcome benefits that have been found in comparison to an open technique. There is, however, a lower incidence of wound infection. Because it can be performed at the bedside, surgeons and non-surgeons alike have adopted the procedure. The indications for PDT are similar to those for standard open tracheostomies, but some special situations require mention. Although there are studies that demonstrate the safety of the procedure in the patient who requires cervical spine immobilization, there may be an increase likelihood of incorrect placement. Previous tracheostomy is not a contraindication to the PDT. Studies on the role of bronchoscopy during PDT have not consistently demonstrated benefit but certain societies have recommended its use Previously, body habitus including morbid obesity and short neck along with recent cervical spine surgery and coagulopathy were thought to be absolute contraindications to PDT. These contraindications have become relative as more experience has been gained with the procedure. An experienced operator is the key to performing the procedure in this cohort of patients.

Answer: C

Cobean R, Beals M, Moss C, *et al.* (1996) Percutaneous dilatational tracheostomy. A safe, cost-effective bedside procedure. *Archives of Surgery* **131**, 265–71.

De Leyn P, Bedert L, Delcroix M, *et al.* (2007) Tracheotomy: clinical review and guidelines. *European Journal of Cardio-thoracic Surgery* **32**, 412–21.

Kluge S, Meyer A, Kuhnell P, *et al.* (2004) Percutaneous tracheostomy is safe in patients with severe thrombocytopenia. Chest **126**, 547–51.

Mayberry JC, Wu IC, Goldman RK (2000) Cervical spine clearance and neck extension during percutaneous tracheostomy in trauma patients. Critical Care Medicine **28** (10), 3436–40.

Yilmaz M, Dosemeci L, Cengiz M, *et al.* (2006) Repeat percutaneous tracheostomy in the neurocritically ill patient. *Neurocritical Care* **5**, 120–3.

6. *All the following statements are correct regarding the current generation inferior vena cava (IVC) filters except:*

A. They are MRI compatible

B. They can be placed either fluoroscopically or via ultrasound guidance

C. The presence of the filter reduces the risk of caval thrombosis

D. The filter should be placed below the level of the renal veins

E. Migration, perforation, and poor retrieval rates are not uncommon

The use of the IVC filter has increased significantly in recent years, likely due to newer technology which allows for removal once the indication for the filter has passed. Indications include: recurrent pulmonary embolism (PE) despite anticoagulation, known deep venous thrombosis (DVT) or PE with contraindication to anticoagulation, and known deep venous thrombosis DVT/PE with complications of anticoagulation. Many filters exist and there seems to be a trend toward placement of retrievable filters despite poor retrieval rates. The majority of IVC filters currently used in the United States are MRI compatible, but individual product information should be sought. They can be placed via transabdominal ultrasound, endovascular ultrasound or fluoroscopically. It is important to understand that the placement of the IVC filter actually carries with it a risk of both deep femoral vein and inferior vena cava thrombosis. For this reason, the standard placement of filter should be below the renal veins to reduce the risk of renal vein thrombosis and subsequent kidney loss should caval thrombosis occur. No therapy is perfect, and IVC filters are not an exception to this rule; there is still a 3–7% risk of pulmonary embolism with the filter in place. Since 2005, the FDA has received approximately 1000 device adverse event reports involving IVC filters. These include: 328 device migrations, 146 embolizations (detachment of device components), 70 perforations of the IVC, and 56 filter fractures. Some of these events led to adverse clinical outcomes in patients. These types of events may be related to a retrievable filter remaining in the body for long periods of time; well beyond when the risk of PE has subsided.

Answer: C

AbuRhama AF, Robinson PA, Boland JP, *et al.* (1993) Therapeutic and prophylactic vena caval interruption for pulmonary embolism: caval and venous insertion site patency. *Annals of Vascular Surgery* **7**, 561–8.

Garrett JV, Passman MA, Guzman RJ (2004) Expanding options for bedside placement of inferior vena cava filters with intravascular ultrasound when transabdominal duplex ultrasound imaging is inadequate. *Annals of Vascular Surgery* **18**, 329–34.

Geisinger MA, Zelch MG, Risius B (1987) Recurrent pulmonary embolism after Greenfield filter placement. *Radiology* **165**, 383–4

Karmy-Jones R, Jurkovich GJ, Velmahos GC, *et al.* (2007) Practice patterns and outcomes of retrievable vena cava filters in trauma patients: An AAST multicenter study. *Journal of Trauma* **62**, 17–25.

US Food and Drug Administration (2010) Removing retrievable inferior vena cava filters: initial communication. August 9, www.fda.gov/MedicalDevices/Safety/AlertsandNotices/ucm221676.htm.

7. *A 24-year-old man who presented after a high-speed motor vehicle collision with a traumatic brain injury and bilateral pulmonary contusions is now requiring pressure control ventilation with an inverse I:E ratio and inspired oxygen fraction 90%. Nursing staff describes a large volume of thick secretions and the patient is now febrile. In regards to fiber-optic bronchoscopy, all the following statements are correct except:*

A. *Hypoxia is a relative contraindication*

B. *Intracranial pressure may spike during the procedure*

C. *Pneumothorax may occur in over 30% of patients*

D. *Can safely be done in unstable cardiac patients*

E. *The FiO_2 should be dialed up to 100% regardless of the patients' saturations*

Flexible bronchoscopy is generally a well tolerated procedure with multiple potential diagnostic and therapeutic indications. As with other interventions, the practitioner must be aware of the possible complications and contraindications. Mortality in experienced hands should not exceed 0.1%. Careful patient selection is the key to keeping the incidence of complications low. Hypoxia should prompt caution given multiple studies that demonstrate a decline in oxygenation that can persist for some time post-procedure. If bronchoscopy is still deemed necessary in a hypoxic patient, minimizing procedure time, withdrawing the bronchoscope frequently, and providing maximal oxygen support will help prevent persistent hypoxia. Bronchoscopy has been noted to raise intracranial pressure but there may not be permanent sequelae. Known complications of flexible bronchoscopy include cardiac arrhythmias, bronchospasm, pneumothorax, and vasovagal reactions. Unless biopsies are being taken, pneumothorax is a rare complication of fiber-optic bronchoscopy (<2%).

Answer: C

Albertini RE, Harrell JH, Kurihara N (1974) Arterial hypoxemia induced by fiberoptic bronchoscopy. *Journal of the American Medical Association* **230**, 1666–7.

Gorman SR, Beamis JF Jr (2005) Complications of flexible bronchoscopy. *Clinical Pulmonary Medicine* **12** (3), 177–83.

Kerwin AJ, Croce MA, Timmons SD (2000) Effects of bronchoscopy on intracranial pressure in patients with brain injury: a prospective clinical study. *Journal of Trauma* **48**, 878–83.

Peerless JR, Snow N, Likavec MJ (1995) The effect of fiberoptic bronchoscopy on cerebral hemodynamics in patients with severe head injury. *Chest* **108**, 962–5.

8. *After a successful PDT performed at the patient's bedside, a discussion ensues with the resident staff about potential complications of tracheostomy. All the following are considered early complications except:*

A. *Tracheostomy tube dislodgement*

B. *Pneumothorax*

C. *Hemorrhage*

D. *Tracheo-inomminate fistula*

E. *Subcutaneous emphysema*

When considering complications of tracheostomy, it may be useful to divide these into early (≤7 days) and late complications (>7 days). Tracheostomy tube dislodgement can occur at any time but is most hazardous in the days after initial placement; the most devastating sequel of tracheostomy tube dislodgement is death secondary to loss of airway. Because the tract between the trachea and skin is not well developed early after tracheostomy, attempting to replace the tracheostomy tube may lead to creation of a false passage without restoration of the airway. For this reason, oral endotracheal intubation is the procedure of choice should the tracheostomy tube be lost in the early postoperative period. Early dislodgement is usually due to a technical problem. There are multiple ways to help prevent this including proper placement of the stoma, avoidance of excessive neck hyperextension, and suturing the tube to the skin along with using tracheostomy tape. Due to the anatomic position of the apices of the lung in the neck, there is a 0–5% risk of pneumothorax with tracheostomy and a postprocedural chest radiograph is widely considered to be standard of care. Hemorrhage can occur in upwards of 37% of patients. Most of this is minor and can be controlled with simple packing. Major hemorrhage occurs in a smaller percentage of patients and may require return to the operating room for exploration and hemorrhage control. Subcutaneous emphysema can occur secondary to positive pressure itself, or a forceful cough against a tightly sutured or packed wound. A pneumothorax can also be a consideration and can be evaluated with a chest x-ray. Subcutaneous emphysema should resolve without intervention over the following days. A rare but devastating late complication of tracheostomy is tracheoinnominate (TI) fistula. In general, it will occur in the first month after the procedure but can happen as late as a year. Pulsation of the tracheostomy tube may be clue. A TI fistula will frequently present with a "herald bleed"; bright red blood from around the tracheostomy site, which abates spontaneously, only to be followed by exanguinating hemorrhage. Should late bleeding occur in a patient with a tracheostomy, it should prompt further diagnostic workup. If bleeding occurs in a patient with a high index of suspicion for a TI fistula, the first step should be overinflation of the tracheostomy tube balloon. Should this work, the patient should be brought to the operating room for definitive repair. If the bleeding continues, the tracheostomy tube should be removed and a finger placed in the tracheal stoma for direct anterior compression of the fistula. A small orotracheal tube should then be passed with its inflated cuff passed the level of the fistula. Finally, the patient should be transported to the operating room for repair.

Answer: D

Conlon AA, Kopec SE (2000) Tracheostomy in the ICU. *Journal of Intensive Care Medicine* **15**, 1–13.

Goldenberg D, Ari EG, Golz, *et al.* (2000) Tracheostomy complications: a retrospective study of 1130 cases. *Otolaryngology Head and Neck Surgery* **123**, 495.

Goldstein SI, Breda SD, Schneider KL (1987) Surgical complication of bedside tracheotomy in an otolaryngology residency program. *Laryngoscope* **97**, 1407–9.

Kirchner JA (1986) Avoiding problems in tracheotomy. *Laryngoscope* **96**, 55.

Mamikunian C (1988) Prevention of delayed hemorrhage after tracheotomy. *Ear Nose and Throat Journal* **67**, 881–2.

Ridley RW, Zwischenberger JB (2006) Tracheoinnominate Fistula: Surgical Management of an iatrogenic disaster. *Journal of Laryngology and Otology* **120**, 676–80.

9. *With regard to the use of lumbar puncture in the ICU, which of the following statements is correct?*

A. *To reduce the risk of adverse events, lumbar puncture must be performed under fluoroscopy*

B. *CSF pressure measurement is accurate no matter the position of the patient when sampling takes place*

C. *Lumbar puncture can safely be performed in most patients without first obtaining a CT scan of the brain*

D. *Irreversible hearing loss is a rare but potentially devastating complication of lumbar puncture*

E. *Utilization of ultrasound to identify landmarks is superior to the palpation technique*

Lumbar puncture can be utilized in the ICU to sample cerebrospinal fluid (CSF) for a variety of reasons. In adults, CSF aspiration can usually be done under local anesthetic. Patients with previous lumbar surgery or congenital abnormal anatomy may require fluoroscopically guided needle placement but, in general, anatomic landmarks can be used. Prior to performing a lumbar puncture, a CT scan of the brain has been recommended in the following patients: immunocompromised states (e.g. HIV, post-transplant), history of central nervous system disease, new onset seizures, pappilledema, abnormal level of consciousness, and focal neurologic deficits. The accuracy of CSF pressure measurement is limited by the patient's position. Cerebrospinal fluid pressure measurements are not accurate if performed when the patient is in a seated position. This can be rectified by reclining the patient into a lateral position. Several complications of lumbar puncture exist. These include spinal headache, hemorrhage, and hearing loss. Hearing loss after lumbar puncture is thought to be due to changes in intracranial pressure. While it is generally reversible, rare cases of long-term hearing loss have been reported. There is mixed literature (mostly in non–ICU patients) regarding the superiority of ultrasound guided LP. Some suggestion exists that it may be beneficial in the morbidly obese patient.

Answer: D

Irwin RS, Rippe JM (eds) (2008) *Intensive Care Medicine*, Lippincott Williams & Wilkins, Philadelphia, PA, p. 155.

Michel O, Brusis T (1992) Hearing loss as a sequel of lumbar puncture. *Annals of Otology Rhinology and Laryngology* **101**, 390–4.

Nomura JT, Leech SJ, Shenbagamurthi S, *et al.* (2007) A randomized controlled trial of ultrasound-assisted lumbar puncture. *Journal of Ultrasound Medicine* **26**, 1341–8.

Tunkel AR, Hartman BJ, Kaplan SL, *et al.* (2004) practice guidelines for the management of bacterial meningitis. Clinical Infectious Disorders **39**, 1267–84.

10. *With regard to paracentesis in the ICU, which of the following statements is correct?*

A. *Paracentesis should never be performed in the presence of coagulopathy*

B. *Ultrasound guided paracentesis has success rates equivalent to landmark-guided paracentesis*

C. *The urinary bladder should be decompressed prior to paracentesis*

D. *Paracentesis-induced circulatory dysfunction (PICD) may occur after the removal of even small volumes of fluid*

E. *Paracentesis should not be performed in the pregnant woman*

Paracentesis has been used in the ICU for both diagnostic and therapeutic purposes. Correction of coagulopathy is not absolutely mandatory but should be considered. The preferred site of access for paracentesis is the anterior abdominal wall, lateral the bladder and epigastric vessels. Because a distended bladder may be at higher risk for inadvertent puncture, decompression of the bladder is recommended prior to paracentesis. Use of ultrasound may increase the success rate of paracentesis relative to the traditional landmark technique (95% versus 61% in one prospective randomized trial). Paracentesis-induced circulatory dysfunction (PCID) is a condition characterized by hyponatremia, azotemia, and increase in plasma rennin activity and typically only occurs after large volume paracentesis. Infusion of albumin has been shown to diminish the chances of this occurring. Caution should be used when performing paracentesis in the pregnant patient. It should only be attempted with an imaging technique such as ultrasound.

Answer: C

Grabau CM, Crago SF, Hoff LK, *et al.* (2004) Performance standards for therapeutic abdominal paracentesis. *Hepatology* **40**, 484.

Nazeer SR, Dewbre H and Miller AH (2005) Ultrasound-assisted paracentesis performed by emergency physicians vs. the traditional technique: a prospective, randomized study. *American Journal of Emergency Medicine* **23** (3), 363–7.

Ruiz-Del-Arbol, L, Monescillo A, Jimenez W, *et al.* (1997) Paracentesis-induced circulatory dysfunction: Mechanism and effect on hepatic hemodynamics in cirrhosis. *Gastroenterology* **113** (2), 579–86.

11. *A 58-year-old man has been on the ventilator for eight days after complicated aortic aneurysm repair. He is now febrile and is noted to have a new infiltrate on chest x-ray. Regarding the use of bronchoscopy for the* *diagnosis of pneumonia, which of the following statements is correct?*

A. *Quantitative protected brush specimens represent the gold standard in ventilator-associated pneumonia diagnosis*

B. *To ensure accurate diagnostic testing, a BAL specimen must be obtained from each lobe of the lung*

C. *To ensure accurate diagnostic testing, at least 100 ml saline should be instilled*

D. *Bronchoscopy should be performed for diagnostic purposes even in patients with severe hypoxia on maximal ventilator settings*

E. *The bronchoscope need only be advanced into the orifice of the desired lobe for appropriate sampling*

Bronchoscopy can be a useful tool in making the diagnosis of pneumonia and in identifying the causative organism(s). Bronchoscopy allows for the performance of either a bronchoalveolar lavage (BAL) or protected brush specimen (PBS) but neither has been definitively accepted as the standard of care for diagnosis of ventilator associated pneumonia. When performing BAL, one need not sample from every lobe but instead attention should be directed to the location of suspected infection. If the disease process is diffuse, there is some controversy as to the location for the best sample but in general, should be taken from the most affected segment. Once chosen, the bronchoscope should be advanced until wedged into a subsegmental bronchus. Saline is then instilled and suctioned into a trap. At least 100–120 ml should be instilled and most advocate discarding the first 35–50 ml as this is likely contaminated from the more proximal airways. One must also be cognizant of the need to retrieve as much as possible as this will increase the yield of the specimen. The risks and benefits must be considered prior to performance of bronchoscopy; caution should be used in patients who may not tolerate further hypoxia as a result of this procedure.

Answer: C

Chastre J, Fagon JY (2002) Ventilator-associated pneumonia. *American Journal of Respiratory Critical Care Medicine* **165**, pp. 867–903.

Combes, A., Luyt, CE, Trouillet JL, Chastre, J. (2010). Controversies in ventilator-associated pneumonia. *Seminars in Respiratory and Critical Care Medicine* **31** (1), 47–54.

Irwin RS, Rippe JM (eds) (2008) *Intensive Care Medicine*, Lippincott Williams & Wilkins, Philadelphia, PA.

12. *A 76-year-old man with significant cardiac and pulmonary history is being treated for septic shock secondary to pneumonia. He has just been placed on his second pressor despite aggressive fluid resuscitation. To rule out a cardiogenic component to his shock, you decide to place a pulmonary artery catheter (PAC). All of the following are true regarding PAC except:*

A. *Pulmonary artery occlusion pressures correlate poorly with volume responsiveness*

B. *Placement is contraindicated in patients with tricuspid or pulmonary valve prostheses*

C. *The catheter should never be pulled back without first inflating the balloon*

D. *Arrhythmia caused by PAC placement usually terminates spontaneously with removal of the catheter*

E. *The PA catheter can be placed through the femoral vein*

Use of pulmonary artery catheters (PAC) has declined in the recent years as contemporary studies have questioned the utility of the procedure. The correlation between pulmonary artery occlusion pressures ("wedge" pressures) and response to volume administration is poor. However, if a PAC is to be used it is important to understand the information it can provide. Indications for which the PAC may be beneficial include: management of complicated myocardial infarctions, assessment of respiratory distress, assessment of shock, management of post-operative open heart patients, and assessment of valvular heart disease.

Contraindications to placement include tricuspid or pulmonary valve prosthetics, right-heart thrombus or tumor, tricuspid/pulmonary valve endocarditis. Caution should be used in the patient with new left bundle branch block as it may precipitate complete heart block. The process of insertion should start with vascular access and can be done from multiple different sites although more difficult from femoral or brachial locations. It is important to recognize that while the balloon needs to be inflated to advance the catheter, it should always be deflated prior to withdrawal. Many complications are possible and include balloon rupture, knotting of the catheter, pulmonary infarction, thrombosis, embolism, arrhythmias, and perforation.

Answer: C

Evans DC, Doraiswamy VA, Proscia MP, *et al.* (2009) Complications associated with pulmonary artery catheters: a comprehensive clinical review. *Scandinavian Journal of Surgery* **98** (4), 199–208.

Gabrielli A, Layon AJ, Yu Mihae (eds) (2009) *Civetta, Taylor, and Kirby's Critical Care,* Lippincott Williams & Wilkins, Philadelphia, PA, p. 42.

Hadian M, Pinsky MR (2007) Functional hemodynamic monitoring. *Current Opinion in Critical Care* **13** (3), 318–23.

Irwin RS, Rippe JM (eds) (2008) Pulmonary Artery Catheters. Intensive Care Medicine. Lippincott Williams & Wilkins, Philadelphia, PA, Table 4-1, pp. 48–65.

13. *Regarding temporary transvenous cardiac pacemakers, which statement is correct?*

A. *Are predominantly used for bradyarrhythmias*

B. *Are preferentially placed via femoral venous access*

C. *Most commonly positioned in the right atrium*

D. *Can result in pacemaker syndrome when using a single atrial pacer*

E. *There is no role for ultrasound guidance in the placement of a transvenous pacemaker*

Temporary transvenous cardiac pacemakers are most often placed for symptomatic bradycardia but can also be used for overdrive pacing in patients with tachyarrhythmias. Although the preferred access approach is through the internal jugular or subclavian vein, transvenous pacemaker may also be placed via the femoral vein using fluoroscopic guidance. The most common cardiac chamber to place the device is the right ventricle. "Pacemaker syndrome" is a condition where dysynchrony occurs between the atria and ventricles, resulting in hemodynamic changes and symptoms of dizziness, throat tightness, neck pulsations, or dyspnea. This occurs with ventricular, not atrial, pacing. With the increasing portability of bedside ultrasound, there is a role for its use in the placement of the pacemaker. As opposed to the blind technique, the ultrasound, in the subxiphoid position, allows the operator to identify the proper placement of the pacer.

Answer: A

Gabrielli A, Layon AJ, Yu Mihae (eds) (2009) *Civetta, Taylor, and Kirby's Critical Care,* Lippincott Williams & Wilkins, Philadelphia, PA, p. 438.

Harrigan RA, Chan TC, Moonblatt S. (2007) Temporary transvenous pacemaker placement in the emergency department. *Journal of Emergency Medicine* **32** (1), pp. 105–11.

14. *For the ICU patient requiring endotracheal intubation, which of the following statements is correct?*

A. *Rapid sequence intubation is the always the best technique for intubation*

B. *Ensuring that the ear and sternal notch are in the same plane greatly facilitates visualization during orotracheal intubation*

C. *In a patient who is able to be oxygenated, repeated attempts at direct laryngoscopy are not associated with worse outcomes*

D. *The nasotracheal intubation approach utilizes the same size endotracheal tubes as orotracheal route*

E. *There is no difference in success rate between direct laryngoscopy and videolaryngoscopy*

Rapid sequence intubation (RSI) is a method of intubating patients in which a sedative agent and short-term paralytic agent are administered prior to intubation. While useful in many situations, eliminating a patient's ability to breathe spontaneously may not always be beneficial. For instance, a patient who is hypoxic but maintaining stable oxygen saturation through spontaneous respiration may be converted to a patient who is progressively hypoxic. If unable to be intubated, adverse events may follow. Whatever method of intubation is selected, preprocedural preparation is imperative.

Correct positioning of the patient (accomplished by aligning the ear and sternal notch in a parallel plane) ensures the best visualization possible and increases the chances of success. Although you can "take your time" securing the airway if the patient is oxygenating and hemodynamically stable, there is some evidence that repetitive laryngoscopy may place the patient at high risk for potentially life-threatening airway and nonairway related complications. When using the nasotracheal approach, it is important to remember that the sizing of the tube should be smaller than the tube that would be used for orotracheal intubation. Videolaryngoscopy has become the latest technique for the difficult and failed intubation. These devices present a magnified image from the tip of the blade onto a video screen. It has been demonstrated that this technique frequently improves intubation success.

Answer: B

Atlas GM, Mort TC (2003) Attempts at emergent tracheal intubation of inpatients: a retrospective practice analysis comparing adjunct sedation with or without neuromuscular blockade. *Internet Journal of Anesthesia* 7.

Jungbauer A, Schumann M, Brunkhorst V, *et al.* (2009) Expected difficult tracheal intubation: a prospective comparison of direct laryngoscopy and video laryngoscopy in 200 patients. *British Journal of Anaesthesia* **102** (4), 546–50.

Mort TC (2004) Emergency tracheal intubation: complications associated with repeated laryngoscopic attempts. *Anesthesia and Analgesia* **99**, 607.

American Society of Anesthesiologists (2003) Practice Guidelines for the management of the difficult airway: an updated report by the American Society of Anesthesiologists Taskforce on Management of the Difficult Airway. *Anesthesiology* **98**, 1269.

15. *With regard to performing endoscopy in the intensive care unit, which of the following statements is correct?*

A. *Orotracheal intubation should be performed prior to upper endoscopy*

B. *Lower gastrointestinal endoscopy for bleeding should not be performed without first ensuring that there is not an upper gastrointestinal source*

C. *Endoscopy is absolutely contraindicated in the presence of coagulopathy*

D. *Lower GI endoscopic decompression is the first line procedure in acute colonic pseudoobstruction (Ogilvie's Syndrome)*

E. *There is no role for endoscopic retrograde cholangiopancreatography (ERCP) in the ICU*

Both upper and lower endoscopies can be carried out safely in the ICU environment. Adequate sedation is needed prior to these procedures but there is no need for orotracheal intubation in many patients unless it is warranted by concern for airway protection or other circumstances. While the majority of bleeding per rectum is from a lower gastrointestinal source (distal to the ligament of Treitz), upwards of 11% of cases will actually have an upper gastrointestinal origin. Coagulopathy is a relative contraindication to performance of endoscopy and the decision to proceed or not must be based on a thorough assessment of the potential risks and benefits of the procedure. After ruling out mechanical causes of obstruction in patients suspected to have acute colonic pseudo-obstruction, neostigmine administration is the initial treatment of choice. Many scenarios exist in which ICU patients are too ill for transport. Multiple procedures, including bedside laparoscopy, ERCP, and abdominal explorations have been shown to be safe in the ICU setting when performed by experienced personnel.

Answer: B

Jensen DM, Machicado GA (1988) Diagnosis and treatment of severe hematochezia: the role of urgent colonoscopy after purge. *Gastroenterology* **95**, 1569–74.

Ponec RJ, Saunders MD, Kimmey MB (1999) Neostigmine for the treatment of acute colonic obstruction. *New England Journal of Medicine* **341**, 137–41.

Saleem A, Gostout CJ, Peterson BT (2011) Outcome of emergency ERCP in the intensive care unit. *Endoscopy* **43** (6), 549–51.

Chapter 25 Diagnostic Imaging, Ultrasound, and Interventional Radiology

Randall S. Friese, MD, MSc, FACS, FCCM and Terence O'Keeffe, MB ChB, MSPH, FACS

1. *All of the following decrease the sensitivity and specificity of the FAST exam (Focused Assessment with Sonography for Trauma) except*

A. *Abdominal tenderness on exam*

B. *Lumbar spine fracture*

C. *Traumatic aortic rupture*

D. *Pelvic fracture*

E. *Ecchymosis/abrasion of the anterior abdominal wall (seatbelt sign)*

The utility of ultrasound as a tool for the evaluation of the trauma patient was pioneered in Europe and Japan. In the early 1990s its use became popularized in the USA after a series of studies reported sensitivity ranging from 79–93% and a specificity ranging from 95–100% for the evaluation of hemoperitoneum after blunt mechanism. These studies also reported that ultrasound techniques can be learned in an expeditious fashion and that ultrasound provides a rapid assessment for hemoperitoneum as a point of care tool.

Several important studies followed highlighting the potential pitfalls of the FAST exam. These studies reported the increased likelihood of false negative and false positive FAST exams in conjunction with certain injuries; specifically, pelvic fracture, thoracolumbar spine fracture, seatbelt sign on the anterior abdominal wall, abdominal tenderness on exam, lower rib fractures, and hematuria. In fact, the sensitivity of the FAST exam was reported to be as low as 26% in patients with pelvic fracture.

Surgical Critical Care and Emergency Surgery: Clinical Questions and Answers, First Edition. Edited by Forrest O. Moore, Peter M. Rhee, Samuel A. Tisherman and Gerard J. Fulda.

Answer: C

Ballard RB, Rozycki GS, Newman PG, *et al.* (1999) An algorithm to reduce the incidence of false-negative FAST examinations in patients at high risk for occult injury. *Journal of the American College of Surgeons* **189** (2), 145–50.

Bode PJ, Niezen A, van Vugt AB, Schipper J (1993) Abdominal ultrasound as a reliable indicator for conclusive laparotomy in blunt abdominal trauma. *Journal of Trauma.* **34** (1), 27–31.

Chiu WC, Cushing BM, Rodriguez A, *et al.* (1997) Abdominal injuries without hemoperitoneum: a potential limitation of focused abdominal sonography for trauma (FAST). *Journal of Trauma* **42** (4), 617–23.

Friese RS, Malekzadeh S, Shafi S, *et al.* (2007) Abdominal ultrasound is an unreliable modality for the detection of hemoperitoneum in patients with pelvic fracture. *Journal of Trauma* **63** (1), 97–102.

Liu M, Lee CH, Peng FK (1993) Prospective comparison of diagnostic peritoneal lavage, computed tomographic scanning, and ultrasonography for the diagnosis of blunt abdominal trauma. *J Trauma* **35** (2), 267–70.

McKenney M, Lentz K, Nunez D, *et al.* (1994) Can ultrasound replace diagnostic peritoneal lavage in the assessment of blunt trauma? *Journal of Trauma* **37** (3), 439–41.

Rozycki GS, Ochsner MG, Jaffin JH, Champion HR (1993) Prospective evaluation of surgeons' use of ultrasound in the evaluation of trauma patients. *Journal of Trauma* **34** (4), 516–26.

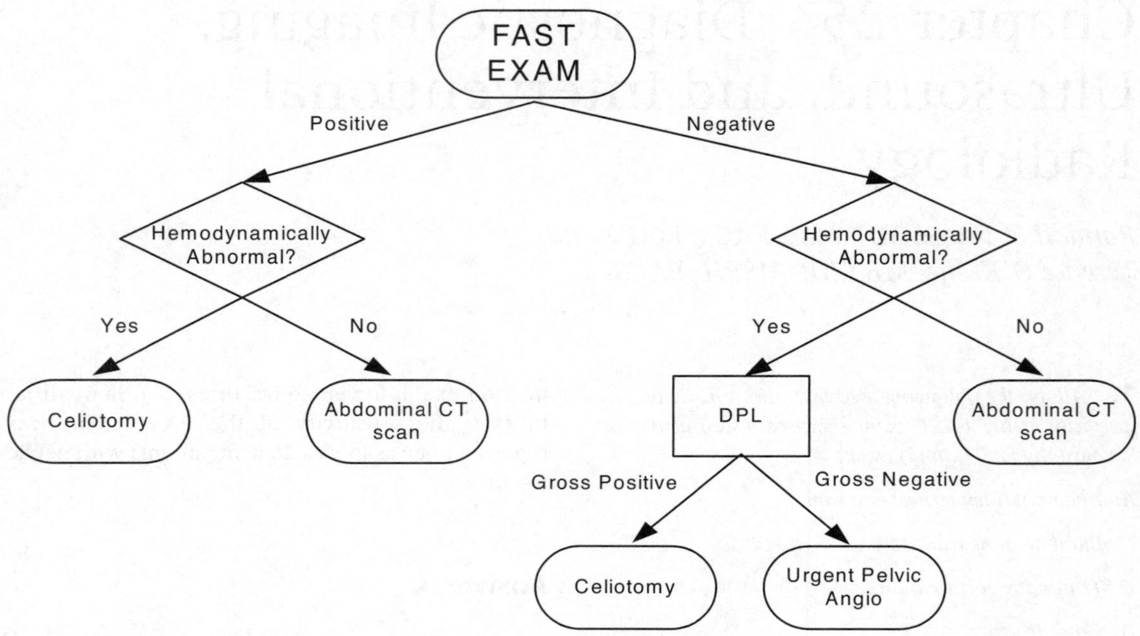

Suggested algorithm for the use of FAST in pelvic fracture

2. *Ultrasound evaluation of the abdomen after anterior abdominal wall stab wounds upon arrival to the emergency room*

A. *Can exclude hemoperitoneum and obviate the need for laparotomy*

B. *Has a high sensitivity for the detection of fascial penetration*

C. *Can identify hemoperitoneum which would mandate laparotomy*

D. *Can identify patients that can be safely discharged from the emergency department*

E. *Should include a high frequency-linear probe in order to exclude fascial penetration*

Ultrasonography is used for the evaluation of injured patients in the vast majority of trauma centers across the USA. Ultrasonography can be performed rapidly at the patient's bedside and is non-invasive, inexpensive, portable, and easily repeated. For these reasons its use in the evaluation of the patient injured by blunt mechanism has become standard of care. However, the use of ultrasound in the evaluation of penetrating abdominal trauma is less widespread.

The sensitivity of abdominal ultrasound for detecting the need for operative intervention, after penetrating injury, is low (28–48%). This low sensitivity may be explained by the fact that the absence of hemoperitoneum does not rule out the presence of injury after penetrating trauma. In fact, patients with penetrating abdominal injury with a negative abdominal ultrasound should not be discharged from the emergency department. They are best managed by further work up including one or more of the following; serial abdominal examination, local wound exploration, or diagnostic peritoneal lavage.

The specificity of abdominal ultrasound for detecting the need for operative intervention, after penetrating injury, is high (94–100%). Although most trauma surgeons recognize that the simple presence of hemoperitoneum does not necessarily correlate with the presence of a significant injury requiring laparotomy and non-therapeutic laparotomy may result. Even though the specificity is high, most studies have found that when the abdominal ultrasound demonstrates hemoperitoneum there is usually enough clinical and anatomical evidence to justify operative exploration and the ultrasound information does not alter the management plan.

Finally, some authors have described the use of ultrasound to evaluate the anterior abdominal wall to rule out potential fascial penetration. In the absence of fascial penetration, intra-peritoneal injury is unlikely. However, the sensitivity of ultrasound for detecting penetration of the fascia is low (59%) with a standard probe, thus a negative exam does not exclude the presence of fascial penetration. When interrogating the fascia for penetration ultrasound examination of the anterior abdominal wall should be performed using a high frequency linear probe (8–10 mHz). The higher frequency allows for better resolution of superficial structures, whereas low frequency probes allow for better tissue penetration.

Answer: E

Biffl WL, Kaups KL, Cothren CC, *et al.* (2009) Management of patients with anterior abdominal stab wounds: A Western Trauma Association Multicenter trial. *Journal of Trauma* **66** (5), 1294–301.

Murphy JT, Hall J, Provost D (2005) Fascial ultrasound for evaluation of anterior abdominal stab wound injury. *Journal of Trauma* **59** (4), 843–6.

Soffer D, McKenney MG, Cohn S, *et al.* (2004) A prospective evaluation of ultrasonography for the diagnosis of penetrating torso injury. *Journal of Trauma* **56** (5), 953–9.

3. *The E-FAST (or Extended FAST) exam has been used in trauma patients to make the diagnosis of all of the following conditions except*

A. *Hemothorax*

B. *Pneumothorax*

C. *Sternal fracture*

D. *Papillary muscle rupture*

E. *Diaphragm injury*

The extended fast exam or E-FAST has been proposed as a useful technique for evaluating thoracic trauma and specific abnormalities that may associated with this. Pneumothorax can be detected by the absence of lung sliding and the absence of comet tail artifacts, and hemothorax can be detected as fluid in the costophrenic angle. Sternal fracture is another diagnosis that can be made using ultrasound, and some reports suggest that ultrasound is more sensitive and specific for this injury than plain radiology. Although the FAST exam does include a pericardial component the detail that is usually evaluated during this examination is not of the quality required to diagnose a papillary muscle rupture. This would usually require more sophisticated machinery and more time, as well as positioning the patient in the left lateral position, something that is usually not possible in the trauma patient. Diaphragmatic rupture, although rare, can sometimes be picked up using thoracic ultrasound in the hands of a skilled and experienced operator, when there is a gross injury with organs migrating from the abdomen into the chest.

Answer: D

Kirkpatrick AW, Sirois M, Laupland KB, *et al.* (2004) Hand-held thoracic sonography for detecting post-traumatic pneumothoraces: the Extended Focused Assessment with Sonography for Trauma (EFAST). *Journal of Trauma* **57** (2), 288–95.

Kirkpatrick AW, Ball CG, Nicolaou S, *et al.* (2006) Ultrasound detection of right-sided diaphragmatic injury; the "liver sliding" sign. *American Journal of Emergency Medicine* **24** (2), 251–2.

You JS, Chung YE, Kim D, *et al.* (2010) Role of sonography in the emergency room to diagnose sternal fractures. *Journal of Clinical Ultrasound* **38** (3), 135–7.

4. *Regarding the use of ultrasound for central venous catheter (CVC) placement, which of the following is false?*

A. *Duplex ultrasound is necessary to be able to tell the difference between arteries and veins.*

B. *Ultrasound identification of the vessel, followed by CVC placement, is more effective than landmark placement alone.*

C. *There is an operator learning curve with the dynamic or "real-time" ultrasound technique for CVC placement.*

D. For internal jugular CVCs, ultrasound increases the "first-stick" success rate.

E. Ultrasound has no role to play in the placement of subclavian CVCs.

Duplex ultrasound combines both pulse echo imaging and Doppler waves, which improves the resolution of vessel images and enables accurate measures of velocity. It is these features that help distinguish the blood flow in arteries as opposed to veins, as this depends on the frequency of the ultrasound as well as the velocity of the blood flow. It is also important to remember that this is dependent on the angle of insonation, and this can be a cause of confusion if the probe was held incorrectly. Ultrasound used in a static technique, that is to say the ultrasound is used solely to map the vessels and then the ultrasound is longer being used when the vein is accessed in a sterile fashion, is not associated with increased success rates compared to the standard landmark technique. However, the disadvantage of the dynamic or real-time technique is that there is a significant operator learning curve, related to using the ultrasound and the needle for access at the same time. It has been shown in multiple studies, particularly for the internal jugular route, that ultrasound can increase the "first-stick" success rate as well as the overall success rate. Although ultrasound has a limited role to play in the placement of subclavian central lines in patients with the appropriate anatomy of sound may still prove useful in imaging the subclavian artery and vein.

Answer: B

Denys BG, Uretsky BF, and Reddy S (1993) Ultrasound-assisted cannulation of the internal jugular vein. A prospective comparison to the external landmark-guided technique. *Circulation* **87**, 1557–62.

Hind D, Calvert N, McWilliams R, *et al.* (2003) Ultrasonic locating devices for central venous cannulation: meta-analysis. *British Medical Journal* **327**, 361–4.

Karakitsos D, Labropoulos N, DeGroot E, *et al.* (2006) Real-time ultrasound-guided catheterization of the internal jugular vein: a prospective comparison with the landmark technique in critical care patients. *Critical Care* **10** (6), R162.

Mansfield PF, Hohn DC, Fornage BD, *et al.* (1994) Complications and failures of subclavian-vein catheterization. *New England Journal of Medicine* **331**, 1735–8.

5. *Surgeon performed cardiac ultrasound in the ICU can be shown to accurately assess all of the following except*

A. Filling status

B. Cardiac output

C. Pericardial effusion

D. Presence of pulmonary hypertension

E. Right ventricular function

There has been increasing interest in echocardiography performed by surgeons and/or intensivists at the bedside in recent years, partly due to the increasingly sophisticated ultrasound machinery that is now available, which is also much more portable. At least two reports have shown that subjective measurements can be taken of global cardiac function as well as accurate assessments of the filling status of the IVC and the heart. Cardiac output can be measured by a number of techniques, but these are limited by the need to obtain adequate images during the examination, which is not always possible in the trauma patient, particularly those with subcutaneous emphysema or other chest trauma. The presence of absence of pericardial effusions has long been part of the FAST exam, and can be easily extended into the ICU. Pulmonary hypertension usually requires more sophisticated machinery and time and is usually not part of the intensivist-performed focused echocardiographic exam. A subjective measure of ventricular function (either right or left) can be made using various different echocardiographic views.

Answer: D

Ferrada P, Murthi S, Anand RJ, *et al.* (2011) Transthoracic focused rapid echocardiographic examination: real-time evaluation of fluid status in critically ill trauma patients. *Journal of Trauma* **70** (1), 56–62; discussion pp. 62–4.

Gunst M, Sperry J, Ghaemmaghami V, *et al.* (2008) Bedside echocardiographic assessment for trauma/critical care: the BEAT exam. *Journal of the American College of Surgeons* **207** (3), e1-3. Epub 2008 July 21.

6. *In which of the following patients, can a pelvic x-ray be safely omitted?*

A. 23-year-old man following a motorcycle crash at high speed, hemodynamically stable but complaining of pain in the left hip

B. 78-year-old woman following a ground level fall

C. 47-year-old man who was ambulatory after a rear-end collision at 45 mph

D. 32-year-old woman, with a BP of 90/60 mm Hg and severe pain over the sacrum

E. 16-year-old boy following a bicycle crash, with blood at the urinary meatus

Pelvic x-rays are notoriously inaccurate for the diagnosis of pelvic fractures, with a false negative rate somewhere between 20 to 30%. However there are a certain group of patients in which they provide useful information as a screening tool, particularly if those patients are not undergoing abdominal and/or pelvic CT scanning. The patient in response A is at risk of either a femur fracture or pubic rami fractures and should therefore be imaged, as should the patient in response B, due to the increased fracture risk in the elderly because of osteoporosis. A patient with significant mechanism for pelvic trauma that is hemodynamically unstable should have a pelvic x-ray performed to help assess whether the patient should go directly to the angiography suite for embolization. Any signs or symptoms of possible urethral trauma mandate a pelvic x-ray as part of the workup prior to placement of Foley catheter as a retrograde urethrogram may be necessary. The 47-year-old man described in response C, who was ambulatory at the scene, is unlikely to have a clinically significant pelvic fracture and as long as a clinical exam is reliable info the x-ray could safely be emitted with a low risk for missed injury. More and more, pelvic x-rays are being omitted in hemodynamically stable patients who are having abdomen and pelvis CT scans as part of their work-up.

Answer: C

Guillamondegui OD, Pryor JP, Gracias VH, *et al.* (2002) Pelvic radiography in blunt trauma resuscitation: a diminishing role. *Journal of Trauma* **53** (6), 1043–7.

Kessel B, Sevi R, Jeroukhimov I, *et al.* (2007) Is routine portable pelvic X-ray in stable multiple trauma patients always justified in a high technology era? *Injury* **38** (5), 559–63.

Obaid AK, Barleben A, Porral D, *et al.* (2006) Utility of plain film pelvic radiographs in blunt trauma patients in the emergency department. *American Surgery* **72** (10) 951–4.

7. *Regarding the need for pelvic angiography in a patient with a significant pelvic fracture, which of the following is true?*

A. The fracture pattern has little bearing on the need for angioembolization

B. In patients without a blush on initial CT scan, the diagnostic yield is so low that pelvic angiography is not indicated

C. Angioembolization must be combined with fixation of the pelvis to be successful, due to the presence of venous bleeding

D. Indications for pelvic angiography are hemodynamic instability, with a significant pelvic fracture, and no identifiable thoracoabdominal source of hemorrhage

E. The presence of a pelvic hematoma in a patient with pelvic fracture mandates angiography

Although the advent of pelvic angiography for the treatment of hemorrhage due to pelvic trauma has been life saving for many patients, the exact indications remain somewhat controversial. Prior studies have shown that the type of fracture, particularly those involving ligamentous disruption of the sacroiliac joint, have an increased risk of bleeding and will more likely require angioembolization. The absence of a contrast blush on CT scanning does not reliably predict absence of active arterial hemorrhage and should not be taken as evidence that angiography will not be required. Likewise, neither the presence nor absence of a pelvic hematoma, nor the size of the pelvic hematoma will reliably exclude the presence of active arterial hemorrhage and should not guide the decision for angiography. Embolization by itself can be definitive treatment without immobilization of the fracture other than bed rest, although placement of an external fixation device or pelvic binder is usually recommended. At this time, the generally accepted indications for pelvic angiography are hemodynamically unstable patients with a significant pelvic fracture, and no thoracic, abdominal or other sources of hemorrhage.

Answer: D

Brown CV, Kasotakis G, Wilcox A, *et al.* (2005) Does pelvic hematoma on admission computed tomography predict active bleeding at angiography for pelvic fracture? *American Journal of Surgery* **71** (9), 759–62.

Hamill J, Holden A, Paice R, Civil I (2000) Pelvic fracture pattern predicts pelvic arterial haemorrhage. *Australian and New Zealand Journal of Surgery* **70** (5), 338–43.

Tanizaki S, Maeda S, Hayashi H, *et al.* (2011) Early embolization without external fixation in pelvic trauma. *American Journal of Emergency Medicine* January 27. Epub ahead of print.

8. *Which of the following is not a possible complication of pelvic angiography:*

A. *Gluteal muscle necrosis*

B. *Impotence*

C. *Poor fracture healing*

D. *Groin hematoma*

E. *Recurrent hemorrhage*

Gluteal muscle necrosis and/or buttock skin sloughing are the most feared complications following pelvic angioembolization. However, the incidence is usually extremely low in most patient groups. Although controversial, bilateral internal iliac artery embolization has been associated with an increased risk of erectile dysfunction due to compromise of the blood supply. To date, there has been no suggestion that embolization of vessels for hemorrhage and severe pelvic trauma has a significant impact on the healing of the fracture site. Groin hematoma of course is a complication of any angiographic procedure, caused by hemorrhage from the arterial puncture site. Thrombosis is also a risk associated with this procedure. There is also a significant rate of recurrent hemorrhage in patients with the most severe pelvic fractures, and this should be taken into account at the time of the original procedure, and it necessary an arterial sheath may be left in place for ease of access for repeat angiography if this becomes necessary.

Answer: C

Travis T, Monsky WL, London J, *et al.* (2008) Evaluation of short-term and long-term complications after emergent internal iliac artery embolization in patients with pelvic trauma. *Journal of Vascular and Interventional Radiology* **19** (6), 840–7.

Yasumura K, Ikegami K, Kamohara T, Nohara Y (2005) High incidence of ischemic necrosis of the gluteal muscle after transcatheter angiographic embolization for severe pelvic fracture. *Journal of Trauma* 58 (5), 985–90.

9. *Which of the following statements is correct regarding the use of visceral angiography?*

A. *Angioembolization has been demonstrated to be safe in adults but should be used with caution in the pediatric population*

B. *In patients with severe liver injuries that are unresponsive to perihepatic packing, angioembolization is unlikely to be successful*

C. *Liver embolization is associated with a high rate of formation of hepatic abscess*

D. *The use of embolization for splenic trauma has achieved reported rates of non-operative management of greater than 90%*

E. *Gelfoam is the preferred embolization technique in superselective embolization of vessels*

Angiography with subsequent embolization has been shown to be safe in both the adult and pediatric population, and the age of the patient should not be consideration when deciding whether a patient is a candidate for the procedure. Angiography is a very useful adjunct to the treatment of severe liver trauma, if perihepatic packing has not been successful. However, it will only work in a setting where any concomitant coagulopathy has been corrected. Although hepatic abscess can form following embolization, this may be related to the liver trauma itself, and not a consequence of the embolization. However, this is more likely if a large branch of the hepatic artery is embolized. Rates of success for no operative management of the spleen have been reported to be over 95% using these techniques. Gelfoam, microcoils, and other small particles used as occlusion devices all form part of the armamentarium of the angiographer. However, in the case of super selective embolization, which is usually permanent, microcoils rather than Gelfoam are preferred.

Answer: D

Kiankhooy A, Sartorelli KH, Vane DW, Bhave AD (2010) Angiographic embolization is safe and effective therapy for blunt abdominal solid organ injury in children. *Journal of Trauma* **68** (3), 526–31.

Wallis A, Kelly MD, Jones L (2010) Angiography and embolisation for solid abdominal organ injury in adults—a current perspective. *World Journal of Emergency Surgery* **5**, 18.

10. *Which of the following is true regarding the use of CT scanning in the workup of a patient with blunt abdominal trauma?*

A. The use of oral contrast will significantly improve the diagnostic yield and should be considered in most trauma patients

B. Sensitivity of CT scans for abdominal injuries is only around 80%

C. CT is a sufficient modality alone for the evaluation of blunt abdominal trauma in all patients

D. Intravenous contrast for an abdominal CT scan should not be given until the patient's blood tests confirm the absence of renal problems

E. Diaphragm injuries cannot be accurately excluded by CT scanning

Although oral contrast may help opacify the bowel, and can be particularly useful in identifying injuries of the pancreatoduodenal complex, it will increase the amount of time taken to perform the scan, and expose the patient to increased risk of aspiration of the material. Neither of these is desirable in the trauma patient, and as most studies show a sensitivity of over 90% for abdominal injuries in emergency CT scans performed in this patient population, it is usually omitted in most trauma centers. CT scanning is not felt to be adequate to rule out the diagnosis of blunt bowel or mesenteric injuries, and in patients with a high suspicion for these injuries, DPL is felt to be a more sensitive test. The consequences of a missed hollow viscous injury can be extremely serious, so it is important that this is ruled out. The risk of inducing a contrast nephropathy is low in the vast majority of trauma patients, and the risk of delayed diagnosis of serious injuries usually outweighs the risk of renal complications. Although certain authors have suggested that diaphragmatic injuries can be picked up on multidetector CT scans, most authorities recommend a policy of diagnostic laparoscopy to definitely rule out injuries to this structure, particularly when it is on the left side.

Answer: E

Friese RS, Coln CE, Gentilello LM (2005) Laparoscopy is sufficient to exclude occult diaphragm injury after penetrating abdominal trauma. *Journal of Trauma* **58** (4), 789–92.

Hoff WS, Holevar M, Nagy KK, *et al.* (2002) Eastern Association for the Surgery of Trauma. Practice management guidelines for the evaluation of blunt abdominal trauma: the East practice management guidelines work group. *Journal of Trauma* **53** (3), 602–15.

Matsushima K, Peng M, Schaefer EW, *et al.* (2011) Posttraumatic contrast-induced acute kidney injury: minimal consequences or significant threat? *J Trauma* **70** (2), 415–19.

Stein DM, York GB, Boswell S, *et al.* (2007) Accuracy of computed tomography (CT) scan in the detection of penetrating diaphragm injury. *Journal of Trauma* **63** (3), 538–43.

11. *In patients with penetrating trauma to zone II of the neck, which of the following would be true regarding the use of CT angiography (CTA) for diagnostic evaluation?*

A. Use of CTA does not reduce the negative operation exploration rate

B. *Violation of the platysma is still an indication for mandatory operation*

C. *CTA can supplant the need for angiography, bronchoscopy and/or endoscopy in patients with penetrating neck trauma*

D. *CT scanning should only be performed in hemodynamically stable patients with no hard signs of injury*

E. *Diagnosis of an injury by CTA always requires an operative intervention*

The use of CT angiography as an initial screening modality in penetrating neck trauma has exploded in recent years, particularly with the advent of multidetector CT scanners. More than one study has shown that the negative exploration rate can be reduced by suing this modality as an initial screening tool for the presence of injury. In fact, some authors have even suggested that violation of the platsyma can no longer be regarded as a mandatory indication for exploration, as significant injuries can be effectively ruled out by CT angiography of the neck. Quoted reports give a CT scanning greater than 90% sensitivity for injuries, even including the aerodigestive tract. However, in select cases CT scanning may indicate the presence of lesions that require further identification by endoscopy, formal angiography or bronchoscopy and it cannot be used to completely eliminate these diagnostic tools. CT angiography of the neck is not appropriate in patients who are hemodynamically unstable, or have a hard sign of neck injury e.g. bubbling, expanding hematoma, hoarseness, stroke; these patients should be taken directly to the OR for operative exploration. Finally, not all injuries seen on CTA will require an intervention. Non-operative management of internal jugular vein injuries for example has been safely performed in patients who were otherwise stable.

Answer: D

Inaba K, Munera F, McKenney M, *et al.* (2006) Prospective evaluation of screening multislice helical computed tomographic angiography in the initial evaluation of penetrating neck injuries. *Journal of Trauma* **61** (1), 144–9.

Osborn TM, Bell RB, Qaisi W, *et al.* (2008) Computed tomographic angiography as an aid to clinical decision making in the selective management of penetrating injuries to the neck: a reduction in the need for operative exploration. *Journal of Trauma* **64** (6), 1466–71.

Brywczynski JJ, Barrett TW, Lyon JA, Cotton BA (2008) Management of penetrating neck injury in the emergency department: a structured literature review. *Emergency Medicine Journal* **25** (11), 711–15.

Inaba K, Munera F, McKenney MG, *et al.* (2006) The nonoperative management of penetrating internal jugular vein injury. *Journal of Vascular Surgery* **43** (1), 77–80.

12. *Which of the following is true regarding the use of CT arteriography in penetrating peripheral vascular trauma?*

A. *Sensitivity for the presence of an arterial injury is less than 75%*

B. *Use of 64-slice multidetector CT scanning allows for the integration of extremity CT angiography into routine thoracoabdominal trauma imaging protocols*

C. *If artifact exists due to bullets or bullet fragments, it will render the study unevaluable*

D. *Poor timing of contrast material bolus is rarely an issue in CTA*

E. *Approximately 15% of extremity CTA studies are non-diagnostic and will require further evaluation by formal angiography*

Most reports evaluating CT angiography in vascular trauma quote sensitivity and specificity of greater than 90% and it has become the first line investigation in many trauma centers for suspected arterial injury. If correctly performed, extremity angiography can be performed using the same contrast bolus that is given for the evaluation of the chest and abdomen that is routinely performed for trauma. Most studies only report a 1–2% nondiagnostic exam rate, most usually due to streak artifact from metallic foreign bodies, although the presence of foreign bodies by no means is a guarantee that the study will be unreadable. In the study by Inaba *et al.*, 19% of studies had streak artifact but only 1 study was nondiagnostic (1.9%). Good diagnostic quality CT angiographic extremity examinations require careful patient preparation, to give images that will provide the necessary information. The extremity to be studied should be immobilized and careful attention to IV contrast bolus timing is necessary to make sure that the arteries are sufficiently opacified or that the CT table does not "overrun" the exam. This has been one of the barriers to the wider implementation of this technology as well as the significant post-processing power that is required to analyze the images.

Answer: B

Inaba K, Potzman J, Munera F, *et al.* (2006) Multi-slice CT angiography for arterial evaluation in the injured lower extremity. *Journal of Trauma* **60**, 502–7.

Peng PD, Spain DA, Tataria M, *et al.* (2008) CT angiography effectively evaluates extremity vascular trauma. *American Journal of Surgery* **74** (2), 103–7.

Pieroni S, Foster BR, Anderson SW, *et al.* (2009) Use of 64-row multidetector CT angiography in blunt and penetrating trauma of the upper and lower extremities. *Radiographics* **29** (3), 863–76.

PART TWO
Emergency Surgery

Chapter 26 Neurotrauma

Bellal Joseph, MD

1. *A 40-year-old man presents two weeks after being discharged from the hospital after an all-terrain-vehicle (ATV) accident in which he suffered a frontal bone fracture and mild traumatic brain injury. He now complains of a "whooshing" sound in his left ear, diplopia, left-eye proptosis, headaches, and fevers. Physical exam revealed conjunctival injection and pulsatile exopthalmos. A computed tomography (CT) scan of the brain showed a known displaced frontal bone fracture. The angiogram is depicted below.*

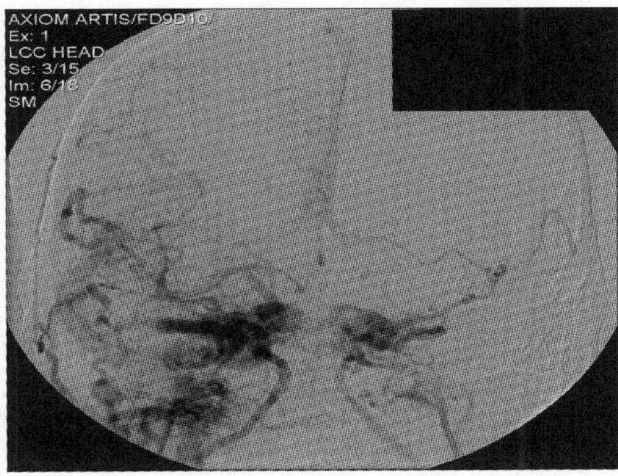

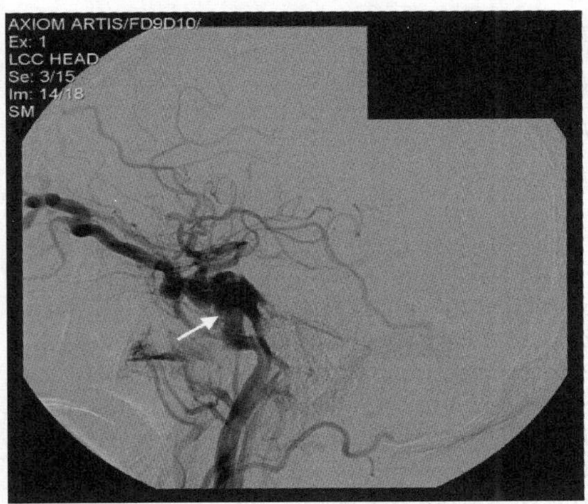

What is the most likely diagnosis?

A. *Cavernous sinus thrombosis*

B. *Occlusion of the internal carotid artery proximal to the ophthalmic artery origin*

C. *Carotid cavernous fistula*

D. *Retrobulbar hematoma*

E. *Unrecognized intraorbital foreign body, with possible cellulitis*

2. *What should be the initial treatment of choice for the patient?*

A. *Anticoagulation*

B. *Two weeks of antibiotics followed by repeat angiography*

C. *Carotid artery ligation*

D. *Transarterial detachable balloon embolization*

E. *Glue embolization of major arterial feeders followed by resection*

Carotid-cavernous fistula (CCF) is an abnormal communication between the carotid artery and the venous plexus of the cavernous sinus. They are divided into two types: spontaneous and post-traumatic or low flow and high flow. Post-traumatic CCFs result from direct flow between the intracavernous carotid artery and the cavernous sinus with high flow and pressure. The most common cause is severe blunt trauma but it can result from penetrating cranial injuries as well. Signs and symptoms usually appear a few weeks after the injury and result from increased venous pressure transmitted through the valveless

Surgical Critical Care and Emergency Surgery: Clinical Questions and Answers, First Edition. Edited by Forrest O. Moore, Peter M. Rhee, Samuel A. Tisherman and Gerard J. Fulda.

ophthalmic veins. Symptoms and signs include headache, orbital bruit, pulsating exopthalmus, chemosis, diplopia, proptosis, dilation of retinal veins, optic disc swelling, and vision loss. Although CT or MRI may reveal enlarged extraocular muscles, dilated ophthalmic veins, and enlarged affected cavernous sinus, the gold standard is cerebral angiography, which reveals direct opacification of an enlarged cavernous sinus, early filling of ophthalmic veins and diminished opacification of the distal arterial system.

The main treatment goal is to occlude the fistula without compromising carotid patency. The treatments of choice are endovascular procedures, which are associated with low morbidity and mortality. Endovascular occlusion using detachable balloons has a success rate of 90–100% with low complication rates (2 to 5%). The overall recurrence rate is 1–3.9%, and recurrence often responds to second embolization.

Answers 1: C, 2: D

Fabian TS, Woody JD, Ciraulo DL, *et al.* (1999) Post-traumatic carotid cavernous fistula: frequency analysis of signs, symptoms, and disability outcomes after angiographic embolization. *Journal of Trauma* **47** (2), 275–81.

Greenberg, M (2005) *Handbook of Neurosurgery*, 5th edn, Thieme Medical Publishers, New York, pp. 811–12.

3. *Basilar skull fractures are associated with ecchymosis of the mastoid process, periorbital ecchymosis, cranial nerve palsy, hemotympanum, and rhinorrhea. The presence of cerebral spinal fluid (CSF) rhinorrhea can be confirmed by which of the following assays?*

A. Hypoglycorrhachia

B. β_2-transferrin

C. α-fetoprotein

D. Sodium level

E. WBC count

Beta-2 transferrin is a protein found only in CSF and perilymph. It was first described in 1979 for its use in the detection of CSF leakage. With a sensitivity of 94%- 100%, and specificity of 98%-100%, this assay has become the gold standard in detection of CSF leakage. The only other source is the vitreous humor of the eye. Other commonly employed tests include measuring the glucose level of the fluid (CSF glucose >30 mg%, whereas lacrimal and mucous secretions are <5 mg%) or placing the fluid on a piece of linen and seeing whether a ring of blood surrounded by a larger concentric ring of clear fluid develops ("halo" sign).

Answer: B

Greenberg, M (2005) *Handbook of Neurosurgery*, 5th edn, Thieme Medical Publishers, New York, pp. 168–9.

Haft G, Mendoza SA, Weinstein SL, *et al.* (2004) Use of beta-2-transferrin to diagnose CSF leakage following spinal surgery. *Iowa Orthopedic Journal* **24**, 115–18.

4. *A 20-year-old man presents to the trauma bay after a motor vehicle accident. He has spontaneous eye opening, is confused and localizes only to pain. His Glasgow Coma Score is*

A. 5

B. 7

C. 9

D. 13

E. 15

The Glasgow Coma Scale (GCS) should be determined for all injured patients (see Table 26.1). It is calculated by adding the scores of the best motor response, best verbal response, and eye opening. Scores range from 3 (the lowest) to 15 (normal). Scores of 13 to 15 indicate mild head injury, 9 to 12 moderate injury and less than 9 sever injury. The GCS is useful for both triage and prognosis. The GCS score has been shown to have a significant correlation with outcome following severe TBI, both as the sum score or as just the motor component.

Table 26.1 Glasgow Coma Scale.

	1	2	3	4	5	6
Eyes	Does not open eyes	Opens eyes to painful stimuli	Opens eyes to response to voice	Opens eyes spontaneously	N/A	N/A
Verbal	Makes no sounds	Incomprehensible sounds	Inappropriate words	Confused, disoriented	Oriented, converses normally	N/A
Motor	Makes no movements	Extension to painful stimuli (decerebrate response)	Abnormal flexion to painful stimuli (decorticate response)	Flexion/ Withdrawal to painful stimuli	Localizes painful stimuli	Obeys commmands

Answer D

Brain Trauma Foundation (2000) *Early Indicators of Prognosis in Traumatic Brain Injury,* Brain Trauma Foundation, New York, NY, p. 163.

Brunicardi, FC (2010) *Schwartz's Principles of Surgery,* 9th edn, McGraw-Hill, New York, pp. 145–1524.

Teasdale G, Jennett B (1974) Assessment of coma and impaired consciousness. A practical scale. *Lancet* **2**, 81–4.

5. *30-year-old man experienced a high-speed motorcycle collision and experienced transient right upper extremity sensory changes. A computed tomography (CT) scan of the head was negative; however, the CT scan of the cervical spine revealed a fracture into the foramen transversarium of the fifth cervical vertebrae. CT angiography of the cervical spine revealed a pseudoaneurysm of the vertebral artery. No other injuries were identified. What would be the most appropriate next step in the management of this patient?*

A. *Antiplatelet agents*

B. *Anticoagulation*

C. *Endovascular treatment*

D. *Surgical intervention*

E. *Repeat angiography*

Blunt vertebral artery injury is associated with complex cervical spine fractures involving subluxation, extension into the foramen transversarium, or upper C1 to C3 fractures. Routine screening should incorporate these findings to maximize yield while limiting the use of invasive procedures. The most appropriate initial treatment of this injury is systemic anticoagulation initially with heparin and subsequent conversion to warfarin. Endovascular treatment is an option when the lesion does not resolve with systemic anticoagulation, however it should not be the initial treatment choice. Acute pseudoaneurysms are unstable lesions and the wall of these structures are weak, making the stent deployment more dangerous in the acute setting. Repeat angiography should be performed. Antiplatelet agents should be reserved for patients who have undergone endovascular stent placement or those in whom systemic anticoagulation is contraindicated.

Answer: B

Cothren CC, Moore EE, Biffl WL, *et al.* (2003) Cervical spine fracture patterns predictive of blunt vertebral artery injury. *Journal of Trauma* **55** (5), pp. 811–13.

Feliciano D, Mattox K, Moore E (2005) *Trauma,* 6th edn,, McGraw-Hill, New York, pp. 467–7.

6. *A 18-year-old boy falls 20 feet from a building and arrives at the trauma bay with a Glasgow Coma Scale (GCS) score of 5, a dilated and non reactive left pupil and a blood pressure of 90/45 mm Hg. After definitive airway management and fluid resuscitation, the patient is also found to have an unstable pelvic fracture and a* *femur fracture. His GCS improves to 8 however his left pupil remains nonreactive. The initial management of this patient is:*

A. *Administer pentobarbital*

B. *Administer mannitol immediately*

C. *Complete the primary survey and, if the patient is stable, obtain a computed tomography (CT) scan and begin hyperventilation*

D. *Complete the primary survey and insert an intracranial monitor and obtain a CT scan*

E. *Take the patient directly to the operating room with no further workup*

Current guidelines of severe traumatic brain injury suggest that mannitol and hyperventilation may exacerbate cerebral ischemia after head injury. However mannitol and hyperventilation are recommended for those patients with acute head injury as a temporary measure to control elevated intracranial pressure. Hyperventilation may be commenced immediately, but mannitol should be withheld until the primary survey is complete and adequate intravascular volume and urine outputs are achieved. The mechanism of action of mannitol is still debated however there are some beneficial effects. First it acts to immediately expand the plasma by reducing hematocrit and blood viscosity (improved rheology). The improved rheology improves cerebral blood flow and O_2 delivery, reducing intracranial pressure quickly. Second, it draws edema from adjacent cerebral parenchyma into the intravascular compartment. Finally, it may act as a free radical scavenger.

Answer: C

Brain Trauma Foundation (2007) *Guidelines for the Management of Severe Traumatic Brain Injury*, 3rd edn, Brain Trauma Foundation, New York, NY, S-14 and S-87.

Feliciano D, Mattox K, Moore E (2005) *Trauma*, 6th edn, McGraw-Hill, New York, NY, pp. 467–7.

7. *Which of the following statements regarding intracranial pressure (ICP) monitoring is true?*

A. *Intraparechymal monitor measurements have better accuracy than ventricular catheters*

B. *ICP monitoring is appropriate in all patients with an abnormal head CT scan and GCS < 12*

C. *ICP monitors carry a 1% risk of hemorrhage and 5% infection risk*

D. *ICP monitoring is indicated in all patients with a GCS 3–8 and a normal CT scan of the head*

E. *Risk factors for elevated intracranial pressure after traumatic brain injury are an age over 40 and systolic blood pressure greater than 90 mm Hg*

Intracranial pressure (ICP) should be monitored in all salvageable patients with a severe traumatic brain injury (TBI; GCS score of 3–8 after resuscitation) and an abnormal CT scan. An abnormal CT scan of the head is one that reveals hematomas, contusions, swelling, herniation, or compressed basal cisterns. ICP monitoring is indicated in patients with severe TBI with a normal CT scan if two or more of the following features are noted at admission: age over 40 years, unilateral or bilateral motor posturing, or systolic blood pressure (BP) < 90 mm Hg. Ventricular catheter ICP measurements are accurate but carry a higher risk of complications than do intraparenchymal monitors. There is a 1% risk of hemorrhage and 5% infection risk with ICP monitoring.

Answer: C

Brain Trauma Foundation (2007) *Guidelines for the Management of Severe Traumatic Brain Injury*, 3rd edn, Brain Trauma Foundation, New York, NY, S-14 and S-87.

Brunicardi, FC (2010) *Schwartz's Principles of Surgery*, 9th edn, McGraw-Hill, New York, pp. 145 and 1524.

8. *A 24-year-old woman was the front seat passenger in a rollover motor vehicle collision. On primary survey the patient was unable to move here lower extremities and had abduction and pronation of the upper extremities. Work up revealed complete transection of the spinal cord at the C7 level. This injury produces all of the following effects except:*

A. *Limited respiratory effort*

B. *Areflexia below the level of the lesion*

C. *Flaccidity below the level of the lesion*

D. Hypotension

E. C6 level root irritation

9. *The use of high-dose steroids after spinal cord injury*

A. Is not routinely recommended

B. Has little risk

C. Is indicated in all patients excluding those who are pregnant or <14 years of age

D. Is indicated in all patients

E. May have improved outcome if steroids are given within 24 h of injury

Injuries to the spinal cord, particularly complete injuries, remain essentially untreatable. The phrenic nerves, which are the motor nerves to the diaphragm, arise from the third, fourth, and fifth cervical roots; therefore, diaphragmatic respiration would not be disturbed by a cord transaction at C7. Anesthesia, areflexia, and flaccidity below this level would be anticipated. Hypotension results from any transaction above T5 because of the loss of sympathetic vascular tone.

A prospective randomized study comparing methlprednisolone with placebo demonstrated a significant improvement in outcome (usually one or two spinal levels) for those who received corticosteroids within 8 h of injury. The National Acute Spinal Cord Injury Study (NASCIS) I and II papers provided basis for the common practice of administering high-dose steroids to patients with acute spinal cord injury. The papers indicate greater motor and sensory recovery at 6 weeks, 6 months, and 1 year after acute spinal cord injury in patients who received steroids. However, the NASCIS trial data have been extensively criticized, as many argue that the selection criteria and study design were flawed, making the results ambiguous. Significant risks of high dose steroids, particularly infectious complications, have been identified. Currently consensus recommendations do not endorse the administration of steroids. Of note, patients with gunshot injuries, or cauda equine injury, as well as those on chronic steroid therapy, who were pregnant, or who were less than 14 years of age were excluded from the trials.

Answers: 8: A, 9: A

Bracken MB, Shepard MJ, Collins WF, *et al.* (1990) A randomized controlled trial of methylprednisolone or naloxone in the treatment of acute spinal cord injury. *New England Journal of Medicine* **322**, 1405.

Brunicardi, FC (2010) *Schwartz's Principles of Surgery*, 9th edn, McGraw-Hill, New York, p. 1530.

10. *A 22-year-old man has a motor vehicle accident and presents with a Glasgow Coma Scale (GCS) of 6. After primary survey and initial resuscitation the patient is found to have a left-side subarachnoid hemorrhage. Appropriate initial treatment of a patient with a severe traumatic brain injury (GCS < 8) injury includes?*

A. Lasix to decrease cerebral swelling

B. Placement of ventriculostomy

C. Hyperventilation to a PCO_2 <30 mm Hg

D. Repeat CT scan within one hour

E. Barbiturate coma

11. *The lowest acceptable cerebral perfusion pressure in a patient with traumatic brain injury is*

A. 110 mm Hg

B. 100 mm Hg

C. 80 mm Hg

D. 60 mm Hg

E. 40 mm Hg

12. *Therapy for increased intracranial pressure (ICP) in a patient with a traumatic brain injury is instituted when the ICP is greater than*

A. 10 mm Hg

B. 20 mm Hg

C. 30 mm Hg

D. 40 mm Hg

E. 50 mm Hg

Attention in the management of severe traumatic brain injuries is now focused on maintaining or enhancing cerebral perfusion rather than merely lowering intracranial pressure (ICP). It has been found that hyperventilation to a $PCO_2 < 30$ mm Hg to induce cerebral vasoconstriction actually exacerbates cerebral ischemia in spite of decreasing ICP. These secondary iatrogenic cerebral injuries cause more harm than previously appreciated. Treatment must avoid the effects of decreased cardiac output due to the excessive use of osmotic diuretics, sedatives, or barbiturates, and hypoxia. Nevertheless, the measurement of ICP is important and is efficiently accomplished with a ventriculostomy catheter. The catheter also allows withdrawal of cerebral spinal fluid, which is the safest method for lowering ICP.

Although an ICP of 10 mm Hg is believed to be the upper limit of normal, therapy is not usually initiated until the ICP reaches 20 mm Hg. Cerebral perfusion pressure (CPP) is an important measurement for assuring adequate cerebral perfusion. CPP is equal to the mean arterial pressure (MAP) minus the ICP; 60 mm Hg is the lowest acceptable pressure. CPP can be altered by either lowering ICP or raising MAP. The goal of fluid therapy is to achieve a euvolemic state. Arbitrary fluid restriction is not indicated as it may increase likelihood for hypotension. Whether boosting MAP with pressors or intropes in patients with an elevated ICP resistant to treatment improves outcome is unclear, although recent data suggest it does. Moderate hypothermia may also be helpful by decreasing metabolic requirements.

Answers: 10: B, 11: D, 12: B

Brain Trauma Foundation (2007) *Guidelines for the Management of Severe Traumatic Brain Injury*, 3rd edn, Brain Trauma Foundation, New York, NY, S-14 and S-87. pp. S-55–59.

Brunicardi, FC (2010) *Schwartz's Principles of Surgery*, 9th edn, McGraw-Hill, New York, pp. 145 and 1524.

13. *A 75-year-old woman is brought to the trauma unit after a motor vehicle crash. She presents with a Glasgow Coma Score of 14. She is alert but confused. After initial evaluation she is found to have an intact airway, and her vital signs and breathing are normal. While a chest and pelvic x-ray are being obtained she is noted to become much more lethargic and is responsive only to pain. Which of the following findings is most likely the cause for her condition?*

A. *Diffuse axonal injury*

B. *Cerebral contusion*

C. *Subdural hematoma*

D. *Epidural hematoma*

E. *Subarachnoid hemorrhage*

Epidural hematoma often presents with a lucid interval followed by sudden neurologic deterioration. After intubation, immediate CT scanning of the head is indicated to identify the site of the lesion and assess the degree of mass effect. If focal signs are present, suggesting a mass effect, empiric therapy with hyperventilation and osmolar therapy (mannitol or hypertonic saline) may be indicated. Acute epidural hematoma is associated with arterial bleeding from the middle meningeal artery. Operative evacuation of the lesion is indicated if significant mass effect is noted, if there is a midline shift of more than 5 mm, or if there is neurologic deterioration.

Answer: D

Greenberg, M (2005) *Handbook of Neurosurgery*, 5th edn, Thieme Medical Publishers, New York, pp. 811–12.

Moore AJ (2005) *Neurosurgery Principles and Practice*, 1st edn, Springer, London, p. 369.

14. *Which of the following statements regarding subdural hematoma is correct?*

A. *Is the least common traumatic extra-axial mass lesion of the brain, occurring in approximately 20–40% of severe injuries*

B. *Is generally a diagnosis of exclusion*

C. *Most commonly occur in the subfrontal and anterior temporal regions of the brain*

D. *Is usually due to shearing of venous sinuses and occurs between the dura and arachnoid layers*

E. *May present with a lucid interval similar to an epidural hematoma*

Subdural hematoma is the commonest traumatic mass lesion of the head, occurring in approximately

20–40 % of severe head injuries. This lesion is usually due to shearing of venous sinuses and occurs between the dura and arachnoid layers. Operative evacuation is necessary if mass effect is present. Intracerebral hematomas most commonly occur in the subfrontal and anterior temporal regions of the brain. Diffuse axonal injury is generally a diagnosis of exclusion. Patients with severe head injury whose CT scan does not reveal significant lesions or those who remain in vegetative or severely disabled despite evacuation of mass lesions are given the diagnosis.

Answers: D

Brunicardi, FC (2010) *Schwartz's Principles of Surgery*, 9th edn, McGraw-Hill, New York, pp. 145 and 1524.

Moore AJ (2005) *Neurosurgery Principles and Practice*, 1st edn, Springer, London, p. 369.

15. *Which of the statements regarding subarachnoid hemorrhage following trauma is correct?*

A. *Mass effect from the subarachnoid blood is a major concern*

B. *They have a characteristic crescent shape on CT of the head*

C. *Usually produces meningismus (stiff neck and headache)*

D. *Subarachanoid hemorrhage is the most common indication for operative intervention after traumatic brain injury*

E. *May produce communicating hydrocephalus as a complication*

Subarachnoid hemorrhage is one of the most common intracranial hemorrhages following head injury. It usually causes signs of headache and changes in the patient's mental status; neck stiffness (meningismus) may occur. The hemorrhage is small and rapidly diluted by the CSF, no localized mass effect occurs. This type of hemorrhage after trauma has little surgical significance. Rarely subarachnoid hemorrhage leads to progressive communicating hydrocephalus that requires shunting.

Answer: C

Brunicardi, FC (2010) *Schwartz's Principles of Surgery*, 9th edn, McGraw-Hill, New York, pp. 145 and 1524.

Moore AJ (2005) *Neurosurgery Principles and Practice*, 1st edn, Springer, London, p. 369.

Chapter 27 Blunt and Penetrating Neck Trauma

Leslie Kobayashi, MD

1. *Regarding zones of the neck, which of the following statements is correct?*

A. Zone I is bounded by the clavicle and cricoid cartilage

B. Zone II injuries require angiography

C. Zone III injuries require surgical exploration

D. Zone of injury is the primary determinant of operative versus non-operative management

E. Zone III is the most easily accessible surgically

Zone I is bounded by the clavicles and cricoid cartilage. Zone II lies between the cricoid cartilage and the angle of the mandible, and is the most easily accessible surgically. Zone III extends from the angle of the mandible to the base of the skull, and is the most difficult area to explore, requiring transection of the mandible, dislocation of the jaw, or drilling into the skull base to expose vital structures Zone I and III injuries are typically investigated with CT scan, endoscopy and, angiography. All Zone II injuries classically underwent mandatory operative exploration, however this resulted in an unacceptably high rate of negative explorations. Currently the primary determinant of operative versus conservative management is clinical presentation. Patients with hard signs of vascular or aerodigestive injury require surgical exploration regardless of location of injury, those with soft signs undergo imaging. Hard signs of vascular injury include arterial bleeding, pulsatile or expanding hematoma, lack of pulse distal to the injury, bruit or thrill at the injury site, unexplained shock or anemia. Hard signs of aerodigestive injury include bubbling from the injury site, large volume hemoptysis or hematemasis, stridor, or massive subcutaneous emphysema. Soft signs of vascular injury include non-expanding and non-pulsatile hematomas or minor bleeding from the injury. Soft signs of aerodigestive injury include odynophagia, small hemoptysis or hematemasis, hoarseness, or minor subcutaneous emphysema.

Surgical Critical Care and Emergency Surgery: Clinical Questions and Answers, First Edition. Edited by Forrest O. Moore, Peter M. Rhee, Samuel A. Tisherman and Gerard J. Fulda.

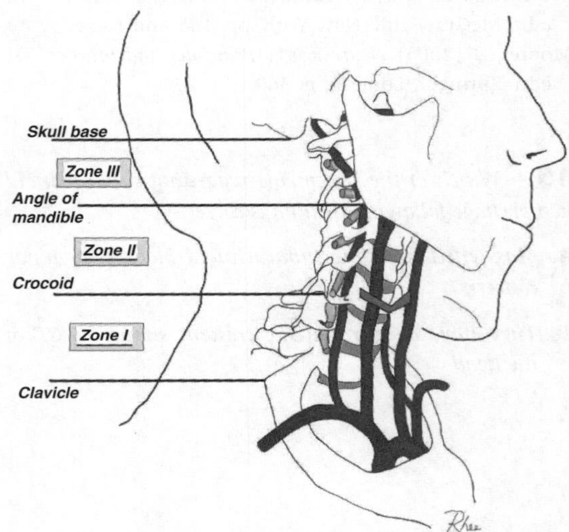

The vascular anatomy and zones of the neck. Figure courtesy of Peter Rhee. A full color version of this figure appears in the plate section of this book.

Answer: A

Britt LD (2007) penetrating neck trauma. In: Fischer JE and Bland KI (eds) *Mastery of Surgery,* 5th edn, Lippincott Williams & Wilkins, Philadelphia, PA, pp. 381–6.

Britt LD, Weireter LJ, Cole FJ (2008) Management of acute neck injuries. In: Feliciano DV, Mattox KL, Moore EE (eds) *Trauma,* 6th edn, McGraw-Hill, New York.

Gale SC and Mattox KL (2009) Trauma to the head, face, and neck. In: Gracias VH, Reilly PM, McKenney MG, Velmahos GC (eds) *Acute Care Surgery: A Guide for General Surgeons*. McGraw-Hill, New York.

2. *A man was stabbed in the neck just above the cricoid. He is hemodynamically stable, however there is a large pulsatile hematoma. What is the next step in management?*

A. *Rapid sequence intubation in the ER followed by surgical exploration*

B. *Emergent cricothyroidotomy in the ER followed by surgical exploration*

C. *Fiberoptic intubation in the operating room followed by surgical exploration*

D. *Observation in the intensive care unit*

E. *Placement of laryngeal mask airway (LMA) followed by surgical exploration*

This patient has a penetrating injury to Zone II with hard signs of vascular injury. Because the patient is stable the best course of action is to proceed immediately to the operating room for definitive airway control with fiberoptic intubation followed by surgical exploration. Direct laryngscopy may not be tolerated well in the awake patient, and medications used in rapid sequence intubation may convert an urgent airway into an emergent airway. Direct laryngoscopy may also be technically challenging due to distortion of the airway from the hematoma. The operating room has several advantages over the ER, it is a controlled environment, and conversion to a surgical airway can occur with the aid of extra personnel, specialized surgical equipment, better positioning, improved lighting, and sterile technique. Cricothyroidotomy is a good option for the unstable patient, but should only be used if endotracheal intubation fails in the stable patient. Additionally, preservation of as much intact airway as possible is important if there is a tracheal injury.

Answer: C

Britt LD (2007) Penetrating neck trauma. In: Fischer JE and Bland KI (eds) *Mastery of Surgery*, 5th edn, Lippincott Williams & Wilkins, Philadelphia, PA, pp. 381–6.

Britt LD, Weireter LJ, Cole FJ (2008) Management of acute neck injuries. In: Feliciano DV, Mattox KL, Moore EE (eds) *Trauma*, 6th edn, McGraw Hill, New York, pp. 467–77.

Gale SC and Mattox KL (2009) Trauma to the head, face, and neck. In: Gracias VH, Reilly PM, McKenney MG, Velmahos GC (eds) *Acute Care Surgery: A Guide for General Surgeons*. McGraw-Hill, New York, pp. 99–108.

3. *In a patient with cervical spinal cord injury, which pulmonary function test best predicts deteriorating lung function?*

A. *Decrease functional residual capacity*

B. *Decreased minute ventilation*

C. *Decreased vital capacity*

D. *Decreased negative inspiratory force*

E. *Decreased diffusion capacity*

Changes in pulmonary physiology after spinal cord injury (SCI) include decreased vital capacity, total lung capacity, end respiratory volume, inspiratory capacity and FEV_1. Residual volume is increased and no change is noted in functional residual capacity. Respiratory complications occur in 36–83% of patients, and a large proportion will require mechanical ventilation. Injury above C5 will result in loss of phrenic nerve function; below C5 loss of accessory muscles inhibit pulmonary function. Because these patients are challenging airways, many advocate early elective intubation. However, mechanical ventilation is not inevitable, and select patients can be observed if carefully monitored. Strong consideration should be given to serial assessment of vital capacity in these patients as decreased vital capacity may precede clinical evidence of respiratory compromise. Vital capacity below 10 mL/kg of ideal body weight is an indication for urgent intubation. Vital capacity is the maximum amount of air expelled after a maximum inspiration. It is equal to the inspiratory reserve volume plus the tidal volume plus the expiratory reserve volume.

Answer: C

Berlly M and Shem K (2007) Respiratory management during the first five days after spinal cord injury. *Journal of Spinal Cord Medicine* 2007; **30**, 309–18.

Schilero GJ, Spungen AM, Bauman WA, *et al.* (2009) Pulmonary function and spinal cord injury. *Respiratory Physiology* **166**, 129–41.

4. *Following a motor vehicle collision, the patient below initially presents with a GCS of 15. CT scan of the head and non-contrast CT of the cervical spine are normal. The patient acutely decompensates to a GCS of 13 and developed weakness in the right arm and leg. What is the next step in diagnosis?*

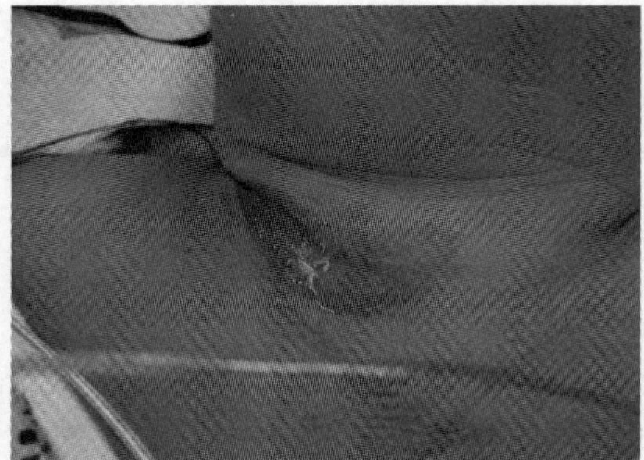

A seat belt sign over the neck in Zone I. A full color version of this figure appears in the plate section of this book.

A. *CT scan of the cervical spine*

B. *Repeat CT scan of the head*

C. *MRI*

D. *CT Angiogram*

E. *Ultrasound*

This patient has a seat belt sign on the neck and now has an unexplained focal neurologic deficit suggesting blunt cerebrovascular injury (BCVI). Angiography remains the gold standard for diagnosis of BCVI. CT angiography with multichannel (16–64) detectors has shown promise as a screening modality. CT angiography has the benefit of being quick, widely available, and easy to perform, and does not require the presence of a specially trained angiography team. It also avoids the morbidity associated with an arterial puncture and uses a lower contrast dose than traditional angiography. Studies have shown detection rates similar to historical controls with four vessel angiography. Sensitivity ranges from 83–100% with negative predictive values of 92–98%. The sensitivity and specificity of ultrasound, MRI/MRA, and CT angiography performed with a four slice or less detector are poor and they have little to no role in diagnosis.

Answer: D

Berne JD, Cook A, Rowe SA, *et al.* (2010) A multivariate logistic regression analysis of risk factors for blunt cerebrovascular injury. *Journal of Vascular Surgery* **51** (1), 57–64.

Biffl WJ, Cothren C, Moore EE, *et al.* (2009) Western Trauma Association Critical decision in Trauma: Screening for and treatment of blunt cerebrovascular injuries. *Journal of Trauma* **67** (6), 1150–3.

Bromberg WJ, Collier BC, Diebel LN, *et al.* (2010) Blunt cerebrovascular injury practice management guidelines: The Eastern Association for the Surgery of Trauma. *Journal of Trauma* **68** (2), 471–7.

5. *A 24-year-old woman presents with an anterior Zone II stab wound. Upon exploration, a laceration to the anterior trachea is noted across the first and second tracheal rings. The next step in her evaluation would include:*

A. *Inspection of the bilateral recurrent laryngeal nerves*

B. *Examination of the superior laryngeal nerve*

C. *Examination of the posterior tracheal wall*

D. *Exploration of the innominate artery*

E. *Exposure of the brachiocephalic vein*

Neck exploration for trauma is performed via a longitudinal incision along the anterior border of the sternocleidomastoid. The presence of an anterior tracheal injury makes evaluation of the posterior wall of the trachea and the esophagus of paramount importance, as concomitant injuries are present in 10-15% of cases. Exploration of the ipsilateal carotid sheath and contents should be performed. Exploration of the innominate artery or brachiocephalic vein are not indicated. Searching for the superior or recurrent laryngeal nerves is not recommended, as dissection can increase the incidence of injury.

Answer: C

Britt LD (2007) Penetrating neck trauma. In: Fischer JE and Bland KI (eds) *Mastery of Surgery*, 5th edn, Lippincott Williams & Wilkins, Philadelphia PA, pp. 381–6.

Gale SC and Mattox KL (2009) Trauma to the head, face, and neck. In: Gracias VH, Reilly PM, McKenney

MG, Velmahos GC (eds) *Acute Care Surgery: A Guide for General Surgeons*. McGraw Hill, New York, pp. 99–108.

Mathisen DJ, Grillo H (1987) Laryngotracheal trauma. *Annals of Thoracic Surgery* **43** (3), 254–62.

6. *Screening for blunt cerebrovascular injury (BCVI) is indicated in which of the following situations?*

A. *Basilar skull fracture*

B. *Seat belt sign on the chest*

C. *Clavicle fracture*

D. *Paraspinal cervical tenderness on exam*

E. *Cephalohematoma*

Blunt cerebrovascular injury is rare following blunt trauma. The overall incidence is <1% even in centers with aggressive screening policies. Injuries can occur as a result of severe hyperextension or rotation, direct force to the vessel, or by injury from adjacent fractures. The majority of patients have minimal to no symptoms at presentation. Indications for screening in asymptomatic patients include: GCS of 8 or less, presence of diffuse axonal injury, basilar skull fracture, cervical spine fracture, Lefort II or III fractures, direct blow to the neck, and hyperextension injuries. The presence of a seat belt sign on the neck is controversial as an indication for screening, and in the absence of other risk factors is unlikely to indicate injury. Seat-belt signs outside of the neck, soft tissue injury to the skull and fractures other than those affecting the base of the skull or cervical spine are not predictive of injury. However, with modern imaging, if the fracture line of the basilar skull fracture is clear and not involving the carotid or vertebral openings, there will be lower yield in the screening process and is probably not indicated.

Answer: A

Biffl WJ, Cothren C, Moore EE, *et al*. (2009) Western Trauma Association critical decision in trauma: Screening for and treatment of blunt cerebrovascular injuries. *Journal of Trauma* **67** (6), 1150–3.

Bromberg WJ, Collier BC, Diebel LN, *et al*. (2010) Blunt cerebrovascular injury practice management guidelines: The Eastern Association for the Surgery of Trauma. *Journal of Trauma* **68** (2), 471–7.

DiPerna CA, Rowe VL, Terramani TT, *et al*. (2002) Clinical importance of the "seat belt sign" in blunt trauma to the neck. *American Journal of Surgery* **66** (5), 441–5.

7. *Regarding blunt cerebrovascular injuries (BCVI), which of the following statements is true?*

A. *Anticoagulation is superior to antiplatelet agents in prevention of stroke*

B. *Plavix is superior to aspirin in prevention of stroke*

C. *Dual therapy with aspirin and plavix is superior to single agent therapy*

D. *Carotid stenting is superior to antiplatelet agents alone in preventing stroke*

E. *Surgery is generally reserved for patients with Grade V injuries*

The optimal type and duration of treatment for BCVI remains unknown, options include anticoagulation, antiplatelet therapy, surgical repair, and endovascular coils or stents. Grade I/II injuries have a low risk of bleeding and barring contraindications, treatment consists of anticoagulation or antiplatelet agents, as these methods have equivalent efficacy. The majority of low grade injuries heal, and repeat imaging is indicated as antithrombotic therapy can be discontinued after healing. Grade III injuries (pseudoaneurysms) are less likely to resolve with antithrombotic therapy alone, and the risk of thromboembolic complications without treatment can be as high as 43–74%; conversely, risk of rupture is very low. Surgery can be considered for accessible lesions, and endovascular treatment for inaccessible lesions. Placement of stents or coils may decrease the risk of enlargement, however there is no evidence that they are superior to antithrombotic agents alone in stroke prevention. Grade IV lesions (occlusions) are unlikely to resolve with antithrombotic therapy, and neither medical nor surgical treatment are likely to reverse symptoms if already present. Follow up imaging is not recommended for Grade IV lesions as they are unlikely to change with time. Grade V lesions (active extravasation) require surgery or endovascular intervention.

Answer: E

Berne JD, Cook A, Rowe SA, *et al.* (2010) A multivariate logistic regression analysis of risk factors for blunt cerebrovascular injury. *Journal of Vascular Surgery* **51** (1), 57–64.

Biffl WJ, Cothren C, Moore EE, *et al.* (2009) Western Trauma Association Critical decision in Trauma: Screening for and treatment of blunt cerebrovascular injuries. *Journal of Trauma* **67** (6), 1150–3.

Bromberg WJ, Collier BC, Diebel LN, *et al.* (2010) Blunt cerebrovasculr injury practice management guidelines: The Eastern Association for the Surgery of Trauma. *Journal of Trauma* **68** (2), 471–7.

8. *The complication seen below can be avoided in patients with craniofacial trauma by which of the following?*

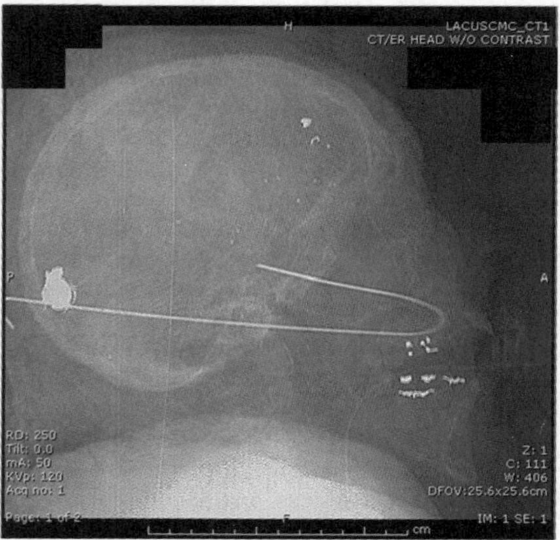

Lateral skull radiograph demonstrating an intracranial nasogastric tube

A. *Placement of an orogastric tube*

B. *Placement of a nasal airway*

C. *Nasotracheal intubation*

D. *Early cricothyroidotomy*

E. *Maxilofacial CT scan*

The lateral radiograph of the skull demonstrates migration of a nasogastric tube into the cranium. This rare complication can be avoided by strict use of the oral route for gastric decompression in patients with evidence of facial or basilar skull fractures. In particular midface instability, epistaxis, hemotympanum, bloody otorrhea, mastoid ecchymosis (Battle's sign), and periorbital ecchymosis (raccoon eyes) should be warning signs to avoid nasal instrumentation including nasal airways, nasotracheal intubation and nasogastric tubes. If these warning signs are not headed, devices may migrate through fractures in the cribiform plate, or sphenoid sinus into the cranial vault. Should this rare complication occur, mortality can be as high as 64%.

Answer: A

Marlow TJ, Goltra DD, Schabel SI (1997) Intracranial placement of a nasotracheal tube after facial fracture: A rare complication. *Journal of Emergency Medicine* **15** (2), 187–91.

Rodrigues P, Moraes de Oliveira D, Vasconcellos RJ, *et al.* (2004) Inadvertent intracranial placement of a nasogastric tube in a patient with severe craniofacial trauma: A case report. *Journal of Oral and Maxillofacial Surgery* **62,** 1435–8.

9. *Which of the following is a known complication of complete spinal cord injury?*

A. *Infertility in women*

B. *Inability to carry a fetus to term*

C. *Inability to deliver vaginally*

D. *Inability to obtain an erection*

E. *Infertility in men*

The reproductive system of both men and women can be affected by spinal cord injury. Women may suffer a temporary interruption of menses, which generally resolves within 6–9 months of injury. However, fertility is preserved and women can carry a fetus to term. Pregnancies of women with SCI can be complicated, most commonly by urinary tract infections, autonomic dysreflexia, and premature labor. Most women can deliver vaginally, although they may require second-stage assistance. In contrast, male fertility is affected at multiple stages. They may suffer from low testosterone, and, while erection is possible, ejaculation is unlikely in the absence of vibrational or electrical stimulation devices. Additionally, spermatogenesis and sperm motility are both decreased after SCI.

Answer: E

Cross LL, Meythaler JM, Tuel SM, *et al.* (1991) Pregnancy following spinal cord injury. *The Western J of Medicine* **154** (5), 607–11.

Schopp LH, Clark M, Mazurek MO, *et al.* (2006) Testosterone levels among men with spinal cord injury admitted to inpatient rehabilitation. *American Journal of Physical Medicine and Rehabilitation* **85** (8), 678–84.

Skowronski E, Hartman K (2008) Obstetric management following traumatic tetraplegia: Case series and literature review. *Australian and New Zealand Journal of Obstetrics and Gynaecology* **48** (5), 485–91.

10. *A 29-year-old man is stabbed in the neck; during exploration you note an esophageal as well as a tracheal laceration. Which of the following is an important principle in repair?*

A. Use of non-absorbable sutures for tracheal repair

B. Use of two-layered closure of the esophageal repair

C. Interposition of healthy tissue between the esophageal and tracheal repairs

D. Identification of the recurrent laryngeal nerve to rule out injury

E. Avoidance of drains to prevent erosion into repairs

Most tracheal injuries can be closed primarily using an absorbable suture in a single layer. Associated injuries of the thyroid or cricoid cartilage can be closed with sutures or plates. Esophageal injuries should be explored to ensure the entire mucosal defect is addressed. Intra-operative esophagoscopy and insufflation of a nasogastric tube with air or dye can aid in the diagnosis of suspected esophageal injury. Once the injury has been identified it can be repaired in one or two layers with absorbable suture. If there has been significant delay in treatment, or severe tissue destruction the repair can be protected with a T-tube; or diversion can be performed with a proximal cervical esophagostomy. All esophageal repairs should be buttressed with healthy tissue; this is of paramount importance if other suture lines are present. Buttressing can be done with one of the strap muscles, or the sternocleidomastoid. Wide drainage of all neck explorations is highly recommended. Drains will help prevent hematoma formation, which can lead to acute airway obstruction, and will control potential esophageal leaks. Careful posterior approach to the esophagus will help prevent recurrent laryngeal nerve injury, but dissection specifically to identify the nerve is discouraged as it can increase the risk of nerve injury.

Answer: C

Britt LD (2007) Penetrating neck trauma. In: Fischer JE, Bland KI (eds) *Mastery of Surgery*, 5th edn, Lippincott Williams & Wilkins, Philadelphia, PA, pp. 381–6.

Gale SC, Mattox KL (2009) Trauma to the head, face, and neck. In: Gracias VH, Reilly PM, McKenney MG, Velmahos GC (eds) *Acute Care Surgery: A Guide for General Surgeons*, McGraw-Hill, New York, pp. 99–108.

11. *Which of the following statements regarding esophageal injury is true?*

A. Delayed surgery results in improved mortality

B. Trauma is the most common etiology of esophageal injury

C. Esophagoscopy is highly sensitive and specific for esophageal injury

D. Cervical injuries have a higher mortality than thoracic or abdominal injuries

E. Conservative management is an acceptable option in the stable patient with a contained perforation

Timing of repair in esophageal injury is an important determinant of outcome, with delay >24 hours significantly decreasing chances of successful primary repair and survival. Iatrogenic perforation is by far the most common cause of esophageal injury; trauma accounts for 5–10% of injuries. Esophagoscopy is widely utilized but may have false negative rates up to 25%. Injuries in the thoracic and abdominal esophagus can freely contaminate the peritoneal, mediastinal and thoracic cavities leading rapidly to sepsis and death. In a recent review, mortality for cervical perforations ranged from 0–20%, with the majority of studies demonstrating zero mortality; in contrast, mortality for thoracic and abdominal injuries ranged from 20–42%. Conservative management is an acceptable strategy in select patients. Indications for nonoperative management include contained perforation, absence of distal obstruction, cervical or thoracic location, and minimal systemic signs of infection. Medical management consists of fasting, antibiotics, and strict monitoring. Follow up imaging is performed in 7–10 days to assess for healing.

Answer: E

Bufkin BL, Miller JI, Mansour KA (1996) Esophageal perforation: emphasis on management. *Annals of Thoracic Surgery* **61** (5), 1447–52.

Onat S, Ulku R, Cigdem KM, *et al.* (2010) Factors affecting the outcome of surgically treated non-iatrogenic traumatic cervical esophageal perforation: 28 years experience at a single center. *Journal of Cardiothoracic Surgery* **5**, 46–50.

Wu, JT, Mattox KL, Wall MJ (2007) Esophageal perforations: New perspectives and treatment paradigms. *Journal of Trauma* **63** (5), 1173–84.

12. *A patient with acute quadriplegia following motor vehicle accident is hypotensive with a heart rate of 55 beats per minute. Physical exam is unremarkable, FAST and diagnostic peritoneal lavage are negative. Pelvis and chest x-rays are unremarkable. Two liters of crystalloid are infused with no change in blood pressure. Which of the following is the most likely cause of hypotension?*

A. Spinal shock

B. Neurogenic shock

C. Hypovolemic shock

D. Cardiogenic shock

E. Obstructive shock

In a trauma patient hemorrhage must be assumed to be the cause of hypotension until proven otherwise. In this case diagnostic maneuvers to search for hemorrhage have been negative. Additionally, bradycardia and lack of response to fluid challenge make hemorrhagic shock less likely. Pneumothorax and tamponade are absent and pulmonary embolus is unlikely in this time frame, making obstructive shock unlikely. Cardiogenic shock is a possibility, but hemdynamically significant dysfunction is rare, especially in the absence of other signs of thoracic trauma. Spinal shock is a neurologic phenomenon resulting in transient loss of reflexes, and does not cause hypotension. The most likely cause of hypotension in this case is neurogenic shock. Neurogenic shock occurs after spinal cord injury to the high thoracic or cervical spine. Loss of sympathetic tone below the level of the injury results in peripheral vasodilation and hypotension. Additionally, in high cervical spine injuries unopposed vagal tone can result in bradycardia and decreased cardiac output. Physical exam may reveal warmth and erythema below the level of the injury due to peripheral vasodilation. Treatment should be aimed at fluid resuscitation to maintain normal central venous pressures (8–10 cm $H_2 0$), and judicious use of vasopressors and inotropes to maintain vascular tone and cardiac output. Neurogenic shock generally resolves in 24–72 hours.

Answer: B

Guly HR, Bouamra O, Lecky FE (2008) Trauma audit and research network. The incidence of neurogenic shock in patients with isolated spinal cord injury in the emergency department. *Resuscitation* **76** (1), 57–62.

Harbrecht BG, Forsythe RM, Peitzman A. (2008) Management of shock. In: Feliciano DV, Mattox KL, Moore EE (eds) *Trauma*, 6th edn. McGraw-Hill, New York, pp. 213–34.

Maull, KI, Letarte P (2009) Spinal cord injury. In: Gracias VH, Reilly PM, McKenney MG, Velmahos GC (eds) *Acute Care Surgery: A Guide for General Surgeons*, McGraw-Hill, New York, 99–108.

13. *Which of the following is a contraindication to percutaneous tracheostomy?*

A. Obesity

B. Coagulopathy

C. *Cervical spine fracture*

D. *Traumatic brain injury*

E. *None of the above*

Several large trials comparing safety profiles of percutaneous tracheostomy (PT) to open tracheostomy revealed equivalent if not improved safety profiles with PT. Percutaneous tracheostomy has also been examined in smaller series of patients previously considered high risk. Current studies reveal excellent safety of PT in the morbidly obese, patients with known or suspected cervical spine injury, anticoagulated or coagulopathic patients, and patients with traumatic brain injury. The decision to perform OT or PT should depend primarily on the comfort level and experience of the provider as well as the local resources of the facility. If performed by experienced surgeons in a monitored setting with proper equipment, PT can be safe in a wide variety of patients.

Answer: E

Mayberry JC, Wu IC, Goldman RK, *et al.* (2000) Cervical spine clearance and neck extension during percutaneous tracheostomy in trauma patients. *Critical Care Medicine* **28** (10), 3436–40.

Milanchi S, Magner D, Wilson MT, *et al.* (2008) Percutaneous tracheostomy in neurosurgical patients with intracranial pressure monitoring is safe. *Journal of Trauma* **65** (1), 73–9.

Pandian V, Vasani RS, Mirski MA, *et al.* (2010) Safety of percutaneous dilational tracheostomy in coagulopathic patients. *Ear Nose Throat Journal* **89** (8), 387–95.

14. *Regarding penetrating trauma to the neck, which of the following signs or symptoms is a contraindication to nonoperative management?*

A. *Dysphagia*

B. *Dysphonia*

C. *Hemoptysis*

D. *Hypotension*

E. *Subcutaneous emphysema*

The decision to explore or expectantly manage injuries is driven by clinical exam, with hard signs of vascular or aerodigestive injury mandating exploration, and soft signs mandating diagnostic imaging. Hard signs of injury include expanding or pulsatile hematoma, bruit/thrill, active bleeding, hypotension, air bubbling through the wound, stridor, unexplained focal neurologic deficit, massive hemoptysis or hematemasis, and airway compromise. Soft signs include minor hemoptysis/hematemesis, dysphagia, dysphonia, subcutaneous emphysema and isolated nerve injury. Patients with soft signs should undergo CT angiography of the neck. This exam gives information on vasculature, bony structures, soft tissue and most importantly the tract of injury in penetrating trauma. If the tract of injury is far from vital structures work up can be considered complete. CT angiography of the neck is diagnostic for vascular injuries with sensitivities approaching 100%. It is less accurate for evaluation of the aerodigestive tract; however, if the tract is suspicious esophagoscopy, bronchoscopy and contrast esophagram can be performed.

Answer: D

Case SJ, Alwis WD (2010) Emergency department assessment and management of stab wounds to the neck. *Emergency Medicine Australasia* **22**, 201–10.

Mazolewski PJ, Curry JD, Browder T, *et al.* (2001) Computed tomographic scan can be used for surgical decision making in zone II penetrating neck injuries. *Journal of Trauma* **51** (2), 315–19.

Osborn Tm, Bell RB, Qaisi W, *et al.* (2008) Computed tomographic angiography as an aid to clinical decision making in selective management of penetrating injuries to the neck: a reduction in the need for operative exploration. *Journal of Trauma* **64** (6), 1466–71.

15. *Which of the following maneuvers can decrease the risk of tracheo-innominate fistula?*

A. *Use of stoma sites no lower than the fourth tracheal ring*

B. *Use of open technique*

C. *Use of percutaneous technique*

D. *Use of bronchoscopy*

E. *Use of high pressure, low volume cuff on the tracheostomy tube*

Tracheo-innominate fistula (TIF) is a rare but devastating complication following tracheostomy. It occurs in less than 1% of cases, with a peak incidence in the first 1–2 weeks. The associated mortality rate is as high as 90%. Risk factors include low placement of the stoma, high-riding innominate artery, overinflated cuffs, and older high-pressure, low-volume cuffs. Preventative measures include avoidance of placing the stoma below the fourth tracheal ring avoidance of neck hyper-extension, maintenance of cuff pressures below 20 mm Hg, and early decannulation. Initial management is to secure an airway, and apply pressure to the bleeding by overinflating the cuff, pulling up on the tracheostomy tube, and direct pressure or packing through the stoma site. Definitive treatment consists of resection of the fistula and ligation or interposition graft of the innominate artery. There is currently no evidence that either open or percutaneous tracheostomy is superior with regard to avoiding TIF. The literature to date on percutaneous tracheostomy reveals few case reports and a single case series consisting of three patients. The single series reported a rate of TIF of 0.3%, comparable to historical rates with open tracheostomy.

Answer: A

Cokis C, Towler S (2000) Tracheo-innominate fistula after initial percutaneous tracheostomy. *Anaesthesia and Intensive Care* **28** (5), 566–9.

Grant CA, Dempsey G, Harrison J, *et al.* (2006) Tracheo-innominate artery fistula after percutaneous tracheostomy: three case reports and a clinical review. *British Journal of Anaestheology* **96**, 127–31.

Jamal-Eddine H, Ayed AK, Al-Moosa A, *et al.* (2008) Graft repair of trachea-innominate artery fistula following percutaneous tracheostomy. *Interactive Cardiovascular and Thoracic Surgery* **7**(4), 654–5.

16. *The vertebral artery enters the vertebral canal at which spinal level?*

A. T1

B. C7

C. C6

D. C5

E. C4

The vertebral arteries originate from the subclavian and enter the neck in Zone III laterally. They enter the transverse foramen at the level of C6, superior to this point they are within the bony vertebral canal before entering the base of the skull with the spinal cord through the foramen magnum. The pharyngeo-esophageal junction also occurs at C6, above this levels is the oropharynx, and below the esophagus. The C5/C6 junction is also at the level of the cricoid cartilage and cricothyroid membrane.

Answer: C

Netter FH (1997) *Atlas of Human Anatomy*, 2nd edn, Novartis, East Hanover, NJ.

17. *A 19-year-old man dives headfirst into a pool, after which he has severe neck pain and presents to the ER. He is neurologically intact. CT scan of his cervical spine is seen below. What is the most likely diagnosis?*

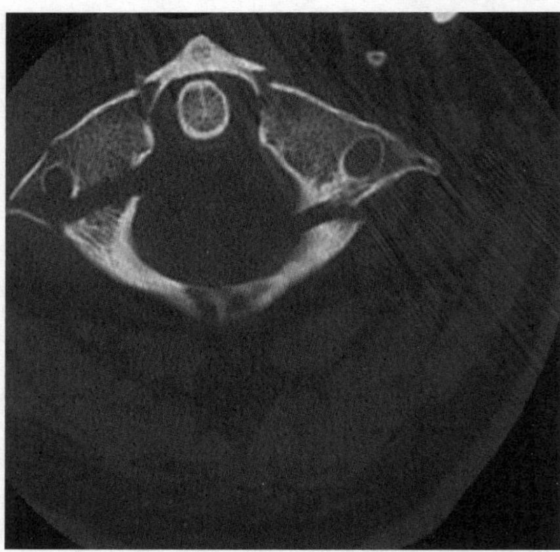

Axial CT scan of a Jefferson fracture with bilateral anterior and posterior ring disruption

A. Hangman's fracture

B. Jefferson fracture

C. Spinal cord injury without radiologic abnormality (SCIWORA)

D. *Atlanto-occipital dissociation (Internal decapitation)*

E. *Chance fracture*

Spinal cord injury without radiologic abnormality is primarily described in pediatric patients, but has been reported in adults. It is associated with flexion/extension and distraction. CT scans are normal and MRI may find disc herniation or ligamentous injury. Atlanto-occipital dissociation is a rare and frequently fatal injury following violent hyperflexion/hyperextension. It is most common after motor vehicle or auto-pedestrian accidents, and occurs when ligamentous disruption between the skull and spine allows distraction between the skull and C1. The hangman's fracture occurs when violent hyperextension combined with distraction results in fracture of both pedicles of C2. Chance fractures occur when hyperflexion around an axis point anterior to the spine results in compression of the anterior vertebral body with a transverse fracture through the posterior vertebral elements. Jefferson fracture occurs when significant axial load results in compression fracture of the bilateral anterior and posterior arches of C1. The classical pattern has four fractures, however it may also present with two or three fractures. Patients complain of neck pain, but are usually neurologically intact. Treatment is stabilization with HALO, collar, or surgery.

Answer: B

Deliganis AV, Mann FA, Grady MS (1998) Rapid diagnosis and treatment of a traumatic atlantooccipital dissociation. *American Journal of Roentgenology* **171**, 986.

Jefferson G. (1919) Fracture of the atlas vertebra. Report of four cases, and a review of those previously recorded. *British Journal of Surgery* **7** (27), 407–22.

Yucesoy K, Yuksel KZ (2008) SCIWORA in MRI era. *Clinical Neurology and Neurosurgery* **10**, 429–33.

18. *Which of the following statements regarding clinical clearance of the cervical spine is incorrect?*

A. *Patients must be awake and able to cooperate with physical examination*

B. *Patients must be free of all neck pain*

C. *Patients must be free of intoxication*

D. *Patients must be free of other painful distracting injuries*

E. *Patients must be free of neurological deficit*

The two most commonly used protocols for cervical spine clearance are the NEXUS and Canadian C-spine criteria. NEXUS—the National Emergency X-radiography Utilization Study—criteria specify that patients must be of normal alertness without intoxication, have no focal neurological deficit, be free of painful distracting injury, and have no midline cervical spinal tenderness. However, anterior, lateral and paraspinal pain are not contraindications to clearance. The Canadian C-spine criteria specify patients must be <65-years-old, have no numbness or tingling in the extremities, and have a low risk mechanism of injury. If they met these criteria and were free of pain at the scene, or free of midline spinal tenderness and could rotate 45 degrees to the left and right patients could be cleared clinically. Nonmidline pain, pain that did not limit rotational range of motion, and late-onset pain were not contraindications to clearance.

Answer: B

Hoffman JR, Mower WR, Wolfson AB, *et al.* (2000) Validity of a set of clinical criteria to rule out injury to the cervical spine in patients with blunt trauma. *New England Journal of Medicine* **343** (2), 94–100.

Stiell IG, Wells GA, Vandemheen KL, *et al.* (2001) The Canadian C-Spine rule for radiography in alert and stable trauma patients. *Journal of the American Medical Association* **288** (15), 1841–8.

19. *A patient in a snowmobile accident suffers a "clothesline" injury with a laceration just above the sternal notch, a moderate hematoma, and subcutaneous emphysema. He is unable to lay flat and has a muffled voice. Initial management of this patient would include all of the following except:*

A. *Maintenance of cervical spine precautions*

B. *Cricothryoidotomy*

C. *Bronchoscopy*

D. *Intubation*

E. *Operative exploration*

This patient has signs of tracheal injury in a location below the cricoid. Given the respiratory distress, airway management is the first priority. This is best accomplished with orotracheal intubation if possible. Orotracheal intubation will allow bronchoscopic evaluation to localize injury and prevent further trauma to the trachea, which is important if complex reconstruction is required. However, endotracheal intubation is likely to be challenging and should be performed in the operating room so that conversion to open surgical tracheostomy can be performed with sterility and proper equipment and lighting. Cricothyroidotomy is likely to be above the level of the injury in this patient and unlikely to result in a satisfactory airway. It is important to maintain cervical spine precautions until injury can be excluded, but work up should not interfere with diagnosis and treatment of injuries to the airway and vasculature.

Answer: B

Britt LD, Weireter LJ, Cole FJ (2008) Management of acute neck injuries. In: Feliciano DV, Mattox KL, Moore EE (eds) *Trauma* 6th edn, McGraw-Hill, New York, pp. 467–77.

Gale SC, Mattox KL (2009) Trauma to the head, face, and neck. In: Gracias VH, Reilly PM, McKenney MG, Velmahos GC (eds) *Acute Care Surgery: A Guide for General Surgeons,* McGraw Hill, New York, pp. 99–108.

20. *Which one of the following is a contraindication to emergent cricothyroidotomy?*

A. *Age less than 12*

B. *Age greater than 65*

C. *Hemodynamic instability*

D. *Hypoxia*

E. *Apnea*

Cricothyroidotomy is a life-saving procedure, indications include hypoxia, apnea or other evidence of respiratory distress in a patient with severe facial and upper airway injury, or if endotracheal intubation is unsuccessful. However, cricothyroidotomy is not recommended for patients under 12 years of age. This is the narrowest portion of the pediatric airway and associated rates of subglottic stenosis are high. Instead, the airway is accessed with percutaneous placement of a large-bore needle into the cricothyroid membrane and jet insufflation is used to temporarily oxygenate the patient. Ventilation is necessarily restricted and carbon dioxide levels will predictably rise over time. Conversion to a tracheostomy or repeated attempt at intubation with advanced airway adjuncts or more experienced personnel should be performed within 45 minutes to prevent accumulation of carbon dioxide. Circothyroidotomy is not contraindicated in the elderly.

Answer: A

Jorden RC, Moore EE, Marx JA, *et al.* (1985) A comparison of PTV and endotracheal ventilation in an acute trauma model. *Journal of Trauma* **25** (10), 978–83.

Toschlog EA, Sagraves SG, Rotondo MF. Airway control. In: Feliciano DV, Mattox KL, Moore EE (eds) *Trauma,* 6th edn, McGraw-Hill, New York, pp. 185–211.

Chapter 28 Cardiothoracic and Thoracic Vascular Injury

Leslie Kobayashi, MD

1. *Which of the following statements regarding traumatic diaphragmatic hernia (TDH) is true?*

A. *TDH is more common on the right than the left*

B. *Left-sided TDHs are associated with a more significant mechanism of injury than the right*

C. *TDHs due to blunt trauma are generally smaller than those due to penetrating trauma*

D. *TDHs are rarely found in association with other injuries*

E. *TDHs can present in a delayed fashion, months to years after the initial trauma*

Traumatic diaphragmatic hernia occurs as a result of high-energy acceleration-deceleration trauma, or as a direct laceration from a weapon or broken rib. Blunt injuries tend to be large avulsions, while penetrating injuries tend to be smaller lacerations. Injuries can grow over time as viscera migrate into the thoracic cavity due to the normal pressure gradient across the diaphragm. Traumatic diaphragmatic hernia is associated with other injuries in 52–100% of cases. Left sided injuries are more common accounting for 70% of cases. This is likely due to several factors: the posterolateral aspect of the diaphragm is structurally weak on the left, the right diaphragm is protected by the liver, and it is more difficult to diagnose injuries on the right side. However right-sided ruptures are associated with more severe injuries and a more significant mechanism. Delay in diagnosis occurs in 30–50% of cases, and the delay can range from seven days to 40 years (average 3–7 years). Mortality ranges from 1–28%, primarily related to associated injuries.

Answer: E

Clarke DL, Greatorex GV, Muckart DJ (2009) The spectrum of diaphragmatic injury in a busy metropolitan surgical service. *Injury* **40**, 932–7.

Murray JA, Weng J, Velmahos G, *et al.* (2008) Abdominal approach to chronic diaphragmatic hernias: Is it safe? *American Journal of Surgery* **70** (10), 897–900.

2. *In a patient sustaining a stab wound to the left parasternal area, which of the following is the most appropriate way to diagnose cardiac tamponade?*

A. *Chest x-ray*

B. *Pulses paradoxus*

C. *FAST (Focused Assessment with Sonography for Trauma)*

D. *Friction rub*

E. *Computed tomography (CT) scan*

Tamponade should be a clinical diagnosis, and a high level of suspicion must be maintained in any penetrating trauma to the parasternal area. The classic (Beck) triad of hypotension, muffled heart sounds and distended neck veins is often missed in the trauma patient because of the noisy ER setting, and concomitant hypovolemia. Pulsus paradoxus, decreased blood pressure with inspiration, can be difficult to appreciate without the benefit of an arterial tracing, and is present in only 10% of cases. Friction rub is more common with pericarditis than tamponade. A globular heart can be seen on chest x-ray but is neither sensitive nor specific for tamponade. CT scan may reveal pericardial fluid, but should not be performed on patients with suspicion of penetrating cardiac injury. If there is clinical concern, careful physical exam and FAST should be used to confirm the diagnosis. FAST is rapid, immediately available, repeatable, and has a sensitivity nearing 100% in most series.

Surgical Critical Care and Emergency Surgery: Clinical Questions and Answers, First Edition. Edited by Forrest O. Moore, Peter M. Rhee, Samuel A. Tisherman and Gerard J. Fulda.

Answer: C

Demetriades D (1986) Cardiac wounds. Experience with 70 patients. *Annals of Surgery* **203** (3), 315–17.

Rozycki GS, Feliciano DV, Ochsner MG, *et al.* (1999) The role of ultrasound in patients with possible penetrating cardiac wounds: a prospective multicenter study. *Journal of Trauma* **46** (4), 543–52.

3. *In a patient with a multiple rib fractures resulting in flail chest which of the following statement is true?*

A. *The majority of patients do not require mechanical ventilation*

B. *Mechanical ventilation is associated with improved mortality*

C. *Age greater than 45 is associated with improved outcome*

D. *PCA is superior to epidural anesthesia*

E. *Mortality is directly related to the flail injury in most patients*

Flail chest occurs when three or more contiguous ribs are fractured in two or more locations, resulting in a segment of chest wall that can move independently. This will result in paradoxical motion of the flail segment with negative pressure respiration. The majority of patients do not require mechanical ventilation. When necessary, mechanical ventilation is associated with worse prognosis and a variety of complications. Pain control and pulmonary toilet are essential in preventing complications associated with flail chest. Several studies have demonstrated the superiority of epidural anesthesia for pain control, prevention of pneumonia, and decreased need for mechanical ventilation. Increasing age is associated with worsened outcomes, with some studies suggesting that age as low as 45 are associated with increased complications and mortality. When mortality does occur, it is most often due to associated injuries.

Answer: A

Bulger EM, Klotz P, Jurkovich GJ. (2004) Epidural anesthesia improves outcomes after multiple rib fractures. *Surgery* **136** (2), 426–30.

Holcomb JB, McMulin NR, Kozar RA, *et al.* (2003) Morbidity from rib fractures increases after age 45. *Journal of the American College of Surgeons* **196** (4), 549–55.

4. *Hypoxia in flail chest is due to:*

A. *Increased shunt from pulmonary contusion*

B. *Paradoxical chest wall movement*

C. *Change in alveolar diffusion*

D. *Associated hemothorax*

E. *Associated pneumothorax*

Many physiologic changes occur with a flail chest, the paradoxical motion can decrease total lung capacity and functional residual capacity, pain associated with rib fractures can result in splinting and atelectasis, and most importantly the associated contusion can lead to ventilation/perfusion mismatch. There is a complex interplay of these pulmonary mechanics that ultimately culminates in increased shunt fraction resulting in hypoxia. While the mechanical injury to the chest wall undoubtedly contributes to respiratory morbidity, the underlying pulmonary contusion is by far the most important determinant of respiratory status.

Answer: A

Athanassiadi, K, Theakos, N, Kalantzi N, *et al.* (2010) Prognostic factors in flail-chest patients. *European Journal of Cardiothoracic Surgery* April 1 Epub ahead of print.

Livingston DH, Hauser CJ. Chest wall and lung. In: Feliciano DV, Mattox KL, Moore EE (eds) *Trauma*, 6th edn, McGraw Hill, New York, pp. 525–52.

5. *A chest tube is placed in a 43-year-old woman after transmediastinal gunshot wound, bloody drainage was minimal, and she is hemodynamically stable. However, you note a continuous air leak. What is the next step in management?*

A. *Place a second chest tube*

B. *Thoracotomy*

C. *Video-assisted thoracoscopic surgery (VATS)*

D. *Bronchoscopy*

E. *Increase the amount of suction on the chest tube*

Air leaks following trauma are common, they may be due to injury of the airways or lung parenchyma, leaks in the drainage system or from chest wall defects, or be due to intraparenchymal placement of the chest tube. The presence of a large or continuous air leak immediately after injury may indicate tracheobronchial injury and should be investigated with bronchoscopy. Persistent leaks should also be investigated with bronchoscopy. Proximal tracheobronchial injury should be addressed surgically, and bronchoscopy will aid in diagnosis, as well as localization for preoperative planning. Smaller distal air leaks will generally seal without intervention and rarely require more than tube thoracostomy drainage. If mechanical ventilation is required care should be taken to minimize airway pressures while maintaining oxygenation. Paradoxically, increased suction on the drainage system may keep air leaks open, and as long as the pneumothorax is adequately drained decreasing suction or water sealing the thoracostomy tube may promote sealing.

Answer: D

Livingston DH, Hauser CJ (2008) Chest wall and lung. In: Feliciano DV, Mattox KL, Moore EE (eds) Trauma, 6th edn, McGraw-Hill, New York, pp. 525–52.

6. *With regards to diaphragmatic injury following penetrating trauma, which of the following exams has the highest sensitivity?*

A. *CT scan*

B. *Magnetic resonance imaging (MRI)*

C. *Laparoscopy*

D. *Diagnostic peritoneal lavage*

E. *Fluoroscopy*

Diaphragmatic injury may complicate as many as 26% of stab and 13% of gunshot wounds. Any patient with penetrating trauma to the area bounded by the nipples superiorly and costal margin inferiorly should be suspected of having a diaphragmatic injury. Injuries are often asymptomatic and radiographic imaging continues to have poor sensitivity and specificity. Chest x-ray may be normal or non-specific in up to 50% of cases and sensitivity for CT scan ranges from 14–61%. MRI and diagnostic peritoneal lavage have poor sensitivity especially after penetrating trauma. Laparoscopy is the most effective means of both diagnosis and treatment of diaphragmatic injury after penetrating trauma. Sensitivity and negative predictive value are 87.5% and 96.8% respectively.

Answer: C

Friese RS, Coln CE, Gentilello LM (2005) Laparoscopy is sufficient to exclude occult diaphragm injury after penetrating abdominal trauma. *Journal of Trauma* **58**, 789–92.

Murray JA, Demetriades D, Asensio JA, *et al.* (1998) Occult injuries to the diaphragm: Prospective evaluation of laparoscopy in penetrating injuries to the lower left chest. *Journal of the American College of Surgeons* **187**, 626–30.

7. *Which of the following statements regarding subclavian artery injuries is true?*

A. *Injuries are more common after blunt trauma*

B. *Injuries are associated with low overall mortality*

C. *There is a concomitant venous injury in approximately 20% of cases*

D. *Arterial injury is associated with significantly worse outcome compared to venous injury*

E. *Associated neurologic or thoracic injuries are rare affecting <5% of cases*

Subclavian artery injuries are rare and affect less than 3% of all penetrating traumas. Injuries associated with blunt trauma are even more uncommon affecting only 0.4% of patients. These injuries are highly lethal with up to 60% of patients expiring prior to, or upon presentation to, the hospital. Because of the close association of vital structures in this area, associated injuries are common. Concomitant brachial plexus injuries can affect up to one-third of patients with axillary or subclavian artery injuries, and intrathoracic injuries up to 28%. Concomitant venous injury is seen in 20% of cases, and isolated venous injury is associated with a higher mortality when compared to isolated arterial injury. There may be many reasons for the increased mortality among victims of venous injury including; inability of the vein to constrict resulting in increased hemorrhage and air embolus in venous injuries, especially in the hypotensive patient with low intravenous pressure.

Answer: C

Demetriades D, Asensio JA (2001) Subclavian and axillary vascular injuries. *Surgical Clinics of North America* **81** (6), 1357–73.

Demetriades D, Chawan S, Gomez H, *et al.* (1999) Penetrating injuries to the subclavian and axillary vessels. *Journal of the American College of Surgeons* **188**, 290–5.

8. *Of the following; which is an acceptable management option for a subclavian artery injury?*

A. *PTFE or vein interposition graft*

B. *Ligation*

C. *Placement of a temporary shunt*

D. *Angiography and covered stent placement*

E. *All of the above*

In repairing subclavian injuries, the operative approach is dictated by the clinical presentation of the patient. Those *in extremis* or in arrest should undergo resuscitative thoracotomy; those who are more stable may undergo median sternotomy with infraclavicular excision for proximal injuries, and infraclavicular incision alone for more distal injuries. In unstable patients, ligation can be considered because of the rich collateral blood supply, however it comes with a significant risk of compartment syndrome and ischemia. The preferred damage-control technique should be temporary arterial shunting. In the stable patient primary repair can be considered in lacerations as a result of stab wounds. However, in most gunshot injuries and in the rare blunt injury tissue loss makes this unfeasible as this vessel has very little mobility and can be very friable. Any existing defect should be bridged with an interposition graft. There is no evidence to suggest superiority of autologous or artificial graft material and the choice of material should depend on surgeon preference, availability, and condition of the patient. There is growing experience with covered stents for treatment of subclavian artery injuries, primarily pseudoaneurysms, and arteriovenous fistulas. This option should only be used in those patients who present in hemodynamically stable condition with minimal chest tube output.

Answer: E

Demetriades D, Asensio JA (2001) Subclavian and axillary vascular injuries. *Surgical Clinics of North America* **81** (6), 1357–73.

du Toit DF, Lambrechts AV, Stark H, *et al.* (2008) Long-term results of stent graft treatment of subclavian artery injuries: management of choice for stable patients? *Journal of Vascular Surgery* **47** (4), 739–43.

9. *Which of the following statements regarding evaluation of a periclavicular gunshot wound is false?*

A. *Complete neurologic exam including cranial nerves should be performed in the stable patient*

B. *Hemodynamically unstable patients should be explored in the OR immediately*

C. *A normal Ankle-Brachial index definitively rules out arterial injury*

D. *Traditional angiography can be both diagnostic and therapeutic*

E. *CT angiography is an acceptable screening modality in stable patients*

Hemodynamic instability is a hard sign of vascular injury in penetrating trauma and should undergo immediate exploration. Although indications for angiography for both diagnosis and treatment continue to expand hemodynamic instability, critical limb ischemia and active hemorrhage remain contraindications. In stable patients lacking hard signs of vascular injury physical examination should include complete neurologic examination of the affected upper extremity as well as cranial nerve examination as there is a high rate of associated injuries to the brachial plexus, sympathetic chain and cervical nerve roots. Additionally, the Ankle-Brachial Index (ABI) can be performed in stable patients, if the ratio is less than 0.9 further imaging should be performed. Unfortunately, the presence of a normal ABI (>0.9) cannot be relied upon to definitively rule out arterial injury as injuries such as pseudoaneurysm, arterio-venous fistula, and intimal flap may be present with a normal ABI. In all stable patients with suspicion of injury, CT angiography is a viable screening modality. CT angiography has the benefit of speed, ease and a low rate of complications. It can be performed without arterial puncture and does not require the presence of an interventional radiology team. It can also be performed with significantly less contrast than traditional angiography and has the benefit of giving additional information on non-vascular structures such as the spine, soft tissues, lungs and aerodigestive tract.

Answer: C

Demetriades D, Asensio JA (2001) Subclavian and axillary vascular injuries. *Surgical Clinics of North America* **81** (6), 1357–73.

Peng PD, Spain DA, Tataria M, *et al.* (2008) CT angiography effectively evaluates extremity vascular trauma. *American Journal of Surgery* **74** (2), 103–7.

10. *In penetrating cardiac trauma, injury to which chamber of the heart is associated with the best chance of survival?*

A. *Left ventricle*

B. *Right ventricle*

C. *Left atrium*

D. *Right atrium*

E. *Intrapericardial aorta*

In penetrating cardiac injuries, there are several favorable prognostic indicators. Stab wounds have a better outcome than gunshot wounds, with mortality ranging from 14–16% compared to 65–81% respectively. Right heart injuries have a better outcome than left-sided injuries presumably due to lower pressures in the right heart, and ventricular injuries have a better prognosis than atrial injuries likely due to the thicker myocardium. The injury with the worst prognosis is the intra-pericardial aorta, likely due to the very high pressure and thin wall. The presence of vital signs or cardiac tamponade upon arrival has also been associated with improved survival.

Answer: B

Alanezi K, Milencoff GS, Baillie FG, *et al.* (2002) Outcome of major cardiac injuries at a Canadian trauma center. *BMC Surgery* **10**, 2–4.

Tyburski JG, Astra L, Wilson RF, *et al.* (2000) Factors affecting prognosis with penetrating wounds of the heart. *Journal of Trauma* **48** (4), 587–90.

11. *Regarding repair of a cardiac laceration, which of the following is true?*

A. *Thoracotomy is preferred over median sternotomy in stable patients*

B. *Closure of the pericardium is always recommended*

C. *When closing the pericardium it is important not to leave any defects*

D. *Failure to close the pericardium will result in increased postoperative complications*

E. *There is generally less postoperative pain and fewer complications after median sternotomy than thoracotomy*

Unstable patients should undergo resuscitative thoracotomy. Patients with suspected cardiac injuries who are stable should be transferred to the operating room immediately. A median sternotomy is the incision of choice because it does not require special positioning, is fast, provides good exposure to the heart, and is associated with less postoperative pain and fewer pulmonary complications than a thoracotomy. Following repair the pericardium is closed, leaving an opening near the base to avoid tamponade in cases of rebleeding. However, acute cardiomegaly may develop due to heart failure or massive fluid resuscitation in many cases, and in these cases the pericardium should be left open. There does not appear to be any increase in complication rates when the pericardium is left open.

Answer: E

Asensio JA, Soto SN, Forno W, *et al.* (2001) Penetrating cardiac injuries: a complex challenge. *Injury* **32** (7), 533–43.

Degiannis E, Loogna P, Doll D, *et al.* (2006) Penetrating cardiac injuries: recent experience in South Africa. *World Journal of Surgery* **30** (7), 1258–64.

12. *In a patient with a stab wound to the epigastrium undergoing laparotomy for peritonitis, which of the following is the most appropriate test to rule out cardiac injury?*

A. Transdiaphramatic window

B. Subxiphoid window

C. Median sternotomy

D. Echocardiogram

E. Pericardiocentesis

Preoperatively FAST can be used to look for pericardial fluid with excellent sensitivity and specificity. However, in the operating room, if there is suspicion of cardiac injury, imaging is not a timely or practical option. Transdiaphragmatic window during laparotomy can be useful and expeditious in ruling out cardiac injury. It is quickly and easily performed with an excellent sensitivity and specificity and is associated with a very low rate of complications. An incision is made in the central tendinous area of the diaphragm, if the pericardial fluid is bloody, the laparotomy is extended into a median sternotomy. If the pericardial fluid is clear cardiac injury is excluded and the window is sutured. Pericardiocentesis has an unacceptably high false negative rate, up to 80%, because of clotting in the pericardial sac, and there is risk of iatrogenic injury, especially in the absence of tamponade. Subxiphoid window is unnecessary if the abdomen is already open for laparotomy.

Answer: A

Brewster SA, Thirlby RC, Snyder WH (1988) Subxiphoid pericardial window and penetrating cardiac trauma. *Archives of Surgery* **123** (8), 937–41.

Fraga GP, Espinola JP, Mantovani M (2008) Pericardial window used in the diagnosis of cardiac injury. *Acta Circurgica Brasileira* **23** (2), 208–15.

13. *Which of the following is an acceptable screening tool for blunt cardiac injury (BCI)?*

A. Trans-esophageal echocardiogram

B. Trans-thoracic echocardiogram

C. 24-hour Holter monitor

D. Dobutamine stress test

E. ECG

The reported incidence of BCI varies widely from 8–71% due primarily to the wide spectrum of disease, which ranges from mild asymptomatic contusion to free wall rupture. The at-risk population is also broad and includes anyone who has sustained blunt chest trauma. In the hemodynamically stable patient with suspicion of BCI ECG is recommended on admission. If this is normal there is little risk of BCI. However, sensitivity is not 100%, and, if abnormal, the chance of clinically significant BCI is still quite low. Several studies have demonstrated the utility of troponin-I (Tn-I) as a biomarker of traumatic myocardial injury. However, elevations in Tn-I can occur after both penetrating and blunt trauma in the absence of cardiac injury. To identify patients at highest risk of clinically significant BCI, it is best to combine both ECG and Tn-I. The sensitivity and specificity of Tn-I and ECG when combined are 100% and 71% respectively.

Answer: E

Pasquale M, Fabian TC (1998) Practice management guidelines for trauma from the Eastern Association for the Surgery of Trauma. *J Trauma* **44** (6), 941–56.

Velmahos GC, Karaiskakis M, Salim A, *et al.* (2003) Normal electrocardiography and serum troponin I levels preclude the presence of clinically significant blunt cardiac injury. *Journal of Trauma* **54** (1), 45–51.

14. *Following blunt trauma, the chest x-ray of a patient reveals a wide mediastinum. Which of the following must be excluded?*

A. Thymoma

B. Thoracic spine fracture

C. Lymphoma

D. Teratoma

E. Mediastinal thyroid gland

A widened mediastinum can be a result of patient body habitus, positioning, and a variety of pathologies including mediastinal masses. However, in the trauma setting, acute injury must be first on the differential diagnosis. The three most common traumatic etiologies of widened mediastinum include; sternal fracture, thoracic spine fracture and aortic disruption. Sternal fracture can be associated with significant blunt cardiac injury, thoracic spine fractures may be unstable, and thoracic aortic injuries are at risk for rupture if not treated. These possible complications mean that diagnosis must be swift and accurate. Errors in technique or positioning or nontraumatic causes of widened mediastinum should be diagnoses of exclusion. The next step in diagnosis should be CT angiography of the chest. This will accurately diagnose aortic injury, associated pulmonary contusion, as well as soft tissue and bony injuries.

Answer: B

Bruckner BA, DiBardino DJ, Cumbie TC, *et al.* (2006) Critical evaluation of chest computed tomography scans for blunt descending thoracic aortic injury. *Annals of Thoracic Surgery* **81** (4), 1339–46.

Rashid MA, Ortenwall P, Wikstrom T (2001) Cardiovascular injuries associated with sternal fractures. *European Journal of Surgery* **167** (4), 243–8.

van Beek EJ, Been HD, Ponsen KK, *et al.* (2003) Upper thoracic spinal fractures in trauma patients-a diagnostic pitfall. *Injury* **31** (4), 219–23.

15. *A resuscitative thoracotomy is indicated in which of the following clinical scenarios?*

A. *Absence of vital signs when paramedics arrive*

B. *Loss of vitals with cardiopulmonary resuscitation time greater than 15 minutes in penetrating trauma*

C. *Loss of vitals with cardiopulmonary resuscitation time greater than 15 minutes in blunt trauma*

D. *Loss of vitals with cardiopulmonary resuscitation time greater than 15 minutes in pediatric trauma*

E. *Loss of vitals on arrival to the hospital in penetrating trauma*

Resuscitative thoracotomy or emergency department thoracotomy (EDT) is performed to address cardiovascular collapse. It will allow evacuation of hemothorax/pneumothorax, release of tamponade, repair of cardiac and intrathoracic vessel injuries, evacuation of air embolus, clamping of hilar injuries, cross clamping of the aorta, and performance of open cardiac massage. Indications for EDT are difficult to clarify and can change from institution to institution. However, in general EDT is indicated for patients with witnessed arrest with cardiopulmonary resuscitation (CPR) less than 15 minutes following penetrating thoracic trauma, witnessed arrest with CPR less than 5 minutes following penetrating non-thoracic trauma, witnessed arrest with CPR less than 5 minutes following blunt trauma, and persistent hypotension due to tamponade or intrathoracic hemorrhage. Outcomes are best with penetrating cardiac injury, followed by penetrating non-cardiac thoracic trauma. Outcomes following penetrating abdominal trauma and blunt trauma are poor. Outcomes in children are similar to adults and indications for pediatric EDT are similar to those for adults.

Answer: E

Rhee PM, Acosta J, Bridgeman A, *et al.* (2000) Survival after emergency department thoracotomy: Review of published date from the past 25 years. *Journal of the American College of Surgeons* **190** (3), 288–98.

Working Group, Ad Hoc Subcommittee on Outcomes, American College of Surgeons-Committee on Trauma (2001) Practice management guidelines for emergency department thoracotomy. *Journal of the American College of Surgeons* **193** (3), 303–9.

16. *Which of the following is not an acceptable treatment for traumatic aortic injury?*

A. *Open repair*

B. *Endovascular stent graft*

C. *Blood pressure control*

D. *Temporary intravascular shunt*

E. *Video-assisted thoracoscopic surgery (VATS)*

The diagnosis and treatment of traumatic aortic injury has undergone a number of changes in recent years. Two multicenter prospective observational studies revealed almost complete conversion from aortography to CT scan for diagnosis and increasing utilization of stent grafts for treatment.

Additionally, when open repair is chosen, bypass is frequently preferred to the clamp-and-sew technique. Open repair is generally performed via posterolateral thoracotomy, although anterolateral thoracotomy may be used for patients who are in extremis, and median sternotomy is used for injuries to the ascending aorta or arch. In addition to open and endovascular repair, nonoperative management with aggressive blood pressure control has become an acceptable treatment option, especially in the elderly patient with multiple co-morbidities, or in patients with minor intimal tears. Shunting is also a viable treatment option in the unstable patient in a damage control situation, although data on patency rates and long term outcomes are lacking.

Answer: E

Demetriades D, Velmahos GC, Scalea TM, *et al.* Diagnosis and treatment of blunt thoracic aortic injuries: Changing perspectives. *Journal of Trauma* 2008; **64** (6), 1415–19.

Ding W, Wu X, Li J (2008) Temporary intravascular shunts used as a damage control surgery adjunct in complex vascular injury: Collective review. *Injury* **39**, 970–7.

17. *Which of the following is an acceptable modality for diagnosis of traumatic aortic injury?*

A. *CT angiography*

B. *Chest x-ray*

C. *FAST*

D. *Transthoracic echocardiography*

E. *PET scan*

Traumatic aortic injury is a rare but potentially lethal complication following thoracic trauma. Chest x-ray has been utilized in the past as a screening exam; however, x-ray can be normal in up to 33% of patients with traumatic aortic injury, and positive findings are nonspecific. While transesophageal echocardiography has a reported sensitivity of 90–100%, transthoracic echocardiography and FAST have low diagnostic yield and accuracy for aortic injury, especially in the presence of chest-wall injuries. MRI can be used for diagnosis with a sensitivity and specificity of 98%. However, MRI has the drawbacks of poor availability and lengthy exam times outside of a monitored critical care setting. The CT scan is increasing in popularity as a screening and diagnostic tool, with sensitivity and specificity ranging from 95–100% in most studies. Additionally, CT scan is widely available in most centers, rapid, easily interpreted and does not require arterial puncture. Aortography was previously the gold standard; however, it is utilized now primarily for therapy as it is invasive and requires the presence of a specialty angiography team.

Answer: A

Bruckner BA, DiBardino DJ, Cumbie TC, *et al.* (2006) Critical evaluation of chest computed tomography scans for blunt descending thoracic aortic injury. *Annals of Thoracic Surgery* **81** (4), 1339–46.

Khalil A, Tarik T, Porembka DT (2007) Aortic pathology: aortic trauma, debris, dissection, and aneurysm. *Critical Care Medicine* **35** (8), (suppl.) S392–S400.

18. *A 37-year-old man sustains blunt chest trauma requiring chest tube for drainage of a hemopneumothorax. After placement of the chest tube there is residual opacification on chest x-ray, subsequent CT scan reveals a retained hemothorax. Which of the following is an acceptable treatment option?*

A. *Systemic thrombolysis*

B. *Intrathoracic thrombolysis*

C. *Postural drainage with chest physiotherapy*

D. *Increasing suction on the chest tube*

E. *Administration of antibiotics*

Retained hemothorax can complicate the hospital course of 3–8% of patients with traumatic hemothorax. Retained blood may occur as a result of delay in presentation, delay in diagnosis/treatment, and thoracostomy tube malposition, migration, or occlusion. Retained blood may result in empyema or fibrothorax. The options for treatment include open drainage, video-assisted thoracoscopic drainage, and intrapleural thrombolysis.

Several studies and a meta-analysis of intrapleural thrombolysis have revealed promising results with complete clinical and radiographic resolution in over 90% of cases in most studies. In contrast, postural drainage, chest physiotherapy and increased suction on the thoracostomy tube are unlikely to resolve retained hemothoraces. Not only is administration of antibiotics unlikely to resolve the hemothorax, but it is also unlikely to prevent infection of retained fluid collections.

Answer: B

Hunt I, Thakar C, Southon R, *et al.* (2009) Establishing a role for intra-pleural fibrinolysis in managing traumatic hemothoraces. *Interactive Journal of Cardiovascular and Thoracic Surgery* **8**, 129–33.

Kimbrell BJ, Yamzon J, Petrone P, *et al.* (2007) Intrapleural thrombolysis for management of undrained traumatic hemothorax: A prospective observational study. *Journal of Trauma* **62** (5), 1175–9.

Chapter 29 Abdominal and Abdominal Vascular Injury

Leslie Kobayashi, MD

1. *Which of the following is a contraindication to a trial of non-operative management in liver injury?*

A. *Pediatric patient*

B. *Grade IV injury*

C. *Elderly patient*

D. *Peritonitis*

E. *Penetrating mechanism*

Initially, criteria for nonoperative management (NOM) included Grade I-III injury, intact mental status, age <65 years, reliable abdominal exam, and transfusion of <2 units of packed red blood cells. Success rates using these criteria were 80–95%. However, current data indicate that age, grade of injury, mechanism, and even comatose state need not be contraindications for NOM in stable patients. Success rates of up to 40% were reported in stable patients with grade IV and V injuries, furthermore, no statistically significant differences could be identified among failure rates in patients with a depressed GCS. A study conducted in patients older than 55 revealed a success rate of 97% with NOM. Current contraindications to NOM include hypotension unresponsive to resuscitation, peritonitis, and concomitant injury requiring surgical repair, although controversial patients with liver injury and hypotension who are responders, meaning they respond to fluid resuscitation and/or transfusion with an increase in blood pressure to acceptable levels, may be candidates for angiographic treatment. However, in these patients there should be a low threshold to convert to laparotomy should they cease responding to resuscitation or have worsening abdominal exam or evidence of ongoing hemorrhage following angiography.

Surgical Critical Care and Emergency Surgery: Clinical Questions and Answers, First Edition. Edited by Forrest O. Moore, Peter M. Rhee, Samuel A. Tisherman and Gerard J. Fulda.

Answer: D

Asensio JA, Roldán G, Petrone P, *et al.* (2003) Operative management and outcomes in 103 AAST-OIS Grades IV and V complex hepatic Injuries: Trauma surgeons still need to operate, but angioembolization helps. *Journal of Trauma* **54** (4), 647–54.

Falmirski ME, Provost D (2000) Nonsurgical management of solid abdominal organ injury in patients over 55 years of age. *The American Surgeon* **66** (7), 631–5.

2. *A 34-year-old man is hypotensive after a motorcycle crash. His abdomen is non-tender, his pelvis is unstable, and x-ray demonstrates a severe open book fracture. After receiving 2 L of ringers lactate he is still hypotensive. What is the most immediate next step in management?*

A. *CT scan of the abdomen and pelvis with IV contrast*

B. *Application of a pelvic binder*

C. *Angiography*

D. *Exploratory laparotomy*

E. *Bilateral needle thoracostomy*

If hypotension is present with pelvic fracture, the pelvic ring should be reapproximated as soon as possible. Stabilization devices include pelvic binders, external fixators, and sheets. Binders or sheets are fitted over the anterior superior iliac spines superiorly, and the femoral heads inferiorly. If orthopedic surgeons are available an external fixation device can be placed to reapproximate the pelvic ring. Stabilization devices close the pelvic ring decreasing pelvic volume to tamponade bleeding. They also stabilize the broken ends of bone preventing further injury to nearby tissues and decrease pain with repositioning and transport. Hemorrhage associated with pelvic fracture can cause significant hypotension and carries a high mortality. The majority of bleeding is from the sacral venous plexus. Occasionally bleeding may be from an arterial source. In stable or semi-stable patients with pelvic hemorrhage, angiography should be considered for diagnostic and therapeutic purposes. If significant arterial bleeding is found, selective embolization can be performed. If no arterial bleeding is found, bilateral internal iliac artery embolization can be performed to decrease pelvic inflow. The rich collateral circulation in the pelvis prevents ischemic complications in most patients. Very rarely, complications such as necrosis of pelvic organs or glutteal compartment syndrome can occur. Transfusion of blood products are also a very important aspect of immediate therapy that can be initiated but stopping bleeding is the highest priority.

Answer: B

Cothren CC, Osborn PM, Moore EE, *et al.* (2007) Preperitoneal pelvic packing for hemodynamically unstable pelvic fractures: a paradigm shift. *Journal of Trauma* **62** (4), 834–9; discussion 839–42.

Velmahos GC, Chahwan S, Hanks SE, *et al.* (2000) Angiographic embolization of bilateral internal iliac arteries to control life-threatening hemorrhage after blunt trauma to the pelvis. *American Journal of Surgery* **66** (9), 858–62.

3. *A patient sustains a liver injury with a blush noted on CT scan as well as a posterior knee dislocation after a motor vehicle crash. Which of the following is the next best step in management?*

A. *Angiography*

B. *Operative repair of the dislocated knee*

C. *Repeat CT scan of the abdomen*

D. *Placement of a traction pin to reduce the knee dislocation*

E. *Laparotomy*

Stable patients with any injury grade and evidence of intraparenchymal extravasation of contrast are candidates for angiography and possible embolization. Angio-embolization can be used before, after, or instead of, surgery. It is required in 5–6% of patients with liver injury and has a success rate of 80–100%. Complications of embolization are not rare and include hepatic necrosis, abscess, and bile leak. Timing of angiography appears to affect morbidity and mortality, with better outcomes observed in patients undergoing early compared with late angiography. In this patient there is a second indication for angiography, as it can also be used to diagnose popliteal artery injury, which is associated with knee dislocation.

Answer: A

Mohr AM, Lavery RF, Barone A, *et al.* (2003) Angiographic embolization for liver injuries: Low mortality, high morbidity. *Journal of Trauma* **55**, 1077–82.

Wahl WL, Ahrns KS, Brandt MM, *et al.* (2002) The need for early angiographic embolization in blunt liver injuries. *Journal of Trauma* **52** (6), 1097–101.

4. *A patient presents after high speed motorcycle crash. Pelvis x-ray reveals bilateral pubic rami fractures and there is blood at the urethral meatus, which of the following should be the next step in management?*

A. *Retrograde urethrogram*

B. *CT cystogram*

C. *Intravenous pyelogram*

D. *Diagnostic peritoneal lavage*

E. *CT of the bony pelvis*

Urethral injury is rare, occurring in 4–10% of patients with pelvic fractures. Blood at the urethral meatus, perineal hematoma, high riding prostate on rectal exam, and inability to void or gross hematuria are all indicators of urethral injury. When present, suspicion for urethral injury should be high and retrograde urethrogram (RUG) should be performed. This can be done by placing a small foley catheter in the fossa navicularis and partially inflating the balloon, or using a non-crushing clamp on the end of the penis to prevent contrast leakage. Approximately 30 mL of full strength contrast is then injected and ideally fluoroscopy is used to assess for extravasation, if not available at least two views using plain radiographs should be taken. Ideally one view will be oblique. While concomitant bladder injury is seen in up to 15% of patients with urethral injury, no attempt should be made to interrogate the bladder or place a foley catheter until a RUG can be performed to rule out urethral injury.

Answer: A

Coburn M (2008) Genitourinary trauma. In: Feliciano DV, Mattox KL, Moore EE (eds) *Trauma,* 6th edn, McGraw Hill, New York, pp. 789–825.

5. *Which of the following is a contraindication to non-operative management of splenic injury?*

A. *Concomitant liver injury*

B. *Peritionitis*

C. *Hemoperitoneum*

D. *Blush on CT scan*

E. *Concomitant pelvic fracture*

Rates of success with splenic nonoperative management (NOM) can be as high as 95% for pediatric an 80% for adult populations. There are two strict contraindications for NOM, peritonitis and hemodynamic instability. Studies have shown acceptable rates of success with NOM in patients with neurologic injury and in patients with concerning CT findings such as high grade injury, blush or hemoperitoneum. While these factors increase the risk for failure they should not be considered strict contraindications to NOM in the stable patient. The addition of angiography with and without embolization has augmented success rates of NOM. Angiography is particularly attractive as an adjunct to NOM in patients with multiple solid organ injuries or concomitant pelvic fracture as it can be diagnostic and therapeutic in these patients with multiple potential sources of hemorrhage.

Answer: B

Jacoby RC, Wisner DH (2008) Injury to the spleen. In: Feliciano DV, Mattox KL, Moore EE (eds) *Trauma,* 6th edn. McGraw Hill, New York, pp. 661–80.

Stein DJ, Scalea TM (2006) Nonoperative management of spleen and liver injuries. *Journal of Intensive Care Medicine* **21** (5), 296–304.

6. *A patient undergoes laparotomy and hepatorraphy for grade IV liver injury. Postoperatively the patient develops bilious output from his drains. He was made nothing per os (NPO), and started on octreotide he is stable and asymptomatic but the drainage persists what is the next step in management?*

A. *Laparotomy*

B. *Endoscopy*

C. *Angiography*

D. *Endoscopic retrograde cholangiopancreatography (ERCP)*

E. *Ultrasound*

Answer: D

Bile leak or biloma formation can complicate the course of 0.5–20% of patients following liver injury. The incidence is slightly higher in operative compared to non-operative patients, and in patients with higher grade injuries. Often these collections are asymptomatic and up to 70% resolve spontaneously. Symptomatic patients with fever, leukocytosis, pain, jaundice, or feeding intolerance, are best treated with image-guided drainage. Percutaneous drainage has a very high success rate. If bilous drainage persists, ERCP with sphincterotomy or stent placement is effective. Surgery can be considered for fluid collections not amenable to percutaneous drainage, or for proximal bile leaks that fail to resolve with ERCP decompression.

Kozar RA, Moore FA, Cothren CC, *et al.* (2006) Risk factors for hepatic morbidity following nonoperative management. *Archives of Surgery* **141**, 451–9.

Marks JM, Ponsky JL, Shillingstad RB, *et al.* (1998) Biliary stenting is more effective than sphincterotomy in the resolution of biliary leaks. *Surgery Endoscopy* **12** (4), 327–30.

7. *Regarding seat belt signs on the abdomen which of the following statements is false?*

A. *They are associated with increased mortality*

B. *They are associated with lumbar spine fractures*

C. *They are associated with pancreatic injury*

D. *They are associated with duodenal injuries*

E. *They are associated with mesenteric injuries*

The presence of a seat belt sign (SBS) on the abdomen is associated with a significant increase in intra-abdominal injuries. In adult populations the presence of a SBS increases the risk of intra-abdominal injury twofold to eightfold. A SBS may be even more concerning in pediatric patients where rates of intra-abdominal injury can be increased as much as twelvefold. Hollow viscous, particularly the duodenum, and mesenteric injuries are markedly increased and the threshold to operate on a patient with free fluid and a SBS should be very low. Additionally, pancreatic injury is increased especially in the pediatric population. Lastly, the use of a lap belt without concomitant use of a shoulder restraint has been associated with chance fracture of the lumbar spine. However, despite increased risk of intra-abdominal injury SBS is not associated with increased mortality. In fact, in a recent study, despite patients with SBS being older, more severely injured and at higher risk of having intra-abdominal injuries, mortality was lower than that of patients without SBS.

Answer: A

Bansal V, Conroy C, Tominaga GT, *et al*. The utility of seat belt signs to predict intra-abdominal injury following motor vehicle crashes. *Traffic Injury Prevention*. 2009; **10**, 567–72.

Sharma OP, Oswanski MJ, Kaminski BP, *et al.* (2009) Clinical implications of the seat belt sign in blunt trauma. *American Journal of Surgery* **75** (9), 822–7.

8. *After falling a patient is found to have a renal artery injury with thrombosis and ischemia. Which of the following statements regarding renal injury is true?*

A. *Hypertension can be an early complication of non-operative management*

B. *Revascularization of the injured kidney generally results in good outcomes*

C. *Complications are more common following nephrectomy than nephrorraphy*

D. *Acute renal failure following nephrectomy is generally permanent*

E. *Non-operative management of renal injuries has a high success rate*

Kidney injury occurs in 1–3% of all trauma patients and up to 10% of abdominal traumas. Blunt mechanisms are far more common than penetrating, accounting for approximately 60% of injuries. Blunt trauma to the renal vessels is more likely to result in thrombosis, whereas penetrating trauma more often results in bleeding. Nonoperative management is successful in >90% of cases. Risk factors for failure include high-grade injuries, large perinephric hematomas, and urinary extravasation. The only absolute contra-indication to non-operative management is hemodynamic instability. In the cases of renal artery thrombosis, warm ischemia time is the most important determining factor in renal salvage rates. Outcomes are generally disappointing following revascularization and are dismal if revascularization is delayed beyond 6–12 hours. Complications, including recurrence of bleeding, abscess, and urine leak are more common following nephrorraphy than nephrectomy. Early complications include re-bleeding, urine leak, and abscess. Late complications include Page kidney, renovasular hypertension and hydronephrosis. Acute renal dysfunction can occur after traumatic nephrectomy, but tends to be transient and self-limited.

Answer: E

Coburn, M (2008) Genitourinary trauma. In: Feliciano DV, Mattox KL, Moore EE (eds) *Trauma*, 6th edn. McGraw Hill, New York, pp. 789–825.

Starnes M, Demetriades D, Hadjizacharia P, *et al.* (2010) Complications following renal trauma. *Archives of Surgery* **145** (4); 377–81.

9. *Which of the following statements regarding blunt pancreatic trauma is true?*

A. *Pancreatic injury is common following motor vehicle accident*

B. *Injury is more common in adults than children*

C. *Associated injuries are uncommon*

D. *Transection following blunt trauma typically occurs near the mesenteric vessels*

E. *Duct disruption is common following blunt injury*

Pancreatic injury following blunt trauma is uncommon, occurring in less than 2% of abdominal trauma cases. Because they tend to have less intraperitoneal and extraperitoneal abdominal fat, children tend to be at increased risk of pancreatic injury. The force required to injure this organ is significant and associated injuries are common, occurring in 70–90% of cases. Anterior-posterior compression of the pancreas against the lumbar spine results in transection at this location in two-thirds of patients, adjacent and just to the left of the superior mesenteric vessels. While duct integrity is the main determinant of intervention and outcome, major duct injury is rare, occurring in less than 15% of pancreatic injuries, and is much more common following penetrating than blunt trauma. Low-grade injuries require drainage and bowel rest only. If the main duct is injured in the pancreatic tail or body distal to the neck, distal pancreatectomy is the best treatment. If the duct injury is more proximal options for management include subtotal pancreatectomy, external drainage with postoperative ERCP, and distal drainage with roux-en-Y pancreaticojejunostomy.

Answer: D

Fabian T, Kudsk K, Croce M, *et al.* (1990) Superiority of closed suction drainage for pancreatic trauma: A randomized prospective study. *Annals of Surgery* **211** (6), 724–8.

Patton JH, Lyden SP, Croce MA, *et al.* (1997) Pancreatic trauma: a simplified management guideline. *Journal of Trauma* **43** (2), 234–9.

10. *Regarding iliac vein injuries, which of the following is true?*

A. *Most blunt injuries can be repaired primarily*

B. *Mortality is low*

C. *Mortality and morbidity increase with concomitant arterial injury*

D. *Compartment syndrome is a common complication following isolated venous injury*

E. *Post-phlebitic syndrome is an early complication*

Iliac vein injury can occur after blunt or penetrating trauma and as a result of iatrogenic injury following pelvic procedures. Mortality can be as high as 70%. Mortality and morbidity are increased with concomitant arterial injury. Minor lacerations can be repaired primarily, however more destructive injuries associated with gunshot wounds and blunt trauma most often require ligation. Complications following ligation include extremity edema, compartment syndrome, thromboembolic complications, and outflow ischemia. Leg edema is common after ligation but compartment syndrome is rare unless there is also arterial injury or prolonged hypotension. Post-phlebitic syndrome characterized by venous hypertension and incompetence, chronic edema, and ulceration can also occur in the late postoperative period.

Answer: C

Pappas PJ, Haser PB, Teehan EP, *et al.* (1997) Outcome of complex venous reconstruction in patients with trauma. *Journal of Vascular Surgery* **25**, 398–404.

Quan RW, Gillespie DL, Stuart RP, *et al.* (2008) The effect of vein repair on the risk of venous thromboembolic events: a review of more than 100 traumatic military venous injuries. *Journal of Vascular Surgery* **47**, 571–7.

11. *Regarding destructive colon injuries, which of the following statements is false?*

A. *Blood transfusion >/= 4 units is associated with increased infectious complications*

B. *Prophylactic antibiotics should be discontinued after 24 hours*

C. *Inappropriate choice of antibiotic is associated with increased infectious complications*

D. *Hypotension is associated with increased infectious complications*

E. *Primary anastamosis is associated with increased complications compared to colostomy*

Destructive colon injuries have a very high rate of postoperative complications ranging from 20–40%. Complications include ileus, abscess, wound infection, and anastamotic leak. Several factors can significantly increase the rate of complications following surgical repair or resection. A large multicenter prospective observational trial identified severe fecal contamination, transfusion of 4 units of blood or greater, and inappropriate antibiotic prophylaxis as independent predictors of postoperative complications. It also found that the method of repair had no effect on the rate of complications. Several other studies have supported these findings, and additionally identified blood loss greater than 1 L, and hypotension as being risk factors for infectious complications. Lastly, several studies have found no additional benefit to continuing antibiotic coverage beyond 24 hours postoperatively regardless of the extent of contamination.

Answer: E

Demetriades D, Murray JA, Chan L, *et al.* (2001) Penetrating colon injuries requiring resection: Diversion or primary anastamosis? An AAST prospective multicenter study. *Journal of Trauma* **50** (5), 765–75.

Murray JA, Demetriades D, Colson M, *et al.* (1999) Colonic resection in trauma: colostomy versus anastamosis. *Journal of Trauma* **46**, 250–4.

12. *Which of the following retroperitoneal hematomas should be surgically explored?*

A. *Zone I hematoma following blunt trauma*

B. *Zone II hematoma following blunt trauma*

C. *Zone III hematoma following blunt trauma*

D. *Retrohepatic hematoma following blunt trauma*

E. *Retrohepatic hematoma following penetrating trauma*

Zone I hematomas are centrally located and contain the major abdominal vessels, because of this vascular injury is highly suspected and Zone I hematomas due to both blunt and penetrating trauma should be explored. Zone II, the lateral upper abdomen, contains the kidneys and renal vessels. Injuries due to blunt trauma in this area are unlikely to require surgical repair and hematomas should be left intact. Zone III is the pelvic retroperitoneum containing the iliac vessels, ureters, rectum and the sacral venous plexus. Following penetrating trauma, major vascular or hollow viscous injuries are common and all hematomas should be explored. However this is less likely following blunt trauma and the risk of releasing venous hemorrhage is high. Most bleeding associated with pelvic fracture following blunt trauma is not amenable to surgical correction and is more likely to respond to interventional techniques or pelvic stabilization. Therefore Zone III blunt hematomas should not be explored. The retrohepatic area contains the inferior vena cava (IVC); this area is difficult to access and injuries to this portion of the IVC are difficult to control. Tamponade is possible even with major vascular injury in this area, and release of tamponade can result in exsanguinating hemorrhage. Stable hematomas resulting from both penetrating and blunt trauma in this area should not be explored.

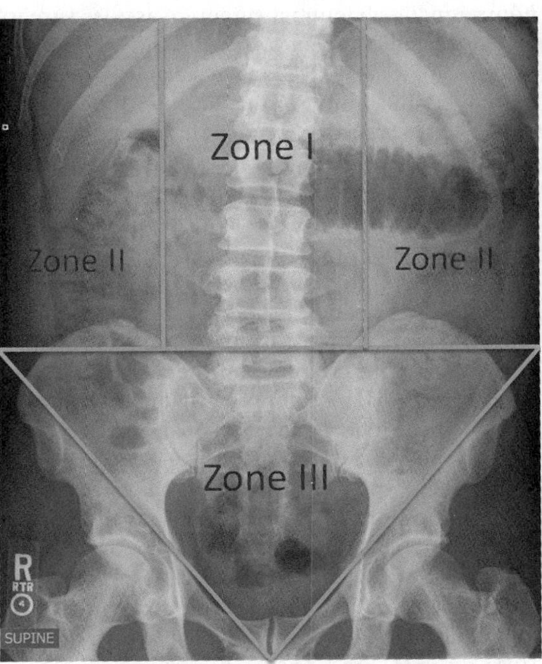

Retroperitoneal zones

Answer: A

Buckman RF, Pathak AS, Badellino MM, *et al.* (2001) Injuries of the inferior vena cava. *Surgical Clinics of North America* **81** (6), 1431–47.

Feliciano DV (1990) Management of traumatic retroperitoneal hematoma. *Annals of Surgery* 1990; **211** (2), 109–23.

13. *Of the following, which is/are taken into account when considering damage-control laparotomy and temporary abdominal closure?*

A. *Physiologic state*

B. *Coagulopathy*

C. *Injury burden*

D. *Fluid/transfusion requirements*

E. *All of the above*

Damage-control surgery (DCS) is a concept originally intended for management of the severely injured exsanguinating trauma patient. It has since been applied to many surgical conditions including nontraumatic abdominal surgery, vascular surgery and orthopedic surgery. The concept of damage-control laparotomy (DCL) is to stage the treatment of catastrophic injuries or insults into three distinct phases. First, control of acute hemorrhage and contamination, second resuscitation, and third planned re-exploration for definitive treatment of surgical pathology. Indications for DCL include hemodynamic instability, severe medical coagulopathy, acidosis (pH <7.2), hypothermia (<35 °C), injuries to multiple body cavities, prohibitively long operative time, and massive transfusion requirements. DCL is not without complication and the decision to convert the goals of laparotomy from definitive care to DCL should not be made based on a single variable, but on the global clinical picture. However, the decision to perform DCL should be made early in the procedure, and ideally will precede actual manifestations of the bloody viscous triad (acidosis, coagulopathy, and bleeding). Severe injury burden, multicavitary injury, and poor physiologic reserve, should also factor into the decision to pursue DCL. This procedure can be controversial as DCL is associated with complications including ventral hernias and enteric fistulas.

Answer: E

Higa G, Friese R, O'Keeffe T, *et al.* (2010) Damage control laparotomy: a vital tool once over utilized. *Journal of Trauma* **69** (1), 53–9.

Rotondo MF, Schwab W, McGonigal MD, *et al.* (1993) Damage control: An approach for improved survival in exsanguinating penetrating abdominal injury. *Journal Trauma* **35** (3), 375–82.

14. *Which of the following methods is an option for temporary abdominal closure in primary damage-control surgery?*

A. *Whip stitching of the skin*

B. *Closure of the skin with towel clips*

C. *Vacuum-assisted wound closure*

D. *Primary fascial closure*

E. *Primary fascial closure with retention sutures*

Any temporary abdominal closure (TAC) must maintain sterility, protect the bowel, prevent evisceration, and prevent adhesions. Additionally as there may be significant drainage from the abdominal cavity the closure method must have a means of collecting, removing and quantifying this drainage. Methods that reapproximate fascia or skin may create abdominal compartment syndrome and should be taken into account. There are some surgeons that prefer to approximate the skin over a suction system as it avoids the loss of domain. Facial closures are usually avoided to preserve it for definitive closure. The two most popular techniques are vacuum-assisted abdominal dressings and the Bogota bag. Vacuum-assisted closure can be performed with commercially available materials, or following the Barker method. The Bogota bag uses sterile plastic sutured to the skin to create an abdominal silo. At the time of repeat laparotomy a number of definitive and TAC methods are available, these include primary closure with or without retention sutures, biologic or artificial graft assisted closure, the previously mentioned TAC methods, as well as devices that attempt to reduce loss of domain. These devices include the Wittmann patch, Zipper, and ABRA dynamic fascial closure device. There is also the option of skin closure, or placement of absorbable mesh with planned ventral hernia. Many physicians also combine methods using a combination of dynamic retention sutures with Barker or other type of vacuum closure system in order to decrease the loss of abdominal domain.

Answer: C

Cothren CC, Moore EE, Johnson JL, *et al.* (2006) One hundred percent fascial approximation with sequential abdominal closure of the open abdomen. *The American Journal of Surgery* **192**, 238–42.

Van Hensbroek PB, Wind J, Dijkgraaf MGW, *et al.* (2009) Temporary closure of the open abdomen: A systematic review on delayed primary fascial closure in patients with an open abdomen. *World Journal of Surgeon* **33**, 199–207.

15. *Following splenectomy for trauma, vaccinations should be sure to include which of the following organisms?*

A. *Enterobacter aerogenes*

B. *Haemophilus influenzae*

C. *Staphlococcus aureus*

D. *Klebsiella pneumonia*

E. *Pseudomonas aeruginosa*

The spleen produces tuftsin and properdin, post-splenectomy patients have diminished immunity and are most at risk for infection from encapsulated organisms. These include *Streptococcus pneumonia, Hemophilus influenzae,* and *Neisseria meningitidis.* Following splenectomy, patients should receive Haemophilus, meningococcal, and pneumococcal vaccinations. Vaccinations are ideally given prior to surgery, however this is not possible in trauma patients. There is evidence to suggest vaccinations should be given 14 days following traumatic splenectomy as immunoglobulin titers are highest following vaccination in this time period. However, as many patients fail to follow up after trauma, vaccinations should be given at 14 days if possible or prior to discharge from the hospital.

Answer: B

Shatz DV, Schinsky MF, Pais LR, *et al.* (1998) Immune responses of splenectomized trauma patients to the 23-valent pneumococcal polysaccharide vaccine at 1 versus 7 versus 14 days after splenectomy. *Journal of Trauma* **44** (5), 760–5.

Vercruysse GA, Feliciano DV (2009) The spleen. In: Gracias VH, Reilly PM, McKenney MG, Velmahos GC (eds) *Acute Care Surgery: A Guide for General Surgeons,* McGraw-Hill, New York, pp. 147–51.

16. *The second stage of damage-control surgery is aimed at correcting which of the following values?*

A. *Acidosis*

B. *Alkalosis*

C. *Hypercarbia*

D. *Hypoxia*

E. *Hypernatremia*

Damage-control surgery (DCS) consists of three phases. The first includes operative control of active hemorrhage and gross contamination. The second phase is resuscitation to correct physiologic derangement. The third phase consists of definitive management of injuries and abdominal closure. Patients with severe trauma often present with extreme physiologic derangements including acidosis due to volume losses, hypoperfusion and anaerobic metabolism; hypothermia; and subsequent coagulopathy. Prolonged surgery with cavitary exposure is likely to exacerbate all of these derangements and contribute to morbidity and mortality. Therefore the initial surgery should be abbreviated and transfer to the ICU for rewarming and resuscitation should occur as soon as possible. The goal of resuscitation is to reverse acidosis with restoration of circulating blood volume using one-to-one plasma-to-red-cell ratios and massive transfusion protocols. Additionally, blankets, forced air warmers, ventilation with warmed humidified air, and warm fluids should be used to correct hypothermia. All of these interventions should help correct hypotension, and reverse coagulopathy. Additionally, evidence of return of normal physiology such as increased urine output or clearance of elevated lactate levels should occur before starting phase 3 of DCS.

Answer: A

Rotondo MF, Schwab W, McGonigal MD, *et al.* (1993) Damage control: An approach for improved survival in exsanguinating penetrating abdominal injury. *Journal of Trauma* **35** (3), 375–82.

Waibel BH, Rotondo MF (2010) Damage control in trauma and abdominal sepsis. *Critical Care Medical* **38** (9 Suppl), S421–S430.

17. *Which of the following is currently recommended for the treatment for extra-peritoneal rectal injury?*

A. *Prolonged antibiotic course*

B. *Pre-sacral drainage*

C. *Diverting colostomy*

D. *Trans-peritoneal repair*

E. *Rectal lavage*

Treatment of extraperitoneal rectal injuries has evolved over the past decades. Traditionally these injuries were treated with the triple approach of diversion, presacral drainage, and rectal lavage. It now appears that this complex and invasive treatment strategy is unnecessary. Comparisons of patients with and without presacral drainage show no benefit in terms of speed of recovery or prevention of abscess or pelvic sepsis. Findings were similar for rectal lavage, with some studies even suggesting worse outcomes with lavage. Similar to other studies of prophylactic antibiotics, prolonged treatment courses do not decrease rates of infectious complications, and most authors only recommend perioperative treatment for 24 hours. While transanal repair may be useful in some patients where injuries are easily accessible, there is no role for trans-peritoneal repair of isolated rectal injuries as this offers no benefit over diversion alone and often results in increased complication rates. Most studies continue to recommend fecal diversion with either open or laparoscopic colostomy.

Answer: C

Gonzalez RP, Falimirski ME, Holevar MR (1998) The role of presacral drainage in the management of penetrating rectal injuries. *Journal of Trauma* **45**, 656–61.

Gonzalez RP, Phelan H, Hassan M, *et al.* (2006) Is fecal diversion necessary for nondestructive penetrating extraperitoneal rectal injuries? *Journal of Trauma* **61** (4), 815–19.

18. *Regarding intra-abdominal hypertension (IAH) and abdominal compartment syndrome (ACS) which of the following statements is true?*

A. *ACS can affect multiple organ systems including neurologic, cardiac, pulmonary, gastrointestinal, hepatic, and renal*

B. *Temporary abdominal closure effectively precludes the diagnosis of ACS*

C. *A bladder pressure of <20 effectively rules out the diagnosis of ACS*

D. *Physical examination is a reliable method for diagnosing IAH and ACS*

E. *Non-invasive therapies rarely succeed in treating IAH or ACS*

Abdominal compartment syndrome is defined by the World Society of the Abdominal Compartment Syndrome as sustained IAH >20 mm Hg associated with new organ dysfunction or failure. Intra-abdominal hypertension is defined as sustained intra-abdominal pressure of 12 mm Hg or greater. Abdominal compartment syndrome can affect many body systems including neurologic, cardiac, pulmonary, gastrointestinal, hepatic, and genitourinary. Risk factors for ACS include severe intra-abdominal trauma, high volume resuscitation, intra-abdominal sepsis, and inflammatory states such as pancreatitis or severe burns. Increasing use of temporary abdominal closure methods may decrease risks of IAH/ACS, however, while ACS is less likely it is not impossible. Patients at high risk for ACS, or those with new onset organ failure should have measurements of their intra-abdominal pressure even if a temporary closure is used. As with other types of compartment syndrome, the absolute value of intra-abdominal pressure is not as important as the perfusion pressure and the clinical picture. A patient may have ACS with organ failure with intra-abdominal pressures below 20 mm Hg, conversely patients with abdominal pressures above 20 mm Hg may not display adverse physiology. The most accurate way to determine intra-abdominal pressure is with intravesicular measurement. Physical examination has a very poor sensitivity even in experienced individuals with sensitivity ranging from 40–60%. Treatment includes adequate sedation, pain control, pharmacologic paralysis, nasogastric decompression, percutaneous catheter decompression, and surgical decompression. Non-invasive methods of treatment especially pharmacologic paralysis and catheter decompression have been shown to be very effective in treating IAH, and even ACS in certain patient populations.

Answer: A

Cheatham MK, Malbrain MLNG, Kirkpatrick A, *et al.* (2007) Results from the international conference of experts on intra-abdominal hypertension and abdominal compartment syndrome. II Recommendations. *Intensive Care Medicine* **33**, 951–62.

Chapter 30 Orthopedic and Hand Trauma

Brett D. Crist, MD, FACS and Gregory J. Della Rocca, MD, PhD, FACS

1. *A 25-year-old man was involved in a high-speed motor-vehicle crash, sustaining an unstable pelvic fracture. Which of the following is associated with the highest risk of mortality?*

A. *Fracture pattern*

B. *Systolic blood pressure of 110 mm Hg*

C. *Revised Trauma Score of 7*

D. *Base deficit of 2.5*

E. *Age <30 years*

Several factors have been identified that predict mortality associated with pelvic fractures. Hypotension, fracture pattern, Revised Trauma Score (RTS), and base deficit are thought to be parameters that are readily available upon arrival, or shortly after arrival, that may predict mortality. Starr *et al.* retrospectively reviewed 325 patients with pelvic fractures to determine which factors predict mortality, transfusion requirements, use of pelvic arteriography, late complications, or associated injuries. Age >50-years-old, shock on arrival (SBP ≤90 mm Hg), base deficit > 6.5, and RTS <11 all significantly predicted mortality.

Answer: C

Hak DJ, Smith WR, Suzuki T (2009) Management of hemorrhage in life-threatening pelvic fracture. *Journal of the American Academy of Orthopedic Surgeons* **17** (7), 447–57.

Starr AJ, Griffin DR, Reinert CM, *et al.* (2002) Pelvic ring disruptions: prediction of associated injuries, transfusion requirement, pelvic arteriography, complications, and mortality. *Journal of Orthopedic Trauma* **16** (8), 553–61.

2. *A 24-year-old man sustains a pelvic fracture. He undergoes ATLS primary survey and fluid resuscitation. No other injuries are identified during the primary and secondary surveys. The type of pelvic ring fracture that is most commonly associated with a need for blood transfusion is a:*

A. *Lateral compression fracture type 1*

B. *Anterior-posterior compression fracture ("open book")*

C. *Vertical shear fracture*

D. *Lateral compression type 2*

E. *Combined mechanism*

Fluid and blood-product requirements for specific pelvic fractures have been associated with either the likelihood of arterial injury or more commonly, with associated injuries. Burgess *et al.* reviewed 210 consecutive patients with pelvic fractures. The anterior-posterior compression (APC) fractures were associated with the highest average number of units of packed red blood cells transfused (mean of 14.8 units). The APC type III injuries are also associated with the highest 24-hour fluid requirements. A higher rate of mortality has been seen in the APC group (20%) when compared with all others. The most common cause of death in the APC group was the combined pelvic fracture and visceral injuries. In the lateral compression group, the most likely cause of mortality was a closed head injury.

Answer: B

Burgess AR, Eastridge BJ, Young JW, *et al.* (1990) Pelvic ring disruptions: effective classification system

Surgical Critical Care and Emergency Surgery: Clinical Questions and Answers, First Edition. Edited by Forrest O. Moore, Peter M. Rhee, Samuel A. Tisherman and Gerard J. Fulda.

and treatment protocols. *Journal of Trauma* **30** (7), 848–56.

Hak DJ, Smith WR, Suzuki T (2009) Management of hemorrhage in life-threatening pelvic fracture. *Journal of the American Academy of Orthopedic Surgeons* **17** (7), 447–57.

3. *A 45-year-old woman sustains a pelvis fracture and is hypotensive with no other injury. Besides adequate fluid resuscitation, the type of pelvis fracture that will benefit most from application of a pelvic binder or sheet in order to reduce pelvic volume is:*

A. *Anterior-posterior compression fracture ("Open Book")*

B. *Lateral compression fracture type 1*

C. *Vertical shear fracture*

D. *Lateral compression fracture type 2*

E. *All of the above*

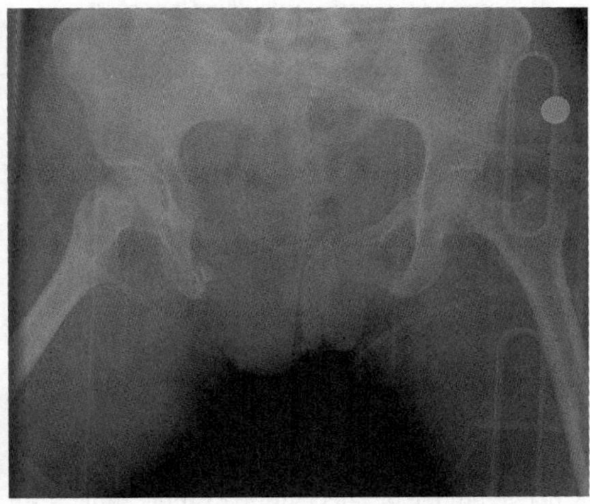

Commercially available pelvic binders or standard bed sheets have been incorporated into the acute management of pelvic fractures to reduce the pelvic volume and aid in patient transport and resuscitation. However, there has been concern about "overcompression" of lateral compression fractures with application of binders or sheets creating increased pelvic deformity. Pelvic binders have been shown to generate more compression than sheets and have been thought to more effectively reduce the pelvic volume. In 16 patients with pelvic fractures, a pelvic circumferential compression device (PCCD) was applied and was able to significantly reduce the pelvic width in anterior-posterior compression (APC) fractures to an amount similar to the reduction obtained with definitive surgical management. Another series showed that the use of pelvic binders reduced transfusion requirements, length of hospital stay and mortality in patients with APC injuries. It is of note that the application of sheets or binders may lead to pressure ulcers when used for prolonged periods without regularly checking the patient's skin.

Answer: A

Hak DJ, Smith WR, Suzuki T (2009) Management of hemorrhage in life-threatening pelvic fracture. *Journal of the American Academy of Orthopedic Surgeons* **17** (7), 447–57.

Krieg JC, Mohr M, Ellis TJ, *et al.* (2005) Emergent stabilization of pelvic ring injuries by controlled circumferential compression: a clinical trial. *Journal of Trauma* **59** (3), 659–64.

White CE, Hsu HR, Holcomb JB (2009) Haemodynamically unstable pelvic fractures. *Injury* **40** (10), 1023–30.

4. *A 32-year-old man has an isolated pelvic fracture involving his left hemi-pelvis. He is able to ambulate with an assistive device with toe-touch weight bearing on the left leg and weight bearing as tolerated on the right leg. He has no other risk factors for venous thromboembolism and is being discharged to home. What is the recommended duration of chemical DVT prophylaxis for this patient?*

A. *48 hours*

B. *Hospital discharge*

C. *Full weight bearing on both extremities*

D. *4 weeks from injury*

E. *6 weeks from injury*

Although it is universal to use DVT prophylaxis in patients with pelvic fractures, the exact protocol used may differ significantly. A systematic review looking at DVT prophylaxis for pelvis and acetabular fractures evaluated 11 studies involving 1760 patients. Due to the limited and poorly controlled data available, no consistent protocol could be recommended except for following published guidelines for the general trauma population. The 2008 CHEST guidelines do not recommend post-hospital discharge chemoprophylaxis in pelvic fracture patients that are able to ambulate (although it may be limited), have no other DVT risk factors, and are not undergoing inpatient rehabilitation.

Answer: B

Geerts WH, Bergqvist D, Pineo GF, *et al.* (2008) Prevention of venous thromboembolism: American College of Chest Physicians evidence-based clinical practice guidelines (8th edition). *Chest* **133** (6 Suppl.), p. 381S–453S.

Rogers FB, Cipolle MD, Velmahos G, *et al.* (2002) Practice management guidelines for the prevention of venous thromboembolism in trauma patients: the EAST practice management guidelines work group. *Journal of Trauma* **53** (1), 142–64.

Slobogean GP, Lefaivre KA, Nicolaou S, *et al.* (2009) A systematic review of thromboprophylaxis for pelvic and acetabular fractures. *Journal of Orthopedic Trauma* **23** (5), 379–84.

5. *What percentage of bleeding from pelvic fractures is normally attributed to arterial bleeding?*

A. 10%

B. 20%

C. 35%

D. 50%

E. 75%

The most common causes of bleeding associated with pelvic fractures are injury to the posterior venous plexus and cancelous fracture surfaces (85–90%). Approximately 10–15% of bleeding is associated with injures to branches of the internal iliac system (superior gluteal or pudendal arteries). In less than 1%, the main iliac trunk may be disrupted by a posterior ring fracture along the SI joint.

Answer: A

Durkin A, Sagi HC, Durham R, *et al.* (2006) Contemporary management of pelvic fractures. *American Journal of Surgery* **192** (2), 211–23.

Huittinen VM, Slatis P (1973) Postmortem angiography and dissection of the hypogastric artery in pelvic fractures. *Surgery* **73** (3), 454–62.

White CE, Hsu JR, Holcomb JB (2009) Haemodynamically unstable pelvic fractures. *Injury* **40** (10), 1023–30.

6. *A 35-year-old man is involved in a head-on motor vehicle crash at highway speeds. He sustains an "open book" pelvic fracture and undergoes nonoperative management of a grade I splenic laceration. Current indications to proceed with pelvic angiography and embolization are:*

A. Hypotension upon arrival to the ER

B. Continued hypotension after 2 L of warmed lactated ringer's solution

C. Continued hypotension after 2 L of warmed lactated ringer's solution and 2 units of pRBC's

D. Continued hypotension after 2 L of warmed lactated ringer's solution, 2 units of pRBC's and 2 units of FFP, and application of pelvic binder or sheet

E. None of the above

Pelvic angiography should be considered in patients with continued unexplained blood loss and hypotension despite pelvic fracture stabilization (sheet, binder, etc.) and adequate fluid resuscitation. Approximately 10% of patients with pelvic fractures require embolization. Eighty-five to 90% of bleeding from pelvic fractures has been shown to be either from the cancelous bone of the fracture surfaces or from injury to the posterior venous plexus. Current protocol recommendations include infusing 2 L of warmed lactated ringer's solution, 2 U pRBC's, 2 units of FFP, and application of a pelvic binder or sheet prior to proceeding with angiography. Angiography may be controversial, secondary to the amount of time that it may take to undergo evaluation and embolization in the angiography suite in an emergent setting, versus directly going to the OR; the fact that most bleeding from pelvic fractures is due to venous or bony bleeding and not amenable to angioembolization; and the potential ischemic complications associated with embolization. Some centers in Europe and in North America have incorporated emergent retroperitoneal packing and pelvic external fixation in the OR when patients have continued hypotension after adequate resuscitation and blood product transfusion to address the more common causes of bleeding (venous or bony bleeding). If continued hypotension occurs after packing and external fixation, then angiography is done to address the probable arterial injury. Following this protocol, only four out of 24 patients with persistent hemodynamic instability required subsequent embolization.

Answer: D

Hak DJ, Smith WR, Suzuki T (2009) Management of hemorrhage in life-threatening pelvic fracture. *Journal of the American Academy of Orthopedic Surgeons* **17** (7), 447–57.

White CE, Hsu JR, Holcomb JB (2009) Haemodynamically unstable pelvic fractures. *Injury* **40** (10), 1023–30.

7. *The incidence of genitourinary injury associated with pelvic fractures is:*

A. 5%

B. 20%

C. 50%

D. 75%

E. 90%

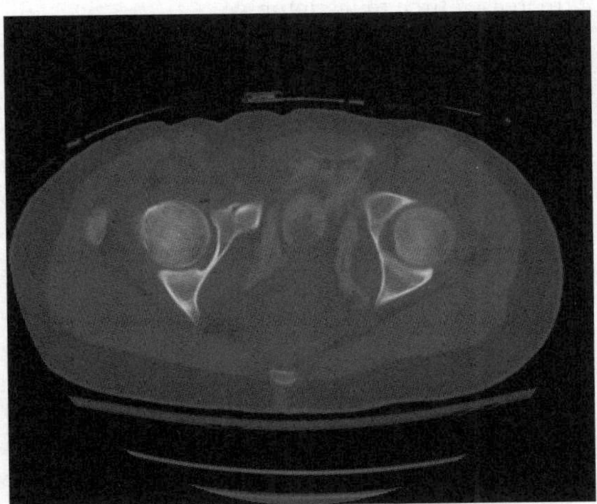

Injuries to the bladder and urethra occur in ~15–20% of patients with pelvic fractures. Bladder injuries are more commonly associated with lateral compression fractures, whereas urethral injuries are more commonly seen in patients with anterior-posterior compression fractures. Mortality may be as high as 34% in patients with bladder ruptures and pelvic fractures. Gross hematuria is the most reliable clinical finding, noted in 95% of pelvic fracture patients with bladder injury, while microscopic hematuria is seen in the remaining 5%.

Answer: B

Durkin A, Sagi HC, Durham R, *et al.* (2006) Contemporary management of pelvic fractures. *American Journal of Surgery* **192** (2), 211–23.

Fallon B, Wendt JC, Hawtrey CE (1984) Urological injury and assessment in patients with fractured pelvis. *Journal of Urology* **131** (4), 712–14.

Palmer JK, Benson GS, Corriere JN (1983) Diagnosis and initial management of urological injuries associated with 200 consecutive pelvic fractures. *Journal of Urology* **130** (4), 712–14.

8. *A 23-year-old man sustains a closed tibial and fibular shaft fracture and is splinted. He has a GCS score of 14 and is complaining of numbness in his leg; has leg pain that is not improved with IV morphine, loosening of his splint, or elevation of his leg; and has increased leg pain with passive flexion and extension of his great toe. His dorsalis pedis pulse is 2+/4. The next step in this patient's management should include:*

A. *Observation and re-examine in 1 hour*

B. *Continued elevation and re-examine in 1 hour*

C. *IV pain medication and re-examine in 1 hour*

D. *Compartment pressure evaluation*

E. *Emergent fasciotomies*

In an awake and alert patient, pain is the earliest and most sensitive clinical sign of compartment syndrome. After the fracture is immobilized in a splint, passive motion of the muscles within the involved compartments (i.e. moving the great toe involves stretching the anterior and deep posterior leg compartments) has been used to correlate with diagnosis of compartment syndrome. Paresthesia is also an early clinical sign. If these signs develop after splinting, the first step should be loosening of any constrictive splint/dressing and elevation of the extremity up to the level of the heart. Elevation above the heart should be avoided in order to maximize perfusion. Since outcomes associated with compartment syndrome are associated with time to fasciotomy, if clinical signs indicate a high likelihood that the patient has a compartment syndrome, compartment pressures should be bypassed and emergent fasciotomies should be performed.

Answer: E

Frink M, Hildebrand F, Krettek C, *et al.* (2010) Compartment syndrome of the lower leg and foot. *Clinical Orthopaedics and Related Research* **468** (4), 940–50.

Olson SA, Glasgow RR (2005) Acute compartment syndrome in lower extremity musculoskeletal trauma. *Journal of the American Academy of Orthopedic Surgeons* **13** (7), 436–44.

9. *With acute compartment syndrome, irreversible anoxic injury to muscle may occur after how many hours of ischemia:*

A. 3

B. 6

C. 8

D. 12

E. 24

Historically, irreversible anoxic injury to muscle was found to occur at 5 to 6 hours, but the most recent clinical series with the largest cohort of 76 patients from four different centers showed that muscle necrosis was identified in two of four cases that underwent fasciotomies within 3 hours of diagnosis.

Answer: A

Frink M, Hildebrand F, Krettek C, *et al.* (2010) Compartment syndrome of the lower leg and foot. *Clinical Orthopaedics and Related Research* **468** (4), 940–50.

Vaillancourt, C., *et al.* (2004) Acute compartment syndrome: how long before muscle necrosis occurs? *Canadian Journal of Emergency Medicine* **6** (3), 147–54.

10. *Successful litigation (indemnity payment) against physicians associated with extremity acute compartment syndrome is most likely associated with:*

A. Upper extremity involvement

B. Presence of an open fracture

C. Associated infection

D. Delay in fasciotomy

E. Associated vascular injury

Compartment syndrome can have devastating complications that can be avoided with early diagnosis and fasciotomy. Bhattacharyya *et al.* reviewed 23 years of closed malpractice claims and identified 16 compartment syndrome malpractice claims and identified risk factors associated with increased physician liability. Risk factors associated with unsuccessful defense and increased liability include:

1 Physician documentation of abnormal findings on neurological exam but no action taken

2 Poor physician communication

3 Increased number of cardinal signs (pain, pallor, pulselessness, paralysis, pain with passive stretch)

4 Increased time to fasciotomy

Answer: D

Bhattacharyya T, Vrahas MS (2004) The medical-legal aspects of compartment syndrome. *Journal of Bone and Joint Surgery, American Volume* **86-A** (4), 864–8.

11. *A 35-year-old man with a closed right tibia fracture has a GCS score of 8 secondary to a closed head injury and is intubated. His right leg compartments continue to become more firm over 2 hours. His blood pressure is 110/80 mm Hg. Compartment pressure monitoring is done to evaluate for compartment syndrome. The anterior compartment pressure was 55 mm Hg. When* *undergoing fasciotomies, what length of a fasciotomy incision is required to adequately decompress the leg compartments?*

A. 5 cm

B. 8 cm

C. 10 cm

D. 12 cm

E. 20 cm

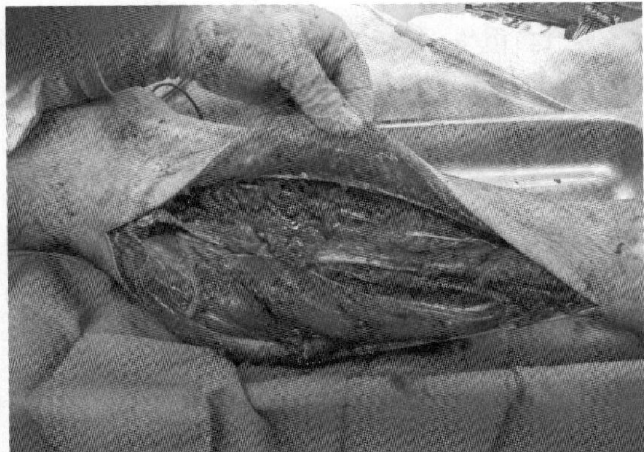

A full color version of this figure appears in the plate section of this book

When using dual incision fasciotomies for acute traumatic leg compartment syndrome, an incision an average of 16 cm long was required to adequately decompress the leg compartments. Although several different compartment pressure thresholds have been used to determine when fasciotomies should be performed, the current pressure used in tibial fractures is less than 30 mm Hg difference from the diastolic blood pressure as shown by McQueen *et al.* in a prospective study. A differential pressure of 30 mm Hg led to no missed cases of acute compartment syndrome and avoided unnecessary fasciotomies. The indication to use invasive compartment pressure monitoring in this patient is the fact that he is obtunded and intubated.

Answer: E

Frink M, Hildebrand F, Krettek C, *et al.* (2010) Compartment syndrome of the lower leg and foot. *Clinical Orthopaedics and Related Research* **468** (4), 940–50.

McQueen MM, Court-Brown CM (1996) Compartment monitoring in tibial fractures. The pressure threshold for decompression. *Journal of Bone and Joint Surgery, British Volume* **78** (1), 99–104.

Olson SA, Glasgow RR (2005) Acute compartment syndrome in lower extremity musculoskeletal trauma. *Journal of the American Academy of Orthopedic Surgery* **13** (7), 436–44.

12. *A 25-year-old man is struck by a motor vehicle and sustains a Gustilo and Anderson type IIIA open tibia fracture. Which of the following will most reliably decrease this patient's risk of infection?*

A. Debridement within 18 hours of injury

B. Debridement within 6 hours of injury

C. Antibiotic administration within 24 hours of injury

D. Antibiotic administration within 3 hours of injury

E. Intramedullary nailing of the tibia within 12 hours

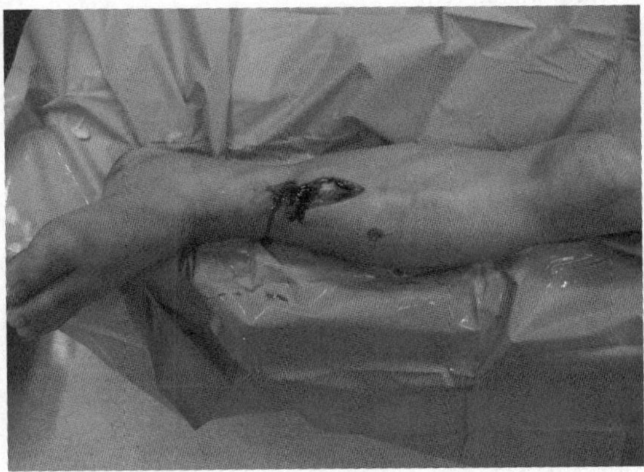

A full color version of this figure appears in the plate section of this book

Several factors have been evaluated to look at risk of infection after open fractures. Of the factors listed, early antibiotic administration is the most appropriate answer. Antibiotic administration within three hours of injury significantly reduced the rate of infection in a series of 1104 open fractures compared to patients receiving antibiotics greater than three hours from injury or no antibiotics at all. Timing of surgical debridement as long as it is within 24 hours has not been shown to reduce infection of open fractures significantly.

Answer: D

Okike K, Bhattacharyya T (2006) Trends in the management of open fractures. A critical analysis. *Journal of Bone and Joint Surgery, American Volume* **88** (12), 2739–48.

Pollak AN (2006) Timing of debridement of open fractures. *Journal of the American Academy of Orthopedic Surgeons* **14** (10, spec no.), S48–51.

Pollak AN, Jones AL, Castillo RC, *et al.* (2010) The relationship between time to surgical debridement and incidence of infection after open high-energy lower extremity trauma. *Journal of Bone and Joint Surgery, American Volume* **92** (1), 7–15.

13. *A 22-year-old man sustains a Gustilo and Anderson type 3A open bi-malleolar ankle fracture. His GCS score is 7 and is noted to have a left-sided intraparenchymal cerebral hemorrhage. Formal operative irrigation and debridement and stabilization of his open ankle fracture should occur:*

A. Emergently

B. Within 6 hours

C. Within 12 hours

D. Within 24 hours

E. As soon as the patient is medically stable

The "6-hour" rule for debridement of open fractures originated from an 1898 presentation by Paul Leopold Frederich where he contaminated guinea pigs with garden mold and stair dust to illustrate the importance of surgical debridement. In this antiquated animal study, debridement of the contaminated wound was less likely to be effective after 6 to 8 hours. Obviously, since this 1898 experiment, patient evaluation and management protocols have changed significantly and the timing of debridement has been questioned. Several studies have shown no association between timing of debridement and infection when debridement occurs within 24 hours. Others have shown a difference between debridement within 6 hours and less than 24 hours. However, all of these studies either have flawed study designs or too small a sample size to gain statistical significance. Therefore, emergent debridement is not necessarily supported, but neither is elective debridement. Current practice is based upon best evidence and includes debridement of open fractures urgently when the patient's medical condition is stabilized and life-threatening emergencies have been addressed, and when the appropriate surgical resources are available.

Answer: E

Pollak AN (2006) Timing of debridement of open fractures. *Journal of the American Academy of Orthopedic Surgeons* **14** (10, spec no.), S48–51.

Werner CM, Pierpont Y, Pollak AN (2008) The urgency of surgical debridement in the management of open fractures. *Journal of the American Academy of Orthopedic Surgeons* **16** (7), 369–75.

14. *A 17-year-old boy sustains a distal one-third Gustilo and Anderson type IIIB open tibia fracture with an associated fibula fracture during a motorcycle accident. He has active flexor hallucis longus, extensor hallucis longus, and ankle plantar and dorsiflexion. He has intact sensation over the dorsum of the foot and in the first dorsal web space, but plantar sensation is absent, consistent with a tibial nerve injury. His posterior tibialis pulse is 2+/4. The patient's absence of plantar sensation should guide treatment toward amputation to improve functional outcome.*

A. True

B. False

The Lower Extremity Assessment Project (LEAP) was a multi-center prospective outcome study that involved 601 patients with severe, limb-threatening lower extremity patients that compared limb salvage versus amputation. Twenty-nine patients in the limb salvage group had absent plantar foot sensation upon admission. These patients were compared with 26 patients that presented with absent plantar sensation and underwent early amputation, and 29 injury-matched control patients that had intact plantar sensation on admission. Only one patient in the insensate salvage group remained insensate at 24 months. Ten of 15 (67%) remaining patients in the salvage group with 24-month follow-up had complete return of plantar sensation. There were no significant outcomes differences found between the insensate salvage, insensate amputation, and the sensate control groups. Although outcomes did not differ between groups, the presence or absence of plantar sensation should not be used to direct treatment.

Answer: B

Bosse MJ, McCarthy ML, Jones AL, *et al.* (2005) The insensate foot following severe lower extremity trauma: an indication for amputation? *Journal of Bone and Joint Surgery, American Volume* **87**, 2601–8.

15. *At 84 months after injury, patients with severe lower extremity trauma distal to the femur that have undergone limb salvage have similar functional outcomes as compared with patients that underwent amputation.*

A. *True*

B. *False*

The Lower Extremity Assessment Program (LEAP) (see question 14) reviewed the Sickness Impact Profile (SIP) outcome data at 84 months and compared it to the 24-month data. Four-hundred-and-sixty-six patients were reviewed at 24 months and 413 patients were reviewed at 84 months. The 24-month data showed that SIP scores were similar in both the amputation and limb salvage groups, but poor compared to the general population. Between 24 and 84 months, the SIP scores increased (worsened) and continued to be significantly worse than the general population. At both time points, patients that underwent through-knee amputations were at the highest risk for poor outcomes.

Answer: A

MacKenzie EJ, Bosse MJ, Pollak AN, *et al.* (2005) Long-term persistence of disability following severe lower-limb trauma. Results of a seven-year follow-up. *Journal of Bone and Joint Surgery, American Volume* **87**, 1801–9.

16. *A 30-year-old man sustains a Gustilo and Anderson type 3B open tibia fracture, which requires free muscle flap coverage. The factor most likely associated with infection is:*

A. *Admission to a tertiary trauma center directly from the scene*

B. *Time to definitive soft tissue coverage*

C. *Fracture pattern*

D. *Size of the open wound*

E. *Delayed transfer from an outside hospital to a tertiary trauma center*

A subgroup analysis of the LEAP study (see questions 14 and 15) investigated the relationship between surgical debridement and incidence of infection in the limb salvage group. The primary outcome was the diagnosis of wound infection or osteomyelitis within the first 3 months. Multiple factors were evaluated in addition to the timing of surgical debridement, including time to arrival to the definitive trauma center, fracture pattern, bone loss, patient education level, type of fixation used, and smoking history. Patients that were transferred from an outside facility to the definitive trauma center greater than 3 hours after admission at the initial hospital had a significant increased risk of infection.

Answer: E

Pollak AN, Jones AL, Castillo RC, *et al.* (2010) The relationship between time to surgical debridement and incidence of infection after open high-energy lower extremity trauma. *Journal of Bone and Joint Surgery, American Volume* **92** (1), 7–15.

17. *A 32-year-old right hand dominant man amputates his right thumb and index and middle fingers through the proximal phalanx while using a table saw. The most appropriate definitive management includes:*

A. *Attempted replantation of all digits*

B. *Attempted replantation of the index finger only and revision amputation of the thumb and middle finger*

C. *Revision amputation of all digits through the metacarpophalangeal joints*

D. *Attempted replantation of the middle finger and revision amputation of the index finger and thumb*

E. *Attempted replantation of the thumb only with revisions amputation of the other digits*

A prospective cohort of 552 patients was followed for 2 years to evaluate the outcomes of digit replantation. Multiple digit amputations are still an absolute indication for replantation. However, single-digit replantation is indicated for sharp-cut amputations only and is not indicated in single digit amputations resulting from avulsion or extensive crush injuries. The thumb is the only exception. An isolated thumb replantation should always be attempted.

Answer: A

Waikakul S, Sakkarnkosol S, Vanadurongwan V, Unnanuntana A (2000) Results of 1018 digital replantations in 552 patients. *Injury* **31**(1), 33–40.

18. *A 20-year-old man was struck by a motor vehicle while walking. He has a large right-knee effusion and has a positive Lachman test (anterior knee laxity at 30° of flexion), posterior drawer test, and is unstable to varus and valgus stress. A lateral knee radiograph shows anterior subluxation of the tibia on the distal femur. His right lower extremity pulse was 1+/4 and is asymmetric. After stabilizing the knee in a long leg splint, his pulse does not change. The next step in management should include:*

A. *Re-evaluation in one hour*

B. *Ankle-brachial index determination*

C. *Duplex ultrasound*

D. *Arteriogram*

E. *Emergent surgery for revascularization of the extremity and external fixation of the knee*

The above patient has clinical exam findings of an ACL tear (positive Lachman test), PCL tear (posterior drawer test), and MCL and LCL tears (unstable to varus and valgus stress). Numerous studies have shown that routine angiography after knee dislocation is no longer necessary. Ten studies, including two prospective trials, evaluated 543 patients with knee dislocations and showed that physical exam alone was sufficient to identify clinically significant vascular injuries. Furthermore, many of the vascular injuries associated with knee dislocations are non-flow-limiting arterial intimal tears. Current management of intimal tears in patients with normal vascular examinations include observation and serial examinations. An arteriogram is indicated in any patient with an abnormal vascular exam. Since this patient had an asymmetric pulse, arteriogram was indicated. The asymmetric pulse also precludes the need for Ankle-Brachial index evaluation.

Answer: D

Levy BA, Fanelli GC, Whelan DB, *et al.* (2009) Controversies in the treatment of knee dislocations and multiligament reconstruction. *Journal of the American Academy of Orthopedic Surgeons* **17** (4), 197–206.

19. *A 50-year-old woman fell 5 feet and has a dorsally displaced distal radius fracture with associated volar index and middle finger numbness that progresses after closed reduction and splinting. The symptoms progress despite loosening the splint and elevating the extremity. In order to avoid permanent neurological deficits, a carpal tunnel release should be performed:*

A. *Emergently*

B. *Within 24 hours*

C. *Within 48 hours*

D. *Within 1 week*

E. *Not at all, it will resolve*

Nerve injury occurs in ~17% of distal radius fractures with the median nerve most commonly involved. Acute carpal tunnel syndrome occurs more frequently in patients with higher energy and comminuted distal radius fractures, and in those patients that undergo multiple closed reductions. If the carpal tunnel symptoms progress after elevation, loosening of the splint, and minimizing flexion of the wrist, a carpal tunnel release should be performed emergently. Patients undergoing early release have better long-term outcomes.

Answer: A

Ford DJ, Ali MS (1986) Acute carpal tunnel syndrome. Complications of delayed decompression. *Journal of Bone and Joint Surgery, British Volume* **68** (5), 758–9.

Mack GR, McPherson SA, Lutz RB (1994) Acute median neuropathy after wrist trauma. The role of emergent carpal tunnel release. *Clinical Orthopedics and Related Research* **300**, 141–6.

Turner RG, Faber KJ, Athwal GS (2007) Complications of distal radius fractures. *Orthopedic Clinics of North America* **38** (2), 217–28.

20. *An 18-year-old boy falls 10 feet off of a ladder. He is complaining of right wrist pain. He has significantly limited range of wrist motion and an obvious deformity. Wrist radiographs show no distal radius fracture. The injury that must be ruled out to avoid a poor outcome if diagnosed in a delayed fashion is:*

A. *Scapholunate ligament injury*

B. *Third and fourth metacarpal base fractures*

C. *Perilunate dislocation*

D. *Scaphoid fracture*

E. *None of the above*

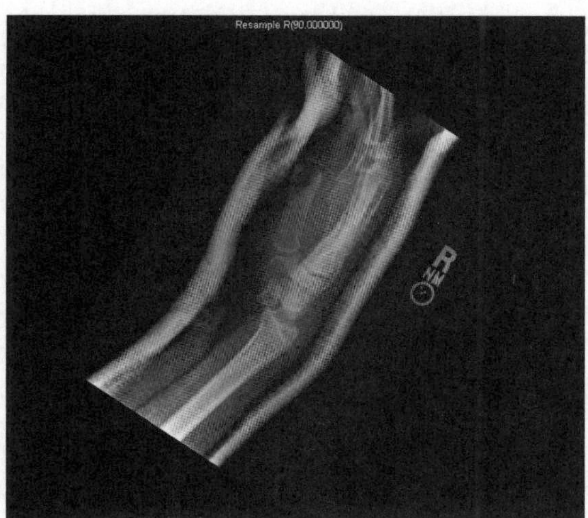

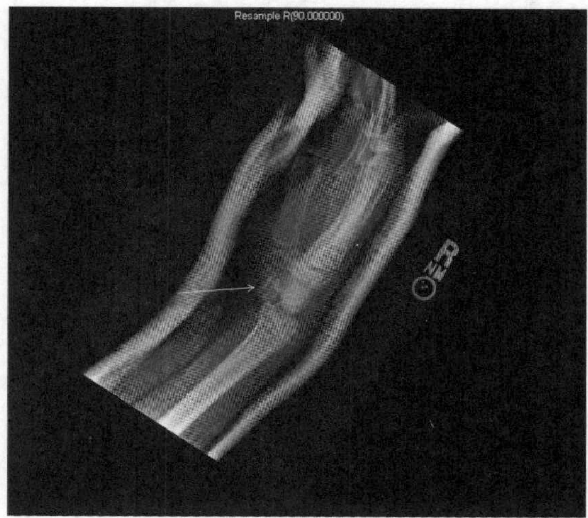

A lateral wrist x-ray with a volarly dislocated lunate (white arrow)

Although any of the diagnoses listed above may cause pain and minor deformity in the wrist/carpal area, only a perilunate dislocation will lead to limited wrist range of motion. Up to 25% of perilunate injuries are missed on initial evaluation. A high-quality lateral wrist radiograph is required for diagnosis. To avoid missing these injuries, a normal lateral wrist radiograph will show the lunate and capitate bones located in their fossa. Delay in diagnosis and management leads to poorer outcomes and are more likely to require salvage procedures including proximal row carpectomy.

Answer: C

Budoff JE (2008) Treatment of acute lunate and perilunate dislocations. *The Journal of Hand Surgery, American Volume* **33** (8), 1424–32.

Chapter 31 Peripheral Vascular Trauma

Daniel N. Holena, MD and Adam D. Fox, DPM, DO

1. *A 19-year-old man arrives by police drop-off with a gunshot wound to the right thigh. He has a history of hypotension in the field, but on arrival at the trauma bay he is hemodynamically stable. His physical examination is notable for a single wound in proximity to the course of the superficial femoral artery and vein, which is not actively bleeding. There is decreased sensation on the anterior and medial aspect of the thigh. Distal pulse evaluation reveals 2+ dorsalis pedis and posterior tibial pulses bilaterally. Plain films reveal no fractures and a retained foreign body in the lateral aspect of the thigh. Which of the following statements is correct?*

A. *The patient can be safely discharged from the trauma bay without further diagnostic because the patient does not have any evidence of vascular "hard signs"*

B. *Further diagnostic testing for vascular trauma is indicated, because the patient has a sensory defect suggestive of femoral nerve injury*

C. *The patient can be safely admitted and observed because the patient has no hard signs and a normal peripheral pulse examination*

D. *Further diagnostic testing for vascular trauma is indicated, because the patient has a history of hypotension in the field*

E. *Further diagnostic testing for vascular trauma is indicated, because the trajectory of the projectile appears to be in proximity to the major vascular structures in the thigh*

The presence of a vascular "hard sign" (pulsatile bleeding, expanding hematoma, palpable thrill, audible bruit, loss of pulse) is specific for major vascular injury and mandates operative exploration, but absence of hard signs does not reliably exclude injury. "Soft signs" of vascular injury (non-expanding hematoma, injury to adjacent nerve, proximity to major blood vessels, unexplained hypotension, or history of prehospital hemorrhage) do not reliably predict major vascular trauma. Because of concern over limb-threatening consequences a result of missed injury, historically there has been a low threshold for operative exploration when the diagnosis of peripheral vascular injury was entertained. High rates of negative exploration lead to liberal use of angiography as an alternative, but this too was associated with a high rate of studies that demonstrated either no injury or injuries that did not require intervention. It is generally accepted that in the absence of hard signs a normal peripheral vascular examination does not require further investigation, even in the presence of vascular soft signs. When angiography is performed under these circumstances, roughly 10% of patients will be found to have an injury, but the natural history of the vast majority of these "minimal vascular injuries" is to resolve without intervention. Physical examination in conjunction with a 24-hour period of observation has been shown to have a false negative rate of less than 1% for major vascular injury, comparable to that of angiography.

Answer: C

Ashworth EM, Dalsing MC, Glover JL, Reilly MK (1988) Lower extremity vascular trauma: A comprehensive, aggressive approach. *Journal of Trauma* **28** (3), 329–36.

Frykberg ER, Crump JM, Dennis JW, *et al.* (1991) Nonoperative observation of clinically occult arterial injuries: A prospective evaluation. *Surgery* **109** (1), 85–96.

Frykberg ER, Dennis JW, Bishop K, *et al.* (1991) The reliability of physical examination in the evaluation of penetrating extremity trauma for vascular injury: Results at one year. *Journal of Trauma* **31** (4), 502–11.

Surgical Critical Care and Emergency Surgery: Clinical Questions and Answers, First Edition. Edited by Forrest O. Moore, Peter M. Rhee, Samuel A. Tisherman and Gerard J. Fulda.

2. *A 44-year-old man presents to the trauma bay with a crush injury to his left lower extremity after being run over by a tractor. On physical examination, there is a contaminated open wound on the left thigh associated with an obvious deformity. No pulses are palpable distal to the level of the injury. A plain radiograph reveals a comminuted femur fracture. Regarding the management of this injury complex, which of the following is correct?*

A. *The addition of skeletal injury to arterial injury does not confer an increased risk of extremity amputation*

B. *Limb salvage rates are equivalent whether revascularization or orthopedic stabilization is performed first*

C. *When definitive vascular repair is performed prior to orthopedic stabilization, manipulation of the extremity leads to need to revise the vascular repair in the majority of cases*

D. *Crush injury but not severe contamination is a risk factor for limb loss*

E. *In limbs at high risk for amputation, limb salvage and amputation are associated with similar functional outcomes at 2 years*

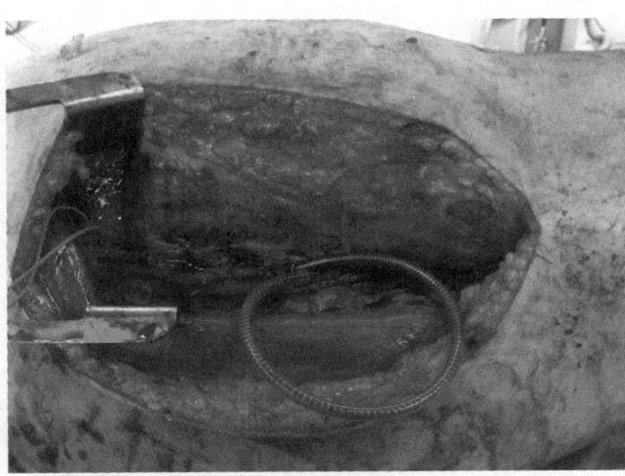

Temporary intravascular shunting of the superficial femoral artery. A full color version of this figure appears in the plate section of this book

Patients with combined skeletal and arterial injuries are much more likely to require amputation than patients with either skeletal or arterial injuries alone (15–35% versus 5%, respectively). Recent series suggest that limb salvage rates are highest when revascularization is performed prior to orthopedic stabilization, but the initial technique of revascularization need not be definitive. In the setting of hemodynamic instability, severely unstable or comminuted fractures, or gross contamination, intraluminal shunting should be considered as bridge to definitive vascular repair. In the absence of these factors definitive vascular repair may be undertaken prior to orthopedic stabilization with a less than 7% need for revision after orthopedic fixation. Factors that are associate with limb loss in combination skeletal and arterial injury include extensive soft tissue loss, severe contamination, associated nerve injury. At 2 years post-injury, patients who underwent limb salvage had similar functional outcomes compared to those who underwent amputation, but with higher rates of complications and hospital admissions.

Answer: E

Bosse MJ, MacKenzie EJ, Kellam JF, *et al.* (2002) An analysis of outcomes of reconstruction or amputation of leg-threatening injuries. *New England Journal of Medicine* **347** (24), 1924–31.

Cakir O, Subasi M, Erdem K, Eren N (2005) Treatment of vascular injuries associated with limb fractures. *Annals of the Royal College of Surgeons of England* **87** (5), 348–52.

Rozycki GS, Tremblay LN, Feliciano DV, McClelland WB (2003) Blunt Vascular Trauma in the Extremity: Diagnosis, Management, and Outcome. *Journal of Trauma—Injury, Infection and Critical Care* **55** (5), 814–24.

Snyder III WH (1982) Vascular injuries near the knee: An updated series and overview of the problem. Surgery **91** (5), 502–6.

3. *Regarding the use diagnostic testing in the evaluation of peripheral vascular trauma, which of which of the following is correct?*

A. *An arterial pressure index (API) <0.9 is an indication for operative exploration*

B. *An normal physical examination and an API >0.9 reliably excludes all vascular injuries*

C. *Compared to CT angiography, conventional angiography is more sensitive and specific*

D. *Compared to CT angiography, conventional angiography is associated with greater costs*

E. *Duplex ultrasound is the single best test for evaluation of peripheral vascular trauma*

The arterial pressure index (API) has gained acceptance in some trauma centers as useful tool in the evaluation of peripheral vascular trauma. Using Doppler ultrasound, the systolic occlusion pressure is measured in the injured limb and compared to an unaffected limb, usually the contralateral extremity. An API < 0.9 has a 95% specificity and 97% specificity for arterial injury, but an abnormal API alone is not an indication for operative exploration but rather for further diagnostic testing. A normal API does not reliably exclude lesions that do not always produce significant interruptions in blood flow, such as intimal flaps and pseudoaneurysms. However, such lesions have a < 10% risk of progression to requiring surgical intervention. The API also does not detect venous injury or muscle bleeding, which may contribute to the development of compartment syndrome. When the API is < 0.9, further imaging is warranted. Traditionally, conventional angiography has been used to evaluate the peripheral vasculature for traumatic injury, but improvements in computed tomography technology have lead to CT angiography largely supplanting this technique. Seamon *et al.* found that the CT angiogram was equal in sensitivity and specificity to formal angiogram, but with substantial decreases in time and cost. While duplex ultrasound is noninvasive, it is less sensitive in the diagnosis of peripheral vascular trauma than angiography. In addition, duplex ultrasound requires the presence of a trained ultrasonographer which may not be available at all times at many institutions.

Answer: D

Edwards JW, Bergstein JM, Karp DL, *et al.* (1993) Penetrating proximity injuries—The role of duplex scanning: A prospective study. *Journal of Vascular Technology* **17** (5), 257–61.

Johansen K, Lynch K, Paun M, Copass M (1991) Noninvasive vascular tests reliably exclude occult arterial trauma in injured extremities. *Journal of Trauma* **31** (4), 515–22.

Sadjadi J, Cureton EL, Dozier KC, *et al.* (2009) Expedited Treatment of Lower Extremity Gunshot Wounds. *Journal of the American College of Surgeons* **209** (6), 740–5.

Seamon MJ, Smoger D, Torres DM, *et al.* (2009) A prospective validation of a current practice: The detection of extremity vascular injury with CT angiography. *Journal of Trauma—Injury, Infection and Critical Care* **67** (2), 238–43.

4. *While trying to stop a crime, a 30-year-old police officer sustains a gunshot wound that enters the left pelvis and exits the right thigh. On arrival to the trauma bay, he is hypotensive and has pulsatile hemorrhage from the right mid-thigh. Which of the following statements is correct?*

A. *If the patient arrests from this injury in the prehospital setting, ED thoracotomy is associated with an approximately 25% chance of survival*

B. *Rapid administration of blood and crystalloid prior with the intent of correcting hypotension prior to operation may be associated with increased survival*

C. *Due to concerns for contamination, interposition grafting with synthetic graft material is contraindicated if the trajectory of the bullet may have included the gastrointestinal tract*

D. *When compared to open repair, endovascular repair of this injury is associated with decreased morbidity and should be considered the first-line treatment*

E. *Completion angiography after repair of vascular injury may reveal technical errors requiring revision in >10% of cases*

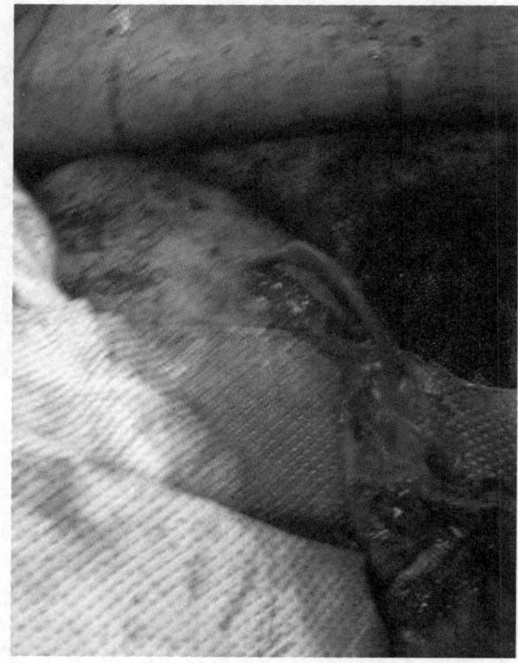

Pulsatile hemorrhage from the right thigh, a vascular "hard sign." A full color version of this figure appears in the plate section of this book

Prehospital arrest is a negative prognostic factor for survival in patients undergoing ED thoracotomy, as is non-cardiothoracic site of injury. A recent review of 25 years of experience on this topic by Rhee *et al.* suggests survival in the scenario described in answer "A" is closer to 5%. Administration of fluid and blood products to treat hypotension prior to definitive control of hemorrhage has been shown in at least one randomized controlled trial to be associated with decreased survival; treatment of hemorrhagic shock is to stop the bleeding as soon as possible. Interposition grafting using synthetic conduit has been shown to be safe in civilian trauma, even in the presence of a contaminated field. Feliciano *et al.* reported a series of 236 synthetic grafts used to repair traumatic vascular injuries; no graft infections were reported in the absence of exposed graft or osteomyelitis. While endovascular repair of penetrating vascular trauma has been reported, it is certainly not the standard of care for patients in hemorrhagic shock and should not be entertained in this situation. Completion angiography reveals technical issues in 10–30% of cases, and in one large series was associated with a decreased rate of amputation.

Answer: E

Bickell WH, Wall Jr MJ, Pepe PE, *et al.* (1994) Immediate versus delayed fluid resuscitation for hypotensive patients with penetrating torso injuries. *New England Journal of Medicine* **331** (17), 1105–19.

Degiannis E, Bowley DM, Bode F, *et al.* (2007) Ballistic arterial trauma to the lower extremity: Recent South African experience. *American Surgeon* **73** (11), 1136–9.

Feliciano DV, Mattox KL, Graham JM, Bitondo CG (1985) Five-year experience with PTFE grafts in vascular wounds. *Journal of Trauma* **25** (1), 71–82.

Rhee PM, Acosta J, Bridgeman A, *et al.* (2000) Survival after emergency department thoracotomy: Review of published data from the past 25 years. *Journal of the American College of Surgeons* **190** (3), 288–98.

5. *A 54-year-old factory worker is hit in the groin by a sharp metal rod, resulting in copious dark red bleeding from the site. At operative exploration, a complete transection of the common femoral vein is discovered. With respect to options for repair for this injury, which of the following statements is correct?*

A. *Ligation of the femoral vein is associated with a >25% rate of limb loss*

B. *When compared to primary repair of this injury, ligation is associated with an equivalent risk of pulmonary thromboembolism*

C. *Temporary intravascular shunting has no role in the treatment of venous injuries*

D. *Primary repair of this injury will require systemic anticoagulation to maintain long-term patency*

E. *Primary repair of this injury is associated with better short-term patency then interposition grafting*

The literature regarding traumatic venous injury is limited to retrospective reviews and a small number of prospective observational studies, but most would agree that primary repair should be performed when possible. Ligation is an option for complex venous injuries as a damage control technique in unstable patients and is generally well tolerated. Approximately 90% of patients will experience lower extremity edema after ligation, but few patients treated postoperatively with venous compression stockings go on to develop severe venous stasis disease. The need for amputation after isolated femoral vein ligation is distinctly uncommon. In the largest series available to date, Quan *et al.* found no difference in pulmonary embolism rates in patients undergoing venous repair versus ligation (3.4% versus 4.2%, P = NS). Temporary intravenous shunting has been employed in both civilian and military settings to allow for life and limb saving procedures to occur prior to undertaking complex repair. No strong data exists supporting the use of systemic anticoagulation to promote patency; short term patency approximates 75% regardless of the type of repair.

Answer: B

Borman KR, Jones GH, Snyder III WH (1987) A decade of lower extremity venous trauma: Patency and outcome. *American Journal of Surgery* **154** (6), 608–12.

Kurtoglu M, Yanar H, Taviloglu K, *et al.* (2007) Serious lower extremity venous injury management with ligation: Prospective overview of 63 patients. American Surgeon **73** (10), 1039–43.

Parry NG, Feliciano DV, Burke RM, *et al.* (2003) Management and short-term patency of lower extremity venous injuries with various repairs. *American Journal of Surgery* **186** (6), 631–5.

Quan RW, Gillespie DL, Stuart RP, *et al.* (2008) The effect of vein repair on the risk of venous thromboembolic events: A review of more than 100 traumatic military venous injuries. *Journal of Vascular Surgery* **47** (3), 571–7.

6. *While working at an international hospital that receives combat injuries after stabilization in the field, you receive a 22-year-old man soldier who sustained a blast injury to the upper extremity. The trauma surgeon who stabilized him initially discovered a brachial artery injury and placed a temporary intravascular shunt. Which of the following statements is correct?*

A. *Placement of a temporary intravascular shunt does not require systemic anticoagulation to maintain patency*

B. *Temporary intravascular shunting requires the use availability of specially manufactured shunting devices*

C. *The upper limit of time that a shunt can remain in place is approximately 12 hours*

D. *While useful under conditions of limited resources, temporary intravascular shunts have not been demonstrated to be of value in civilian trauma*

E. *While temporary intravascular shunts may be useful as a damage control technique, up to 25% of shunts will become dislodged with patient transport*

First described for traumatic injury in 1971, temporary intravascular shunt (TIVS) placement has become an invaluable addition to the toolkit of the trauma surgeon. Shunt placement simultaneously arrests hemorrhage and restores distal perfusion, allowing time to triage other life and limb threatening injuries. Because most patients undergoing damage control techniques such as shunting are not candidates for systemic anticoagulation, heparinization is not generally an option. The use of virtually any available flexible tubing has been described in TIVS placement, from those devices specifically designed for this purpose (such as commercially available Argyle and Javid shunts) to peripheral IV tubing and even nasogastric tubes. The upper limit of time that a shunt may remain patent is unknown, but case reports exist in which shunts remained patent for up to 10 days. Beyond the military theatre, temporary intravascular shunts have been employed in civilian trauma. Subramanian *et al.* reported the use of 101 temporary intravascular shunts in 67 patients, with an overall limb salvage rate of 83%. While dislodgement of temporary intravascular shunts is possible this is a rare event, even in combat casualties transported great distances with shunts in place.

Answer: A

Dente CJ, Rasmussen TE, Schiller HJ, *et al.* (2006) The use of temporary vascular shunts as a damage control adjunct in the management of wartime vascular injury. *Journal of Trauma—Injury, Infection and Critical Care* **61** (1), 12–15.

Feliciano DV, Accola KD, Burch JM, Spjut-Patrinely V (1989) Extraanatomic bypass for peripheral arterial injuries. *American Journal of Surgery* **158** (6), 506–10.

Granchi T, Schmittling Z, Vasquez Jr J, *et al.* (2000) Prolonged use of intraluminal arterial shunts without systemic anticoagulation. *American Journal of Surgery* **180** (6), 493–7.

Khalil IM, Livingston DH (1986) Intravascular shunts in complex lower limb trauma. *Journal of Vascular Surgery* **4** (6), 582–7.

Subramanian A, Vercruysse G, Dente C, *et al.* (2008) A decade's experience with temporary intravascular shunts at a civilian level I trauma center. *Journal of Trauma—Injury, Infection and Critical Care* **65** (2), 316–24.

7. *Regarding fasciotomy for peripheral vascular trauma, which of the following is correct?*

A. *Combined arterial and venous injury requires therapeutic fasciotomy*

B. *A compartment pressure of >30 mm Hg is a standard indication for a therapeutic decompressive fasciotomy*

C. *Coolness (poikilothermia) of the affected extremity is the most frequently occurring clinical indicator in compartment syndrome*

D. *Compartment syndrome can be reliably diagnosed based on physical examination findings*

E. *Fasciotomy after peripheral vascular injury is associated with up to a 60% non-closure rate*

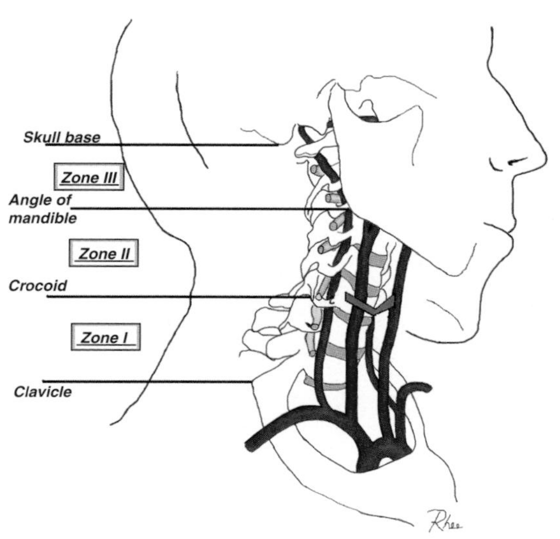

Chapter 27 Question 1.

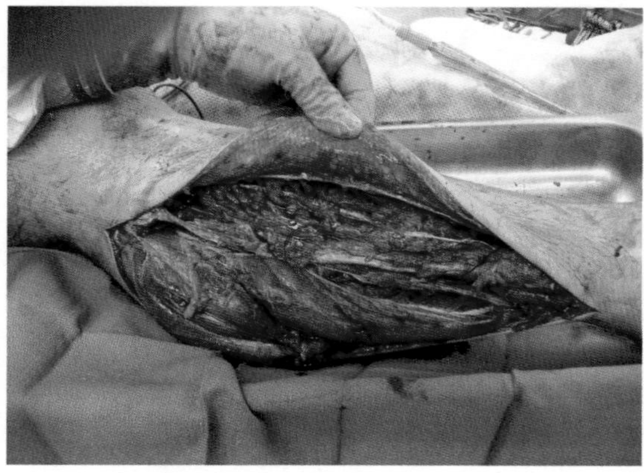

Chapter 30 Question 11.

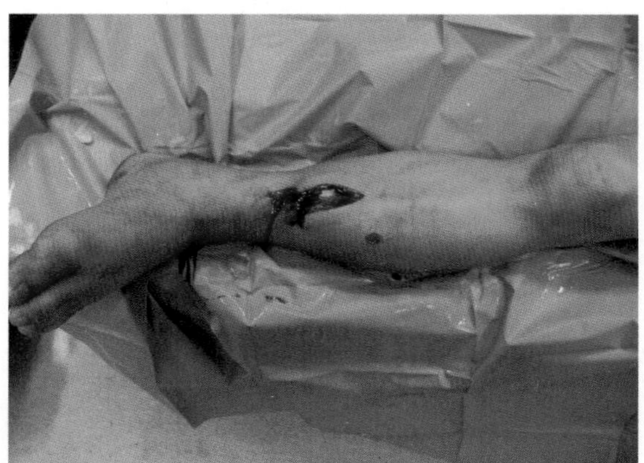

Chapter 30 Question 12.

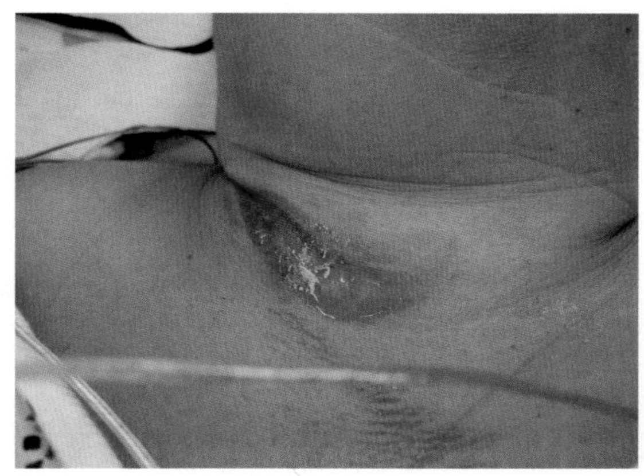

Chapter 27 Question 4.

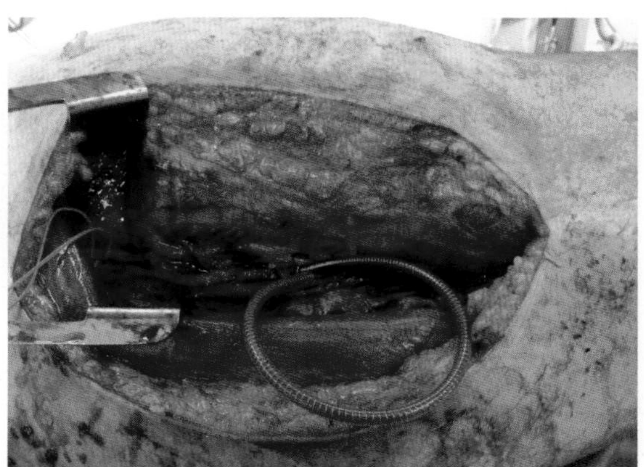

Chapter 31 Question 2.

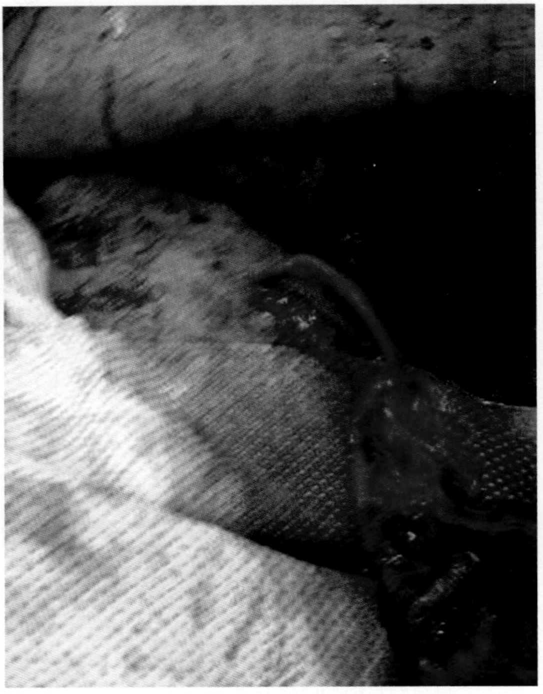

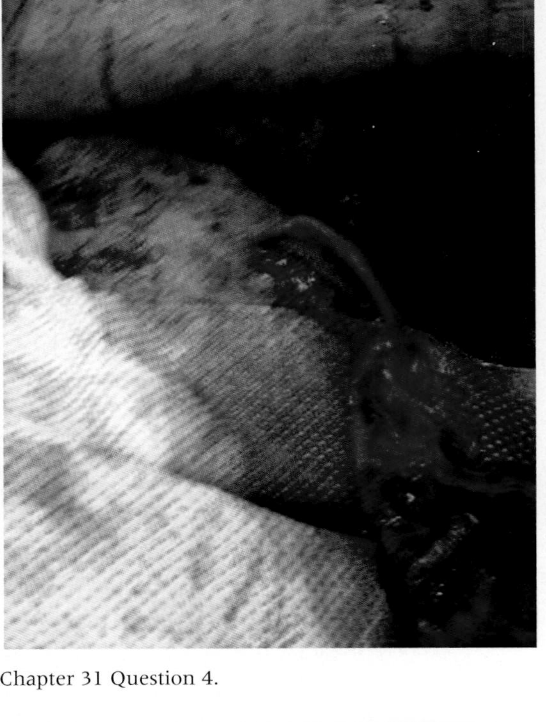

Chapter 31 Question 4.

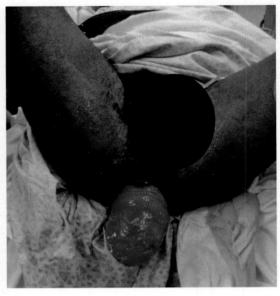

Chapter 35 Question 11.

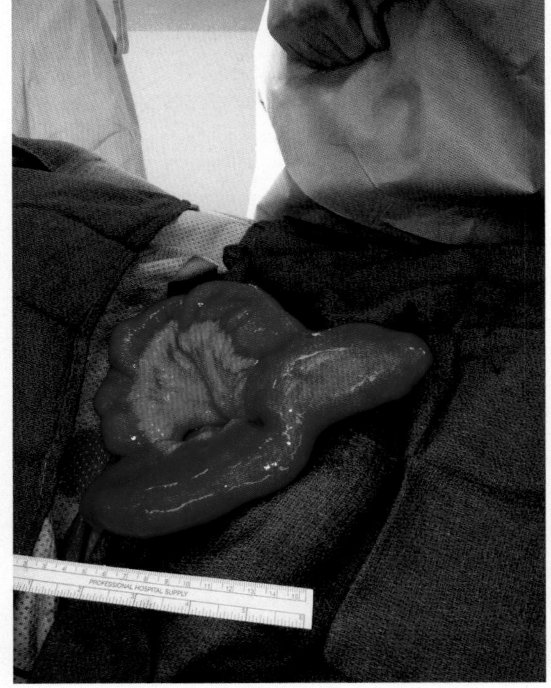

Chapter 35 Question 9.

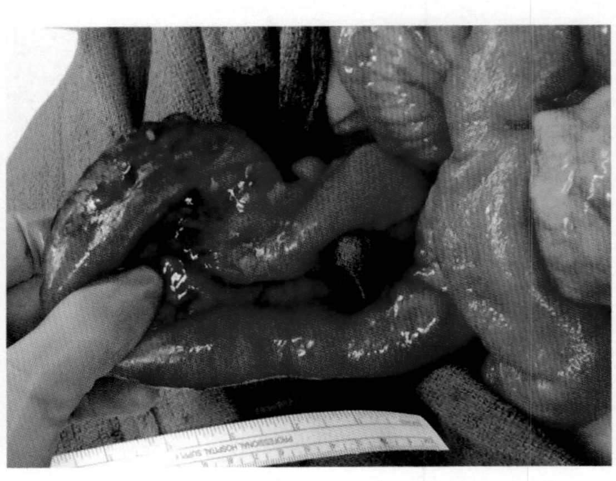

Chapter 35 Question 12.

Early diagnosis of compartment syndrome after peripheral vascular injury is of great importance because delays in treatment can lead to increased complications and mortality. While not all patients with peripheral vascular trauma will require fasciotomy, specific clinical scenarios associated with high rates of developing compartment syndrome have led some authors to propose guidelines for *prophylactic* fasciotomies. These situations include combined arterial and venous injury, arterial injury and systemic hypotension, and prolonged (>6 hours) of ischemic time. Direct measurement of intracompartmental pressure has been used to test for compartment syndrome, and a pressure of >30 mm Hg would be an indication for a *therapeutic* fasciotomy. When considering the clinical diagnosis of compartment syndrome, pain has been shown to be the most frequently occurring symptom but obviously lacks specificity in patients with injured extremities. A high index of suspicion is required for diagnosis, as the sensitivity of clinical indicators alone ranges from 13–19%. Regardless of the indication, it is important to recognize that fasciotomy is not a risk-free procedure; overall, approximately one-third of lower extremity fasciotomies will not be able to be closed by delayed primary intention.

Answer: B

Ulmer T (2002) The clinical diagnosis of compartment syndrome of the lower leg: Are clinical findings predictive of the disorder? *Journal of Orthopaedic Trauma* **16** (8), 572–7.

Velmahos GC, Theodorou D, Demetriades D, *et al.* (1997) Complications and nonclosure rates of fasciotomy for trauma and related risk factors. *World Journal of Surgery* **21** (3), 247–53.

Velmahos GC, Toutouzas KG (2002) Vascular trauma and compartment syndromes. *Surgical Clinics of North America* **82** (1), 125–41.

8. *Concerning popliteal artery injuries, which of the following statements is not correct?*

A. *The rate of amputation after popliteal artery injury has declined in both military and civilian series over the past century*

B. *Delay to revascularization, blunt mechanism of injury, and associated injuries to other body regions are risk factors for amputation in popliteal artery injury*

C. *An ABI > 0.9 reliably excludes clinically significant popliteal artery injury after knee dislocation*

D. *Due to excellent collateral circulation, popliteal artery injury is associated with a lower rate of amputation when compared to other peripheral arterial injuries*

E. *In the case of hard signs associated with blunt or complex trauma to the popliteal region, angiography or CT angiography is warranted prior to operative exploration*

Popliteal artery injuries have long been recognized as a condition meriting special consideration because of their unforgiving nature. The rate of limb salvage after these injuries has improved throughout the past century, with reported amputation rates of 12% in recent conflicts compared to ~70% during the first and second world wars. Prior to 1980, the rate of amputation after civilian injuries was 30%; after 1980, the rate was closer to 15%. Risk factors associated with amputation after popliteal artery injuries include delay to revascularization, blunt mechanism of injury, and concomitant injuries to other body regions. Blunt force injuries to the knee are associated with popliteal artery injury; knee dislocation is associated with ~10–40% incidence of popliteal artery injury, mandating a high index of suspicion. In a small prospective study by Mills *et al.*, an API > 0.9 was been shown to reliably exclude clinically significant popliteal artery injury with a sensitivity of 100%. An API < 0.9 is an indication for angiography or CTA, but only ~30% of these patients will require operative intervention. While the popliteal artery is collateralized by the geniculate network around the knee, this generally not sufficient to maintain perfusion in the absence of popliteal flow; this may in part explain why popliteal artery injuries are associated with higher rates of amputation relative to peripheral vascular injuries at other locations. Although hard signs of vascular injury generally mandate immediate operative intervention, Frykberg *et al.* have advocated imaging of the popliteal artery even in the presence of hard signs associated with blunt or complex trauma, because physical examination may be false positive in up to 87% of these cases.

Answer: D

Frykberg ER (2002) Popliteal vascular injuries. *Surgical Clinics of North America* **82** (1), 67–89.

Levin PM, Rich NM, Hutton JE (1971) Collateral circulation in arterial injuries. *American Journal of Surgery* **102**, 592–9.

Mills WJ, Barei DP, McNair P (2004) The value of the ankle-brachial index for diagnosing arterial injury after knee dislocation: A prospective study. *Journal of Trauma—Injury, Infection and Critical Care* **56** (6), 1261–5.

Thomas DD, Wilson RF, Wiencek RG (1989) Vascular injury about the knee. Improved outcome. *American Surgeon* **55** (6), 370–7.

9. *A 24-year-old man sustained a single stab wound to the right thigh and pulsatile hemorrhage ensued. A prehospital tourniquet was applied to the right lower extremity above the level of the injury and he was rapidly transported to the trauma center. Speaking with the patient's family after a successful operative repair, they have concerns about the use of the tourniquet. Which of the following is correct?*

A. *Current advanced trauma life support (ATLS) protocol recommends tourniquet application as the first line of treatment for exanguinating extremity wounds*

B. *Successful control of hemorrhage with tourniquets is greater with lower extremity wounds than upper extremity wounds*

C. *Tourniquet application with pressures of 200–250 mm Hg is associated with increased venous bleeding*

D. *Tourniquet application for exanguinating extremity injury is associated with an amputation rate of nearly 30%*

E. *Neurologic injury is a potential complication of tourniquet application, but is unlikely to occur with tourniquet duration less than 2 hours*

There has been a recent resurgence in interest in the use of tourniquets to control active bleeding from extremity wounds, but the first line of treatment according to current ATLS protocol remains direct pressure. If a tourniquet is applied, it is important that the arterial occlusion is assured, typically with pressures between 200–250 mm Hg. Lower pressures may lead to venous outflow occlusion without arterial inflow occlusion, leading to increased venous bleeding. Tourniquets are more successful at controlling hemorrhage from upper extremity wounds than lower extremity wounds (94% versus 71%). The risk of peripheral nerve injury as a result of tourniquet application is low appears to be related to the duration of ischemia. In a study of 110 tourniquet applications, Lakestein *et al.* found an overall incidence of peripheral nerve injury of 5.5%, with only one case occurred when the tourniquet time was less than two hours. A more recent study by Kragh *et al.* reported a ~2% risk of neuropathy in 651 limbs. The amputation rate in this series was ~15%.

Answer: E

American College of Surgeons. Advanced Trauma Life Support Course for Doctors, Student Course Manual, ed 8. Chicago, American College of Surgeons, 2008.

Kragh Jr JF, Littrel ML, Jones JA, *et al.* (2009) battle casualty survival with emergency tourniquet use to stop limb bleeding. *Journal of Emergency Medicine*. Epub ahead of print.

Lakstein D, Blumenfeld A, Sokolov T, *et al.* (2003) Tourniquets for hemorrhage control on the battlefield: a 4-year accumulated experience. *The Journal of Trauma* **54** (5 Suppl.), 221–5.

10. *You receive notice that prehospital providers are en-route to your trauma center with a 24-year-old woman with multiple stab wounds the lower extremities. She is hypotensive and has pulsatile bleeding from the right groin. Which of the following is not a 'key concept' in her operative management?*

A. *Temporary control of bleeding*

B. *Extensile exposure*

C. *Proximal and distal control of bleeding vessels*

D. *Local heparinization*

E. *Definitive repair of vascular injury*

Reports of hypotension or copious bleeding in the prehospital setting should prompt providers to secure uncrossmatched blood products and consider the activation of a massive transfusion protocol, if one is available. Upon arrival to the trauma bay, assessment should proceed along ATLS protocol guidelines. Temporary control of bleeding refers to arresting hemorrhage prior to operative intervention. Bleeding should be controlled with direct pressure where possible; tourniquets may be useful in cases where direct pressure is not an option secondary to massive tissue destruction. Pulsatile hemorrhage from deep wounds may on occasion be temporized by insertion of a Foley catheter into the tract and inflating the balloon until the bleeding stops. Ultimate management of these injuries necessitates operative intervention. Extensile exposure refers to the technique of choosing incisions which may be extended proximally or distally along the course of a vessel, even as this vessel courses through different anatomic regions (e.g. chest to upper extremity). Proximal and distal control of bleeding vessels allows for inspection and repair while hemorrhage is arrested; it is often safest to obtain proximal and distal control outside of the zone of injury using extensile exposure. While systemic heparinization prior to clamping vessels is the ideal, this is often not possible in trauma patients who may have other sources of bleeding. Therefore, local heparinization of the extremity prior to application of the distal occlusion must usually suffice. Definitive repair of vascular injures at index operation may not be the best option in all patients; the patient's physiology and concomitant injuries must be considered. For patients with competing injury priorities or severely deranged physiology, "damage control" options must be considered. In these situations, temporary intraluminal shunting or even arterial ligation ("life over limb") may be the most appropriate option.

Answer: E

Feliciano DV (2010) Management of peripheral arterial injury. *Current Opinion in Critical Care* **16** (6), 602–8.

Hirschberg A, Mattlox K (2005) *Top Knife*, tfm Publishing Ltd; Castle Hill Barnes.

11. *A 17-year-old boy presents at the trauma bay with a slash wound that extends from the antecubital fossa proximally onto the forearm. Which of the following statements is not correct?*

A. While vascular hard signs mandate immediate surgical operation, the absence of hard signs does not preclude a major vascular injury.

B. When possible, a thorough neurologic examination of the affected extremity should be performed and documented prior to operation.

C. If at operation a brachial artery transection is discovered, synthetic graft is the material of choice for interposition grafting.

D. If at operation the ulnar artery is discovered to be transected but the radial artery is intact, ligation of the ulnar artery is an acceptable treatment.

E. When brachial artery injury is associated with complex orthopedic injury, revascularization prior to orthopedic stabilization is the treatment of choice.

The brachial artery is the most commonly injured artery of the upper extremity, constituting 15%–30% of all peripheral arterial artery injuries. While patients with brachial artery injuries typically present with vascular hard signs, because of a rich network of collaterals around the elbow it is possible to have complete transection of the brachial artery with a palpable radial pulse and a well perfused hand. In patients where the diagnosis is uncertain, imaging of the vessel is indicated. Because of the density of nervous structures in the upper extremity and the morbidity associated with loss of function, it is extremely important to perform and document a complete neurologic assessment of the upper extremity prior to operative exploration. This helps assure that neurologic deficits occurring as a result of the extremity injury are not attributed to operative intervention. The most commonly used techniques used for upper extremity arterial injuries are primary end-to-end repairs and interposition grafting with saphenous vein; size-matched synthetic graft has poor 30-day patency. Isolated radial or ulnar artery injuries may be ligated with relative impunity provided the ipsilateral ulnar or radial vessel is intact. Even when repair is undertaken, ultrasound studies demonstrate that only ~50% of repairs remain patent at 30 days. Approximately 50% of patients with injuries to the radial or ulnar artery have postoperative weakness and 12% have postoperative temperature sensitivity, but these morbidity rates appear to associated with concomitant nerve injury rather than method of treatment for arterial injury. Similar to lower extremity vascular injuries associated with complex orthopedic injuries, revascularization of the extremity is the first priority. Intraluminal shunting should be considered as a temporizing measure prior to orthopedic stabilization; once the extremity is stable, definitive vascular repair can occur. Ligation of the brachial artery should not be considered as it is associated with unacceptably high amputation rates.

Answer: C

Feliciano DV, Mattox KL, Graham JM, Bitondo CG (1985) Five-year experience with PTFE grafts in vascular wounds. *Journal of Trauma* **25** (1), 71–82.

Johnson M, Ford M, Johansen K, *et al.* (1993) Radial or ulnar artery laceration: Repair or ligate? *Archives of Surgery* **128** (9), 971–5.

Rich N, Mattox K, Hirshberg A (2004) *Vascular Trauma,* 2nd edn. Philadelphia, PA: Elsevier Saunders.

12. *A 22-year-old man presents to the trauma bay with a shotgun wound to the left lower extremity. On physical examination there are multiple punctuate wounds from the mid-thigh to the mid calf; there is no evidence of active bleeding but there are no pulses in the left foot. Plain films demonstrate no fractures and innumerable radiopaque foreign bodies consistent with shotgun pellets. Which of the following is not correct?*

A. *Arterial injuries caused by shotgun wounds are associated with a high rate of concomitant venous injuries*

B. *Because of the possibility of multi-level injury, angiography should be performed prior to definitive operation*

C. *This patient is more likely to require multiple operations and have a longer length of stay when compared to patients with handgun wounds*

D. *Vascular injuries associated with shotgun wounds are associated with a lower rate of amputation than other low-velocity gunshot wounds*

E. *Pellet embolism via both venous and arterial routes is a known sequelae of vascular injury caused by shotgun wounds*

Shotgun wounds represent a special class of injuries that must be considered separately from other gunshot wounds. Close range shotgun injuries produce multiple trajectories across the affected body region and are capable of producing massive soft tissue damage. Combined venous and arterial injures are common with shotgun woundings; a small case series by Bongard *et al.* reported a 100% incidence of venous injuries associated with arterial injuries. A single shotgun blast can create arterial injuries at multiple levels, and delineating the extent of injury before undertaking repair can obviate the need to perform multiple repairs. CT angiography may have distinct limitations in the evaluation of shotgun wounds due to beam scatter effect from the plethora of retained radiopaque foreign bodies. For this reason conventional angiography may be more useful in this situation. Patients with shotgun wounds require more operative interventions and have longer lengths of stay compared to those with wounds from other types of guns. Vascular injuries caused by shotgun wounds are associated with a higher rate of amputation than those caused by other low-velocity gunshot wounds (~20% versus 11%). While the overall incidence is unknown, there are dozens of case reports of shotgun pellets embolizing through the venous and arterial circulation. Clinical presentation can range from stroke with hemiparesis to asymptomatic radiographic findings, depending on the ultimate resting site of the pellet embolism.

Answer: D

Bongard FS, Klein SR (1989) The problem of vascular shotgun injuries: Diagnostic and management strategy. *Annals of Vascular Surgery* **3** (4), 299–303.

Dozier KC, Miranda MA, Kwan RO, *et al.* (2009) Despite the increasing use of nonoperative management of firearm trauma, shotgun injuries still require aggressive operative management. *Journal of Surgical Research* **156** (1), 173–6.

Hafez HM, Woolgar J, Robbs JV (2001) Lower extremity arterial injury: Results of 550 cases and review of risk factors associated with limb loss. *Journal of Vascular Surgery* **33** (6), 1212–19.

Yoshioka H, Seibel RW, Pillai K, Luchette FA (1995) Shotgun wounds and pellet emboli: Case reports and review of the literature. *Journal of Trauma—Injury, Infection and Critical Care* **39** (3), 596–601.

Chapter 32 Urologic Trauma

Hoylan Fernandez, MD, MPH and Scott Petersen, MD, FACS

1. *A 29-year-old man presents to the emergency room with suprapubic pain after a motor vehicle collision. Examination reveals slight abdominal distention and inability to void. The prostate is felt to be in its normal position. Appropriate treatment of the findings after a retrograde cystogram may include which of the following?*

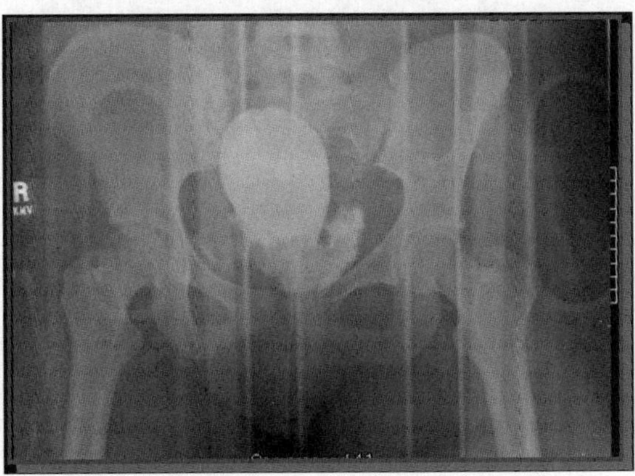

A. *Exploratory laparotomy*

B. *Percutaneous retroperitoneal drainage*

C. *Urinary catheter placement*

D. *Observation*

E. *Repeat cystogram in six weeks*

Bladder injuries occur frequently in association with pelvic fractures. They have also been found in patients with blunt abdominal trauma, or patients who sustained lower abdominal trauma with a distended bladder. Extraperitoneal bladder ruptures comprise the majority of bladder trauma, approximately 55%, while intraperitoneal and extraperitoneal bladder ruptures occur about 38% of the time. A combination of intraperitoneal and extraperitoneal bladder ruptures comprise a small minority of bladder injuries associated with trauma.

Presence of gross hematuria with a pelvic fracture mandates the performance of a retrograde cystogram, which is considered the gold standard diagnostic study. CT cystograms have been used, and are considered an accurate method of identifying bladder injuries in blunt trauma, if additional CT evaluation is needed.

Bladder injury should be suspected with suprapubic pain, inability to void, hematuria, blood at the urethral meatus, or increased BUN/Cr.

Extraperitoneal bladder injuries, such as demonstrated in the image, are mainly managed by urinary catheter drainage and rarely required surgical intervention. The majority of these injuries are healed within 10–14 days. However, some studies suggest that these injuries can be primarily repaired if an exploratory laparotomy is mandated for associated trauma injuries. Surgical intervention is also performed if the urinary catheter is not adequately draining the injury, and if an extraperitoneal bladder injury is encountered with the presence of a vaginal or rectal injury, bladder neck injury or avulsion, or pelvic fracture requiring internal or external fixation.

Answer: C

Deck A, Shaves S, Talner L, Porter J (2001) Current experience with computed tomographic cystography and blunt trauma. *World Journal of Surgery* **25**, 1592–6.

Iverson A, Morey A (2001) Radiographic evaluation of suspected bladder rupture following blunt trauma: critical review. *World Journal of Surgery* **25**, 1588–91.

Tezval H, Tezval M, von Klot C, *et al.* (2007) Urinary tract injuries in patients with multiple trauma. *World Journal of Urology* **25**, 177–84.

Surgical Critical Care and Emergency Surgery: Clinical Questions and Answers, First Edition. Edited by Forrest O. Moore, Peter M. Rhee, Samuel A. Tisherman and Gerard J. Fulda.

2. *A 29-year-old man is seen in the ER after a boiling pot of water accidently spills across his genital region. On physical examination, he is in profound pain and noted to have an erythematous penile shaft with enlarging blisters. This wound is initially treated conservatively with removal of blisters, copious irrigation, and topical antimicrobials. However, a few days later, the penile shaft confirms full-thickness tissue loss and requires surgical attention. The procedure of choice in treatment of this genital burn is:*

A. *Debridement with primary closure*

B. *Debridement with full-thickness skin graft*

C. *Debridement with split-thickness skin graft*

D. *Debridement with meshed split-thickness skin graft*

E. *Debridement with application of negative pressure wound therapy*

Genital burns are infrequent injuries that are usually found in conjunction with greater surface injuries. These injuries are commonly caused by fire, hot liquids, chemical agents, or electricity. Most burns sustained to the genital region are caused by direct contact.

Urinary diversion should be performed if a catheter-free approach cannot be met due to immobilization or urinary soiling. Catheter or suprapubic cystostomy increases the probability of urinary tract colonization, increasing risk of infection by approximately 4% per day.

Burns are initially managed by removing any foreign debris or necrotic tissue, cleansing with copious water, and topical antimicrobials. Surgical debridement of necrotic tissue may be necessary in second or third degree burns. Full-thickness grafts are used in penile shaft injuries to prevent contractures. Split-thickness grafts to this area may form hypertrophic scars, which can be treated with multiple Z-plasties. Deep scrotal injuries may be treated with split-thickness grafts.

Answer: B

Michielsen D, Lafaire C (2010) Management of genital burns: A review. *International Journal of Urology* **15**, 755–8.

Michielsen D, Van Hee R, Neetens C, *et al.* (1988) Burns to the genitalia and the perineum. Journal of Urology **159**, 418–19.

Peck M, Boileau M, Grube B, Heimback D (1990) The management of burns to the perineum and genitals. *Journal of Burn Care and Rehabilitation* **11**, 54–6.

3. *A 9-year-old boy is a passenger in a rollover vehicle. He presents to the ED with abdominal pain, and on physical exam is noted to have suprapubic tenderness and blood at the urethral meatus. His retrograde urethrogram is shown below:*

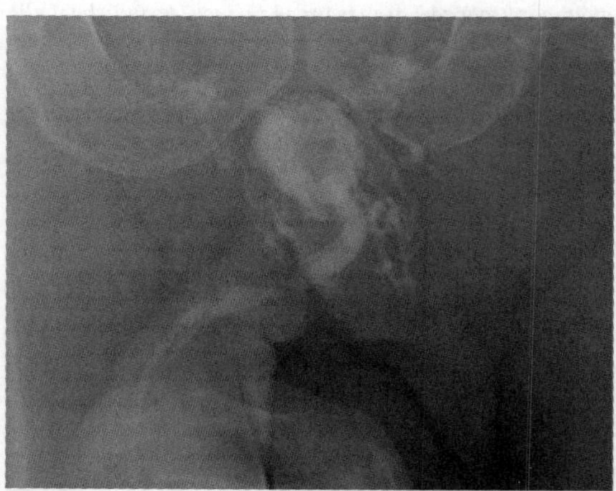

Which of the following diagnostic tests should be performed next for further evaluation of this patient, prior to surgical intervention?

A. *Fast exam*

B. *CT cystogram*

C. *CT abdomen/pelvis*

D. *Intravenous pyelography*

E. *Diagnostic peritoneal lavage*

Urethral injuries may be observed with blunt, penetrating or iatrogenic injuries. Urethral injuries are more common in men, and are usually seen in combination with pelvic fractures. If present in women, these injuries are usually partial, ventral, and can cause incontinence. On presentation, these patients may have blood at the meatus, a high-riding prostate, voiding difficulty, and co-existing rectal injuries may be apparent.

The diagnosis of these injuries should occur prior to placement of a Foley. The gold standard diagnostic test is a retrograde urethrogram. Once identified, a computed tomogram cystourethrogram, especially in stable patients who require further imaging of the abdomen and pelvis, should be performed to gather information regarding the location, length and severity of the injury. An intravenous pyelogram will not add to the urethral or bladder evaluation. Treatment of urethral disruption is controversial and depends on the stability of the patient and the severity and location of the urethral injury. Suprapubic cystostomy with delayed urethral reconstruction is the traditional mode of therapy. Endoscopic realignment of the urethra especially in patients with posterior membranous urethral tears is gaining favor. Urethral stenting with careful Foley catheter placement may be the only therapy required for partial injuries.

Answer: B

Koraitim M (1996) Risk factors and mechanism of urethral injury in pelvic fractures. *British Journal of Urology* **77**, 876–80.

Moore FO, Petersen SR, Norwood SH (2010) Diagnosis of blunt urethral injuries with computed tomogram retrograde urethrography. *Journal of Trauma* **68** (5), 1264.

Moudouni SM, Patard JJ, Manunta A, *et al.* (2001) Early endoscopic realignment of post-traumatic posterior urethral disruption. *Urology* **57** (4), 628–32.

Sandler C, Goldman S, Kawashima A (1998) Lower urinary tract trauma. *World Journal of Urology* **16**, 69–75.

Tezval H, Tezval M, von Klot C, *et al.* (2007) Urinary tract injuries in patients with multiple trauma. *World Journal of Urology* **25**, 177–84.

4. *A 25-year-old woman is thrown from her horse while attempting to jump a fence. She is hemodynamically stable, and found to have left chest wall pain and ecchymosis on physical exam. Her urinalysis demonstrates microscopic hematuria. The next step in assessment of her injury is:*

A. *Ultrasound*

B. *CT abdomen/pelvis*

C. *Intravenous pyelogram*

D. *Retrograde urethrogram*

E. *CT cystogram*

The most common genitourinary injury is renal trauma, usually resulting from the application of an external force. The majority of renal injuries are found in conjunction with multiple associated injuries. Rapid deceleration, such as that experienced in motor vehicle collisions, are associated with vascular injury, renal artery thrombosis, or renal pedicle avulsion.

Suspicion for renal trauma can be raised by the presence of lower rib fractures, ecchymosis in thoracic or lumbar region, or gross/microscopic hematuria. The gold standard to assess stable patients is a contrast enhanced CT scan. An intravenous pyelogram (IVP) can be considered in unstable patients, those requiring immediate surgical intervention, or intraoperatively to evaluate extent of renal trauma or assess viability of contralateral kidney. Ultrasound can be used to assess renal injury, but inexperienced health care providers may be unable to clearly identify the presence or type of renal injury by this modality. Angiography allows for the identification of vascular injuries, while at the same time permitting endoluminal access to treat these injuries.

Answer: B

Broghammer J, Fisher M, Santucci R (2007) Conservative management of renal trauma: a review. *Urology* **70**, 623–9.

Heyns C (2004) Renal trauma: indications for imaging and surgical exploration. *British Journal of Urology International* **93**, 1165–70.

Tezval H, Tezval M, von Klot C, *et al.* (2007) Urinary tract injuries in patients with multiple trauma. *World Journal of Urology* **25**, 177–84.

Voelzke B, Mcaninch J (2008) The current management of renal injuries. *American Surgeon* **74**, 667–8.

5. *A 45-year-old man is a driver in a head on collision in which he is ejected from the vehicle. His vitals in the trauma bay have been stable. CT demonstrates a right perinephric hematoma, with absence of contrast* *in the right renal vasculature. He underwent a renal angiogram, which demonstrates the findings below.*

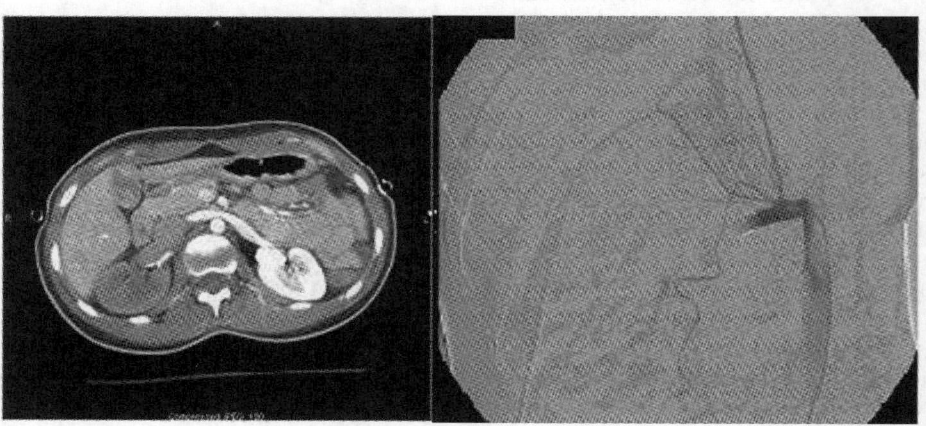

The next step in management involves:

A. Nephrectomy

B. Open revascularization

C. Endovascular embolization

D. Endovascular stent placement

E. Repeat CT in 2–4 days

Renal staging is now classically conducted with the use of CT. Angiography has the disadvantage of leading to delays in treatment due to the greater amount of time required and exposure to an invasive procedure. However, angiography does allow for specific localization of the renal lacerations, vascular injuries, active extravasation, and pedicle injuries, with the opportunity to treat these injuries with endovascular techniques.

A nonenhanced kidney on CT, such as demonstrated in the figure, should alert physicians to the possibility of a renal pedicle injury. The most common injuries sustained with a non-visualized kidney include total avulsion of renal vasculature, renal artery thrombosis, or severe renal contusion. This patient had an intimal flap with complete occlusion of the main renal artery.

Nonoperative management has become the treatment of choice for the majority of renal injuries, including grades 1, 2, and 3. Grade 3 injuries are expectantly managed with bed rest, and hydration in hemodynamically stable patients.

Grade 4 and 5 injuries are often seen in conjunction with other intra-abdominal injuries necessitating exploration. However, there are multiple reports of grade 4 or 5 vascular injuries in hemodynamically stable patients being managed with observation, delayed nephrectomy, vascular repair, or endovascular stenting. Endovascular stent use in the treatment of renal artery dissection has been reported, and offers an alternative to open revascularization, with better results. Absolute indications for renal exploration include severe hemodynamic instability due to renal hemorrhage and expanding or pulsatile hematoma encountered during exploratory laparotomy for associated intra-abdominal injury, and grade 5 renal injuries.

Answer: D

Broghammer J, Fisher M, Santucci R (2007) Conservative management of renal trauma: a review. *Urology* **70**, 623–9.

Heyns C (2004) Renal trauma: indications for imaging and surgical exploration. *British Journal of Urology International* **93**, 1165–70.

Tezval H, Tezval M, von Klot C, *et al.* (2007) Urinary tract injuries in patients with multiple trauma. *World Journal of Urology* **25**, 177–84.

Voelzke B, Mcaninch J (2008) The current management of renal injuries. *American Surgeon* **74**, 667–8.

6. *A 33-year-old woman is evaluated in the trauma bay after she was stabbed in the right flank during a robbery. A CT demonstrates a large perinephric hematoma with active ongoing blood loss. Her arteriogram is shown below.*

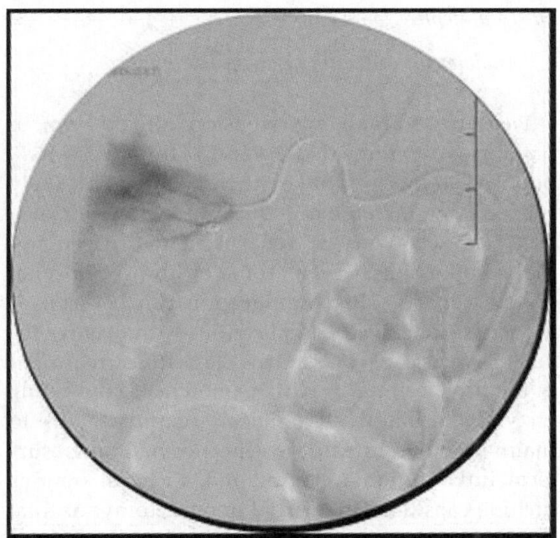

The next step in management of this patient is:

A. *Endovascular embolization*

B. *Endovascular stent placement*

C. *Partial nephrectomy*

D. *Renorrhaphy*

E. *Open revascularization*

The arteriogram demonstrates a cortical branch bleed. Renovascular injuries are uncommon, and usually associated with multiple sites of trauma and intra-abdominal injuries. Blunt trauma, attempted open revascularization, and grade 5 injuries have been associated with greater morbidity and mortality.

Arteriography with endovascular renal embolization is attempted if there is no other operative indication. Success rates (70–80%) are equivalent for vascular injuries sustained in blunt or penetrating trauma. Surgical intervention is pursued if endovascular techniques fail.

Renorrhaphy is the primary surgical technique attempted, but at times a partial nephrectomy is required if nonviable tissue is present. Repairs are usually supported with omentum, perinephric fat, or polyglycolic acid mesh. Nephrectomy is indicated in patients with hypothermia, coagulopathy, and hemodynamic instability. Penetrating trauma, high-velocity weapons and severe injuries have been associated with higher nephrectomy rates. Significant renal vascular injuries are most quickly resolved with a nephrectomy.

Answer: A

Broghammer J, Fisher M, Santucci R (2007) Conservative management of renal trauma: a review. *Urology* **70**, 623–9.

Heyns C (2004) Renal trauma: indications for imaging and surgical exploration. *British Journal of Urology International* **93**, 1165–70.

Tezval H, Tezval M, von Klot C, *et al.* (2007) Urinary tract injuries in patients with multiple trauma. *World Journal of Urology* **25**, 177–84.

Voelzke B, Mcaninch J (2008) The current management of renal injuries. *American Surgeon* **74**, 667–8.

7. *A 27-year-old man is seen the ED after sustaining a right flank stab wound, and is found to have a 2cm renal laceration through the corticomedullary junction on CT scan, with no other injuries. He is treated conservatively, and four days later complains of vague abdominal and right flank discomfort and develops a low-grade fever with a normal WBC count. A repeat CT scan demonstrates a right perirenal low density fluid collection. The next appropriate step in management of this patient is:*

A. *Observation alone*

B. *Percutaneous drainage*

C. *Percutaneous nephrostomy*

D. *Retrograde ureteral stenting*

E. *Anterograde ureteral stenting*

Complications after renal injury can be categorized as early or delayed complications. Early complications typically occur within the first month following injury and can include bleeding, infection, perinephric abscess, sepsis, urinary fistula, hypertension, urinary extravasation and urinoma. Delayed complications can include bleeding, nephrolithiasis, chronic pyelonephritis, hypertension, AV fistula, hydronephrosis and pseudoaneurysms. Retroperitoneal bleeding can occur within weeks of injury, and is most commonly treated by endovascular embolization. Abscess formation is preferentially managed by percutaneous drainage.

Urinary extravasation is observed in renal reconstruction or in transected kidney from blunt or penetrating trauma, and appears as a low density fluid collection on CT scan. This complication is usually treated by observation alone, with success rates of 74–87%. Percutaneous drainage or nephrostomy, and stenting are only necessary in particular circumstances. Extravasation of urine in the face of ureteral obstruction or presence of infection may necessitate surgical intervention. Persistent extravasation may be treated with ureteral retrograde stent placement, or percutaneous nephrostomy. Percutaneous drainage of a urinoma may be necessary in rare cases. Since this patient does not appear to have an infected urinoma (normal WBC and a low-grade fever is expected with the urinoma) observation would be the initial course of action.

Answer: A

Broghammer J, Fisher M, Santucci R (2007) Conservative management of renal trauma: a review. *Urology* **70**, 623–9.

Heyns C (2004) Renal trauma: indications for imaging and surgical exploration. *British Journal of Urology International* **93**, 1165–70.

Tezval H, Tezval M, von Klot C, *et al.* (2007) Urinary tract injuries in patients with multiple trauma. *World Journal of Urology* **25**, 177–84.

Voelzke B, Mcaninch J (2008) The current management of renal injuries. *American Surgeon* **74**, 667–8.

8. *A 54-year-old man is seen in the emergency room following a motor vehicle collision. He is hemodynamically stable, and is found to have a 1.5 cm cortical laceration with no noted urinary extravasation on CT scan. After undergoing bed rest, he is discharged from the hospital. He is seen for follow up 1 year later. His blood pressure in the office is 184/95 mm Hg. Which of the following should be considered for this patient?*

A. 24 hour urinary assay for metanephrines

B. Capsulotomy

C. Partial nephrectomy

D. Total nephrectomy

E. Angiotensin-converting enzyme inhibitor

Postrenal trauma hypertension can be seen in patients with an incidence varying from 0.25–55% of cases. Hypertension in these patients is likely related to an increase in renin (not metanephrines) secretion secondary to renal ischemia, parenchymal compression by hematoma or fibrosis, or renal artery stenosis. This complication can be seen as an acute or delayed complication, with occurrence at an average of 34 months. First line treatment is medical, primarily with angiotensin-converting enzyme inhibitors. If medical treatment fails to maintain blood pressure within normal limits, surgical intervention is considered. Surgical options include capsulotomy, partial nephrectomy, or total nephrectomy. Hypertension may also result from the presence of an AV fistula, which can be managed with endovascular embolization or open vascular repair.

Answer: E

Broghammer J, Fisher M, Santucci R (2007) Conservative management of renal trauma: a review. *Urology* **70**, 623–9.

Heyns C (2004) Renal trauma: indications for imaging and surgical exploration. *British Journal of Urology International* **93**, 1165–70.

Tezval H, Tezval M, von Klot C, *et al.* (2007) Urinary tract injuries in patients with multiple trauma. *World Journal of Urology* **25**, 177–84.

Voelzke B, Mcaninch J (2008) The current management of renal injuries. *American Surgeon* **74**, 667–8.

9. *A 52-year-old intoxicated man is involved in a motor vehicle collision while driving home from the bar. He was wearing his seat belt, and now complains of suprapubic tenderness and an inability to void. A retrograde urethrogram is performed and is shown below.*

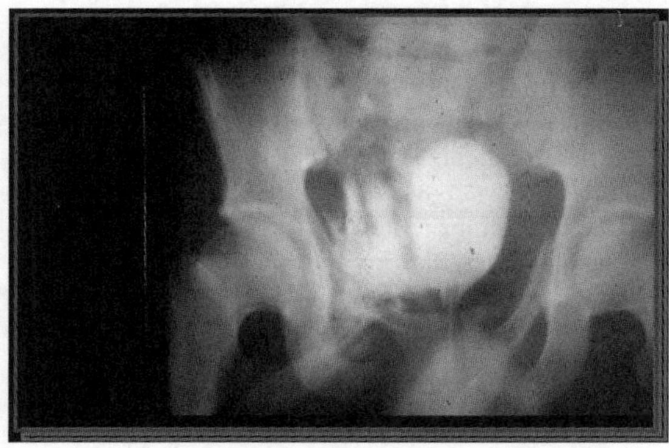

The next step in management of this patient is:

A. *Exploratory laparotomy*

B. *Placement of Foley catheter*

C. *Percutaneous drainage*

D. *Insertion of suprapubic catheter*

E. *Angiography*

This patient has an intraperitoneal bladder rupture. Retrograde cystography or CT cystography are the diagnostic procedures of choice. CT cystography can be used in patients who are undergoing CT evaluation for other traumatic injuries. This must be performed with retrograde filling of the bladder with at least 350 mL of diluted contrast to achieve high specificity and sensitivity.

Intraperitoneal bladder ruptures must always be surgically explored, and large dome lacerations are usually found upon exploration. If these injuries are observed without intervention, they will result in urinary extravasation and development of severe peritonitis. These injuries are primarily repaired in layers with absorbable sutures.

Answer: A

Deck A, Shaves S, Talner L, Porter J (2001) Current experience with computed tomographic cystography and blunt trauma. *World Journal of Surgery* **25**, 1592–6.

Iverson A, Morey A (2001) Radiographic evaluation of suspected bladder rupture following blunt trauma: critical review. *World Journal of Surgery* **25**, 1588–91.

Tezval H, Tezval M, von Klot C, *et al.* (2007) Urinary tract injuries in patients with multiple trauma. *World Journal of Urology* **25**, 177–84.

10. *A 12-year-old boy is seen in the emergency department following a football game. He states he was tackled hard after receiving the ball following a kickoff, and received most of the impact to the left flank. He is hemodynamically stable but is noted to have gross hematuria. Which of the following is the most appropriate screening study in the evaluation of this patient?*

A. *MRI*

B. *Dimercaptosuccinic acid scan*

C. *Ultrasound*

D. *CT scan*

E. *Retrograde urethrogram*

Pediatric renal injuries are most commonly caused by blunt trauma. Children are more likely than adults to sustain renal injury due to the location of the kidneys lower in the abdomen, less protection provided by ribs, increased mobility of kidneys, less perirenal fat, and are larger proportionally in the abdomen than adults. Hypotension is not always present in children who have significant volume losses, or severe injuries. Hematuria is a crucial clinical sign to the presence of renal injury, and in the presence of stable vital signs in children may still represent a significant renal injury.

Diagnostic imaging is undertaken in children with the following criteria: blunt or penetrating trauma with hematuria, associated abdominal injury, rapid deceleration, direct flank trauma, fall from height. Ultrasound is considered a screening method for those children with suspected minimal blunt trauma or stable cases. CT scans should be used in patients with multiple injuries and is the modality of choice for staging renal injuries.

Nonoperative management is the mainstay of treatment. Surgical intervention is indicated in the presence of hemodynamic instability or grade 5 injuries. Stable patients with urinary extravasation are managed conservatively. Mild renal injuries do not require repeat imaging, although major renal injuries should be reevaluated as these patients are likely to develop delayed complications and are more susceptible to renal insufficiency. All patients with hematuria should have follow up 6–8 weeks after injury to confirm resolution of hematuria and to identify any subsequent development of hypertension.

Answer: C

Broghammer J, Fisher M, Santucci R (2007) Conservative management of renal trauma: a review. *Urology* **70**, 623–9.

Heyns C (2004) Renal trauma: indications for imaging and surgical exploration. *British Journal of Urology International* **93**, 1165–70.

Tezval H, Tezval M, von Klot C, *et al.* (2007) Urinary tract injuries in patients with multiple trauma. *World Journal of Urology* **25**, 177–84.

Voelzke B, Mcaninch J (2008) The current management of renal injuries. *American Surgeon* **74**, 667–8.

Chapter 33 Care of the Pregnant Trauma Patient

Julie L. Wynne, MD, MPH, FACS and Terence O'Keeffe, MB ChB, MSPH, FACS

1. *Regarding uterine rupture from trauma, which of the following is false?*

A. *Only occurs after the first trimester, when the uterus has risen out of the pelvis*

B. *Typically involves the uterine fundus*

C. *Clinical presentation varies from uterine tenderness to hypovolemic shock*

D. *Can be diagnosed with ultrasonography*

E. *Most common presentation in laboring patients is an abnormal fetal heart rate pattern*

Traumatic uterine rupture has been reported at all gestational ages. The extent of injury ranges from serosal hemorrhage to complete disruption of the myometrial wall and extrusion of the fetus. Approximately three-quarters of cases involve the uterine fundus. Overall, this injury is associated with fetal mortality rates as high as 100%. Presenting signs and symptoms include uterine tenderness, abnormal fetal heart rate patterns, and frank shock, but the most common sign in an already laboring patient is an abnormal fetal heart rate pattern. Disruption of the uterus can be diagnosed with ultrasonography.

Answer: A

Mirza FG, Devine PC, Gaddipati S (2010) Trauma in pregnancy: a systematic approach. *Am J Perinatol*. **27** (7), 579–86.

Mirza FG, Gaddipati S (2009) Obstetric emergencies. *Semin Perinatol* **33** (2), 97–103.

Surgical Critical Care and Emergency Surgery: Clinical Questions and Answers, First Edition. Edited by Forrest O. Moore, Peter M. Rhee, Samuel A. Tisherman and Gerard J. Fulda.

2. *Regarding pelvic fractures sustained during pregnancy, which of the following is false?*

A. *Rarity of the event makes it difficult to establish management guidelines*

B. *Any pelvic fracture is an absolute contraindication to subsequent vaginal delivery*

C. *Compared to all other classes of orthopedic injuries, carries the highest risk of placental abruption*

D. *It is a significant independent risk factor for fetal loss*

E. *It has long term impact on fetal, neonatal, and infant death rates*

While the most recently published data from the CDC reports that pulmonary embolism is the most common cause of pregnancy-related mortality, traumatic injury is the most common nonobstetric cause of pregnancy-related mortality. Within the subgroup of pregnant trauma patients, pelvic fractures are rare events, and it is difficult to draw conclusions regarding their specific management in the pregnant patient. However, pelvic fracture carries the highest risk of placental abruption, as well as maternal and fetal death. It is independently a risk factor for fetal loss. American College of Obstetrics and Gynecology guidelines suggest that a pelvic fracture is not a contraindication to vaginal delivery.

Answer: B

Cannada LK, Pan P, Casey BM, *et al.* (2010) Pregnancy outcomes after orthopedic trauma. *Journal of Trauma* **69**, 694–8.

Ikossi DG, Lazar AA, Morabito D, *et al.* (2005) Profile of mothers at risk: an analysis of injury and pregnancy loss in 1195 trauma patients. *Journal of the American College of Surgeons* **200**, 49–56.

3. *Which of the following is false regarding the supine hypotensive syndrome of pregnancy?*

A. *Effects may be more pronounced in patients with mitral or aortic stenosis*

B. *It is typically not observed before 24 weeks of gestation*

C. *The decrease in cardiac output can be as much as 25–30%*

D. *It principally results from the compressive effect of the gravid uterus on the maternal inferior vena cava*

E. *Relief of this syndrome by left lateral tilting of the patient is contraindicated in patients with spinal injuries*

While the blood volume in a healthy patient with uncomplicated pregnancy increases as much as 50% during the pregnancy, cardiac output can be compromised as the gravid uterus enlarges and compresses the maternal inferior vena cava. This effect is typically not noted prior to 24 weeks gestation, and has its greatest effect during the late third trimester. Cardiac output can be decreased as much as 25–30%. The effect may be magnified in patients with mitral stenosis, who have a fixed cardiac output, and patients with aortic stenosis, who are prone to sudden death with any decrease in cardiac output. A second effect of compression on the maternal aorta may reduce flow to the uterine arteries and thus compromise the fetus. Maneuvers to ameliorate this syndrome include left lateral position, left lateral tilt to 15°, and manual displacement of the uterus to the left. All of the above can be performed in conjunction with maintenance of spinal precautions.

Answer: E

Fujitani S, Baldisseri MR (2005) Hemodynamic assessment in a pregnant and peripartum patient. *Critical Care Medicine* **33** (10), S354–61.

Knudson MM, Wan JJ (2008) Reproductive system trauma. In: Feliciano DV, Mattox KL, Moor EE (eds) *Trauma*, 6th edn, McGraw-Hill, New York, pp. 827–50.

4. *Which of the following is not a physiologic change that occurs during pregnancy?*

A. *Patients with preeclampsia have an exaggerated anemia of pregnancy*

B. *Enlargement of all four chambers of the heart, with resulting development of new murmurs and increased risk of arrhythmia*

C. *Mild compensated respiratory alkalosis due to increased tidal volume*

D. *Increased glomerular filtration rate up to 50%, with upper limit of normal creatinine of 0.8 mg/dL*

E. *Increased alkaline phosphatase secondary to placental production*

The blood volume in a healthy pregnant patient expands up to 50%, and this includes an increase in both plasma volume as well as erythrocytes. It should be noted that this phenomenon is not noted in pre-eclamptic patients, who actually manifest decrease in both plasma volume and erythrocyte mass, increasing their risk of shock from blood loss.

Answer: A

Fujitani S, Baldisseri MR (2005) Hemodynamic Assessment in a pregnant and peripartum patient. *Critical Care Medicine* **33** (10), S354–61.

Yeomans ER, Gilstrap LC (2005) Physiologic Changes in Pregnancy and their impact on Critical Care. *Critical Care Medicine* **33** (10), S256–8.

5. *Correct statements regarding fetal assessment in the context of maternal traumatic injury include all of the following except:*

A. *Ultrasound*

B. *Clinical examination of the mother*

C. *External monitoring of fetal heart rate tracings*

D. *Only indicated after the first trimester*

E. *External tocographic monitoring*

Optimization of the maternal clinical status is paramount, and includes avoidance of hypotension, hypoxia, and acidosis. Specifically, abdominal or uterine tenderness or presence of vaginal bleeding can lead to the diagnoses of uterine or placental abnormalities, or maternal intra-abdominal injury. Cardiotocographic monitoring, which monitors both uterine contractions and fetal heart rate tracings, is mandatory following trauma if the fetus is of a viable age. Fetal bradycardia (<110 bpm), tachycardia (>160 bpm), decelerations, and lack of variability suggest fetal distress. Uterine contractions in excess of one per ten minutes are abnormal and mandate further evaluation. Ultrasound is useful for determining gestational age, placental location, amount of amniotic fluid, fetal viability, fetal biophysical profile, as well as presence or absence of maternal intra-abdominal hemorrhage. The duration of fetal monitoring is debated, but several authors suggest 4–6 hours of continuous monitoring, with extension to 24 hours if the above described cardiotocographic parameters are concerning, or if the mother has demonstrated abdominal pain, vaginal bleeding, or hypotension.

Answer: D

Knudson MM, Wan JJ (2008) Reproductive system trauma. In: Feliciano DV, Mattox KL, Moor EE (eds) *Trauma*, 6th edn, McGraw-Hill, New York, pp. 827–50.

6. *Risk factors for fetal loss following maternal trauma include all of the following except:*

A. *Maternal tachycardia*

B. *Orthopedic trauma including extremity and pelvic fractures*

C. *Isolated head injury*

D. *Motor vehicle collision with ejection, motorcycle crash, and pedestrian struck*

E. *Injury Severity Score (ISS) > 15 or Abbreviated Injury Scale (AIS) $\geq$ 3 for head, abdomen, thorax, or lower extremity*

Characteristics of maternal trauma that prognosticate for fetal loss have been difficult to determine, partially due to issues with case finding and data collection. The mechanisms of MVC with ejection, motorcycle crash, and pedestrian struck are frequently cited as risk factors. It is largely agreed that pelvic fracture is a risk factor for fetal loss, and several studies have also identified an association of fetal mortality with any orthopedic injury. Isolated head injury as a risk factor was identified in an NTDB analysis. This analysis also identified ISS > 15 and AIS $\geq$ 3 as predictors of fetal loss. Maternal heart rate does not reliably predict fetal loss.

Answer: A

Cannada LK, Pan P, Casey BM, *et al.* (2010) Pregnancy outcomes after orthopedic trauma. *Journal of Trauma* **69**, 694–8.

Curet MJ, Schermer CR, Demarest GB, *et al.* (2000) Predictors of outcome in trauma during pregnancy: identification of patients who can be monitored for less than 6 hours. *Journal of Trauma* **49**, 18–25.

Ikossi DG, Lazar AA, Morabito D, *et al.* (2005) Profile of mothers at risk: an analysis of injury and pregnancy loss in 1.195 trauma patients. *Journal of the American College of Surgeons* **200**, 49–56.

7. *Which of the following laboratories would be abnormal in the pregnant trauma patient:*

A. *PCO_2 45 mm Hg*

B. *Fibrinogen 450 mg/dL*

C. *Hematocrit 32%*

D. *WBC 15,000/μL*

E. *HCO_3 19 mEq/L*

Due to the physiologic anemia of pregnancy, hematocrit between 32 and 42 mg/dL is considered normal, and a relative leukocytosis exists. As well, pregnancy is a hypercoagulable state, and nearly all coagulation factors are increased, including fibrinogen, which may increase as much as 50%. Low levels of fibrinogen may be consistent with disseminated intravascular coagulopathy (DIC), and suggest placental abruption or other type of hemorrhage. Progesterone-mediated stimulation of tidal volume results in increased minute ventilation, and a state of mild hypocarbia, with mean pCO_2 of 30 mm Hg. Lower than normal serum bicarbonate results as compensation for the hypocarbia.

Answer: A

Yeomans ER, Gilstrap LC (2005) Physiologic changes in pregnancy and their impact on critical care. *Critical Care Medicine* **33** (10), S256–8.

8. *Which of the following statements is true regarding the use of Kleihauer–Betke testing in pregnant trauma patients?*

A. It is indicated in all patients

B. It is indicated in all patients of gestational age >24 weeks

C. Its utility may be as an independent predictor of preterm labor

D. The routine use of RhIG in all Rh(−) patients has rendered the use of this test obsolete

E. A positive test is a marker for placental abruption or uterine rupture

The utility of Kleihauer–Betke testing is much discussed. This test allows for calculation of the amount of fetal Hgb transferred from a fetus to the mother's bloodstream (fetomaternal hemorrhage, or FMH), but does not identify the acuity of the hemorrhage. The test is generally not useful in the severely injured trauma patient, for whom clinical manifestations such as abdominal tenderness, vaginal bleeding, and abnormal cardiotocography are more likely to identify catastrophes such as placental abruption or uterine rupture. The correlation between a positive test result and placental abruption is poor. Several studies have suggested a lack of benefit of this test in minor trauma as well. In contrast, one study suggested that Kleihauer–Betke testing accurately predicts uterine contractions and preterm labor in trauma patients, suggesting that fetal monitoring may then be warranted.

Answer: C

Muench MV, Baschat AA, Reddy UM, *et al.* (2004) Kleihauer–Betke testing is important in all cases of maternal trauma. *Journal of Trauma* **57**, 1094–8.

Van Hook JW, Gei AF, Pacheco LD (2004) Trauma in pregnancy. In: Dildy G, Clark SL, Hankins GDV, *et al.* (eds) *Critical Care Obstetrics*, Blackwell Science, Oxford, pp. 484–505.

9. *Regarding abdominal trauma in pregnancy, which of the following is false?*

A. All patients taken for exploratory laparotomy should undergo concomitant Cesarean section

B. In the context of penetrating trauma, a uterus enlarged above the pelvic brim may be protective of maternal viscera

C. Fetal mortality in the context of penetrating abdominal trauma exceeds 70%

D. The most common complication following blunt abdominal trauma is fetal loss

E. The most common complication following penetrating abdominal trauma is ileus

The fundus of a 20-week uterus is palpable at the umbilicus, while a fundus palpated between the umbilicus and the costal margin is typically ≥24 weeks, suggesting viability. Third-trimester pregnancies may absorb the kinetic energy in penetrating trauma, with resultant protection of maternal viscera. A recent multicenter study of abdominal trauma in pregnancy reported 73% fetal mortality in penetrating trauma, consistent with earlier studies, and a 7% maternal mortality rate. Fetal loss was the most commonly identified complication following blunt abdominal trauma, while ileus was the most frequent morbidity in the cohort of penetrating trauma patients. Patients taken to the operating room for laparotomy for either blunt or penetrating trauma should be monitored with sterile sonography, and the decision for Cesarean section rests on the hemodynamic status of the mother, the condition of the fetus, or the inability to repair uterine injury.

Answer: A

Oxford CM, Ludmir J (2009) Trauma in pregnancy. *Clinical Obstetrics and Gynecology* **52** (4), 611–29.

Petrone P, Talving P, Browder T, *et al.* (2011) Abdominal injuries in pregnancy: a 155 month study at two level 1 trauma centers. *Injury* **42**, 47–9.

10. *A safe algorithm for evaluation and management of a hemodynamically normal pregnant patient s/p blunt traumatic injury includes all of the following except:*

A. Following completion of the primary survey, the uterine size is palpated to estimate gestational age; fundus below the umbilicus suggests gestational age <20 weeks, and this patient does not require any further investigations regarding the pregnancy

B. Focused assessment by sonography for trauma (FAST) scan precedes fetal ultrasound

C. Fetal ultrasound without evidence for fetal heart activity, in a fetus of viable gestational age, mandates induction of labor following stabilization of maternal condition

D. Fetal ultrasound with evidence for fetal heart activity mandates initiation of cardiotocography; contractions <4 per hour obligate the trauma team to initiate aggressive volume resuscitation and minimum of 24 hours fetal monitoring

E. Sterile speculum examination is recommended following stabilization of pregnant trauma patients >20 weeks gestational age

Prioritizing the status of the pregnant patient as the best means of optimizing the status of the fetus cannot be overemphasized. The gestational age is then estimated based on fundal height, and pregnancies less than 20 weeks do not require any further specific interventions. FAST exam can be useful in detecting maternal hemorrhage, and this study should precede the obstetric ultrasound. If the obstetric ultrasound reveals absence of fetal heart activity, a catastrophic condition such as placental abruption or uterine rupture may be present, and labor should be induced as allowed by the status of the mother. The presence of fetal heart activity in a viable fetus mandates initiation of cardiotocographic monitoring, and contractions *greater than* 4–6 per hour correlate with a high risk of preterm labor, and extended monitoring is required. The perineum should be visually inspected for vaginal bleeding; in the absence of bleeding, a sterile speculum exam should be performed. The purpose of the speculum exam is to determine if rupture of membranes has occurred, and the presence and degree of cervical effacement and dilation. Amniotic fluid, and thus rupture of membranes, is diagnosed by color change on nitrazine paper, or by the presence of ferning on microscopic exam. Rupture of membranes in conjunction with cervical effacement >3–4 cm is consistent with active labor.

Answer: D

Knudson MM, Wan JJ (2008) Reproductive system trauma. In: Feliciano DV, Mattox KL, Moor EE (eds) *Trauma*, 6th edn, McGraw-Hill, New York, pp. 827–50.

Muench MV, Canterino JC (2007) Trauma in pregnancy. *Obstetrics and Gynecology Clinics of North America* **34**, 555–83.

11. *Imaging the pregnant trauma patient can be challenging. Which statement is true regarding radiation exposure during pregnancy?*

A. The maximum permissible radiation dose for fetal exposure is 500 mSv.

B. Fetal radiation exposure from a single maternal pelvic CT scan increases the risk of fatal childhood cancer by approximately twofold.

C. Exposure during the first eight weeks does not increase the risk of spontaneous abortion, malformations and mental retardation.

D. The radiation risks to the fetus during the first trimester of pregnancy are so high that they outweigh the benefit of timely and accurate diagnosis.

E. Three percent of trauma patients who are undergoing CT scanning will have an unidentified pregnancy.

The National Council on Radiation Protection and Measurements has recommended that the maximal permissible radiation dose for fetal exposure during pregnancy is 5 mSv. The dose exposure from a pelvic CT scan is well within the permissible guidelines, even though it has been estimated to increase the likelihood of fatal childhood cancer by a factor of two. Early exposure will indeed increase the risk of spontaneous abortion, malformations and mental retardation in the fetus. Although there is significant concern regarding fetal exposure to radiation during investigation for trauma by plain radiography or computed tomographic scanning, it is important to remember that the priority is the mother, and without maternal survival, the fetus will also perish. The benefits of accurate diagnosis always outweigh the fetal risks, in ANY trimester. Although 3% of trauma patients are estimated to be pregnant, only 0.3% will be diagnosed during their trauma evaluation.

Answer: B

ACR (2008) ACR practice guideline for imaging pregnant or potentially pregnant adolescents and women with ionizing radiation. *American College of Radiology* **26**, 1–15.

Chen MM, Coakley FV, Kaimal A, *et al.* (2008) Guidelines for computed tomography and magnetic resonance imaging use during pregnancy and lactation. *Obstetrics and Gynecology* **112**, 333–40.

12. *Which of the following is true regarding placental abruption?*

A. *Placental abruption following trauma frequently presents without any symptoms.*

B. *Placental abruption must be ruled out in pregnant trauma patients with abdominal pain and vaginal bleeding.*

C. *A positive Kleihauer-Betke test is highly diagnostic in cases of placental abruption.*

D. *The risk of placental abruption is lower if the placenta is located posteriorly.*

E. *The management in all cases of placental abruption following trauma is delivery of the fetus if over 24 weeks gestational age.*

Trauma is one of the many risk factors that can lead to placental abruption, which is defined as premature separation of a normally implanted placenta. The range of presentation is very wide, from completely asymptomatic to fetal demise with significant maternal morbidity. In all cases where there is vaginal bleeding and abdominal pain, the diagnosis of abruption should be considered and aggressively investigated. Unfortunately, there is no correlation between a Kleihauer–Betke test and the existence of a placental abruption. Likewise, there is no difference in the risk of abruption following trauma in pregnancy and the location of the placenta on the uterine wall. Management depends on the gestational age of the fetus, and other associated factors such as bleeding or DIC. Abruption at term or near term with a live fetus is generally managed with delivery of the fetus, but earlier than this, it may be possible to manage the condition nonoperatively with steroids and tocolytics.

Answer: B

Oyelese Y, Ananth CV (2006) Placental abruption. *Obstetrics Gynecology* **108** (4), 1005–16.

13. *Which of the following below is not an indication for emergency Caesarean section in a pregnant trauma patient?*

A. *After 10 minutes of maternal cardiac arrest*

B. *After 3 minutes of maternal cardiac arrest with ongoing CPR*

C. *Stable mother with worrisome fetal heart tracing, fetal age 32 weeks*

D. *Penetrating trauma to the abdomen causing uterine injury in a pregnant patient with a viable, near-term fetus*

E. *The onset of labor in a pregnant patient with a term (>36 weeks) fetus, in the presence of pelvic fractures related to blunt abdominal trauma*

An emergency caesarean section can be accomplished extremely quickly by a skilled operator, and may be used to improve both maternal and fetal mortality and morbidity. Outcomes are optimal in neonates delivered within four minutes after cardiac arrest, as long as delivery can be achieved within one minute for a total time of five minutes following maternal death. Survival is 70% when delivery is achieved in less than five minutes, and survivors are usually neurologically intact, as opposed to 13% survival with 100% neurological morbidity after 5 minutes. Caesarean section should be performed in a viable fetus if there is concern for fetal distress, as this will give good outcomes. Penetrating trauma to the abdomen in the pregnant woman is rare, but may affect up to 8% of all pregnancies. An emergency caesarian section should be performed in the presence of maternal shock, uterine injury or concern for intra-abdominal injury if the fetus is near term. Pelvic fractures are not a contraindication for vaginal delivery, according to the American College of Gynecologists although they acknowledge that a severe, dislocated or unstable fracture may preclude vaginal delivery.

Answer: A

Mirza FG, Devine PC, Gaddipati S (2010) Trauma in pregnancy: a systematic approach. *American Journal of Perinatology* **27** (7), 579–86

Oxford CM, Ludmir J (2009) Trauma in pregnancy. *Clinical Obstetrics and Gynecology* **52** (4), 611–29.

14. *Regarding pregnancy-induced hypertension:*

A. *The goal of treatment of severe hypertension in the pregnant patient should be to normalize the blood pressure*

B. *Labetalol is the most commonly used first line treatment for acute severe hypertension in pregnancy*

C. *Pre-eclampsia is defined by hypertension (>140 mm Hg systolic or >90 mm Hg diastolic) and peripheral edema*

D. *It is a rare condition, responsible for less than 2% of maternal deaths in the US*

E. *Induction of labor in near-term fetuses (>36 weeks) is not associated with an improvement in maternal outcome*

Acute hypertension of pregnancy is defined as a systolic pressure of 140 mm Hg or a diastolic pressure of >90 mm Hg. Pre-eclampsia is defined as hypertension with proteinuria. It is a complication of approximately 12% of pregnancies and causes 18% of the maternal deaths in the US. Treatment should be initiated with labetalol as first line therapy. One of the advantages of this drug is the lack of fetal side effects. The aim should be to reduce the diastolic blood pressure to less than 100 mm Hg, and not normalize the BP, due to potentially deleterious effects on the fetus.

Answer: B

Koopmans CM, Bijlenga D, Groen H, *et al.* (2009) Induction of labour versus expectant monitoring for gestational hypertension or mild pre-eclampsia after 36 weeks' gestation (HYPITAT): a multicentre, open-label randomised controlled trial. *Lancet* **374** (9694), 979–88.

Vidaeff AC, Carroll MA, Ramin SM (2005) Acute hypertensive emergencies in pregnancy. *Critical Care Medicine* **33**(10 Suppl), S307–12.

15. *Amniotic fluid embolism is a potentially fatal complication of pregnancy that usually occurs during labor, but can also be associated with abdominal trauma. Which of the following is true regarding this condition?*

A. *Disseminated intravascular coagulation is a rare (<10%) consequence*

B. *It is the cause of 30–40% of the maternal mortality in the US*

C. *Neonatal survival is 70–80%*

D. *Most survivors do not have permanent neurologic impairment*

E. *Treatment with prostaglandin F2 has dramatically improved survival*

Amniotic fluid embolism is thought to occur secondary to the entry of amniotic fluid and fetal cells into the maternal circulation, although current data suggests that the process is more similar to anaphylaxis than to embolism, and the term *anaphylactoid syndrome of pregnancy* has been proposed. It often presents with a significant coagulopathy. Disseminated intravascular coagulation is present in up to 80% of cases, and most patients require transfusion with blood and coagulation factors. Although maternal mortality from amniotic fluid embolism ranges from 60–80%, it is only responsible for 5–10% of overall maternal mortality in the USA. However, permanent neurologic sequelae are present in the majority of survivors. Prostaglandin F2 has a role in reducing post-partum bleeding by stimulating myometrial contractions, but no medication has been shown to effectively impact survival. The only positive note for this disease is the high fetal survival rate, which is 79% in the USA and 78% in the UK.

Answer: C

Moore J, Baldisseri, MR Amniotic Fluid Embolism (2005) *Critical Care Medicine* **33** (10 Suppl), S279–85.

Moore LE (n.d.) Amniotic Fluid embolism, http://emedicine.medscape.com/article/253068-overview (accessed February 2011).

16. *Which of the following is true regarding hypercoagulability of pregnancy?*

A. *Pregnancy increases the risk of thrombosis by a factor of ten times*

B. *The risk of arterial thromboembolism is the same as the risk of venous thromboembolism*

C. *Normal pregnancy causes an increase in Factors VII, VIII, X and von Willebrand*

D. *Heparin and Low-molecular weight heparin can cross the placenta and therefore are not considered safe in pregnancy*

E. *Warfarin is transmitted via breast milk and should not be used in a woman developing a peripartum DVT or PE*

Pregnancy increases the risk of thromboembolism by only three to four times, although this is somewhat higher for venous disease at four to five times. The hypercoagulability associated with pregnancy likely has a mechanical component due to the mechanical obstruction caused by the gravid uterus, as well as increased venous capacitance with decreased venous outflow. However, there are also increases in Factors VII, VIII, X and von Willebrand factor, and increases in fibrinogen. Heparin and LMWH do not cross the placenta and are therefore considered the treatment of choice for thromboembolic disease in the pregnant patient, unlike warfarin, which is associated with abortion and hemorrhage. However, warfarin is not secreted in the breast milk, and can be considered safe in the post-partum period.

Answer: C

James AH (2010) Pregnancy and thrombotic risk. *Critical Care Medicine* **38** (2 Suppl), S57–63.

17. *Which of the following treatments is not useful in the management of preterm labor?*

A. *Bed rest and hydration*

B. *Amniocentesis to assess fetal lung maturity*

C. *The administration of corticosteroids to improve fetal lung maturity*

D. *Short term treatment with tocolytic drugs to prolong pregnancy by 2 to 7 days*

E. *Antibiotic prophylaxis for Group B streptococcus*

Preterm labor is defined as the presence of uterine contractions of sufficient frequency and intensity to effect progressive effacement and dilation of the cervix prior to term gestation (20–37 weeks). Neither bed rest nor hydration has been proven to be effective treatment regimens for preterm labor. Amniocentesis has a role in assessing the degree of fetal lung maturity and amniotic fluid infection. Steroids should be administered to improve lung maturity and decrease respiratory distress syndrome. Tocolytic therapy should be short-term only to allow pregnancy to be prolonged and steroids given to reduce respiratory distress. Antibiotics should be used to prevent group B streptococcal prophylaxis in patients in whom delivery is imminent.

Answer: A

American College of Obstetricians and Gynecologists (ACOG) (n.d.) Management of Preterm Labor, www.guideline.gov/content.aspx?id=3993 (accessed February 2011).

Ross, MG. Eden, RD (n.d.) Preterm Labor, http://emedicine.medscape.com/article/260998-overview (accessed February 2011).

18. *Regarding seatbelt use by pregnant women, which of the following statements is correct?*

A. *Studies have not demonstrated any significant decline in maternal mortality with the use of seatbelts*

B. *Appropriate education has not been demonstrated to improve the use of seatbelts by pregnant woman, as they find the seatbelts too uncomfortable*

C. *The correct position for seatbelts in the pregnant woman is under the abdomen, over both anterior superior iliac spines and the pubic symphysis, with the shoulder belt left behind the left shoulder*

D. *Even if a seatbelt is appropriately applied, there is increased force transmitted to the fetus*

E. *Placing the lap belt over the dome of the uterus is associated with uterine and fetal injury*

Pregnant women cite a number of reasons not to use seatbelts in cars, from lack of comfort, fear of injuring the fetus in a crash to forgetfulness. Nevertheless the risk of maternal mortality was reduced from 33% to 5% in one early study on seatbelt use in pregnant women, and education has been shown to improve compliance. The correct position for a seatbelt in a pregnant woman is under the abdomen, over both anterior superior iliac spines and the pubic symphysis, with the shoulder belt positioned between the breasts. There is no evidence that there is significant force transmission to the gravid uterus when the seatbelt is properly applied; however, if the lap belt is placed over the dome of the uterus, this is associated with significant morbidity in the event of a crash.

Answer: E

Crosby WM, Costiloe JP (1971) Safety of lap-belt restraint for pregnant victims of automobile collisions. *New England Journal of Medicine* **284** (12), 632–6.

19. *In the evaluation of suspected abdominal trauma in the pregnant patient, which of the following is correct?*

A. *Kleihauer–Betke test is not necessary as part of the laboratory investigations.*

B. *Direct fetal injury is rare, with an incidence of less than 1%*

C. *Fetal monitoring should be performed for a minimum of 12 hours in ALL patients with a potentially viable fetus*

D. *MRI is the recommended second line investigation after ultrasound to assess for intra-abdominal injury due to the lack of radiation risk to the fetus*

E. *Diagnostic peritoneal lavage is contra-indicated in the first trimester due to possible teratogenic effects*

All pregnant patients should receive the same initial labwork as any other trauma patient, with the addition of a Kleihauer-Betke test. Rhesus immunoglobulin is given if the test is positive for fetal cells in the maternal circulation. Direct fetal injury is luckily very rare, at 1% with uterine rupture even rarer at 0.6%. Fetal monitoring is recommended for 6 hours for those at low risk—i.e. low injury severity, absence of maternal tachycardia and/or fetal brady or tachycardia—but 24 hours of monitoring is recommended in those at higher risk. The CT scan remains the main stay of investigation following abdominal trauma, AFTER ultrasound. MRI is too time consuming to be of significant use. Diagnostic peritoneal lavage can be performed safely in the first trimester, with a supra-umbilical approach, but is contra-indicated in the third trimester due to increased uterine size.

Answer: B

Curet MJ, Schermer CR, Demarest GB, *et al.* (2000) Predictors of outcome in trauma during pregnancy: identification of patients who can be monitored for less than 6 hours. *Journal of Trauma* **49** (1), 18–24; discussion 24–5.

Mirza FG, Devine PC, Gaddipati S (2010) Trauma in pregnancy: a systematic approach. *American Journal of Perinatology* **27** (7), 579–86.

20. *In the pregnant trauma patient, which one of the following statements is correct regarding the focused assessment by sonography for trauma (FAST) exam?*

A. *The FAST exam in the pregnant trauma patient should be performed by an ultrasonographer or obstetrician experienced in pelvic ultrasound*

B. *The sensitivity of the FAST exam is highest in the third trimester*

C. *Ultrasound for assessment of the pregnant trauma patient can easily pick up other conditions of pregnancy, such as placental abruption*

D. *The FAST exam has been shown to be as sensitive in pregnancy as in the general trauma population*

E. *The diagnostic yield of the FAST is limited by increasing gestational age*

Sonography, and specifically the FAST exam, are well established in pregnancy, and ultrasound has the advantage of avoiding ionizing radiation, with no side effects for the fetus. However, the sensitivity of the FAST exam is reduced, particularly with advancing gestational age. Sensitivity is between 60–80% in this patient population, across all trimesters, although it can be as high as 90% in the first trimester. It has poor sensitivity for accurately diagnosing placental abruption, and between 50–60% of cases can be missed. The FAST exam can easily be performed by an experienced operator, without the necessity of waiting for an ultrasonographer or obstetrician.

Answer: E

Brown MA, Sirlin CB, Farahmand N (2005) Screening sonography in pregnant patients with blunt abdominal trauma. *Journal of Ultrasound Medicine* **24** (2), 175–81.

Dahmus MA, Sibai BM (1993) Blunt abdominal trauma: are there any predictive factors for abruptio placentae or maternal-fetal distress? *American Journal of Obstetrics and Gynecology* **169** (4), 1054–9.

Chapter 34 Esophagus, Stomach, and Duodenum

Andrew Tang, MD

1. *Which statement regarding esophageal anatomy is false?*

A. *There are three predictable areas of narrowing: the cricopharyngeus muscle, the aortic arch, and the diaphragm*

B. *The cervical and most distal esophagus lie to the left of midline*

C. *The left gastric vein provides the principle venous drainage when esophageal varices develop*

D. *The segmental blood supplies to the esophagus arise from the superior thyroid, the intercostals and the left gastric artery*

E. *The lower esophageal sphincter is a physiological rather than an anatomical entity*

The esophagus is approximately 25 cm long with an inner circular and outer longitudinal muscular layer, and no serosal covering. The upper 2/3 of the esophagus is lined by squamous epithelium, which transitions to columnar epithelium distally. The esophagus is divided into four segments: the pharyngoesophageal segment is between the pharynx and the cervical esophagus. It consists of the superior, middle and inferior constrictors. The cricopharyngeus muscle is believed to be part of the inferior constrictor, and serves as the upper esophageal sphincter. The potential space between the inferior constrictor and the cricopharyngeus muscle is the site of Zenker's diverticulum development. The cervical esophagus is approximately 5 cm long. It begins at the cricopharyngeus muscle and ends at T1. The recurrent laryngeal nerves lie in the groove between the esophagus and the trachea. The right recurrent laryngeal nerve has a more oblique course and is more prone to anatomic variants. Consequently, surgical access to the cervical esophagus is typically chosen from the left. The thoracic esophagus begins at T1 and ends at the hiatus. It lies directly posterior to the trachea. Above the level of the tracheal bifurcation, the esophagus courses to the left, behind the bifurcation and the left main-stem bronchus, and descends to the diaphragmatic hiatus left of midline. The left mainstem bronchus and aortic arch creates a narrowing of the thoracic esophagus at the level of T4. The bronchoaortic constriction can be visualized during endoscopy as a subtle pulsation along the posterior wall of the esophagus. The lower thoracic esophagus is covered by a flimsy layer of mediastinal pleura to the left, and this location is commonly associated with Boerhaave's perforation. The abdominal esophagus begins at the diaphragmatic hiatus, which is the third location of anatomical narrowing. The lower esophageal sphincter is a physiologic entity that does not correspond to any particular anatomical structures. Manometrically, it is detected as a high-pressure zone 3–5 cm long with both an intra-abdominal and thoracic component. Blood supply to the esophagus is segmental. The inferior thyroid artery is the main supply of the cervical esophagus. The proximal thoracic esophagus is largely supplied by the bronchial arteries where as branches arising directly from the aorta supply the distal esophagus. The left gastric and inferior phrenic arteries supply the abdominal esophagus. The superior thyroid artery is the first branch of the external carotid artery and along with the inferior thyroid artery comprises the vascular supply to the thyroid gland. The anterior and posterior intercostal arteries are the main blood supply to the thoracic cage. The first two posterior intercostal arteries arise from the subclavian artery, and the remaining arise from the thoracic aorta.

Surgical Critical Care and Emergency Surgery: Clinical Questions and Answers, First Edition. Edited by Forrest O. Moore, Peter M. Rhee, Samuel A. Tisherman and Gerard J. Fulda.

The posterior intercostal arteries anastomose with the anterior intercostal arteries, which are branches of the internal mammary arteries.

Answer: D

Patti MG, Gantert W, Way LW (1997) Surgery of the esophagus; anatomy and physiology. *Surgical Clinics of North America* **77**, 959.

2. *Which of the following statements regarding Boerhaave's syndrome is false?*

A. *Endoscopic evaluation of the esophageal tear is an integral component of diagnosis*

B. *The esophageal full-thickness tear is typically located in the left posterolateral aspect of the lower esophagus approximately 2–3 cm above the gastroesophageal junction*

C. *The classic Mackler's triad of vomiting, lower chest pain and subcutaneous emphysema has a sensitivity of 60% in diagnosing Boerhaave's syndrome*

D. *The underlying pathophysiology involves uncoordinated esophageal contraction against a closed pylorus distally and cricopharyngeus muscle proximally*

E. *Upper GI bleeding frequently accompanies Boerhaave's syndrome*

Boerhaave's syndrome is postulated to result from forceful esophageal contractions against a closed cricopharyngeus muscle and pylorus. The resultant sudden increase in intraluminal pressure creates the transmural esophageal tear, typically located in the left posterolateral aspect of the distal esophagus, 2–3 cm above the GEJ. Meckler's triad of vomiting, lower chest pain and subcutaneous emphysema is only present in up to 2/3 of patients, and therefore cannot be heavily relied on for diagnosis. The diagnostic test of choice is an esophagram. When a perforation is suspected, water-soluble contrast such as gastrograffin is the initial agent used. It has a sensitivity of 80% in detecting intrathoracic esophageal perforations. If a perforation is not identified by gastrografin, the study should be repeated with thin barium, which has a sensitivity of 90% for intrathoracic perforations. Should gastrograffin identify an intraperitoneal leak, then it obviates the need for barium which poses the risk of barium peritonitis. Endoscopic evaluation of the esophageal tear adds little additional diagnostic value, and air insufflation can potentially enlarge the injury and further spread bacterial contamination. The treatment of choice in Boerhaave's syndrome identified within twenty-four hours in a stable patient is primary repair in two layers with tissue buttressing through a laparotomy or left thoracotomy. Boerhaave's syndrome, in contrast to Mallory Weiss tears, is not typically associated with massive upper GI bleeding.

Answer: A

Lawrence DR, Ohri SK, Moxon RE, *et al.* (1999) Primary esophageal repair for Boerhaave's syndrome. *Annals of Thoracic Surgery* **67**, 818–20.

Vial CM, Whyte RI (2005) Boerhaave's syndrome: diagnosis and treatment. *Surgical Clinics of North America* **85** (3), 515–24.

3. *Which statement regarding esophageal perforation is most accurate?*

A. *The incidence of spontaneous perforation has increased since the early 2000s*

B. *Isolated penetrating esophageal injuries that are untreated are associated with 80% mortality due to the severe mediastinitis*

C. *Iatrogenic injury to the esophagus accounts for approximately 60% of esophageal perforations*

D. *Esophageal perforation from food bolus impedance is frequently associated with untreated achalasia*

E. *In hemodynamically stable patients, small thoracic esophageal free perforations demonstrated on esophagram can be successfully managed with chest drainage and antibiotics alone*

Since the early 1990s, the incidence of spontaneous esophageal perforation has decreased, now accounting for approximately 10–15% of all cases. The majority of esophageal perforations nowadays are iatrogenic in nature, most commonly resulting from diagnostic and therapeutic endoscopies. The exact mortality contributable to esophageal disruption in the setting of blunt or penetrating trauma is unknown due to its rarity, and the influence of the associated mediastinal and thoracic injuries on outcome. In general, free esophageal perforation is a contraindication to conservative management due to the uncontrolled source of sepsis. Criteria for nonoperative management of esophageal perforations include: intraluminal dissection; transmural dissection that drains back into the esophagus; no associated distal obstruction; the perforation is not in the abdominal cavity and no evidence of sepsis. Achalasia is an esophageal motility disorder characterized by a hypertensive lower esophageal sphincter that does not relax in response to bolus transport, and esophageal aperistalsis. Esophageal pneumatic dilatation for achalasia carries a perforation risk of 4–6%. The presence of the disease alone without therapeutic interventions, however, is not commonly associated with perforations.

Answer: C

Brinster CJ, Singhal S, Lawrence L, *et al.* (2004) Evolving options in the management of esophageal perforation. *Annals of Thoracic Surgery* **77**, 1475–83.

4. *What is the antibiotic regimen of choice for a patient with suspected esophageal perforation from balloon dilation for achalsia?*

A. *Cefazolin, piperacillin and tazobactam*

B. *Cefazolin, piperacillin and tazobactam, fluconazole*

C. *Vancomycin, piperacillin and tazobactam*

D. *Vancomycin, piperacillin and tazobactam, fluconazole*

E. *Cefazolin, gentamicin and flagyl*

Esophageal perforation is associated with mortality rates of 20–40%, largely secondary to the overwhelming mediastinal sepsis and ensuing multisystem organ failure. Appropriate antibiotic administration is of paramount importance in addition to prompt therapeutic interventions. Normally, the bacterial count of the esophagus and stomach is less than 1000 organisms per mL of fluid. The flora is chiefly composed of alpha-hemolytic streptococci, lactobacilli, yeast and some swallowed bacteria. There are no obligate anaerobes. Measures taken to decrease gastric acidity such as acid reduction surgeries and the use of agents such as proton pump inhibitors and H_2-blockers increase the bacterial and fungal counts significantly. Anesthesia likewise reduces gastric acidity and permits increase in the bacterial count. This particular patient who is presumed to have had previous hospital based therapeutic procedures due to his achalasia is also at higher risk for methicillin-resistant *Saphylococcus aureus* colonization. Therefore, in light of the high infectious lethality of inadequate antibiosis and the patient's increased risk for MRSA colonization, wide spectrum antibiotic and antifungal coverage is recommended.

Answer: D

Wittmann DH, Condon RE (2004) Approach to the patient with intraabdominal infections. In: Gorbach SL, Bartlett JG, Blacklow NR (eds) *Infectious Diseases*, 3rd edn, Lipincott Williams & Wilkins, Philadelphia, PA, pp. 717.

5. *Which of the following statements most accurately describes the treatment for Mallory–Weiss syndrome?*

A. *The primary treatment modality for bleeding associated with Mallory–Weiss syndrome is arteriography with selective epinephrine infusion*

B. *Sixty percent of Mallory–Weiss syndrome cases will stop bleeding with resuscitation and observation alone*

C. *Sclerosants is contraindicated in Mallory–Weiss syndrome due to the increased risk of perforation*

D. *Rebleeding in Mallory–Weiss syndrome has been reported in up to 5% of patients after successful initial endoscopic therapy*

E. *Endoscopic electrocoagulation is less effective in hemorrhage control than sclerotherapy*

Mallory–Weiss syndrome occurs as a result of abrupt and forceful increase in the gradient between intragastric and intrathoracic pressure, leading to an acute linear mucosal tear near the gastroesophageal junction. The rich submucosal blood supply produces arterial bleeding. It is classically described in the setting of retching, hematemesis and alcohol abuse. Although it accounts for 5–15% of patients hospitalized for upper GI bleeding, up to 90% of patients will resolve with resuscitation and observation alone. Definitive diagnosis is confirmed by flexible upper endoscopy, which reveals a single mucosal tear in 80–90% of cases. Endoscopic therapies that employ injection therapy, electrocoagulation, band ligation and hemoclipping have all been used with excellent success. Although electrocoagulation is the most prevalent therapeutic intervention for Mallory–Weiss tears, injection therapy consisting of either or a combination of vasoconstrictors (epinephrine) and sclerosants (ethanol, polidocanol) have been well documented to be equally effective. Esophageal perforation is an unusual complication of sclerotherapy and occurs in less than 1% of patients. Rebleeding is observed in up to 5% of patients after initial endoscopic therapy. Angiotherapy, which selectively delivers vasoconstrictive or embolizing agents, have achieved hemostasis in up to 94% of cases. However, it is not the first line therapy due to the increased cost and higher local (hematoma, bleeding, arteriovenous fistulas) and systemic (vasopressin associated myocardial infarction) complications. Surgery for hemorrhage refractory to endoscopic therapies accounts for less than 3% of cases. It is performed through a longitudinal proximal anterior gastrotomy with oversewing the tear with absorbable sutures. Ligation of the descending branch of the left gastric artery should be considered.

Answer: D

British Society of Gastroenterology Endoscopy Committee (2002) Non-variceal upper gastrointestinal hemorrhage: guidelines. *Gut* **51** (suppl 4), iv1–iv6.

Harbison SP, Dempsey DT. Mallory–Weiss syndrome. In: Cameron JL (ed.) *Current Surgical Therapy,* 9th edn, Mosby Elsevier, Philadelphia, PA, pp. 98–103.

6. *Which of the following statement about duodenal ulcer is true?*

A. *Endoscopic balloon dilatation achieves 80% short-term relief from ulcer related obstructive symptoms*

B. *Unlike gastric ulcer, the pathophysiology of duodenal ulcer lies in acid hypersecretion rather than Helicobacter pylori*

C. *Intractability is the most common indication for acid reduction surgeries*

D. *Lifetime risk for duodenal ulcer is 30%*

E. *Age over 60 is a risk factor for failure of non-operative management for duodenal ulcer bleeding*

Approximately 90% of patients with duodenal ulcers have *H. pylori* infection of the gastric antrum. In a prospective randomized controlled trial comparing the bismuth therapy consisting of amoxicillin, metronidazole and ranitidine to ranitidine alone, duodenal ulcer healing was achieved in 90% of the antibiotic group in six weeks versus 75% in the ranitidine and placebo group. Ulcer recurrence was 2% in the group that had *H. pylori* eradication versus 85% in the group that had *H. pylori* persistence. Nonsteroidal anti-inflammatory drugs are also an increasingly common reason for duodenal ulcers, particularly in the elderly. The lifetime risk for development of duodenal ulcer is approximately 10%. The frequency of operative indications has decreased with the advent of the bismuth therapy; however, the classic indications of bleeding, perforation, intractability and obstruction remain valid. Of these, bleeding accounts for 90% of the procedures performed for duodenal ulcers. Upper endoscopy will establish the diagnosis and exclude other sources of bleeding. Factors predicting failure of nonoperative management for bleeding include ongoing hemodynamic instability, significant morbidities, and transfusion requirements exceeding 6 units in 24 hours. Intractability in cases of non-healing ulcers or recurrence despite maximal medical therapy is now a rare surgical indication. Ulcer related gastric outlet obstruction account for less than 5% of all surgical indications. Endoscopic dilatation may transiently achieve symptom relief in 80% of patients; however, long-term success is estimated at less than 50%.

Answer: A

Hentschel E, Brandstätter G, Dragosics B, *et al.* (1993) Effect of ranitidine and amoxicillin plus metronidazole on the eradication of *Helicobacter pylori* and the recurrence of duodenal ulcer. *New England Journal of Medicine* **328** (5), 308–12.

Jamieson GG (2000) Current status of indications for surgery in peptic ulcer disease. *World Journal of Surgery* **24**, 256–8.

7. *A 35-year-old man presents with 10 hours of severe epigastric pain that has progressed to diffuse abdominal tenderness. His vitals are temp 101.7°F, HR 115 beats/minute, BP 110/65 mm Hg. A CT scan demonstrates periduodenal inflammation with free air and free fluid. Which statement about his treatment is false?*

A. *Surgical options include simple patch closure and postoperative H. pylori eradication*

B. *Surgical options include simple patch closure and proximal gastric vagotomy*

C. *Simple patch closure is sufficient for patients whose duodenal perforation is clearly associated with NSAID use*

D. *Laparoscopic repair of duodenal ulcer is associated with a 20% conversion rate*

E. *Nonoperative management consisting of nil per os, nasogastric decompression and wide spectrum antibiotics is the safest option in patients with hemodynamic instability from sepsis*

Perforation is the second most common complication of duodenal ulcer after bleeding. Pneumoperitoneum is demonstrated in 80% of upright chest X-rays, and therefore its absence should not exclude this diagnosis. Surgical options for duodenal perforation include simple patch closure alone if the underlying pathophysiology does not involve *H. pylori* or acid hypersecretion, as in the case of NSAID use. If *H. pylori* or hypersecretion is suspected, an acid reduction procedure is not always necessary, particularly in patients who have not been placed on *H. pylori* or acid reduction therapies. In the current era, proton pump inhibitors and H_2 blockers have been shown to achieve over 90% symptom resolution. *H. pylori* treatment is an imperative component of therapy. Complete eradication with the bismuth therapy expedites ulcer healing as well as reduces the likelihood of ulcer recurrence. An acid-reduction procedure is appropriate in stable patients who are medically noncompliant or refractory to medical therapy. Nonresective procedures such as highly selective vagotomy or truncal vagotomy and pyloroplasty have higher recurrence rates when compared to resective procedures, however they are also associated with lower morbidity and mortality rates. In the setting of duodenal perforations, resective procedures such as antrectomies are discouraged due to the duodenal inflammation and the resultant increased risk of duodenal stump leak in the case of Billroth II or anastomotic leak in the case of Billroth I. Recent reports indicate that in the era of effective acid suppression and *H. pylori* treatment, definitive ulcer surgery in the emergent setting may not be necessary. In a retrospective review performed at a Veteran's Administration medical center, only 36% of 42 patients underwent definitive ulcer surgery at the time of operation for complications of peptic ulcer disease. At a median follow up of 18 months, only one patient had ulcer recurrence. In recent years, minimally invasive techniques for the management of duodenal ulcer disease and its complications have been shown to be safe and technically feasible. Several studies have demonstrated decreased postoperative analgesia requirements, decreased incidence of wound infection, shorter hospital stays, and earlier return to work. Laparoscopy is associated with a 20% conversion rate. Hemodynamic instability in the setting of perforated viscus is an indication for urgent resuscitation and surgical septic source control, not nonoperative management.

Answer: E

Lunevicius R, Morkevicius M (2005) Systematic review comparing laparoscopic and open repair for perforated peptic ulcer. *British Journal of Surgery* **92** (10), 1195–207.

Sarosi GA Jr, Jaiswal KR, Nwariaku FE, *et al.* (2005) Surgical therapy of peptic ulcers in the 21st century: more common than you think. *American Journal of Surgery* **190** (5), 775–9.

8. *After repair of several small bowel enterotomies in a 35-year-old victim of multiple gunshot wounds, you are left with a 60% disruption of the GEJ. The patient remains hemodynamically stable throughout the operation requiring two units of pRBC transfusions. What is the optimal management of the GEJ injury?*

A. *Left anterolateral thoracotomy, resection of the gastroesophageal segment, intrathoracic esophago-gastric anastomosis*

B. *Debridement of injury with primary closure*

C. *Segmental resection with intraabdominal anastomosis*

D. *Segmental resection, intraabdominal anastomosis and Nissen fundoplication*

E. *Staple off the distal esophagus, gastrostomy and jejunostomy*

Esophageal injuries account for less than 1% of patients admitted following trauma. The majority of traumatic perforations require operative management with the intention of primary repair. However, in the presence of hemodynamic instability or delayed diagnosis where intense inflammation precludes safe primary anastomosis, simple drainage with or without stapling above and below the esophageal injury is most prudent. Primary repair of a destructive injury involving more than 50% of luminal circumference will result in stricture. In such cases segmental resection with tissue buttressing provides the most leakproof anastomosis. The cervical esophagus can be buttressed with the sternocleidomastoid or other strap muscles. Pleura, intercostal muscles or the pericardium can buttress the thoracic esophagus. Of note, it is not advisable to circumferentially wrap the esophagus as the scar tissue formation will lead to an unyielding extrinsic stricture. In the abdomen, the omentum or various forms of fundoplications are options. In this case of a destructive GEJ disruption, the injury can be relatively easily accessed through the hiatus. Further mobilization can be achieved through blunt transhiatal dissection in order to gain adequate length for a tension-free anastomosis.

Answer: D

Gouge TH, Depan GH, Spencer FC (1989) Experience with the Grillo pleural wrap procedure in 18 patients with perforation of the thoracic esophagus. *Annals of Surgery* **209**, 612.

Richardson JD, Tobin GR (1994) Closure of the esophageal defects with muscle flaps. *Archives of Surgery* 129, 541.

9. *With regard to corrosive substance ingestion, which of the following statement is true?*

A. *After caustic ingestion, the esophagus is at the highest risk for perforation within the first 24 hours*

B. *Blind passage of nasogastric tube with gastric lavage should be immediately performed in order to reduce gastric exposure to the caustic substance*

C. *Racemic epinephrine and steroids have been shown to decrease the need for intubation in patients presenting with stridor after caustic substance ingestion*

D. *Steroids have been shown to decrease esophageal stricture rate in Grade III injuries*

E. *Early endoscopy is the gold standard in evaluating esophageal caustic injuries and should be performed with 24 hours*

Caustic ingestion is the leading toxic exposure in children and the second most common in adults after analgesic ingestion. The extent of tissue damage depends on the type, quantity and concentration of ingested substance, and the duration of exposure. Acids cause coagulative necrosis, which limits its penetration by the formation of a protective eschar over the undamaged tissues. By contrast, alkaline agents typically produce more extensive damage by liquefactive necrosis in which the process continues through protein denaturation until all alkaline substances have been neutralized by the host tissue. In fact, most mortality is associated with ingestion of strong alkali such as liquid lye or button batteries. The esophageal perforation associated with full-thickness penetration is bimodal. Most early perforations occur on the second to third day after exposure when the tissue is most friable. As a result endoscopy should be performed in the first 12–24 hours to avoid the risk of causing iatrogenic perforation. For the same reason, the blind passage of nasogastric tube is contraindicated. Patients with laryngeal injury manifesting as stridor should be immediately intubated. Attempts at temporizing the situation with racemic epinephrine and steroids is dangerous and can turn a controlled intubation into an airway emergency. Steroids have been theorized to reduce the incidence of esophageal stricture formation, however, scientific evidence does not supported its use.

Answer: E

Hugh TB, Kelly MD (1999) Corrosive ingestion and the surgeon. *Journal of the American College of Surgeons* **189**, 508.

Mamede RC, De Mello Filho FV (2002) Treatment of caustic ingestion: an analysis of 239 cases. *Diseases of the Esophagus* **15** (3), 210–13.

10. *Which of the following statements correctly describes the treatment of a hemodynamically stable, asymptomatic 5-year-old child who presents one hour after accidental ingestion of a liquid cleaning substance?*

A. *Upper endoscopy should be performed within 24 hours to evaluate the extent of injury*

B. *If he remains asymptomatic, it is safe to discharge the child after 24 hours of monitoring*

C. *In lieu of upper endoscopy, this patient can undergo contrast radiography performed with water-soluble contrast followed by thin barium to evaluate for esophageal injury*

D. *The patient should be placed on a proton pump inhibitor drip for three days*

E. *Due to the high risk of stricture formation, a gastrostomy should be performed for enteral nutrition and retrograde dilations*

As a general rule, caustic ingestions are accidental in children and suicidal attempts in adults. Initial assessment should follow the algorithm outlined by advanced trauma life support beginning with determining airway patency. Indications for endoscopy include any patient with stridor, all intended suicidal ingestions, any symptomatic patient, and those with oropharyngeal burns. Endoscopy is not necessary in asymptomatic children who have ingested only small amounts of caustic material. They can be safely discharged after 24 hours of close monitoring. The classification of caustic injury is based on endoscopic findings. First-degree injury is limited to the mucosa and is associated with very low immediate and long-term complication rates. Second-degree injury is transmucosal and further subclassified into IIA and IIB based on patchy ulcerations versus circumferential injury. As in first-degree injury, Grade IIA is not associated with stricture formation. However, Grade IIB will have invariable rates of progression to strictures. Third-degree injury is managed with a low threshold for aggressive operative intervention as the transmural injury may result in mediastinitis or peritonitis. The management algorithm for Grade IIB and III injuries consist of *nil per os*, antibiotics to reduce oropharyngeal flora, gastric acid suppression and either intravenous or enteral nutrition. In addition, gastrostomies should be considered as a conduit for enteral feeding and future retrograde dilations.

Answer: B

Anderson KD, Rouse TM, Randolph JF (1990) A controlled trial of corticosteroids in children with corrosive injury of the esophagus. *New England Journal of Medicine* **323**, 637.

Fischer A (2008) Chemical esophageal injuries. In: Cameron JL (ed.) *Current Surgical Therapy*, 9th edn, Mosby Elsevier, Philadelphia, PA, pp. 49–52.

11. *A 50-year-old man presents to the ED with severe chest pain, nausea but with the inability to vomit. Attempts at passing a NGT fail due to resistance at 35 cm from the incisors. Which statement regarding the patient's condition is true?*

A. *Endoscopic detorsion of the incarcerated paraesophageal hernia should be attempted*

B. *Acute strangulation can be expected in over 30% of patients with paraesophageal hernias*

C. *Mesh closure of the hiatal repair have been associated with erosion and fibrotic strictures*

D. *Repair of strangulated paraesophageal hernias performed through a left thoracotomy yields superior results than the transabdominal approach*

E. *The addition of an antireflux procedure to paraesophageal hernia repair is associated with high rates of dysphagia*

Paraesophageal hernias develop due to attenuation of the phrenoesophageal ligament thus allowing for the intrathoracic migration of abdominal contents. The location of the gastroesophageal junction serves as the reference point for determining the four types of hiatal hernias. Type I hiatal hernia is the most common and involves herniation of the GEJ into the mediastinum. Most patients are asymptomatic, however, surgical repair should be offered to symptomatic patients. Type II is a true paraesophageal hernia in which the GEJ is in its anatomical subdiaphragmatic location; however, the gastric fundus herniates through the patulous hiatus alongside the esophagus. Type III is a combination of Types I and II with herniation of the GEJ and stomach into the chest. Type IV hernia is a complex entity where the herniation encompasses the stomach as well as other abdominal organs. In contrast to previous teachings that all paraesophageal hernias should undergo elective repair regardless of symptom, new studies suggest that the risk of strangulation is around 1% per year, and the mortality associated with emergency repair is less than 20% as opposed to the previously believed 30% mortality rate published by Skinner and Belsey. Currently, it is acceptable to offer surgical correction only on the basis of significant symptoms and perhaps younger age (<60 years). Chest pain, the inability to vomit and failure to pass a nasogastric tube are suggestive of an incarcerated intrathoracic stomach. In this surgical emergency, endoscopy shares no diagnostic or therapeutic roles. Transthoracic, transabdominal or laparoscopic approaches have all been described with similar long-term results in the elective setting, the caveat being that thoracotomy is associated with higher postoperative morbidities and laparoscopy should be reserved for experienced surgeons due to the higher technical difficulty. In the setting of strangulated paraesophageal hernias, the transabdominal approach is most prudent given the shorter operative time and possible need for subtotal gastrectomy. The patulous esophageal hiatus should be closed with nonabsorbable sutures and a fundoplication added as over 30% of patients will have gastroesophageal reflux disease after the extensive hiatal dissection. The reinforcement of prosthetic mesh is gaining popularity as some studies have shown the practice to reduces the incidence of recurrence. However, it is associated with complications including erosions, fibrotic strictures and dysphagia. These risks are theoretically reduced by the usage of bioprosthetic mesh although the long-term data are lacking.

Answer: C

Schieman C, Grondin SC (2009) Paraesophageal hernia: clinical presentation, evaluation, and management controversies. *Thoracic Surgery Clinics* **19** (4), 473–84.

Stylopoulos N, Gazelle GS, Rattner DW (2002) Paraesophageal hernias: Operation or observation? *Annals of Surgery* **236**, 492–501.

12. *A hemodynamically stable 16-year-old boy is found to have an obstructive duodenal hematoma on CT performed for blunt assault. He remains NPO and continues to have bilious NG output of 2.5L per day 4 days after admission. What is the most accepted management of his duodenal obstruction?*

A. *Continue conservative management consisting of nil per os, nasogastric suctioning and intravenous fluid for up to 2 weeks*

B. *Operative duodenal hematoma evacuation*

C. *CT guided percutaneous hematoma aspiration*

D. *Gastrostomy and jejunostomy with expectant management of the duodenal hematoma*

E. *Endoscopically placed self expanding duodenal stent*

Although the incidence of duodenal hematomas is unclear, it is recognized as a rare complication, particularly following blunt trauma, endoscopic biopsies or peptic ulcer disease. Much of the data regarding this subject are limited to small case series in the pediatric population; however, extrapolations are made for the treatment of adults. It is believed that the rich blood supply of the duodenum accelerates hematoma resorption and protects against the late development of fibrosis and stenosis. Available data suggest that most of the symptomatic duodenal hematomas resolve in 7 to 10 days. Therefore expectant management is advocated for up to two weeks, after which operative hematoma evacuation is considered. More recently, case reports of ultrasound or CT guided percutaneous drainage have shown that these techniques can be safe and effective alternatives to operative evacuation. There is one case report of a successful endoscopic incision and drainage.

Answer: A

Clendenon JN, Meyers RL, Nance ML, *et al.* (2004) Management of duodenal injuries in children. *J Pediatric Surgery* **39**, 964–8.

Yang JC, Rivard DC, Morello FP, *et al.* (2008) Successful percutaneous drainage of duodenal hematoma after blunt trauma. *Journal of Pediatric Surgery* **43**, e13–5.

13. *Which statement about Helicobacter pylori testing is true?*

A. *Serologic testing is the most expensive of the nonendoscopic tests*

B. *The use of proton pump inhibitors does not reduce the sensitivity of the urease breath test*

C. *The monoclonal antibody test detects serum Helicobacter pylori antigens*

D. *Urea breath test can be used to confirm Helicobacter pylori eradication*

E. *Random biopsies are taken from the stomach for culture and histologic assessment*

Testing for *Helicobacter pylori* fall into two categories: endoscopic or nonendoscopic. Among the three nonendoscopic methods, serologic testing which examines for serum IgG antibody to *H. pylori* is the most widely available and cheapest. However, the overall sensitivity and specificity of the several commercially available quantitative assays is 85% and 70% respectively. In addition, the presence of IgG antibody for months after *H. pylori* eradication makes this test suboptimal for assessing treatment response. The urea breath test utilizes *H. pylori*'s intrinsic urease activity in converting orally administered ^{13}C-labeld or ^{14}C-labeled urea into measurable radiolabeled carbon dioxide. The test is 95% sensitive and specific. The fecal antigen test detects *H. pylori* specific antigen in the stool with the use of either monoclonal or polyclonal antibodies. For both the urea breath test and the fecal stool antigen test, the patient should be off proton pump inhibitors for 2 weeks, H_2 blockers for 24 hours, and avoid antimicrobials for four weeks before testing because these medications may suppress the infection and reduce the test sensitivity. All endoscopic methods begin with biopsy of the gastric antrum. The tissue can then be processed for histologic evaluation for the presence of *H. pylori* and associated gastritis. *H. pylori* can also be cultured from the antral tissue, although facilities with such capabilities are not widely available. Lastly, the urease-based method entails placing the biopsy specimen in a solution of urea and pH-sensitive dye. In the presence of active infection, the urease converts urea into ammonium, which alkalinizes the solution and changes its color. The test is 95% sensitive and 90% specific, but the aforementioned medications should be avoided. In the United States, the recommended treatment of *H. pylori* infection consists of a 10–14 day course of two antibiotics plus a proton-pump inhibitor or a bismuth preparation.

Answer: D

Suerbaum S, Michetti P (2002) *Helicobacter pylori* infection. *New England Journal of Medicine* **347**, 1175–86.

14. *Which statement regarding gastric Dieulafoy's lesion is true?*

A. *Dieulafoy's lesions are associated with up to 20% of nonvariceal upper GI hemorrhages*

B. *It is caused by erosion of a submucosal arteriovenous malformation*

C. *Epigastric pain is a common finding among patients with bleeding gastric Dieulafoy's lesions*

D. *Sucralfate has been shown to decrease the incidence of hemorrhage from Dieulafoy's lesion*

E. *The gastric erosions associated with Dieulafoy's lesions are usually less than 5 mm*

Dieulafoy's lesions account for 0.3–7% of nonvariceal upper GI hemorrhages. It is caused by an abnormally large, tortuous submucosal artery (1–3 mm) that erodes through the gastric mucosa. Patients typically present with painless and massive, but intermittent hematemesis. The diagnosis of Dieulafoy's lesion can be difficult due to the relative small size of the mucosal erosion (2–5 mm) that is surrounded by normal appearing gastric mucosa. Esophagogastroduodenoscopy is the diagnostic and treatment modality of choice, and can identify 80% of lesions. The various modalities used to treat variceal bleeding can be used for Dieulafoy's lesions, including multipolar electrocoagulation, injection sclerotherapy, band ligation and endoscopic clipping. In cases refractory to endoscopic therapy, angioembolization have been shown to yield success, though most of the experience is through case reports. Traditionally the difficulty in surgical approach is the difficulty in identifying the location of the intraluminal lesion. However, endoscopic tattooing and intraoperative endoscopic transillumination of the lesions can facilitate both open and laparoscopic gastric wedge resection.

Answer: E

Mercer D, Robinson E (2008) Stomach. In: Townsend C, Beachamp R, Evers B, Mattox K (eds) *Sabiston Textbook of Surgery*, 18th edn, Saunders Elsevier, Philadelphia, PA, pp. 1272–3 .

Rollhauser C, Fleischer DE (2002) Nonvariceal upper gastrointestinal bleeding. *Endoscopy* **34** (2), 111–8.

15. *A 34-year-old woman who is 24 hours from an uneventful laparoscopic Roux-en-Y gastric bypass is found to be persistently tachycardic at 130 BPM, BP 115/70 mm Hg and RR 25 breaths/minuts. Her abdomen is mildly tender. An ABG obtained on room air is 7.32/32/98/25/−0.5. A routine post-operative upper GI series with gastrografin and thin barium did not demonstrate a leak. What is the next step in management?*

A. *Continue observation for another 24 hours*

B. *Discharge the patient with follow up in 2 weeks*

C. *Repeat upper GI swallow with full strength barium*

D. *Operative exploration to rule out a leak*

E. *CTPA to rule out pulmonary embolism*

One of the most detrimental complications of Roux-en-Y gastric bypass is an anastomotic leak. The incidence of anastomotic leaks after Roux-en-Y gastric bypass is 1 to 5.6%, and appears similar between open and laparoscopic approaches. According to large series, 50% of the leaks occur at the gastrojejunostomy anastomosis with the rest affecting the excluded stomach staple line, the jejunojejunostomy, the staple line of the gastric pouch or from enterotomies elsewhere along the GI tract. Identified risk factors include male gender, increased weight, multiple comorbidities and revisional surgery. Symptoms of leak range from mild abdominal pain to frank peritonitis; however, in general the clinical presentation in bariatric patients tends to be subtler. Studies have consistently identified tachycardia and tachypnea to be one of the earliest signs associated with anastomotic leaks. In a retrospective series of 210 laparoscopic Roux-en-Y gastric bypass operations, patients with the combination of heart rate over 120 BPM and respiratory rate over 24 had a 20% chance of harboring a leak. Routine postoperative UGI studies with gastrografin are associated with a sensitivity of 22% of detecting a leak, and the sensitivity of CT scans is around 40%. The subset of patients with contained leaks who are hemodynamically stable can be managed nonoperatively. However, the mainstay of diagnosis and treatment for patients whose presentation is highly suggestive of an anastomotic leak despite negative radiographic studies is operative exploration. In the majority of cases where the leak is detected early, simple repair of the enterotomy will suffice. However, in cases of delayed diagnosis where the inflamed tissue prevent secure suture repairs, wide drainage is the most prudent intervention.

Answer: D

Gonzalez R, Sarr MG, Smith CD, *et al.* (2007) Diagnosis and contemporary management of anastomotic leaks after gastric bypass for obesity. *Journal of the American College of Surgeons* **204** (1), 47–55.

Hamilton EC, Sims TL, Hamilton TT, *et al.* (2003) Clinical predictors of leak after laparoscopic Roux-en-Y gastric bypass for morbid obesity. *Surgical Endoscopy* **17**, 679–84.

Chapter 35 Small Intestine, Appendix, and Colorectal

Jay J. Doucet, MD, MSc, FRCSC, FACS and Vishal Bansal, MD

1. *A 72-year-old woman presents to the ED with acute left lower quadrant abdominal pain. Her past medical history is significant only for mild hypertension. On exam, she is febrile to 38.2 °C with focal rebound tenderness in her left lower quadrant. She has a WBC of 12 000/mm³. Abdominal CT imaging reveals a thickened sigmoid with a 3.0 cm × 3.0 cm perisigmoid colon abscess with a very small pocket of extraluminal air in the pelvis. The next step in management should be:*

A. *Exploration, sigmoidectomy with descending end colostomy (Hartmann's procedure)*

B. *Exploration with sigmoidectomy, primary colorectal anastamosis*

C. *Exploration with sigmoidectomy, primary colorectal anastamosis, and loop ileosotomy*

D. *Resuscitation, broad spectrum IV antibiotics and percutaneous drainage of the abscess*

E. *Resuscitation, broad spectrum IV antibiotics, colonoscopy for likely colon carcinoma on this admission*

Complicated diverticulitis will often require operative intervention and, depending on the Hinchey staging system, a morbid two-stage procedure may be avoided. Hinchey I is defined as colonic inflammation with associated pericolic abscess; stage II includes inflammation with pelvic abscess; stage III is purulent peritonitis, and stage IV is fecal peritonitis. This patient is a Hinchey I, where IV antibiotics with percutaneous abscess drainage offers a chance for a future colonoscopy to rule out malignancy (four to six weeks later) and a planned one-stage sigmoidectomy with primary anastomosis. For patients with persistent, unresolving symptoms, pelvic sepsis or patients who are immunocompromised, sigmoidectomy and diversion should be considered, although a single-stage operation with intraoperative colonic lavage and primary anastomosis has been reported in these patients.

Answer: D

Aydin HN, Tekkis PP, Remzi FH, *et al.* (2006) Evaluation of the risk of a nonrestorative resection for the treatment of diverticular disease: the Cleveland Clinic diverticular disease propensity score. *Diseases of the Colon and Rectum* **49** (5), 629–39.

Schilling MK, Maurer CA, Kollmar O, Büchler MW (2001) Primary vs. secondary anastomosis after sigmoid resection for perforated diverticulitis (Hinchey Stage II and IV): A prospective outcome and cost analysis. *Diseases of the Colon and Rectum* **44** (5), 699–703.

2. *An 86-year-old male nursing home resident with severe dementia presents to the ER with a four-day history of constipation and a distended abdomen. His vital signs and laboratory studies are unremarkable. His abdominal x-ray reveals a "coffee-bean" sign of his sigmoid colon with a dilated transverse and descending colon. The patient underwent successful endoscopic decompression of his sigmoid volvulus and was observed in the hospital. On the second hospital day the patient had return of abdominal distention with evidence of a recurrent sigmoid volvulus. The patient should undergo:*

A. *Exploration, sigmoidectomy with descending end-colostomy (Hartmann's procedure)*

B. *Exploration with detorsion of the sigmoid and sigmoidopexy*

C. *Repeat endoscopic decompression through rigid proctoscopy*

Surgical Critical Care and Emergency Surgery: Clinical Questions and Answers, First Edition. Edited by Forrest O. Moore, Peter M. Rhee, Samuel A. Tisherman and Gerard J. Fulda.

D. *Exploration with sigmoidectomy and primary colorectal anastamosis*

E. *Laparoscopic detorsion of the sigmoid with sigmoidopexy*

In a stable patient without evidence of bowel ischemia, endoscopic decompression is the first-line therapy for a sigmoid volvulus. However, a 40–50% recurrence rate is expected and the timing can vary from immediate to a recurrence several years following the initial volvulus. In the face of a recurrent sigmoid volvulus, operative intervention is the treatment of choice. Even though there are several reports in the literature documenting the possibility of sigmoidectomy with primary anastomosis, in this institutionalized patient with evidence of a dilated descending colon without the ability for preoperative colonic cleansing, a Hartmann's procedure with end colostomy is the best therapeutic option offering the quickest chance of recovery and minimal complications.

Answer: A

Grossmann EM, Longo WE, Stratton MD, *et al.* (2000) Sigmoid volvulus in Department of Veterans Affairs Medical Centers. Diseases of the Colon and Rectum **43** (3), 414–18.

Oren D, Atamanalp SS, Aydinli B, *et al.* (2007) An algorithm for the management of sigmoid colon volvulus and the safety of primary resection: Experience with 827 cases. *Diseases of the Colon and Rectum* **50**, 489–97.

3. *A 48-year-old man undergoes successful renal transplantation for end-stage renal disease. He is maintained on prednisone and tacrolimus for immune suppression. Four weeks post-transplant he developed diarrhea, increasing pain, abdominal distention and presents to the ED. He denied any history of nausea, vomiting, but continues to have diarrhea. He has a temperature of 38.0 °C, a pulse of 96 beats per minute and blood pressure of 129/64 mm Hg. His abdomen was markedly distended and minimally tender to palpation with a white cell count of 21 000/mm^3. A CT of the abdomen and pelvis reveals very dilated large bowel from cecum to splenic flexure, with a cecal diameter of 9 cm and pneumatosis within the cecal wall. The next best step in management is:*

A. *Admit, resuscitate, empiric IV metronidazole, and send stool for C. difficile toxin*

B. *Exploratory laparotomy and right hemicolectomy and primary anastamosis*

C. *Exploratory laparotomy and subtotal colectomy with end ileostomy*

D. *Exploratory laparoscopy*

E. *Admit, resuscitate, NPO, send stool for C. difficile toxin and begin metronidazole pending results*

Clostridium difficile colitis has increased in incidence and severity since the early 2000s. Most *C. difficile* colitis can be treated with oral or IV metronidazole with or without the addition of oral vancomycin. More severe disease may require operative intervention. The operation of choice remains a subtotal colectomy, however, the timing of operation is often difficult and controversial. In general, patients not responsive to medical therapy with worsening organ dysfunction or patients with signs or symptoms of toxic megacolon should undergo operative exploration. This patient has radiologic evidence of toxic megacolon and moreover, is highly immune suppressed, which may blunt peritoneal signs and abdominal tenderness. Laparoscopic exploration is not an effective option since the external appearance of the colon often times seems normal.

Answer: C

Berman L, Carling T, Fitzgerald TN, *et al.* (2008) Defining surgical therapy for pseudomembranous colitis with toxic megacolon. *Journal of Clinical Gastroenterology* **42** (5), 476–80.

Dallal RM, Harbrecht BG, Boujoukas AJ, *et al.* (2002) Fulminant Clostridium difficile: an underappreciated and increasing cause of death and complications. *Annals of Surgery* 235 (3), 363–72.

4. *A 28-year-old man undergoes a laparoscopic appendectomy secondary to suspected appendicitis. The patient is discharged home post-operative day one without complication. Final pathology of the appendix reveals an 0.8 cm* *carcinoid tumor at the tip of the appendix. The next step in management is:*

A. *Exploratory laparotomy, omentectomy, right hemicolectomy, intraoperative hyperthermic chemotherapy*

B. *Completion right hemicolectomy*

C. *Observation, no additional operation is required*

D. *Six-month imatinib (Gleevac) adjuvant therapy followed by completion right hemicolectomy*

E. *Six-month adjuvant therapy with imatinib only*

Carcinoid tumors are rare gastrointestinal tumors, the majority of which are found on the appendix. These tumors may appear as a dense mass on CT imaging, resembling a fecolith, and thus are often found incidentally on pathology when the suspected diagnosis is appendicitis. Malignant potential as well as risk of metastasis is directly related to size. Carcinoid tumors of the appendix <1 cm are treated by simple appendectomy. Tumors >1 cm should also undergo an extended right hemicolectomy. In this patient, with an 0.8 cm carcinoid of the appendix, no additional operation besides an appendectomy is needed, since there is a low probability of recurrence in this lower stage. Imatinib therapy may be effective in gastrointestinal stromal tumors but does not have a role in treating carcinoid tumors.

Answer: C

Landry CS, Woodall C, Scoggins CR, *et al*. (2008) Analysis of 900 appendiceal carcinoid tumors for a proposed predictive staging system. *Archives of Surgery* **143** (7), 664–70.

Roggo A, Wood WC, Ottinger LW (1993) Carcinoid tumors of the appendix. *Annals of Surgery* **217** (4), 476–80.

5. *A 91-year-old man with severe dementia presents to the ED from his nursing home with constipation and abdominal distention for the last eight days. The patient's past medical history is remarkable for hypertension and dementia. His abdomen is distended but non-tender. His laboratory studies are unremarkable. Abdominal x-ray reveals a markedly distended ascending, transverse and descending colon with no visible air in the sigmoid or rectum. The next step in management is:*

A. *Urgent exploratory laparotomy for toxic megacolon*

B. *Loop sigmoid ostomy for managing chronic pseudo-obstruction*

C. *Decompressive rectal tube*

D. *IV neostigmine for colonic pseudo-obstruction*

E. *Gastrograffin enema*

Colonic pseudo-obstruction (Ogilvie's syndrome) commonly occurs in hospitalized or immobilized patients. Narcotic use, prolonged bed rest, electrolyte abnormalities and other medications can contribute to developing this adynamic condition. These patients rarely require operative intervention. A rectal tube usually does not help with decompression since the adynamic colon is usually proximal. Endoscopic colonoscopy may be helpful to decompress the dilation. Neostigmine has been also shown to induce colonic motility and relieve the pseudo-obstruction. However, because of significant bradycardia and transient asystole, neostigmine should not be used in patients with known heart block or significant cardiovascular disease. All medical and endoscopic treatment should only be utilized when a mechanical obstruction, such as tumor, can be ruled out. Of the choices above, this is best accomplished by gastrograffin enema.

Answer: E

Ponec RJ, Saunders MD, Kimmey MB (1999) Neostigmine for the treatment of acute colonic pseudo-obstruction. *New England Journal of Medicine* **341** (3), 137–41.

Strodel WE, Brothers T (1989) Colonoscopic decompression of pseudo-obstruction and volvulus. *Surgical Clinics of North America* **69** (6), 1327–35.

6. *A 63-year-old woman is undergoing chemotherapy for lymphoma. She presents to the emergency department with severe right sided abdominal pain. She has no previous surgical history. On exam she is tender on the right side of her abdomen with mild guarding. She is febrile to 38.2 °C and her white count is 0.9/mm^3*

with 30% neutrophils. All other laboratory values are unremarkable. A CT scan reveals a moderately dilated and thickened ileum, right and transverse colon. What is the most appropriate management?

A. *Urgent exploratory laparotomy for toxic megacolon*

B. *Colonoscopy to rule out colonic ischemia*

C. *Ileo-cecectomy with illeostomy and mucus fistula*

D. *IV fluid resuscitation, NPO, and IV gram negative, gram positive and anaerobic antibiotic coverage.*

E. *Outpatient management with oral broad spectrum antibiotics*

Neutropenic enterocolitis, or typhlitis, is a rare yet well described complication of chemotherapy causing transmural bowel wall inflammation of the ileum, and commonly the right colon. The exact pathophysiology of this condition is not completely known. Typical presentation is right-sided abdominal pain with peritoneal signs, fever, and neutropenia. Diagnosis is made clinically and should be confirmed using abdominal CT, which usually shows bowel-wall edema and thickening of the terminal ileum and ascending colon. Treatment should entail cessation of chemotherapy, aggressive fluid resuscitation, bowel rest and broad spectrum antibiotics targeting colonic flora. Granulocyte-colony stimulating factor may play a role to improve the neutropenia. Surgical exploration in these cases is usually not indicated unless the patient has evidence of colonic perforation or sepsis.

Answer: D

Kirkpatrick ID, Greenberg HM (2003) Gastrointestinal complications in the neutropenic patient: characterization and differentiation with abdominal CT. *Radiology* **226** (3), 668–74.

Kunkel JM, Rosenthal D (1986) Management of the ileocecal syndrome. Neutropenic enterocolotis. Diseases of the Colon and Rectum **29** (3), 196–9.

7. *A 64-year-old otherwise healthy woman presents with significant lower GI bleeding for the last 12 hours. Her systolic blood pressure is 80 mm Hg, pulse of 100 beats per minute, and her physical exam is unremarkable except for gross blood per rectum. Her current hematocrit is 28%. What is the next step in management?*

A. *Urgent exploration, subtotal colectomy and illeostomy*

B. *Urgent exploration, procto-colectomy and illeostomy*

C. *Resuscitation with IV fluid, blood and nasogastric lavage*

D. *Urgent colonoscopy*

E. *Resuscitation with IV fluid, blood and abdominal CT scan*

Severe lower GI bleeding can lead to profound shock and circulatory collapse. The first line therapy is aggressive resuscitation and appropriate transfusion with correction of coagulopathy as needed. Nearly 15% of lower GI bleeding is caused by upper GI sources, therefore expeditious gastric lavage is important. More than 70% of lower GI bleeding ceases spontaneously, therefore urgent laparotomy without localization of the source of hemorrhage should only be undertaken when the patient is in extremis. In hemodynamically stable patients, colonoscopy is the procedure of choice following resuscitation. If the source of bleeding cannot be localized, nuclear RBC scanning or angiography may be useful followed possibly by capsule endoscopy.

Answer: C

Elta GH (2001) Urgent colonoscopy for acute lower-GI bleeding. *Gastrointestinal Endoscopy* **29**, 227–34.

Laine L, Shah A (2010) Randomized trial of urgent vs. elective colonoscopy in patients hospitalized with lower GI bleeding. *American Journal of Gastroenterology* **105** (12), 2636–41.

8. *A 45-year-old male Jehovah's Witness with diabetes presents to the ED with right lower quadrant pain for three days and tenderness to abdominal palpation, fever to 38.2 °C and a WBC of 12 000/mm^3. An abdominal CT scan shows a thickened appendix, appendiceal fecolith, and small amount of pelvic fluid. A diagnosis of appendicitis is made. What is the next step in management?*

A. *Broad spectrum IV antibiotics, non-operative observation, interval appendectomy in 6 weeks*

B. *Broad spectrum IV antibiotics, with percutaneous drainage of pelvic fluid, interval appendectomy in 6 weeks*

C. *Appendectomy*

D. *Oral ciprofloxacin and metronidazole, inpatient observation*

E. *Outpatient therapy with oral ciprofloxacin and metronidazole*

The emergence of percutaneous drainage techniques and data suggesting that antibiotic therapy is as efficacious as operative management for appendicitis, one may be confused with these various management strategies. Data supporting antibiotic treatment for appendicitis must be taken with caution, since these reports exclude septic patients and patients with known early perforation. There is also a 15% reported failure rate of nonoperative management, ultimately requiring appendectomy. Given the free pelvic fluid in this patient's CT scan, a partial perforation of the appendix is likely. In this case, operative appendectomy is the treatment of choice. Percutaneous drainage should be reserved for perforation without a visible appendix and adequate fluid or abscess for drainage. The operative approach is either laparoscopic or an open approach with mostly equivalent outcomes.

Answer: C

Styrud J, Eriksson S, Nilsson I, *et al.* (2006) Appendectomy versus antibiotic treatment in acute appendicitis. a prospective multicenter randomized controlled trial. *World Journal of Surgery* **30** (6), 1033–7.

Varadhan KK, Humes DJ, Neal KR, Lobo DN (2010) Antibiotic therapy versus appendectomy for acute appendicitis: a meta-analysis. *World Journal of Surgery* **34** (2), 199–209.

9. *A 23-year-old man presents with a 24-hour history of increasing crampy abdominal pain, nausea, vomiting and a CT scan showing dilated small bowel with a transition point in the terminal ileum. Past medical history is unremarkable; he has had no previous surgery. On examination, he has mild abdominal distension, no peritoneal signs and frequent bowel sounds. He has a while blood cell count (WBC) of 12,300/mm^3. After explanation of likely diagnoses and informed consent, he is taken to the operating room for laparotomy. The operative findings are shown below, with food impacted in the large diverticulum. This congenital condition is associated with what other mechanical cause of bowel obstruction?*

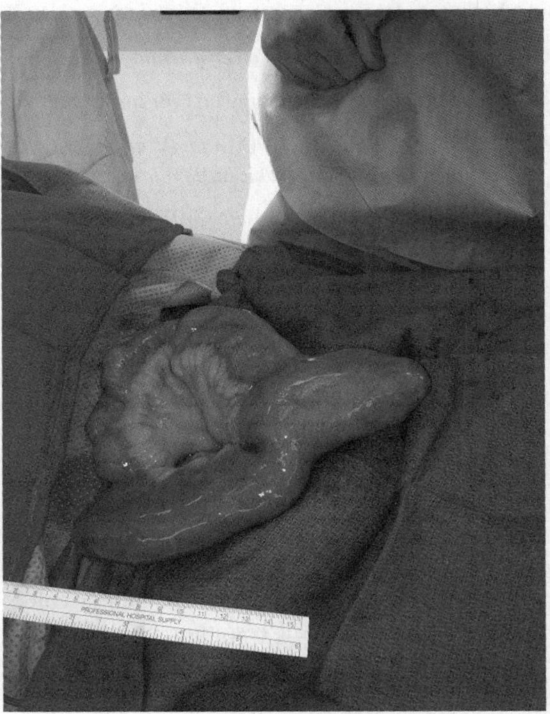

A full color version of this figure appears in the plate section of this book

A. *Mesodiverticular band*

B. *Ileocecal intussuception*

C. *Terminal ileitis*

D. *Hirschsprung's disease*

E. *Cecal volvulus*

The operative photograph shows a large Meckel's diverticulum with obstruction due to impaction with food. Meckel's diverticulum can also present with bowel obstruction due to internal hernia caused by interposition of a small bowel loop between the diverticulum and a persistent mesodiverticular band. Meckel's diverticulum is an embryologic remnant of the omphalovitelline duct and its features can be recalled by the "rule of 2s": Present in 2% of the population, usually about

2 feet (60 cm) proximal to the ileocecal valve and malignancy is present in 2% of specimens. Meckel's diverticulum can also present with other symptoms, most notably upper gastrointestinal bleeding caused by the presence of ectopic gastric, pancreatic or other mucosa with leads to ulceration and bleeding, and this diagnosis should be entertained in patients with an obscure source of gastrointestinal bleeding. Management is by resection of the diverticulum and adjacent intestinal segment. Meckel's diverticulum does not increase the risk of ileocecal intussuception. Terminal ileitis may cause obstructive symptoms but is readily identified by contrast CT scanning. Hirschsprung's disease can cause colonic obstruction due to a distal colonic aperistaltic segment with aganglionosis; this is not associated with Meckel's diverticulum. There is no association between Meckel's diverticulum and cecal volvulus.

Answer: A

Sagar J, Kumar V, Shah DK (2006) Meckel's diverticulum: a systematic review. *Journal of the Royal Society Medicine* **99** (10), 501–5.

Tavakkolizadeh A, Whang E, Ashley SW, Zinner MJ (2010) Small intestine. In: Brunicardi FC, Andersen DK, Billiar TR, *et al.* (eds) *Schwartz's Principles of Surgery*, 9th edn, McGraw-Hill, New York.

10. *A 52-year-old man with a history of hepatocellular carcinoma presents with a three-day history of nausea, vomiting and crampy abdominal pain. He has had no bowel movements since the onset of symptoms. On examination he has diffuse, mild abdominal tenderness, no peritoneal signs and obvious abdominal distension. Bowel sounds are infrequent. His past medical history is remarkable only for a liver resection two years ago and a course of transarterial chemoembolization (TACE) of a recurrent liver tumor four weeks ago. Labwork shows a white blood cell (WBC) count of 9200/mm^3, ALT of 192 units/L, AST of 178 units/L and is otherwise unremarkable. Representative abdominal imaging studies are shown. What is the best initial management of this patient?*

A. *Placement of a nasogastric tube, NPO status and observation with serial abdominal examinations*

B. *Colonoscopy*

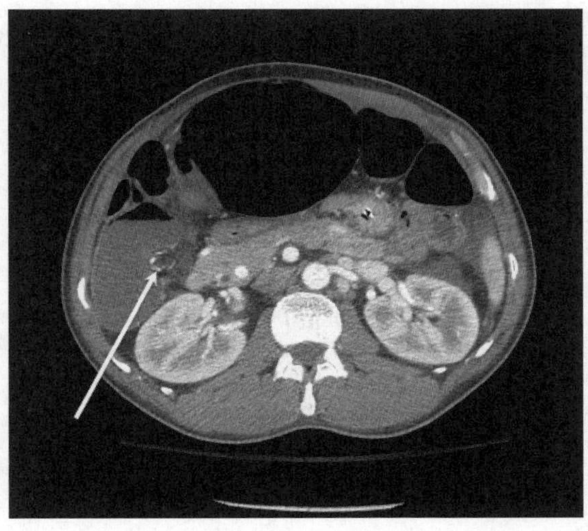

C. *Laparoscopic cecopexy*

D. *Laparotomy and cecostomy*

E. *Laparotomy and ileocecal resection*

The imaging shows a cecal volvulus. Cecal volvulus occurs in younger patients who are less debilitated than those presenting with sigmoid volvulus. The acute presentation is best treated by resection of the redundant segment of colon in those patients that can tolerate the procedure and may be required if ischemic intestine is discovered. Flexible sigmoidoscopy is successful in over 50% cases of sigmoid volvulus, but decompressive colonoscopy is almost never successful in cecal volvulus. Cecopexy would appear to have less risk as no colonic resection or anastomosis would be required, however the recurrence rate is high and would place the patient at risk of recurrent volvulus with risk of perforation or reoperation. Cecostomy has been performed as a percutaneous, laparoscopic, endoscopic or open procedure. It is associated with a high rate of serious complications such as leak, perforation or missed intestinal ischemia and has no advantage over colostomy or ileostomy at laparotomy.

Answer: E

Bullard DKM, Rothenberger DA (2010) Colon, rectum, and anus. In: Brunicardi FC, Andersen DK, Billiar

TR, *et al.* (eds) *Schwartz's Principles of Surgery*, 9th edn, McGraw-Hill, New York.

Madiba TE, Thomson SR (2002) The management of cecal volvulus. *Diseases of the Colon and Rectum* **45** (2), 264–7.

11. *A 62-year-old man presents to the emergency department with the condition shown below. He is a resident of a nursing home due to cognitive defects after a disabling traumatic brain injury that occurred six years previously. Other medical history reveals Type II diabetes managed with oral antihyperglycemic agents. According to his attendants, this condition also occurred about six weeks ago. The nursing home physician was able to reduce the mass into the rectum the mass after pouring sugar on it. This therapy was repeated with this episode and was unsuccessful. The mass is dusky in color and has an area of ulceration. It has apparently been present for more than 18 hours on this occasion. The patient has normal vital signs and appears to be in moderate distress with perineal pain. Laboratory results are unremarkable. What is the next best step in management of this condition, if attempted reduction in the emergency department is unsuccessful?*

A. *Operating room reduction under general anesthesia*

B. *Altemeier procedure*

C. *Laparotomy and sigmoidopexy (Ripstein procedure)*

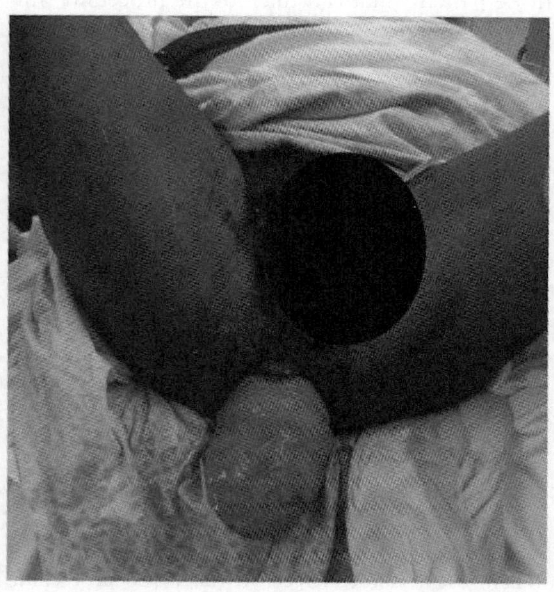

A full color version of this figure appears in the plate section of this book

D. *Laparoscopic sigmoid resection*

E. *Sigmoid colostomy*

This patient has a large rectal prolapse. Reduction of the prolapse can allow conversion of a surgical emergency into a delayed procedure. Prolonged prolapse and dependency of the prolapsed segment can lead to congestion of the exposed rectum, which can make reduction impossible. Gentle circumferential pressure usually allows reduction, however use of topically osmotically active agents such as powdered sugar may allow a previously irreducible prolapse to be reduced. If monitored sedation does not allow reduction, then general anesthesia may allow reduction. Irreducible rectal prolapse is uncommon and leads to a decision for an emergent perineal versus abdominal procedure. The Altemeier procedure is a perineal proctocolectomy, which avoids a laparotomy but has a higher recurrence rate than abdominal procedures. The perineal incision of the Altemeier can also cause complications such as bleeding, infection and dehiscence. If the patient can tolerate a laparotomy, abdominal procedures have the lowest rates of recurrence when the excess colon is resected rather than simply retaining with sacral sutures or a mesh sling (Ripstein procedure). Colostomy is reserved for complications such as bowel necrosis, perforation or failure of prior procedures. It is important to recognize that this condition is associated with pelvic floor dysfunction, and the associated incontinence is not managed by resection of bowel alone.

Answer: A

Bullard DKM, Rothenberger DA (2010) Colon, rectum, and anus. In: Brunicardi FC, Andersen DK, Billiar TR, *et al.* (eds) *Schwartz's Principles of Surgery*, 9th edn, McGraw-Hill, New York.

Jones OM, Cunningham C, Lindsey I (2011) The assessment and management of rectal prolapse, rectal intussusception, rectocoele, and enterocoele in adults. *British Medical Journal* **342**, c7099.

12. *A 54-year-old female nurse practitioner presents with crampy abdominal pain of 60 hours duration, associated with nausea and vomiting. Her last bowel movement was 24 hours ago. She has a past history of* *being admitted 22 days ago after a freeway motor vehicle collision. She recalls that she had a seat-belt mark across her mid-abdomen and significant abdominal pain. A CT scan of the abdomen was done during that admission. She is unsure of the CT scan findings but was told she had "minor internal bleeding." Her abdominal pain gradually improved and she was discharged five days later. She undergoes laparotomy and the intraoperative findings are seen below. What is the diagnosis?*

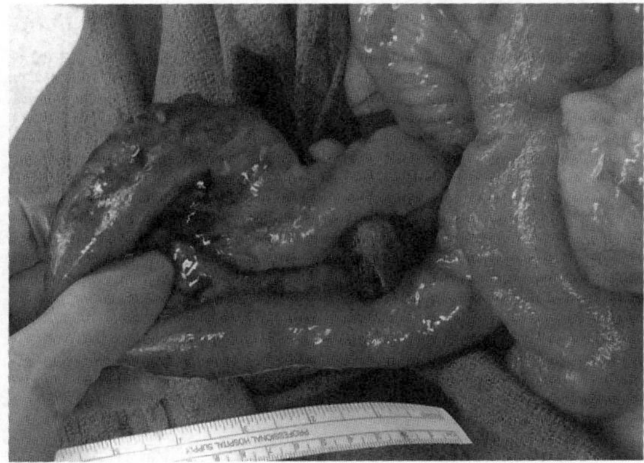

A full color version of this figure appears in the plate section of this book

A. *A "bucket handle" tear of the small bowel mesentery which has led to a segment of ischemic ileum and internal small bowel hernia*

B. *Mesenteric ischemia caused by arterial embolism from an aortic injury*

C. *Antibiotic-associated enteritis caused by recent administration of broad spectrum antibiotics*

D. *Small bowel perforation caused by compression of a closed loop of small bowel by the seat belt*

E. *Regional enteritis, consistent with Crohn's disease in the terminal ileum*

After blunt abdominal trauma, a CT scan revealing intraperitoneal fluid without an attributable solid organ source should be considered evidence of a mesenteric injury. When blunt trauma is associated with an abdominal seat belt mark, the diagnosis should also be considered. Multidetector CT scan with IV contrast may show the mesenteric injuries and small bowel ischemia and/or edema, but is reader dependent. Early exploration is the optimal management. Seat belts, while reducing traffic accident fatalities and serious injuries, can cause mesenteric injuries by shearing forces that may tear the small bowel from its supporting mesentery. The small bowel may then become ischemic, which may lead to perforation or stricture, which may present in a delayed fashion. The mesenteric defect is a possible source for an internal hernia as small bowel may become trapped or twisted within the fenestration. The photograph shows a strictured segment of ischemic ileum with a mesenteric defect that caused bowel obstruction due to internal hernia. Perforation from seat belt injury can also occur, but would be associated with peritonitis, abdominal sepsis or abscess. Antibiotic-associated enteritis is typically a colitis; the small bowel is usually not inflamed although it may become edematous with severe pancolitis. Aortic injuries from trauma are most commonly associated with delayed aortic rupture, not embolism.

Answer: A

Cothren CC, Biffl WL, Moore EE (2010) Trauma. In: Brunicardi FC, Andersen DK, Billiar TR, *et al.* (2010) *Schwartz's Principles of Surgery*, 9th edn, McGraw-Hill, New York.

Ng AK, Simons RK, Torreggiani WC, *et al.* (2002) Intra-abdominal free fluid without solid organ injury in blunt abdominal trauma: an indication for laparotomy. *Journal of Trauma* **52** (6), 1134–40.

13. *A 54-year-old man presents with a history of one week of increasing abdominal pain, which is made worse with meals. He notes some abdominal bloating and his bowel movements have been normal. On examination he has mild diffuse abdominal tenderness without peritoneal signs. He relates no prior abdominal surgery, and he has a past history of non-traumatic deep venous thrombosis of his left leg 3 years ago for which he took coumadin for six months. A CT scan was obtained and is shown. What is the appropriate initial therapy for this condition?*

A. *Intravenous heparin, followed by coumadin*

B. *Mesenteric angiography*

C. *Exploratory laparotomy*

D. *Low-molecular-weight heparin*

E. *Transjugular intrahepatic portal-caval shunt (TIPS)*

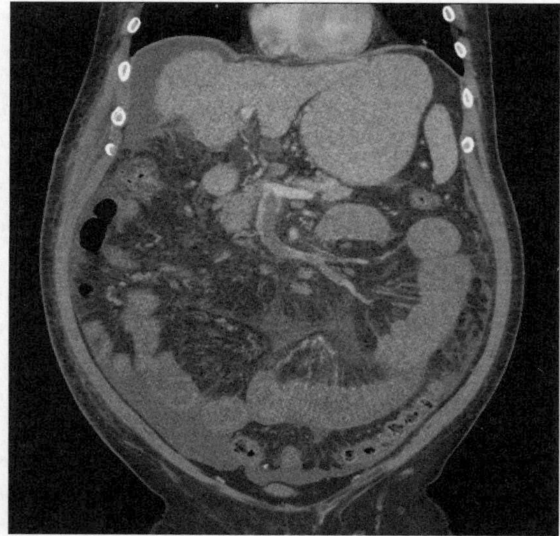

This patient has mesenteric venous ischemia, associated with portal vein and superior mesenteric vein thrombosis. While this condition has a slower progression than mesenteric arterial ischemia, the diagnosis is typically delayed, and may lead to extensive intestinal infarction, short-gut syndrome or death. The condition is usually associated with portal or mesenteric vein thrombosis. Patients may have cirrhosis or a thrombotic disorder such as protein C or S deficiency, factor V Leiden or anti-thrombin III deficiency. Hematologic workup for a prothrombotic condition is indicated. Management in cases when bowel infarction is not suspected is by anticoagulation, intravenous heparin being the first choice in case of non-response and subsequent need for an urgent procedure. Angiography will not show the mesenteric venous anatomy significantly better than CT scanning with intravenous contrast. Laparotomy is performed when peritonitis and bowel infarction are suspected. TIPS is used to reduce risk of variceal bleeding from portal hypertension, but its use in mesenteric venous ischemia is not defined.

Answer: A

Harnik IG, Brandt LJ (2010) Mesenteric venous thrombosis. *Vascular Medicine* **15** (5), 407–18.

Tavakkolizadeh A, Whang EE, Ashley S, *et al.* (2010) Small intestine. In: Brunicardi FC, Andersen DK, Billiar TR, *et al.*, *Schwartz's Principles of Surgery*, 9th edn, McGraw-Hill, New York.

14. *You are consulted regarding a 78-year-old woman who presented with left lower quadrant pain and a single episode of dark red blood per rectum 4 hours ago. She is afebrile and is hemodynamically stable in normal sinus rhythm. Labwork reveals a WBC count of 13000/mm^3 with 80% segmented neutrophils and a hemoglobin of 11 g/dl.Her past medical history reveals a remote cholecystectomy, type II diabetes, and she takes clopidogrel for a suspected transient ischemic attack three years ago. Abdominal examination reveals tenderness in the left lower quadrant without peritoneal signs. On rectal examination, dark red blood is seen on a gloved finger. Pulses are palpable all extremities. A CT scan with intravenous contrast was obtained, which reveals a 4 cm infrarenal aortic aneurysm, and some bowel wall thickening in the sigmoid colon. The inferior mesenteric artery is not visualized. What is the appropriate initial management?*

A. *Intravenous antibiotics, observation*

B. *Colonoscopy*

C. *Mesenteric angiogram*

D. *Vascular surgery consult for endovascular stenting*

E. *Laparotomy and sigmoid resection*

This patient has a presentation typical of ischemic colitis, which is typified by abdominal pain accompanied by lower gastrointestinal bleeding. Most mild to moderate cases will resolve under observation as the affected sigmoid colon develops collateral circulation. Severe cases resemble small bowel mesenteric ischemia with abdominal pain out-of-proportion to findings on examination. Some patients may develop frank necrosis of colon and therefore close follow-up examinations are required. Antibiotics reduce pain and fever symptoms caused by poor gut wall integrity. CT scans with intravenous contrast will reveal mucosal edema, and "thumbprinting" of the affected colon. Colonoscopy will confirm the diagnosis, but is unnecessary in this case. Mesenteric angiography will not add significantly to the CT findings. A late complication is ischemic stricture (10–15%), which can be confirmed by a contrast study or colonoscopy, and may require sigmoid resection.

Answer: A

Bullard DKM, Rothenberger DA (2010) Colon, rectum, and anus. In: Brunicardi FC, Andersen DK, Billiar TR, *et al.* (eds) *Schwartz's Principles of Surgery*, 9e:

Feuerstadt P, Brandt LJ (2010) Colon ischemia: recent insights and advances. *Current Gastroenterology Reports* **12** (5), 383–90.

15. *A 61-year-old man presents to the ED with pain at the umbilicus for one day, nausea, and he has vomited twice today. He is known to be cirrhotic with a history of hepatitis C and alcoholism, and he has had ascites for which he takes sprinolactone. He has had two prior transjugular intrahepatic portocaval shunt (TIPS) procedures. On examination, he has a protuberant umbilicus and some erythema around the umbilicus. The ED resident states she attempted to reduce the mass but was unsuccessful. The patient has a white blood cell count of 14,000/mm^3, hemoglobin of 11 g/dl platelets of 72000/mm^3, AST and ALT are within normal limits, INR of 1.6, total bilirubin of 1.9 mg/dL, and albumin of 2.9 g/dl. A CT scan shows a proximal bowel obstruction with a transition point at the umbilicus, and there appears to be bowel within the umbilicus. Moderate ascites is also noted. Reduction of the umbilical mass with moderate pressure fails. What is the optimal management of this patient provided no bowel resection is required?*

A. *Laparoscopy, reduction of hernia, intraperitoneal composite mesh umbilical repair*

B. *Open umbilical hernia repair with polypropylene mesh*

C. *Open umbilical hernia with biologic mesh*

D. *Open umbilical hernia repair without mesh*

E. *Open umbilical hernia repair, without mesh, and placement of paracentesis catheter*

This is a patient with advanced cirrhosis and ascites. These patients typically have umbilical hernias and little omentum, which is a setup for incarcerated or strangulated umbilical hernias with trapped bowel. Laparotomy in such patients is associated with significant mortality. Umbilical hernia repair in these patients has a high failure rate, and indeed the objective is often to reduce subsequent complications rather than obtain definitive hernia repair. Breakdown of the umbilical repair and uncontrolled ascites leakage from the wound is a morbid complication. Mesh repair has not shown to lessen hernia recurrence rates in such patients, and may risk mesh-related complications such as mesh infection and bowel perforation. Placement of a paracentesis catheter or drain in the peritoneal space may prevent the postoperative reaccumulation of tense ascites, allowing the umbilical wound an opportunity to heal without tension. Refractory cases may need a functioning TIPS prior to attempted repair.

Answer: E

Deveney KE (2009) Hernias and other lesions of the abdominal wall. In: Doherty GM (ed.) *Current Diagnosis and Treatment: Surgery*, 13th edition, McGraw-Hill, New York.

Telem DA, Schiano T, Divino CM (2010) Complicated hernia presentation in patients with advanced cirrhosis and refractory ascites: management and outcome. *Surgery* **148** (3), 538–43.

Chapter 36 Gallbladder and Pancreas

Andrew Tang, MD

1. *A hepaticojejunostomy is performed immediately after intraoperative realization of a transected common bile duct during laparoscopic cholecystectomy (Strasberg-Soper E1). Which of the following statement is most accurate?*

A. In experienced hands, the patient has a 90% long-term patency rate at long-term follow-up

B. The patient will likely require anastomotic revision within three years due to stricture

C. Emergency bile duct reconstruction increases the patient's immediate postoperative complication rate to 50%

D. An end-to-end anastomosis has a lower stricture rate than a hepaticojejunostomy

E. Immediate bile duct reconstruction should be delayed for 72 hours to allow for proximal bile duct dilation

Over 750 000 cholecystectomies are performed annually, making it one of the most commonly performed operations worldwide. The laparoscopic approach is associated with a slightly higher incidence of bile duct injury than open cholecystectomies, approximately 0.6% as compared to 0.2%. Large retrospective reviews have found that less than one-third of iatrogenic injuries are identified at the time of the cholecystectomy. Keys to intraoperative recognition of bile-duct injuries include persistent bile leakage from near the porta hepatis or liver, or the finding of a "second" unidentified ductal structure. Immediate cholangiography is imperative to clarify the anatomy should a ductal injury be suspected. Several studies have shown that bile duct reconstruction performed by experienced hepatobiliary surgeons have up to a 90% long-term patency rate. Debridement and primary anastomosis can be attempted for common bile duct injuries less than 1 cm in length. However, in the vast majority of such cases, the undiseased common bile duct is narrow, which makes the anastomosis challenging and prone to a higher stricture rate. Otherwise, a hepaticojejunostomy should be performed both for injuries longer than 1 cm and for proximal ductal injuries near the hepatic bifurcation. External transanastomotic drainage in the form of a T-tube should be used in all emergent bile duct reconstructions. A retrospective review of 200 patients with major bile duct injuries found the mean interval from bile duct injury to referral was 29 weeks. Hepaticojejunostomies were performed in 98% of patients. Postoperative mortality was 1.7%, and 42.9% of patients sustained at least one postoperative complication, most commonly wound infection (8%), cholangitis (5.7%), and intra-abdominal abscess/biloma (2.9%). In cases where the injury is promptly identified and followed by immediate reconstruction such as the scenario presented here, the infectious complications are much lower.

Answer: A

Kapoor VK (2009) Management of bile duct injuries: a practical approach. *American Journal of Surgery* **75** (12), 1157–60.

Sicklick JK, Camp MS, Lillemoe KD, *et al.* (2005) Surgical management of bile duct injuries sustained during laparoscopic cholecystectomy: perioperative results in 200 patients. *Annals of Surgery* **241** (5), 786–92.

2. *Which of these patients should not undergo prophylactic cholecystectomy for asymptomatic gallstones?*

A. 55-year-old man with end-stage ischemic cardiomyopathy on the heart transplant waiting list

B. 25-year-old African-American man with sickle cell anemia

Surgical Critical Care and Emergency Surgery: Clinical Questions and Answers, First Edition. Edited by Forrest O. Moore, Peter M. Rhee, Samuel A. Tisherman and Gerard J. Fulda.

C. *35-year-old woman with a BMI of 50 who is to undergo laparoscopic Roux-en-Y gastric bypass*

D. *50-year-old with short bowel syndrome who is long-term TPN dependent*

E. *85-year-old retiree with an active lifestyle*

Gallstones develop in 10–20% of the population. Nearly 80% of these patients remain asymptomatic throughout their lives, with only 1–4% progressing to symptoms or develop gallstone related complications. Prophylactic cholecystectomy in the general population is therefore not justified. Special cases exist in which prophylactic cholecystectomy for asymptomatic patients have been proposed to reduce the long-term complications. Heart transplant patients have been shown to have higher rate of gallstone formation and complication related morbidity and mortality. The 42% incidence of gallstone formation in transplant patients as reported by Peterseim is attributed to cyclosporine. Hemoglobinopathies such as sickle-cell anemia, hereditary spherocytosis and thalassemia are associated with gallstones in the range of 70%, 85% and 24%. Such patients are also at higher risk of stone-related complications largely due to delay in diagnosis because of the difficulty in distinguishing symptomatic cholelithiasis from abdominal sickling crisis. Morbidly obese patients who undergo rapid weight loss after gastric bypass procedures have up to a 40% incidence of harboring asymptomatic gallstones. Although concomitant laparoscopic cholecystectomy at the time of gastric bypass increases the operative time and adds to the technical difficulty, there is no increase in postoperative morbidity or mortality. It is therefore recommended by some bariatric experts that cholecystectomies be performed either before or during obesity surgeries. Patients who are TPN dependent have a nearly 35% incidence of gallstone formation and are at an increased risk for gallstone related complications due to bile stasis and changes in bile composition. Due to the chronic debilitated and immunocompromised state of TPN-dependent patients, emergent cholecystectomies are associated with an overall operative morbidity of 54% and mortality of 11%. Surveillance ultrasound is therefore recommended and cholecystectomies performed when gallstones are detected.

Answer: E

Garwood RA, Hanks FB (2008) Asymptomatic (silent) gallstones. In: Cameron JL (ed.) *Current Surgical Therapy*, 9th edn, Mosby Elsevier, Philadelphia, PA, pp. 405–8.

Milas M, Ricketts RR, Amerson JR, *et al.* (1996) Management of biliary tract stones in heart transplant patients. *Annals of Surgery* **223**, 747.

3. *Which statement is most accurate regarding early (<7 days) versus late cholecystectomy for acute cholecystitis?*

A. *Delayed laparoscopic cholecystectomy has a higher conversion rate*

B. *Delayed laparoscopic cholecystectomy has a higher incidence of bile-duct injuries*

C. *Patients who undergo early laparoscopic cholecystectomy are discharged faster compared to late cholecystectomy*

D. *Delayed laparoscopic cholecystectomy has significantly more blood loss*

E. *A higher incidence of wound infection is associated with delayed laparoscopic cholecystectomy*

Much controversy exists between the timing of cholecystectomy for acute cholecystitis. Some surgeons advocate "cooling down" patients with acute cholecystitis who present beyond seven days with antibiotics, fluid maintenance and *nil per os*. They cite the theoretical increased risk of inflammation-induced obliteration of anatomy, which increases the likelihood of bile-duct injury, operative blood loss, and is potentially associated with a higher conversion rate. However, such concerns are unsubstantiated in several randomized clinical trials comparing the outcomes between the two approaches. A Cochrane Review that examined five studies of high methodological quality found no difference in conversion rate or bile-duct injury rate between cholecystectomies performed within or beyond seven days. The author then published a meta-analysis using the same five randomized clinical trials, which in addition to the same findings as the Cochrane Review, also found the total hospital stay to be shorter by four days for the early cholecystectomy group.

Answer: C

Gurusamy KS, Samraj K (2006) Early versus delayed laparoscopic cholecystectomy for acute cholecystitis. *Cochrane Database of Systematic Review* **18** (4), CD005440.

Gurusamy K, Samraj K, Gluud C, *et al.* (2010) Meta-analysis of randomized controlled trials on the safety and effectiveness of early versus delayed laparoscopic cholecystectomy for acute cholecystitis. *British Journal of Surgery* **97** (2), 141–50.

4. *A 45-year-old man has been hospitalized for alcohol-induced pancreatitis for 3 days. His temperature is 100.3 degrees Celsius, heart rate 110 beats/minute, blood pressure 140/70 mm Hg. His abdominal exam reveals unchanged mild epigastric tenderness. WBC has been persistently elevated at 14,300/mm³ amylase and lipase high. What is the optimal route of nutritional support for him?*

A. *Immediately begin TPN, begin enteral nutrition only after his abdomen is nontender*

B. *Immediately begin TPN, begin enteral nutrition only after his amylase and lipase have normalized*

C. *Begin nasogastric tube feeding*

D. *Begin postpyloric feeding via a Dobb-Hoff tube*

E. *Wait for up to 7 days of NPO, then begin TPN if the patient still has abdominal pain*

Acute pancreatitis affects 220 000 patients in the USA annually. It is a hypermetabolic, hyperdynamic systemic inflammatory syndrome that results in a highly catabolic state. Despite the lack of prospective evidence, "gut rest" consisting of *nil per os*, intravenous fluid with or without total parenteral nutrition had become common practice. However, recent data from critically ill trauma and burn patients have indicated that septic complications can be reduced by the early introduction of enteral nutrition, possibly due to the maintenance of intestinal mucosal integrity and function and the resultant decrease in bacterial translocation. The dictum of avoiding pancreatic stimulation can still be satisfied if enteral nutrition is delivered past the ligament of Treitz. A Cochrane review of eight randomized clinical trials comparing enteral to parenteral nutrition in acute pancreatitis have found the relative risk for death was 0.5, for multisystem organ failure was 0.55, and for systemic infection was 0.39. Other findings include less need for operative interventions for the management of pancreatitis, decreased local septic complications, and the mean hospital length of stay reduced by 2.37 days. An abundance of evidence suggests that the use of TPN is associated with increased catheter-related septic complications, electrolyte abnormalities and overall cost. It should not be relied upon in patients who are able to tolerate enteral feeding.

Answer: D

Al-Omran M, Albalawi ZH, Tashkandi MF, *et al.* (2010) Enteral versus parenteral nutrition for acute pancreatitis. *Cochrane Database Systematic Reviews* **20** (1), CD002837.

Marik PE, Zaloga GP (2004) Meta-analysis of parenteral nutrition versus enteral nutrition in patients with acute pancreatitis. *British Medical Journal* **328** (7453), 1407.

Rhee P, Hadjizacharia P, Trankeim C, *et al.* (2007) What happened to total parenteral nutrition? The disappearance of its use in a trauma intensive care unit. *Journal of Trauma* **63** (6), 1215.

5. *Which of the following statements regarding antibiotic selection for biliary disease is correct?*

A. *Antibiotics should be continued for 48 hours after biliary stent placement for benign strictures*

B. *Empiric pseudomonal coverage in biliary sepsis has been shown to significantly decrease mortality*

C. *Carbapenem coverage should be considered for nursing home residents and hospitalized patients with biliary sepsis*

D. *Antimicrobial therapy is the mainstay of therapy in AIDS-associated cholangiopathy*

E. *Aerobic and anaerobic enteric organisms are equally common in biliary sepsis*

The biliary tract maintains its sterility in the absence of disease or instrumentation. The mechanism by which bacteria infect the biliary tree has been poorly defined. Existing hypothesis include the retrograde reflux of duodenal bacteria through the sphincter of Oddi, or the translocation of bacteria through lymphatic and portal venous channels from the intestinal tract. The most commonly identified bacteria in the biliary tree are aerobic enteric organisms such as *Escherichia coli* and *Klebsiella pneumoniae*.

Enterococcus is the third most commonly cultured bacteria from bile. However, it tends to be less virulent and affects mostly the elderly and immunocompromised patients. Pseudomonal infection of the biliary tract is uncommon, therefore it is generally not necessary to institute empiric antipseudomonal coverage unless compelling reasons exist. Culture and sensitivity is particularly important in patients residing in nursing homes, with recent hospitalizations, or antecedent antibiotic usage. A carbapenem should be considered in these cases involving potential resistant gram-negative rods. Anaerobic organisms such as *Clostridium* or *Bacteroides fragilis* are rarely seen in bile. When present, it is usually in the setting of the immunocompromised or elderly. Patients with acquired immunodeficiency syndrome are subject to opportunistic infections of the biliary tract by unusual organisms such as *Cytomegalovirus, Cryptosporidium* and *Microsporidia*. Antimicrobials are adjuncts to the primary treatment consisting of highly active antiretroviral therapy to boost the host immune response. Diagnostic and therapeutic manipulations of the biliary tree should be preceded by a single dose of antibiotics to cover *E. coli* and *Klebsiella pneumoniae*. However, continued antimicrobial usage even in the setting of biliary stents or catheters is of no benefit.

Answer: C

Fry D (2008) Antibiotic selection in biliary surgery. In: Cameron JL (ed.) *Current Surgical Therapy*. 9th edn, Mosby Elsevier, Philadelphia, PA, p. 4536.

Lillemoe KD (2000) Surgical treatment of biliary tract infections. *American Journal of Surgery* **66**, 138.

6. *Which of the following is not a risk factor for cholesterol stone formation?*

A. Total parenteral nutrition

B. Age

C. Cirrhosis

D. Rapid weight loss

E. Pregnancy

The incidence of gallstones increases by 1–3% per year with the highest cumulative incidence occurring in the first four decades of life. Total parenteral nutrition is associated with gallbladder hypomotility and biliary stasis. Comparing patients on TPN with normal controls, Pitt and colleagues have shown the TPN cohort to have a much higher propensity for stone formation (45% versus 12%). Patients who have undergone rapid weight loss, particularly through morbid obesity surgeries have a 40% incidence of developing stones within the immediate six months. Pregnancy increases the risk of cholesterol stone formation through two proposed mechanisms. One involves the estrogen induced change in bile composition, particularly an increase in cholesterol secretion. The other mechanism involves biliary stasis secondary to gallbladder hypokinesia, a result of pregnancy induced smooth-muscle relaxation. Cirrhosis is associated with a 30% increase in pigment stone formation.

Answer: C

Lambou-Gianoukos S, Heller SJ (2008) Lithogenesis and bile metabolism. *Surgical Clinics of North America* **88** (6), 1175–94.

7. *Which statement regarding biliary anatomy is false?*

A. The right hepatic artery arises from the superior mesenteric artery in 20% of the cases

B. The most common hepatic arterial variant is a replaced right hepatic artery

C. The common bile duct and the pancreatic duct form a common channel in 70% of cases

D. The 3 and 9 o'clock arteries, which supply the common bile duct, are branches of the proper hepatic artery

E. The right anterior sectoral duct drains Couinaud's segments 5 and 8

The right and left lobes of the liver are defined by Cantelie's line, which corresponds to an imaginary line between the gallbladder fossa and the inferior vena cava. The left lobe is then divided into medial (segment 4) and lateral sections (segments 2 and 3), separated by the umbilical fissure that is in continuity with the falciform ligament. The right lobe is divided into the anterior (segment 5 and 8) and the posterior sections (6 and 7). Each section is subdivided into the inferior (segments 5 and 6) and superior (7 and 8) segments. Normally, the cystic artery branches from the right hepatic artery. Its location is fairly constant within Calot's triangle, which is bordered medially by the common hepatic duct, the cystic duct inferiorly and the inferior edge of the right lobe superiorly. The 3 and 9 o'clock arteries are major axial vessels that run along the medial and lateral borders of the supraduodenal common bile duct in locations implied by their names. They arise inferiorly from the anterior and posterior superior pancreaticoduodenal, gastroduodenal and retroportal arteries, and above from the right and left hepatic and cystic arteries. Given the locations of the 3 and 9 o'clock arteries, choledochotomies should be created longitudinally through an area devoid of vessels, leaving the fascial envelope intact. The CBD invariably lies to the right of the proper hepatic artery, and both structures lie anterior to the portal vein. In most cases, the right hepatic artery then courses posterior to the common hepatic duct as it ascends to supply Couinaud's segments 5–8. The most common hepatic vascular variant occurring in 20% of patients is a replaced or accessory right hepatic artery arising from the superior mesenteric artery. The variant right hepatic artery can be palpated in the hepatoduodenal ligament posterior to the CBD and portal vein. In 15% of patients, a replaced or accessory left hepatic artery courses through the gastrohepatic ligament as it branches from the left gastric artery.

Answer: D

Hiatt JR, Gabbay J, Busuttil RW (1994) Surgical anatomy of the hepatic arteries in 1000 cases. *Annals of Surgery* **220** (1), 50–2.

Vakili K, Pomfret EA (2008) Biliary anatomy and embryology. *Surgical Clinics of North America* **88** (6), 1159–74.

8. *A 75-year-old nursing home resident presents with 2 days of nausea, vomiting and abdominal pain. His vitals are temp 100.2 degrees Celsius, HR 110 beats/minute, BP 159/90 mm Hg. An abdominal series reveals pneumobilia, small bowel air fluid levels and a 5cm opacification in the right lower quadrant. Which statement regarding his treatment is true?*

A. *Enterolithotomy alone predisposes the patient to a 30% chance of recurrence*

B. *The cholecystenteric fistula should be repaired either at the time of the enterolithotomy or as a second stage operation due to the rare spontaneous closure rate*

C. *The patient should be conservatively managed given the gallstone size and the likelihood of spontaneous passage*

D. *Resection of the obstructed small bowel segment and enterolithotomy have similar complication rates*

E. *The one stage procedure is associated with a higher morbidity and mortality than enterolithotomy alone*

Gallstone ileus accounts for 1–4% of mechanical small bowel obstructions and up to 25% of bowel obstructions in patients over 65 years. The process starts with gallstone impaction which leads to ischemia and pressure necrosis at the interface between the gallbladder and adjacent viscera. The duodenum is involved with cholecystoenteric fistula formation in over 80% of cases. The passage of stone is dependent on the size of the stone and the intestinal luminal diameter. It is generally believed that stones less than 2 cm will spontaneously pass. Those greater than 5 cm are likely to be impacted, typically in the terminal ileum in cases of small bowel fistulas, or the sigmoid colon in cases of colonic fistulas. The clinical presentation is characteristic of bowel obstruction. Most gallstones are not radiopaque enough to be easily detected on plain abdominal radiographs. The classic Rigler's triad of pneumobilia, small bowel air fluid levels and an ectopic gallstone is only present in 50% of patients. The sensitivity and specificity of CT scan for the detection of gallstone ileus are 93% and 100% respectively. Controversy exists regarding the optimal management of gallstone ileus. Three options exist: enterolithotomy alone, a one-stage procedure consisting of enterolithotomy, cholecystectomy and fistula repair, or the two-stage procedure of separating the enterolithotomy and the cholecystoenteric fistula takedown by 4–6 weeks to allow for patient optimization. Enterolithotomy alone is increasingly being offered to patients with gallstone ileus as the recurrence rate is only 5%

and spontaneous fistula closure rate of 50% have been reported. In the largest review to date, Reisner and Cohen found the associated mortality of the one-stage procedure to be 17% as compared to 12% for enterolithotomy alone. Enterolithotomy is performed by milking the obstructing stone proximally to unaffected bowel where the longitudinal enterotomy and stone extraction take place. Small bowel resection and anastomosis is another option when the impacted stone has created irreversible damage to the bowel wall. However, this approach is associated with particularly high anastomotic leak rates.

Answer: E

Ayantunde AA, Agrawal A (2007) Gallstone ileus: diagnosis and management. *World Journal of Surgery* **31** (6), 1292–7.

Reisner RM, Cohen JR (1994) Gallstone ileus: a review of 1001 reported cases. *American Journal of Surgery* **60**, 441–6

9. *Which statement regarding the treatment of gallstone related disease during pregnancy is true?*

A. *Symptomatic cholelithiasis should be managed non-operatively during pregnancy*

B. *Cholecystitis during the first trimester should be "cooled off" with antibiotics, followed by cholecystectomy in the second trimester*

C. *All pregnant patients should undergo tocodynamometer monitoring during cholecystectomy*

D. *Common bile duct exploration is preferred over ERCP in the management of choledocholithiasis during pregnancy due to the risk of radiation exposure*

E. *Laparoscopic cholecystectomy is associated with decreased risk of spontaneous abortion and preterm labor when compared to open cholecystectomy*

Gallstone-related disease affects 0.5–0.8% of pregnancies. Patients with symptomatic cholelithiasis can undergo laparoscopic cholecystectomy during any semester. Studies have shown that conservative management is associated with a readmission rate of 38–70%, and about a quarter of these patients will undergo surgery for debilitating symptoms or complications of cholelithiasis. The traditional dictum of avoiding cholecystectomies in the first and third trimester was largely based on data for open surgical procedures where spontaneous abortion rate of 12% during the first trimester and preterm labor rate of 40% during the third trimester have been reported. Available data support laparoscopic cholecystectomy's safety during all trimesters with little appreciable increase in maternal and fetal complications. In addition to the well-established benefits of laparoscopy, post cholecystectomy patients are also protected from the high likelihood of further gallstone related complications. Tocodynamometry is typically used in patients who are past the age of fetal viability of 24 weeks. Intraoperative fetal heart rate monitoring was believed to be the most accurate method of detecting fetal distress during laparoscopy. However, given the safety data accumulated over the past two decades, many institutions now perform only pre and postoperative fetal heart monitoring with no increase in fetal mortality. In the non-pregnant patients who undergo ERCP, the risk of bleeding and pancreatitis is 1.3% and 3.5% respectively. This risk is further compounded by the added risk of radiation, although in general, the radiation dose used during ERCP fluoroscopy is less than the harm threshold of 5 rad or 50 mGy as suggested by the American College of Obstetricians and Gynecologists. Nonetheless, fetal protective measure such as lead shielding and limiting fluoroscopy time should be practiced.

Answer: E

Date RS, Kaushal M, Ramesh A (2008) A review of the management of gallstone disease and its complications in pregnancy. *American Journal of Surgery* **196** (4), 599–608.

Jackson H, Granger S, Price R, *et al.* (2008) Diagnosis and laparoscopic treatment of surgical diseases during pregnancy: an evidence-based review **22**, 1917–27.

10. *An abdominal ultrasound incidentally identifies a 0.9 cm polypoid gallbladder lesion in a 45-year-old man. What is the next step in management?*

A. *Laparoscopic cholecystectomy*

B. *Open cholecystectomy with intraoperative frozen section*

C. Extended cholecystectomy with hepatic segment IVB and V resection and portal lymphadenectomy

D. CT scan with IV contrast

E. Observation with serial ultrasounds in 3 months

Polypoid lesions of the gallbladder are present in 5% of the population, most of which are identified incidentally during workup for other indications. The benign lesions account for 85% of gallbladder polyps and can be further divided into lesion with malignant potential such as adenoma and adenomyoma, and those with no malignant potential such as cholesterol polyps or adenomyomatous hyperplasia. Comparative analysis between benign and malignant lesions have found that 94% of benign lesions are smaller than 1 cm, whereas 88% of malignant lesions are larger than 1 cm. It is therefore recommended that patients with lesions larger than 1 cm with no malignant features on imaging should undergo laparoscopic cholecystectomy. In addition to polyp size, other factors associated with the development of malignancy include age over 50 years and coexistent gallstones. No standard guidelines exist regarding the surveillance of gallbladder polyps less than 1 cm. However, serial abdominal ultrasound in 3 to 6 months is a reasonable approach. Lesions that are found to be stable in size over a year can then be followed over longer intervals.

Answer: E

Lee KF, Wong J (2004) Polypoid lesions of the gallbladder. *American Journal of Surgery* **188** (2), 186–90.

Mainprize KS, Gould SW, Gilbert JM (2000) Surgical management of polypoid lesions of the gallbladder. *British Journal of Surgery* **87** (4), 414–7.

11. *A 45-year-old immigrant from Southeast Asia presents with cholangitis and jaundice. Ultrasound reveals multiple intrahepatic stones. Which of the following is not an advisable treatment option?*

A. Hepaticocutaneous jejunostomy (Hudson Loop)

B. Roux-en-Y hepaticojejunostomy

C. Percutaneous transhepatic cholangiocatheterization with biliary drainage and choledoscopic stone removal

D. Hepatic resection if stones are confined to one anatomical region

E. Endoscopic retrograde cholangiopancreatography (ERCP)

Hepatolithiasis is infrequently encountered in the Western population, but accounts for approximately 3–10% of all gallstone disease in Asia. These are typically brown pigment stones formed in association with states of prolonged partial biliary tract obstruction such as sclerosing cholangitis, benign or malignant biliary strictures and biliary parasites. Endoscopic retrograde cholangiopancreatography is associated with a high failure rate due to biliary stricture imposed access difficulty and the extensive nature of stone formation. Percutaneous transhepatic cholangiography allows for repeated fluoroscopically guided stone extraction with steerable stone baskets, or with percutaneous choledochoscopy. Surgical options include Roux-en-Y hepaticojejunostomy after intraoperative choledochoscopic guided stone clearance. A hepaticocutaneous jejunostomy, otherwise known as a Hudson Loop, involves a long Roux limb that extends from the hepaticojejunostomy to the anterior abdominal wall. This construct allows for future endoscopic access to the biliary tree should stone disease recur or for treatment of biliary strictures. If the hepatolithiasis is limited to a single lobe or segment of the liver, and associated with significant biliary stricture or atrophy, then hepatic resection may be indicated.

Answer: E

Neuhaus H (1999) Intrahepatic stones: the percutaneous approach. *Canadian Journal of Gastroenterology* **13** (6), 467–72.

Pitt HA, Venbrux AC, Coleman J, *et al.* (1994) Intrahepatic stones. The transhepatic team approach. *Annals of Surgery* **219** (5), 527–35.

12. *Gallbladder cancer limited to the lamina propria (Stage T1a) was found in the cholecystectomy specimen. What is the next step?*

A. Referral to radiation and medical oncology

B. Re-operation for radical cholecystectomy

C. *CT of the abdomen and pelvis for cancer staging*

D. *ERCP and endoscopic ultrasound*

E. *Observation*

Surgery is the only potentially curative treatment for gallbladder cancer. A majority of early stage gallbladder cancers (Tis or T1a) are identified by pathological examination of specimens removed for symptomatic cholelithiasis and cholecystitis. Simple cholecystectomy is adequate oncological treatment for such tumors as there is minimal chance of lymph node involvement. The five-year survival rate with simple cholecystectomy approaches 85–100% whether the procedure is performed open or laparoscopically. However, if preoperative suspicion of cancer exists such as in the case of large polyps, then open cholecystectomy is recommended in order to minimize gallbladder perforation with tumor spillage and port site metastasis.

Answer: E

Gourgiotis S, Kocher HM, Solaini L, *et al.* (2008) Gallbladder cancer. *American Journal of Surgery* **196** (2), 252–64.

Mainprize KS, Gould SW, Gilbert JM (2000) Surgical management of polypoid lesions of the gallbladder. British Journal of Surgery **87** (4), 414–17.

13. *A 45-year-old woman is recovering from a three week ICU course complicated by ARDS and acute renal failure secondary to necrotizing pancreatitis. A CT of the abdomen demonstrates an 8 cm fluid collection around a contrast non-enhancing pancreatic tail with no extraluminal air. Which statement regarding the next step in management is correct?*

A. *CT guided aspiration of the fluid collection for culture and sensitivity*

B. *Operative debridement of the necrotic pancreas and peripancreatic collection*

C. *CT guided percutaneous drainage of the fluid collection*

D. *Antimicrobial administration with gram positive, gram negative and fungal coverage*

E. *Observation with repeat CT scan in four weeks*

Ten percent of patients who develop acute pancreatitis will be afflicted by pancreatic fluid collections. This can be a non-enzymatic collection of fluid developed in response to the localized inflammation or the result of extravasated pancreatic enzymes from a disrupted pancreatic duct. Eighty-five to 90% of this group of patients will have spontaneous resolution of the fluid collection without intervention. Attempts to drain these collections either percutaneously or surgically should be discouraged due to the high recurrence rate and the risk of secondarily infecting a previously sterile environment. Pancreatic debridement in the acute setting is reserved only for patients with infected pancreatic necrosis as evidenced by gas in the retroperitoneum or by documentation of bacteria on Gram's stain or culture from aspirations of suspected fluid collections. The routine use of antibiotics for sterile peripancreatic collections have not been shown to reduce the incidence of infectious complications. Collections that persist for longer than six weeks will be covered by a nonepithelialized wall of fibrous or granulation tissue, at which time it is termed a pancreatic pseudocyst.

Answer: E

Cannon JW, Callery MP, Vollmer CM Jr. (2009) Diagnosis and management of pancreatic pseudocysts: what is the evidence? *Journal of the American College of Surgeons* **3**, 385–93.

Cheruvu CV, Clarke MG, Prentice M, *et al.* (2003) Conservative treatment as an option in the management of pancreatic pseudocyst. *Annals of the Royal College of Surgeons of England* **85** (5), 313–16.

14. *A 45-year-old man is admitted for severe alcohol induced pancreatitis. A CT scan demonstrates non-enhancement in 45% of the pancreatic body and tail. Which statement regarding antibiotic prophylaxis in necrotizing pancreatitis is most accurate?*

A. *Antibiotic prophylaxis used in conjunction with an antifungal agent is associated with the least infectious complications*

B. *Prophylactic antibiotics should be started on all patients with pancreatic necrosis*

C. *Prophylactic antibiotics should be started within 24 hours of admission*

D. *Antibiotic prophylaxis should be started in patients who demonstrate progression of pancreatic necrosis on serial contrast enhanced CTs*

E. *Antibiotic prophylaxis does not decrease the infectious complications associated with necrotizing pancreatitis*

Necrotizing pancreatitis develops in about 15% of patients with pancreatitis and accounts for mortality ranging from 12–35%. The associated mortality has a bimodal distribution with multisystem organ failure implicated in the early phase while pancreatic or peripancreatic infections account for much of the late deaths. The prevalent practice of antibiotic prophylaxis directed against common causative enteric organisms such as *E. coli*, Klebsiella, Enterobacter and Bacteroides does not appear to reduce the incidence of late infectious complications. Rather, several recent studies have documented an increase in gram-positive and Candida isolates from infected pancreatic aspirates, possibly due to the prevalent use of prophylactic antibiotics. A multicenter prospective randomized, double-blinded, placebo-controlled trial with 100 participants with greater than 30% pancreatic necrosis showed no difference in the incidence of pancreatic and peripancreatic infections, the number of surgical interventions, or mortality between those who received Meropenem and placebo. A Cochrane review of seven studies involving 404 patients randomly assigned to receive prophylactic antibiotics or placebo likewise concluded that there is no difference in the rate of infectious complications. The preponderance of available evidence does not support antibiotic prophylaxis for pancreatic necrosis.

Answer: E

Dellinger EP, Tellado JM, Soto NE, *et al.* (2007) Early antibiotic treatment for severe acute necrotizing pancreatitis: randomized, double-blind, placebo-controlled study. *Annals of Surgery* **245**, 674–83.

Villatoro E, Mulla M, Larvin M (2010) Antibiotic therapy for prophylaxis against infection of pancreatic necrosis in acute pancreatitis. *Cochrane Database Systematic Reviews* 5, CD002941.

Chapter 37 Liver and Spleen

Narong Kulvatunyou, MD, FACS

1. *Which of the following statements about the current management of blunt liver trauma is not true?*

A. *Nonoperative management is appropriate*

B. *Operative management is indicated for hemodynamic abnormality and associated organ injury*

C. *Patient with grade V injury usually require operation*

D. *Angiographic embolization is useful as an adjunct in both operative and non-operative management*

E. *Anatomic lobar resection is not required for most injuries*

Nonoperative management is appropriate and often can be performed with 90% success rate, as long as the patient remains hemodynamically within a normal range and does not have any other associated intra-abdominal injuries. Although the failure rate of nonoperativemanagement is increased with higher grade injuries, most grade IV and V injuries may still be successfully managed nonoperatively. In a nonoperative patient, angiographic embolization (AE) can be an adjunct in liver injury that contains arterio-venous fistula, ongoing bleeding. Angiographic embolization can also be of assistance in operative cases with difficulty where bleeding may be difficult to access and control. Lobar resection is rarely required for blunt hepatic trauma.

Answer: C

Asensio JA, Demetriades D, Chahwan S, *et al.* (2000) Approach to the management of complex hepatic injuries. *Journal of Trauma* **48** (1), 66–9.

Malhotra AK, Fabian TC, Croce MA, *et al.* (2000) Blunt hepatic injury: A paradigm shift from operative to non-operative management in the 1990s. *Annals of Surgery* **231** (6), 804–13.

2. *Which of the following is incorrect regarding liver abscess?*

A. *Both pyogenic and amoebic abscess have similar clinical presentation*

B. *Both pyogenic and amoebic abscess require drainage*

C. *Amoebic abscess is caused by Entamoeba histolytica*

D. *The most common source of pyogenic liver abscess is biliary source*

E. *Antibiotic of choice for amoebic abscess is metronidazole*

In the USA, pyogenic liver abscess is much more common than amoebic; however, the clinical presentation for both is similar. One must obtain a thorough history of traveling to the endemic areas—central America, southeast Asia, etc.—and diagnosis is confirmed by serologic test. Pyogenic treatment requires drainage, antibiotic, and identifying the possible source. Amoebic abscess is caused by *Entamoeba histolytica* and does not require drainage because it responds effectively to metronidazole. Ascending suppurative cholangitis is the most common identifiable cause of pyogenic abscess.

Answer: B

Cameron JL (2008) *Current Surgical Therapy*, 9th edn, Mosby, Philadelphia, PA.

3. *An 8-year-old girl is taken to the emergency department after being struck by a car. She landed on her right side. On arrival she is alert with a systolic blood pressure of 110 after 500 ml of crystalloids. She has bilateral breath sounds. Her vital signs*

Surgical Critical Care and Emergency Surgery: Clinical Questions and Answers, First Edition. Edited by Forrest O. Moore, Peter M. Rhee, Samuel A. Tisherman and Gerard J. Fulda.

have remained normal. The computed tomography (CT) scan below is obtained. The most appropriate next step would be:

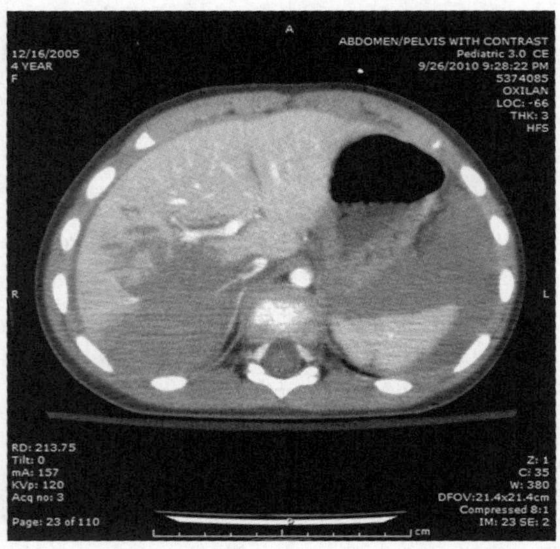

A. *Laparotomy*

B. *Diagnostic peritoneal lavage (DPL)*

C. *Angiography*

D. *Admission for observation*

E. *Laparoscopy*

Abdominal computed tomography (CT) shows a grade IV liver injury. A nonoperative management of blunt liver injuries with normal hemodynamics is recommended with greater than 90% success. Diagnostic peritoneal lavage will confirm the presence of blood but will not add any information helpful in the management of this patient. Laparoscopy may benefit this patient later in her course if he develops significant hemoperitoneum or biliary ascites but has no role in initial management once the diagnosis has been made. While some authors recommend angiography in all high-grade liver injury it is not an absolute indication especially when the CT does not show any evidence of active bleeding or arterio-venous fistula, "blush." While the CT looks as if the liver injury is severe and there is a lot of blood in the abdomen, in hemodynamically stable and normal patients, observation is the first course of action. However the CT should make one cautious and careful monitoring and follow up is required.

Answer: D

Duane TM, Como JJ, Bochicchio GV, *et al.* (2004) Reevaluating the management and outcomes of severe blunt liver injury. *Journal of Trauma* **57**, 494–500.

Kozar RA, Moore JB, Niles SE, *et al.* (2005) Complications of non-operative management of high-grade blunt hepatic injuries. *Journal of Trauma* **59**, 1066–71.

4. *Which of the following is incorrect regarding hydatid disease of the liver?*

A. *It is caused by parasitic Echinococcus whose definitive host is cat*

B. *Unique ultrasound or computed tomography characteristic is a calcified wall of the cyst, but diagnosis can be confirmed by serology*

C. *Chemotherapeutic with benzimidazole compound should be given 1–4 days preoperatively before and continued post-procedurally*

D. *Percutaneous aspiration, injection, and reaspiration (PAIR) is a possible treatment option*

E. *Before surgically entering the cyst, the operative field should be protected with scolicidal agent-soaked gauzes to prevent contamination*

Hydatid disease of the liver is uncommon. It is caused by parasitic *Echinococcus,* which has dogs as its definitive hosts. Humans come in contact by ingesting contaminated food infested with parasites. Signs and symptoms are vague but ultrasound and computed tomography has its unique characteristic of a cyst with a calcified wall. Medical therapy alone with benzimidazole agent results in incomplete resolution as 70% will have recurrence. So treatment must be combined with PAIR (percutaneous aspiration, injection, and reaspiration) or surgical cystectomy. It is important that operative field be protected with scolicidal agent-soaked gauzes, usually 20% normal saline, to prevent spillage and contamination.

Answer: A

Alonso CO, Moreno GE, Loinaz SC, *et al.* (2001) Results of 22 years of experience in radical surgical treatment of hepatic hydatid cyst. *Hepatogastroenterology* **48**, 235–9.

Gil-Grande LA, Rodriguez-Caabeiro F, Prieto JG, *et al.* (1993) Randomized controlled trial of efficacy of albendazole in intra-abdominal hydatid disease. *Lancet* **342**, 1269–75.

5. *A 24-year-old woman continues to have persistent abdominal pain one month after her motor vehicle collision in which she suffered a liver injury. The computed tomography (CT) shows a biloma. Attempted CT-guided drainage was unsuccessful. What would be the next step of management?*

A. *Exploratory laparotomy and hepatectomy*

B. *Exploratory laparotomy and debridement of necrotic parenchyma*

C. *Laproscopy with drainage*

D. *drainage and endoscopic retrograde cholangiopancreatography (ERCP) with sphincterotomy*

E. *Somatostatin and observe*

Patients with high-grade liver injuries have increased risk of developing postinjury biloma complication. In general, CT-guided drainage is the initial treatment of choice for patient who is asymptomatic and it is usually successful. However, if unsuccessful, endoscopic retrograde cholangiopancreatography (ERCP) with sphincterotomy and stent insertion reduces the biliary ductal pressure, and shorten the time of the resolution of the biloma. Laparoscopic insertion of a drain has been described for early management of grade III and IV liver injury, but not for the management of biloma. Hepatectomy and debridement are not indicated for this patient and is probably too radical an option at this time. Somatostatin use for this indication has not been shown to be effective.

Answer: D

Duane TM, Como JJ, Bochicchio GV, *et al.* (2004) Reevaluating the management and outcomes of severe blunt liver injury. *Journal of Trauma* **57**, 494–500.

Kozar RA, Moore JB, Niles SE, *et al.* (2005) Complications of non-operative management of high-grade blunt hepatic injuries. *Journal of Trauma* **59**, 1066–71.

6. *A 13-year-old girl suffered a grade V liver injury for a motor vehicle collision. Three weeks later she presents to the emergency department complaining of abdominal pain and hematesis. Her vital signs are stable and her abdominal exam is unremarkable. Upper endoscopy showed no obvious bleeding source. What would be the most appropriate next step for the management of this patient?*

A. *Assure the mother of the patient that her symptoms will pass*

B. *Prescribe H_2-blocker and ask her to see her primary physician the following day*

C. *Obtain serial ultrasound examinations*

D. *Laparotomy*

E. *Angiography*

Fifty percent of high-grade (IV–V) blunt liver injuries may develop delayed complications such as those seen in this patient. This patient developed hemobilia as a cause of her upper gastrointestinal bleed. The diagnosis and treatment option of choice is angiography and embolization. Prescribing of H_2 blockers will not treat the pseudoaneurysm that is causing the hemobillia. Ultrasound will not definitively diagnose the problem and while it is not invasive, it will not treat the underlying problem. Because angiography can be curative and is relatively less invasive then surgery, the first approach should be angiography.

Answer: E

Carrillo EH, Spain DA, Wohltmann CD (1999) Interventional techniques are useful adjuncts in non-operative management of hepatic injuries. *Journal of Trauma* **46**, 619–22.

Carrillo EH, Wohltmann C, Richardson JD (2001) Evolution in the treatment of complex blunt liver injuries. *Current Problems in Surgery* **38**, 1–60.

7. *A 47-year-old patient was involved in a motorcycle collision. On arrival to the trauma bay, he was hypotensive with a positive FAST (focused assessment by sonography for trauma). He was emergently taken to the operating room for laparotomy. Intra-operatively he was found to have liver cirrhosis. Which of the following statements is not true concerning patients with cirrhosis in trauma in comparison to those with noncirrhosis?*

A. *They have double the complication rate in comparison to noncirrhotic patients*

B. *They have prolonged intensive care unit and hospital stay*

C. *Their mortality is not affected by the presence of cirrhosis*

D. *The mortality is higher in subset of cirrhotic patients who undergo abdominal surgery*

E. *The presence of cirrhosis is a criterion for a trauma team activation*

Cirrhosis probably represents 1% of all trauma admission annually. Literature on cirrhosis and trauma is, however, limited. A study by Georgiou *et al.*, which represents the largest series, demonstrates mortality and morbidity rate are significantly increased (12% versus 6%, 10% versus 4%), respectively. The hospital stay and intensive care-unit stay is also increased. A subset of patients who underwent abdominal surgery in this series has a 40% mortality rate, in comparison to 15% noncirrhotic patient. The wide-ranging systemic abnormalities in the physiology mean that a minor trauma can be significant; hence, a trauma patient who has a known history of cirrhosis is a criterion for a transfer to the trauma center with trauma team activation.

Answer: C

Georgiou C, Inaba K, Teixeira PG, *et al.* (2009) Cirrhosis and trauma are a lethal combination. *World Journal of Surgery* 1087–92.

Wahlstrom K, Ney AL, Jacobson S, *et al.* (2000) Trauma in cirrhotics: survival and hospital sequelae in patients requiring abdominal exploration. *American Surgery* **66**, 1071–6.

8. *With regard to liver anatomy, which of the following statement is not true?*

A. *Morphologic anatomy, liver is divided into two lobes divided by the falsiform ligament*

B. *Functional anatomy, liver is divided into segments based on the distribution of portal pedicles and hepatic veins*

C. *Right liver is divided into anteromedial and posterolateral by the plane drawn by the right hepatic vein*

D. *Left liver is divided into anterior and posterior by the plane drawn by the left hepatic vein*

E. *Quadrate lobe (segment IV) is a part of the left lobe*

To deal successfully with liver surgery one must understand the liver anatomy. Liver anatomy can be described by a morphologic and a functional anatomy. Morphologically, the line is drawn between the gallbladder and the inferior vena cava, giving rise to the anatomical right and left lobe. The functional anatomy is divided based on hepatic veins and portal pedicles distribution, giving rise to the Couinaud's eight segmental anatomy. The

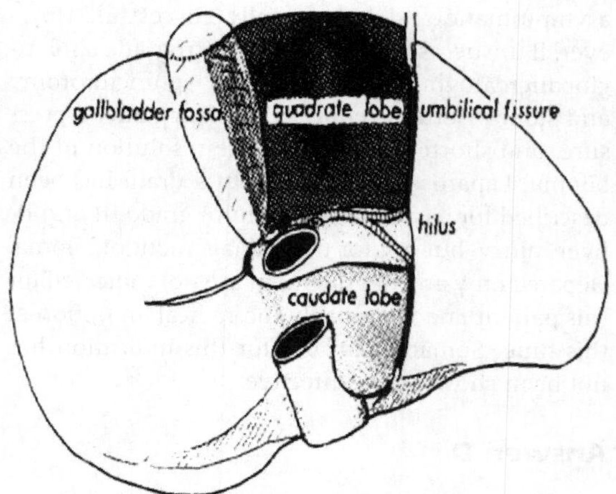

Source: Reproduced from Bismuth H (1982) Surgical anatomy and anatomical surgery of the liver. *World Journal of Surgery* **6**, 3–9 with kind permission of Spring Science and Business Media.

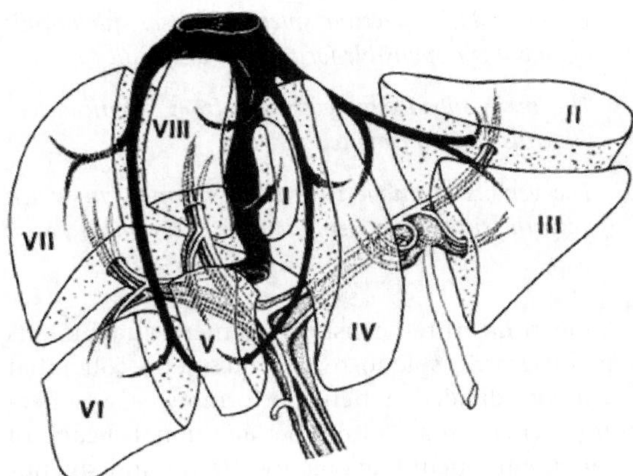

Source: Reproduced from Tsugawa K, *et al.* (2002) Anatomical resection for severe blunt liver trauma in 100 patients: significant differences between young and elderly. *World Journal of Surgery* **26,** 544–9 with kind permission of Spring Science and Business Media.

middle hepatic vein runs along the main fissure, which divides the liver into the right and left liver (not lobe, to prevent confusion with anatomical lobe). The right hepatic vein runs and divides the right liver into the anteromedial (segment V, VIII) and the posterolateral (segment VI, VII) segments. Similarly, the left hepatic vein runs and divides the left liver into anterior (segment IV, III) and posterior (II) segments. Quadrate lobe (segment IV) is a part of the left lobe and lies to the right of the falsiform ligament.

Answer: A

9. *Which of the following statement is not true regarding liver tumor?*

A. *Hepatic adenoma is a benign tumor and often associated with women of child-bearing age who are taking oral contraceptives*

B. *Focal nodular hyperplasia (FNH) is a malignant tumor that is characterized by central scarring*

C. *Hepatic hemagioma is the most common hepatic benign tumor and characterized by early enhancement of the periphery*

D. *Hepatic angiosarcoma is a rare malignant tumor seen in children*

E. *Hepatocellular carcinoma is associated with history of viral or alcohol hepatitis and elevated alpha-fetoprotein is diagnostic*

Distinguishing hepatic tumors as benign or malignant is important in liver management. History and radiographic findings will help guide the diagnosis and management. Hepatic adenoma is a benign tumor that is seen in women with child-bearing age and who are taking oral contraceptives. They often present with abdominal pain because of their size. They require resection because of symptomatic pain and they can degenerate into hepatocellular carcinoma. Focal nodular hyperplasia (FNH) is a benign tumor that is sometimes difficult to distinguish from hepatic adenoma, except the radiographic characteristics central scarring. They do not require resection. Hepatic hemangioma is the most common benign hepatic lesion. It has a CT scan characteristic of early enhancement of periphery. It may require resection when it is associated with large size and abdominal pain. Hepatic angiosarcoma is a rare malignant tumor seen primarily in children. It is highly vascular on CT scan and treatment is resection. Finally, hepatocellular carcinoma is a malignant tumor that is frequently seen in patient with hepatitis. It requires surgical resection and elevated alpha-fetoprotein is diagnostic.

Benign	Malignant
Hepatic adenoma	Hepatocellular carcinoma
Focal nodular hyperplasia	Hepatic angiosarcoma
Hemangioma	Hepatic metastasis
	Hepatic cholangiocarcinoma

Answer: B

Cameron JL (2008) *Current Surgical Therapy,* 9th edn, Mosby, Philadelphia, PA.

Yun EJ, Choi BI, Han JK, *et al.* (1999) Hepatic hemangioma: contrast-enhancement pattern during arterial and portal venous phases of spiral CT. *Abdominal Imaging* **24**, 262–6.

10. *Which of the following has not been shown to be a reliable criterion predicting increased* *mortality for a nontransplanted surgery in a patient with cirrhosis?*

A. *Age*

B. *American Society of Anesthesiologists (ASA) physician status*

C. *Emergency operation*

D. *Model end-stage liver disease (MELD) score*

E. *APACHE II score*

Cirrhosis of the liver is associated with increased morbidity and mortality when the patient must undergo an operation. Appreciating the risk factor may help clinicians make better decisions if the risk outweighs the benefit. Several studies have shown that increasing age, ASA class IV and V, emergency operation, and MELD score are reliable risk factors predicting peri-operative morbidity and mortality. APACHEII score, although used for predicting prognosis of a broad range of critically ill patients, has not performed well in cirrhotic patients because of the lack the liver function components (bilirubin, albumin). The MELD score, calculated from serum creatinine, total serum bilirubin, and international normalized ratio (INR) for prothrombin time, and etiology of cirrhosis, has been found to be reliable not only just in allocation of livers for transplantation, but also for risk assessment of non-transplant elective and emergency operation as well.

Answer: E

Teh SH, Nagorney DM, Stevens SR, *et al.* (2007) Risk factors for mortality after surgery in patients with cirrhosis. *Gastroenterology* **132**, 1261–9.

Ziser A, Plevak DJ, Wiesner RH (1999) Morbidity and mortality in cirrhotic patients undergoing anesthesia and surgery. *Anesthesiology* **90**, 42–53.

11. *Which of the following statement is incorrect regarding splenic anatomy?*

A. *It has three constant ligament attachments including spleno-gastric, spleno-renal, and spleno-colic ligament*

B. *Spleno-reno ligament contains the short gastric vessels that need to be ligated when performing the splenectomy*

C. *When mobilizing colon splenic flexure, spleno-colic ligament is responsible for the tear of splenic capsule*

D. *The main blood supply derives from splenic artery which is derived from celiac artery*

E. *The venous drainage is through splenic vein which joins the superior mesenteric vein to become a portal vein*

Spleen has three constant ligament attachments (spleno-gastric, spleno-renal, and spleno-colic) that must be divided when performing a splenectomy. There may often be additional ligament attachments including spleno-phreno and spleno-omental. Most ligament attachments are avascularized except the spleno-gastric, which contains the short-gastric vessels. Spleno-colic can sometimes be vascularized. The spleen derives dual blood supplies from the main splenic artery and the short gastric. The venous drainage follows the same arterial path.

Answer: B

Fraker DL (2006) Splenic disorders, in Mulholland MW, Lillemore KD, Doherty GM, Maier RV, Upchurch GR. (eds): Greenfield's Surgery: Scientific Principles and Practice, Philadelphia, PA, Lippincott Williams & Wilkins, pp 1220–1250.

12. *A 26-year-old man with autoimmune hemolytic anemia has failed medical therapy and needs to have a splenectomy. The most likely location for an accessory spleen would be the*

A. *Greater omentum*

B. *Splenic hilum*

C. *Small bowel mesentery*

D. *Tail of the pancreas*

E. *Spleno-colic ligament*

Accessory spleen is a common anomaly, occurring in up to 20% of the population. However, it can occur in up to 30% of patients with a hematologic disorder. If splenectomy is indicated as treatment for hemolytic anemia, then a thorough search for accessory spleens must be accomplished;

otherwise, it can lead to a relapse. Approximately 80% of accessory spleens are located within the splenic hilum or its vascular pedicle. Other areas include the greater omentum, tail of the pancreas, spleno-colic ligament, small bowel mesentery, and ovary.

Answer: B

Fraker DL (2006) Splenic disorders, in Mulholland MW, Lillemore KD, Doherty GM, Maier RV, Upchurch GR. (eds): Greenfield's Surgery: Scientific Principles and Practice, Philadelphia, PA, Lippincott Williams & Wilkins, pp 1220–1250.

13. *A 23-year-old man diagnosed with idiopathic thrombocypenic purpura (ITP) failed medical therapy and has a platelet count of 20 000/mm³. He now requires a splenectomy. Which of the following BEST predicts that he will have a favorable response to a splenectomy?*

A. *Time since diagnosis*

B. *Response to glucocorticoids*

C. *HIV status*

D. *Age*

E. *Platelet count*

Idiopathic thrombocytopenic purpura (ITP) is an autoimmune disorder resulting in low platelets counts secondary to the development of IgG antiplatelets antibodies. In adults, it tends to affect more women than men. It is usually a diagnosis of exclusion after other causes have been ruled out. It can be associated with other chronic immune conditions such as HIV infection. Initial therapy consists of oral glucocorticoids. Intravenous immunoglobulin is usually reserved for refractory cases associated with bleeding. Splenectomy is indicated for failure of medical management. Several preoperative indicators have been suggested for predicting a positive response to splenectomy, including short interval between diagnosis and operation, initial response to glucocorticoid therapy, positive HIV status, high preoperative platelet count, and young age. However, young age was the strongest predictor of positive response.

Answer: D

Duperier T, Brody F, Feisher J, *et al.* (2004) Predictive factors for successful laparoscopic splenectomy in patients with immune thrombocytopenic purpura. *Archives of Surgery* **139**, 61–6.

Kojouri K, Vesely SK, Terrell DR, *et al.* (2004) Splenectomy for adults patients with idiopathic thrombocytopenic purpura: a systemic review to assess long-term platelet count responses, prediction of response, and surgical complication. *Blood* **104**, 2623–34.

14. *A 17-year-old boy presents with several months of increasing left upper quadrant discomfort. Computed tomography (CT) demonstrates a large 7-cm splenic cyst. The single best treatment would be:*

A. *Non-steroidal anti-inflammatory agents*

B. *Percutaneous aspiration*

C. *Angiographic embolization*

D. *Partial splenectomy*

E. *Total splenectomy*

Splenic cysts overall are uncommon. Approximately 75% of all splenic cysts are post-traumatic in nature, and are truly pseudocysts. Primary cysts are generally classified as parasitic, congenital, and neoplastic, and the treatment is based on the type. Parasitic cysts (*Echinococcus*) are treated medically, followed by resection. Neoplastic requires splenectomy. The congenital or posttraumatic can be observed if they are asymptomatic. However, if they are symptomatic, they should be treated with partial splenectomy. Asymptomatic cysts over 5 cm in diameter should also be treated with partial splenectomy, primarily to rule out neoplasm. The patient in this question is symptomatic and has a cyst greater than 5 cm.

Answer: D

Hansen MB, Moller AC (2004) Splenic Cysts. *Surg Laporosc Endosc Percutan Tech.* **14**, 316–22.

Morgenstern L (2002) Nonparasitic splenic cysts: pathogenesis, classification, and treatment. *Journal of the American College of Surgeons* 306–14.

15. *A 26-year-old woman presents with two weeks increasing vague left upper quadrant abdominal pain. A computed tomography (CT) shows a 2-cm splenic aneurysm. Which of the following is true about this medical condition?*

A. *This condition is best observed in this patient*

B. *Artery embolization offers the most definitive treatment*

C. *Surgical splenectomy should be considered in this patient as there is increasing risk of rupture*

D. *This condition is more common in men*

E. *The treatment is the same for a 65-year-old who lacks any symptoms*

Splenic artery aneurysm is very uncommon but it is the second most frequent abdominal artery to undergo aneurismal changes. It is twice as common in women as men. There is an increasing risk of rupture at this young childbearing age and surgical splenectomy with aneurismal ligation is recommended. The recommendation is not true in an elderly patient whose pathophysiology is related to atherosclerotic changes and, if the patient is asymptomatic, no surgical intervention is required. Arterial embolization will not be effective. A less invasive intervention, such as an intravascular stent, is probable an option but it is not well studied in this area.

Answer: C

Lambert CJ, Williamson JW (1990) Splenic artery aneurysm: a rare cause of upper gastrointestinal bleeding. *American Journal of Surgery* **56**, 543–5.

16. *A 34-year-old man was involved in a motorcycle accident. On arrival, his initial systolic blood pressure (SBP) was 80/50 mm Hg but subsequently improved to 120/65 mm Hg after a 2 L of normal saline bolus. His Glasgow coma scale (GCS) was 13. He was taken to the computerized scan (CT). His head CT showed depressed skull fracture with subdural hematoma. While being transported back to the trauma bay, he again became hypotensive with SBP 85/50 mm Hg. His abdominal CT scan is shown. What would be the most appropriate treatment for this patient?*

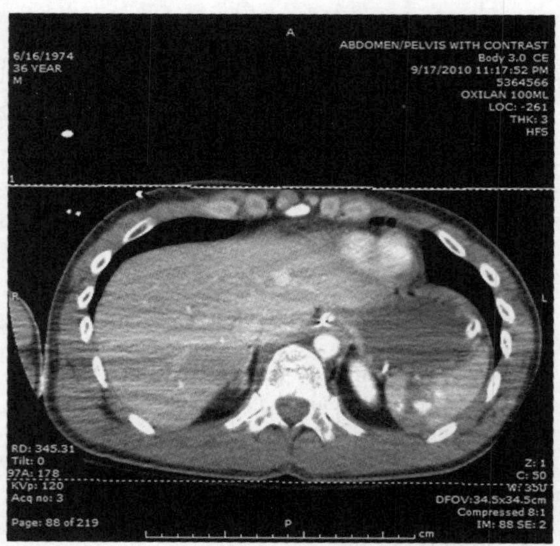

A. *Administer 2 L of normal saline and continue observe*

B. *Administer 2 units of O- and continue observe*

C. *Arterial embolization by interventional radiologist*

D. *Administer 2 units of O- and take the patient directly to surgery*

E. *Type and cross and wait for radiologist report*

This patient has a blush (arrow) on the CT scan, which indicates an active contrast extravasation. In view of his transient response to fluid resuscitation, he should be taken emergently to surgery after two units of O– have been given. Any further delay may further compromise his traumatic brain injury. Contacting and mobilizing an interventional radiology team would take time and is usually not as expedient as the surgical approach. Although the patient's blood pressure normalized, in order to prevent secondary traumatic brain injury from any future episodes of hypotension, rapid definitive treatment is wise and does not put the patient at risk of bleeding due to the splenic injury. If the patient does not have a concomitant head injury and the patient's blood pressure always remained normal, and the institution has rapid access to interventional radiology, then embolization may be an alternative.

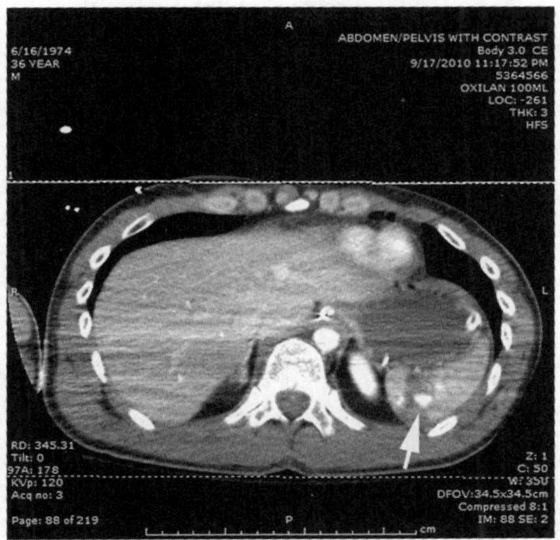

Answer: D

Haan JM, Bochicchio GV, Kramer N, *et al.* (2005) Non-operative management of blunt splenic injury: a 5-year experience. *Journal of Trauma* **58**, 492–8.

Thompson BE, Munera F, Cohn SM, *et al.* (2006) Novel computed tomography scan scoring system predicts the need for intervention after splenic injury. *Journal of Trauma* **60**, 1083–6.

17. *Which of the following is true regarding angioembolization and splenic injury?*

A. AAST splenic injury grading system has a high correlation with success and failure of non-operative management

B. Angioembolization does not alter the success rate of non-operative management

C. Superselective distal embolization is associated with less splenic infarct, as compared to the proximal embolization

D. The absence of a blush on a delay or "wash-out" phase of the CT scan is indicative of pseudo-aneurysm

E. Angioembolization has a success rate of 60%

Blunt splenic injury nonoperative management has a success rate of approximately 90% in the modern series. However, the AAST splenic injury grading system does not take into account the presence of splenic vascular injury, which manifests itself as a blush on a modern CT scan. As a result, there is a poor correlation within the grading system. The presence of a "blush" implies an active extravasation or a post-traumatic pseudoaneurysm or arterio-venous malformation. However, unlike active hemorrhage, pseudoaneurysms or arteriovenous fistula has a "wash-out" from the parenchyma and becomes isodense relative to normal parenchyma during the delay or "washout" phase. The addition of angioembolization in the management of blunt splenic injury has improved the success rate of non-operative management, especially in the group who is hemodynamically stable. The proximal embolization is associated with lower incidence of splenic infarct because of collateralization for the short gastric, and overall the success rate of angioembolization has improved into a range of 73–100% in the most current series.

Answer: D

Gavant ML, Schurr M, Flick PA (1997) Predicting clinical outcome of non-surgical management of blunt splenic injury: using CT to reveal abnormalities of splenic vasculature. *American Journal of Roentgenology* **168**, 207–12.

Raikhlin A, Baerlocher MO, Asch MR, Myers A (2008) Imaging and transcatheter arterial embolization for traumatic splenic injuries: review of the literature. *Canadian Journal of Surgery* **51** (6), 464–72.

18. *Which of the following is a contraindication to non-operative management of splenic trauma?*

A. Contrast extravasation

B. Associated intra-abdominal injuries

C. Abnormal hemodynamic status

D. Patient is a Jehovah's Witness

E. Subcapsular splenic hematoma

Abnormal hemodynamic status that is unresponsive to resuscitation is an indication that this patient must go to the operating room. On the other hand, the presence of contrast extravasation may be amendable to angiographic embolization just as long as patient remains hemodynamically within normal and there is ample time to mobilize angiographic team. The presence of other associated intra-abdominal injuries is not contraindicated for a nonoperative management but serial abdominal exam must be performed to exclude blunt hollow viscus injury. A Jehovah's Witness with splenic injury is not treated differently from other patients.

Answer: C

Peitzman AB, Heil B, Rivera L, *et al.* (2000) Blunt splenic injury in adults: multi-institutional study of the Eastern Association for the Surgery of Trauma. *Journal of Trauma* **49**, 177–87.

Peitzman AB, Harbrecht BG, Rivera L, *et al.* (2005) Failure of observation of blunt splenic injury in adults: variability in practice and adverse consequences. *Journal of the American College of Surgeons* **201**, 179–87.

19. *Splenectomy is not the treatment of choice in the following disease?*

A. *Immune (idiopathic) thrombocytopenic purpura (ITP)*

B. *Thrombotic thrombocytopenic purpura (TTP)*

C. *Felty's syndrome*

D. *B-Thalassemia*

E. *Spherocytosis*

Immune (idiopathic) thrombocytopenic purpura (ITP) is a diagnosis of exclusion. HIV, pregnancy, drugs, and systemic lupus erythematosis can produce a similar syndromes. Platelets are normally produced. Primary treatment is glucocorticoid or gamma globulin. However, if medical therapy fails, splenectomy is performed.

Thrombotic thrombocytopenic purpura (TTP) classically presents with thrombocytopenia, fever, a hemolytic anemia, renal disease, and central nervous system dysfunction, and is quite similar to hemolytic uremic syndrome. Plasmapheresis is the treatment of choice.

Felty's syndrome is the clinical triad of thrombocytopenia, cutaneous leg ulcers, and rheumatoid arthritis. The syndrome is not well understood but sometimes patients will benefit from splenectomy if medical therapy fails.

Both B-thalassemia and spherocytosis are genetic disorders that result in abnormal red blood cells. Splenctomy can provide the treatment of choice if medical therapy fails.

Answer: B

Swain JM, Schlinkert RT (2004) Thrombocytopenia and other hematologic disorders. In Kelly KA, Sarr MG, Hinder RA (eds) *Mayo Clinic Gastrointestinal Surgery*, WB Saunders, Philadelphia PA, pp. 365–74.

20. *Which of the following statement is not true about overwhelming post-splenectomy infection (OPSI)?*

A. *The risk occurs within the first two to three years after the splenectomy*

B. *The risk affects patient of any ages*

C. *It is more common after splenectomy for the underlying hematological diseases*

D. *The vaccination is targeted against encapsulated organisms such as pneumococcus, H. Influenza, and N. meningococcus*

E. *Hyposplenic diseases like sickle cell disease, celiac disease, and dermatitis herpetiformis can result in impaired immunity just like post-splenectomy*

In the early 1950s it was noticed that neonates with hematological disease who required splenectomy had a very high subsequent risk of serious infection. However, the actual incidence is not really known. Initially it was believed that it only occurred within the first two to three years but, as shown in a study by Waghorn *et al.*, it could occur from as early as 24 days to a late 59 years after splenectomy, and it can affect patients of any age, from 18-months old to 85 years old. It is more common in hematological patients, probably because of their underlying suppressed immunity. Currently, a vaccination against encapsulated agents like *Pneumococcus, H. influenzae, N. meningococcus,* as well as viral influenza, is given, usually before the patient is being discharged from the hospital. Several medical conditions including sickle disease, celiac disease, and dermatitis herpetiformis behave like an asplenic condition; hence, the clinician must beware of the same risk.

Answer: A

Waghorn DJ, Mayon-White RT (1997) A study of 42 episodes of overwhelming post-splenectomy infection: is current guidance for asplenic individuals being followed? *Journal of Infection* **35**, 289–94.

Wisner DH (2004) Injury to the Spleen. In: Moore EE, Feliciano DV, Mattox KL (eds) *Trauma,* 5th edn, McGraw-Hill, New York, p. 681.

Chapter 38 Incarcerated Hernias

Narong Kulvatunyou, MD, FACS

1. *A 34-year-old man presents to the emergency department with an acute onset of a right groin pain, nausea, and vomiting. This occurred after he tries to lift a heavy box. Physical examination shows abdominal distension and a right groin mass that is tender to palpation. What is the most appropriate management for this patient?*

A. *Prescribe motrin for pain and ask him to see his primary physician the following day*

B. *Attempt to reduce the hernia and then discharge home*

C. *Premedicate prior to attempt to reduce the hernia, and then instruct never to lift any more heavy boxes*

D. *Premedicate prior to attempt to reduce the hernia, and then scheduled for an elective hernia repair*

E. *Surgical evaluation for an emergency repair*

There is no consensus whether one should ever attempt to reduce a hernia. However, in the setting where patient shows signs and symptoms suggesting intestinal obstruction, to discharge this patient would be unsafe. The hernia can be repaired in many different ways as well as at different times but the main focus should be the possible incarceration and bowel obstruction. He has an increased risk of recurrence with possible strangulation and its associated morbidity.

Answer: E

Akinci M, Ergul Z, Kulah B, *et al.* (2010) Risk factors related with unfavorable outcomes in groin repairs. *Hernia* **14,** 489–93.

Harissis HV, Douitsis E, Fatouros M (2009) Incarcerated hernia: to reduce or not to reduce. *Hernia* **13**, 263–6.

Kulah B, Kulacoglu IH, Oruc MT, *et al.* (2001) Presentation and outcome of incarcerated external hernias in adults. *American Journal of Surgery* 101–4.

Surgical Critical Care and Emergency Surgery: Clinical Questions and Answers, First Edition. Edited by Forrest O. Moore, Peter M. Rhee, Samuel A. Tisherman and Gerard J. Fulda.

2. *A 62-year-old woman presents to the emergency department with acute onset of umbilical pain. She has nausea but no vomiting. Examination of the umbilicus shows the overlying skin to have reddish discoloration and it is associated with tenderness to palpation. The most appropriate management is:*

A. *Prescribe pain mediation and then discharge*

B. *Prescribe antibiotic and then discharge*

C. *Obtain ultrasound to rule out urachal cyst*

D. *Obtain CT-guided biopsy since this is probably a Sister Mary Joseph node*

E. *Surgical repair*

Because of the sudden onset of periumbilical pain in association with discoloration of skin and tenderness, the differential diagnosis of skin cellulitis, infected urachal cyst, or other benign conditions are unlikely. Reduction of incarceration and repair of the umbilical hernia should be considered immediately.

Answer: E

Kulah B, Kulacoglu IH, Oruc MT, *et al.* (2001) Presentation and outcome of incarcerated external hernias in adults. *American Journal of Surgery* 101–4.

Tufaro AP, Campbell AK (2008) Incisional, epigastric, and umbilical hernias. In: Cameron JL (2008) *Current Surgical Therapy,* 9th edn, Mosby, Philadelphia, PA, pp. 573–6.

3. *Three borders that define the femoral ring (hernia) are:*

A. *Inferior epigastric vessels, inguinal ligament, conjoined tendon*

B. *Inferior epigastric vessels, inguinal ligament, spermatic cord*

C. *Inferior epigastric vessels, inguinal ligament, femoral vessels*

D. *Lacunar ligament, inguinal ligament, femoral vessels*

E. *Conjoined tendon, inguinal ligament, femoral vessels*

Femoral hernia is bordered superiorly by an inguinal ligament, laterally by a femoral vein, and medially by the lacuna ligament. The lacuna ligament is just a reflection of the conjoined tendon that ends on the pubic symphysis and becomes the line of Cooper ligament. Understanding this anatomy is important for the repair and to prevent recurrence. The repair may be performed by suturing the conjoined tendon to the Cooper ligament (McVay), by using the mesh plug technique, or by open versus laparoscopic pre-peritoneal repair technique.

The inferior epigastric vessel, conjoined tendon, and inguinal ligament actually define the border that represents the direct hernia. Often direct hernia is more obvious and femoral hernia is easily missed.

Answer: D

Alimoglu O, Okan KI, Dasiran F, *et al.* (2006) Femoral hernia: a review of 83 cases. *Hernia* **10**, 70–3.

Sandblom G, Haapaniemi S, Nilsson E (1999) Femoral hernias: a register analysis of 588 repairs. *Hernia* **3**, 131–4.

4. *In contrast to inguinal hernia, femoral hernia*

A. *Is often associated with an elective operation*

B. *Is more common in men*

C. *Is often associated with intestinal resection*

D. *Age is not the risk factor associated with increased morbidity*

E. *Clinical presentation is always obvious*

Dahlstand *et al.* studied 3980 femoral hernias from the national Swedish Hernia Registry and found that femoral hernia, in comparison to inguinal hernia, is more commonly associated with an emergency operation (36% versus 5%), and a bowel resection (23% versus 5%). In both the Dahlstand *et al.* and Alimoglu *et al.* series, femoral hernia is more common in woman (60–70%). Femoral hernia often presents as a mass below the inguinal ligament, which can often be confused with lymph node, lipoma, etc. Increasing age is a risk factor for perioperative morbidity and mortality for both femoral and inguinal hernia, particularly under an emergency operation.

Answer: C

Alimoglu O, Okan Ki, Dasiran F, *et al.* (2006) Femoral hernia: a review of 83 cases. *Hernia* **10**, 70–3.

Dahlstand U, Wollert S, Nordin P, *et al.* (2009) Emergency femoral hernia repair: A study based on a national register. *Annals of Surgery* **249**, 672–6.

5. *A 50-year-old man with advanced hepatitis C cirrhosis with Child–Turcotte–Pugh class C and a model of end-stage liver disease (MELD) score of 15 presents to the emergency department complaining of fluid leaking from his umbilicus. Examination shows an umbilical hernia with skin excoriation and fluid leakage but no evidence of infection. His abdominal exam is benign. Which is incorrect regarding the management of this patient?*

A. *He should not undergo operative repair due to his high perioperative risk*

B. *He should undergo operative repair with a preoperative transjugular intrahepatic portosystemic shunt (TIPS) placement*

C. *Intraoperative drain does not prevent wound complication*

D. *He should be evaluated for a possible liver transplant*

E. *His postoperative complication includes worsening encephalopathy*

Operative repair should be considered; however, the definitive guideline for the management of this condition is lacking. Regardless, it has an associated high short-term and long-term mortality. Several experts suggest a preoperative TIPS placement to help control the ascites, and minimize the wound complication. However, there is a lack of level-1 evidence. Several authors also recommend leaving a drain, but then again there is no level-1 evidence to support or reject this approach.

Worsening encephalopathy, wound complications, liver decompensation are all among the usual post-operative complications. As a result, this patient should be considered for a possible liver transplant.

Answer: A

Belghiti J, Durand F (1997) Abdominal wall hernia in the setting of cirrhosis. *Seminars in Liver Disease* **17**, 219–26.

Telem DA, Schiano T, Divino CM (2010) Complicated hernia presentation in patients with advanced cirrhosis and refractory ascites: management and outcome. *Surgery* **148** (3), 538–43.

6. *Which of the following is not considered a principle for the repair of incisional hernia?*

A. *Patient optimization by improving nutrition and ceasing smoking*

B. *Wound preparation by reducing the wound bioburden*

C. *Midline wound reapproximation if possible using a component separation*

D. *Immediate reconstruction should always be considered*

E. *Use of appropriate reinforcement material in a patient at increased risk of recurrence*

The Ventral Hernia Working Group (VHWG) convened in September 2008 to develop principles and guidelines for the management of ventral hernia, using an evidence-based approach. Four guideline principles include optimizing the patient's condition, which includes improving nutrition and quitting smoking, preparing the wound by reduction of wound bioburden, reapproximating the midline if possible using the component separation, and using appropriate reinforcement material in high risk ventral hernia. Reduction of bioburden means excision of all devitalized or infected tissue. If it cannot be done in one stage, immediate reconstruction should be delayed.

Answer: D

Breuing K, Butler CE, Ferzoco S, *et al.* (2010) Incisional ventral hernias: review of the literature and recommendations regarding the grading and technique of repair. *Surgery* **148,** 544–58.

7. *Which of the following regarding component separation is not true?*

A. *The steps consist of an incision and release of the posterior rectus sheath as well as the lateral external oblique release*

B. *The steps always requires lateral skin and subcutaneous tissue mobilization*

C. *Achieving midline approximation is the goal*

D. *It is often associated with an increased incidence of skin and fat necrosis*

E. *To minimize the recurrence at the epigastrium, the rectus muscle should be mobilized above the costal margin*

Ramirez *et al.* first described the component separation in 1990 and it consists of the posterior rectal sheath release (not commonly performed) and the lateral external oblique release. In order to perform the external oblique release, one often has to mobilize the skin and subcutaneous tissue laterally. This maneuver often leads to a disruption of the blood supply to skin and fat, which results in an increased postoperative wound complication.

Several modifications of technique to preserve these "peri-umbilical perforators" to preserve the blood supply below the umbilicus have risen. This includes a bilateral inguinal approach subfascial dissection. The maneuver allows the avoidance of an excessive lateral mobilization of the skin and subcutaneous and hence minimizes the disruption of the blood supply and postoperative wound complications

Answer: B

Clarke JM (2010) Incisional hernia repair by fascial component separation: results in 128 cases and evolution of technique. *American Journal of Surgery* **200**, 2–8.

Ramirez OM, Ruas E, Dellon AL (1990) Component separation method for closure of abdominal wall defects: an anatomic and clinical study. *Plastic and Reconstructive Surgery* **86**, 519–26.

8. *Which of the following is not true regarding parastomal hernia?*

A. *A higher incidence is associated with loop colostomy compared to end-colostomy*

B. *Repair includes relocation, aponeurotic repair, or repair with prosthetic mesh*

C. *Incidence may be as high as 50%*

D. *A new large pore light weight with decreasing polypropylene content has shown promise in decreasing paracolostomy hernia in a recent randomized trial*

E. *A "sublay" technique has been proposed to decrease the incidence of intestinal obstruction*

A paracolostomy hernia is a complicated issue with which an acute care surgeon may have to deal. The incidence can be as high as 50% and is higher with an end-colostomy. Just like the incisional hernia problems, it often has to do with patient's several poor risk factors like obesity, smoking, and tissue factor. Several recent randomized studies have suggested utilization of a new lightweight large pore with decrease polypropylene content prosthetic mesh in a "sublay" position (between peritoneum and posterior fascia) may help decrease the incidence of paracolostomy hernia.

Answer: A

Reinhard K, Klinge U, Schumpelick V (2000) The repair of large parastomal hernias using a midline approach and a prosthetic mesh in the sublay position. *American Journal of Surgery* **179**, 186–8.

Serra-Aracil X, Moreno-Matias J, Darnell A, *et al.* (2009) Randomized, controlled, prospective trial of the use of a mesh to prevent parastomal hernia. *Annals of Surgery* **249**, 583–7.

9. *A 32-year-old man underwent multiple small bowel resections with primary anastomosis and a left colectomy with an end-colostomy after a gunshot wound to the abdomen. He has been doing relatively well until post-operative day 17 in which he develops abdominal pain, nausea, and vomiting. His colostomy is no producing stool. He is afebrile and his abdominal exam shows distension and fullness around the colostomy. Computed tomography (CT) scan of the abdomen is obtained and is shown. What is the diagnosis?*

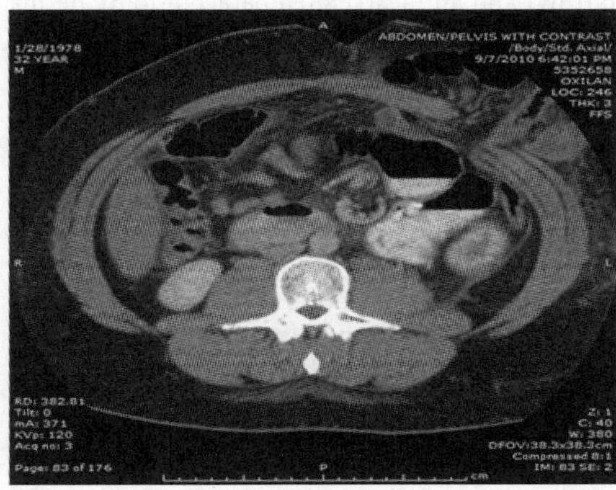

A. *Intra-abdominal abscess*

B. *Small bowel obstruction secondary to adhesion*

C. *Small bowel obstruction secondary to paracolostomy hernia*

D. *Large bowel obstruction secondary to mal-function colostomy*

E. *CT scan showed no abnormality*

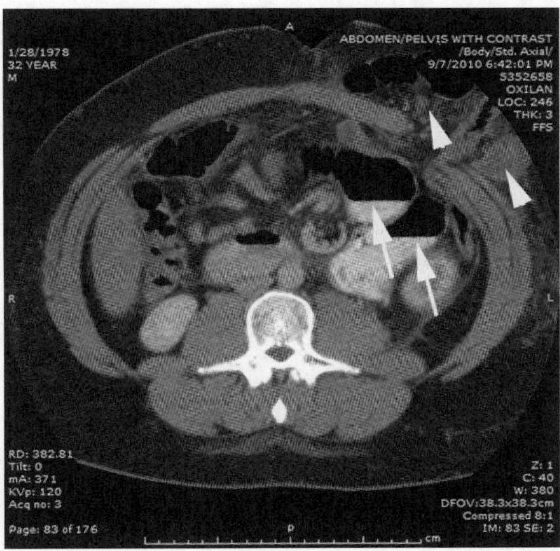

This patient developed clinical signs and symptoms of a postoperative small-bowel obstruction. The CT showed distended small-bowel loops (arrow) and an incarcerated paracolostomy hernia (arrow head). Clinical exam of fullness around the colostomy and this CT finding should prompt a re-exploration and repair of the paracolostomy hernia. An intraoperative finding showed a 20 cm of incarcerated paracolostomy hernia with a proximal small-bowel obstruction. An early paracolostomy hernia, especially with incarceration, as in this case, is quite unusual. It was a technical error of the initial operation for creating a too large a stoma that allowed small bowel to herniate through. A large-bowel obstruction is unlikely as the CT showed normal colon. Small-bowel obstruction secondary to adhesion is also unlikely considering that patient has been doing relatively well and acutely developed a small bowel obstruction picture. The CT scan did not show an obvious fluid collection, so intra-abdominal abscess is also unlikely.

Answer: C

Serra-Aracil X, Moreno-Matias J, Darnell A, *et al.* (2009) Randomized, controlled, prospective trial of the use of a mesh to prevent parastomal hernia. *Annals of Surgery* **249**, 583–7.

Tam KW, Wei PL, Kuo LJ, Wu CH (2010) Systemic review of the use of a mesh to prevent parastomal hernia. *World Journal of Surgery* **34**, 2723–9.

10. *A 69-year-old man with history of COPD presents with 24-hour history of abdominal distension and emesis. Physical examination reveals abdominal distension with hypoactive bowel sounds and a tender mass in the left groin below the inguinal ligament. During groin exploration, an incarcerated femoral hernia is found. Bowel is not viable and required resection. The preferred repair of the hernia would be*

A. *Bassini repair*

B. *Lichenstein repair*

C. *Shouldice repair*

D. *Cooper's ligament repair*

E. *Mesh plug in femoral canal*

A Bassini repair involves reconstruction of the floor by suturing the transversalis fascia, the transverses abdominis, and the internal oblique muscle to the inguinal ligament. The Shouldice, which used to be the standard repair, is similar but is done in multiple layers. Both are tension repair. The Lichenstein repair uses mesh and is considered a tension-free repair, which is viewed as a gold standard. These repairs, however, do not address the femoral canal defect.

The mesh plug technique was developed by Gilbert and then modified by Rutkow and Robbins, Milikan, and others. The technique involves a premade mesh shaped like a mushroom or self-made rolled up mesh that was placed in the defect like internal ring for indirect hernia, or the neck of the defect for direct hernia, or into the femoral canal in femoral hernia and secured in place by stitches. However, it is not recommended in this case because of the contamination and a possible mesh infection.

A Cooper ligament repair is similar to Bassini repair, except that Cooper's ligament instead of the inguinal ligament is used for the medial portion of the repair. This addresses the femoral defect and is indicated for this patient.

Answer: D

Deveney KE (2006) Hernias and other lesions of abdominal wall. In Doherty GM (ed.) *Current Surgical Diagnosis and Treatment,* 12th edn, New York, McGraw-Hill, pp. 765–78.

Chapter 39 Soft-tissue and Necrotizing Infection

Joseph J. DuBose, MD, FACS

1. *Which of the following signs or symptoms of necrotizing soft-tissue infection (NSTI) are present in the vast majority of patients?*

A. *Bullae*

B. *Crepitus*

C. *Gas on radiograph*

D. *Skin necrosis*

E. *None of the above*

Proposed "hard signs" of necrotizing soft-tissue infection include bullae, crepitus, gas in the tissues on radiographic imaging, hypotension with systolic blood pressure less than 90 mm Hg or skin necrosis. The presence of these signs or symptoms certainly aids a rapid diagnosis of this infectious process. Hard signs of NSTI are often absent on presentation, however, with studies documenting that less than 50% of patients who have had definitive diagnosis of NSTI established actually presented with hard signs of these infections.

Answer: E

Chan T, Yaghoubian A, Rosing D, *et al.* (2008) Low sensitivity of physical examination findings in necrotizing soft-tissue infection is improved with laboratory values: a prospective study. *American Journal of Surgery* **196** (6), 926–30 (discussion: 930).

2. *Which statement is most true of complicated skin and soft-tissue infections (cSSTIs):*

A. *They are associated with very low risk for life- or limb-threatening infection*

B. *They can best be treated by surgical incision alone*

C. *They can be treated on an outpatient basis with careful follow-up*

D. *They require initial emperic antimicrobial therapy with coverage for MRSA*

E. *They are rarely associated with co-morbid conditions*

As opposed to uncomplicated SSTIs such as simple abscesses, cellulitis or furuncles, which are associated with low risk for life- or limb-threatening infection, complicated SSTIs include infections of the deep soft tissue requiring significant surgical intervention, infected ulcers, infected burns and major abscesses. Patients with complicated SSTIs require hospitalization for treatment and commonly have significant underlying disease conditions that complicate response to treatment. Early initial emperic antibiotic coverage for these patients should include coverage for MRSA.

Answer: D

Napolitano LM (2009) Severe soft-tissue infections. *Infectious Disease Clinics of North America* **23** (3), 571–91.

Ruhe JJ, Smith N, Bradsher RW, *et al.* (2007) Community onset methicillin-resistant Staphylococcus aureus skin and soft-tissue infections: impact of antimicrobial therapy on outcome. *Clinical Infectious Diseases* **44**, 777–84.

3. *The most definitive method available to accurately diagnose the presence of necrotizing soft-tissue infection (NSTI) is:*

A. *Erythema and pain*

B. *Magnetic resonance imaging*

Surgical Critical Care and Emergency Surgery: Clinical Questions and Answers, First Edition. Edited by Forrest O. Moore, Peter M. Rhee, Samuel A. Tisherman and Gerard J. Fulda.

C. *The presence of elevated WBC count and hyponatremia*

D. *Surgical exploration*

E. *Hyponatremia in the setting of fever and an elevated WBC*

Erythema and pain may be present, but are not specific to necrotizing infections. Magnetic resonance imaging may demonstrate soft-tissue edema or fluid, but these findings do not prove the presence of NSTI and may also occur in any condition causing edema. The presence of an elevated WBC and hyponatremia, even in the setting of fever, are not specific to NSTI. The definitive diagnosis requires surgical incision carried down to the fascial and muscle levels.

Answer: D

Napolitano LM (2008) Introduction: the diagnosis and treatment of skin and soft-tissue infections (SSTIs). *Surgical Infections* **9** (suppl 1), s1.

Napolitano LM (2009) Severe soft-tissue infections. *Infectious Disease Clinics of North America* **23** (3), 571–91.

4. *What factor has been identified as an independent predictor of both treatment failure and hospital mortality among MRSA soft-tissue infections?*

A. *Type I diabetes mellitus*

B. *Failure to initiate early and appropriate antibiotics*

C. *Delay of initial surgical intervention*

D. *Patient age*

E. *None of the above*

Appropriate and timely antibiotic therapy improves treatment outcomes for SSTIs caused by MRSA. Studies have demonstrated that initiation of therapy within 48 hours improves treatment outcomes and failure to initiate antimicrobial therapy within 48 hours of presentation is an independent predictor of treatment failure. Additionally, among patients admitted to the hospital for MRSA sterile-site infections, it has been shown that inappropriate antibiotics are an independent risk factor for hospital mortality.

All of the other factors—diabetes, delay in surgical intervention, and patient age—are likely to be contributory, but have not been identified as independent predictors of treatment failure and hospital mortality.

Answer: B

Ruhe JJ, Smith N, Bradsher RW, *et al.* (2007) Community-onset methicillin-resistant Staphylococcus aureus skin and soft-tissue infections: impact of antimicrobial therapy on outcome. *Clinical Infectious Diseases* **44**, 777–84.

Schramm GE, Johnson JA, Doherty JA, *et al.* (2006) Methicillin-resistant Staphylococcus aureus sterile-site infection: the importance of appropriate initial antimicrobial treatment. *Critical Care Medicine* **34** (8), 2069–74.

5. *Which antibiotic choice is least appropriate for patients with complicated severe skin and soft-tissue infections (cSSTIs) and evidence of toxic shock syndrome?*

A. *Vancomycin*

B. *Linezolid*

C. *Clindamycin*

D. *Amoxicillin*

E. *Daptomycin*

The selection of antimicrobials to treat cSSTIs should include those that inhibit toxin production, particularly among patients with evidence of toxic shock syndrome. Toxic shock syndrome is commonly present in patients with streptococcal and staphylococcal infections. Beta lactams, such as amoxicillin, may actually enhance the toxin production of some classes of secreted staphylococcal peptides and should be avoided. In contrast, clindamycin and linozelid have the ability to inhibit toxin production by suppressing translation of toxin genes for *S. aureus* and by directly inhibiting synthesis of group A streptococcal toxins. Vancomycin and Daptomycin are other appropriate choices for utilization, but do not have the same demonstrated ability to inhibit toxin production.

Answer: D

Filbin MR, Ring DC, Wessels MR, *et al.* (2009) Case 2-2009: a 25-year-old man with pain and swelling of the right hand and hypotension. *New England Journal of Medicine* **360**, 281–90.

Stevens DL, May Y, Salmi DB, *et al.* (2007) Impact of antibiotics on expression of virulence-associated exotoxin genes in methicillin-sensitive and methicillin-resistant Staphylococcus aureus. *Journal of Infectious Diseases* **195**, 202–11.

Wang R, Braughton KR, Kretschmer D, *et al.* (2007) Identification of novel cytolytic peptides as key virulence determinants for community-associated MRSA. *Nature Medicine* **13** (12), 1510–4.

6. *What laboratory values have been identified as risk indicators for necrotizing fascitis?*

A. *Total white blood cell count*

B. *Hemoglobin*

C. *Glucose*

D. *Sodium*

E. *All of the above*

The laboratory risk indicator for necrotizing fascitis (LRINEC) score was initially developed in a retrospective observational study of 145 patients with necrotizing fascitis and 309 patients with cellulitis. This score uses C-reactive protein, total white blood cell count, hemoglobin, sodium, creatinine and glucose levels. In the initial study, a score of ≥6 had a positive predictive value of 92% for the detection of necrotizing fascitis. Several subsequent cohort studies have validated the utility of the LRINEC in diagnosing necrotizing soft-tissue infections.

The Laboratory Risk Indicator for Necrotizing Fascitis (LRINEC) score.

Variable, Units	Score
C-reactive protein, mg/L	
<150	0
≥150	4
Total white cell count, per mm³	
<15	0
15–25	1
>25	2
Hemoglobin, g/dL	
>13.5	0
11–13.5	1
<11	2
Sodium, mmol/L	
≥135	0
<135	2
Creatinine μmol/L	
≤141	0
>141	2
Glucose, mmol/L	
≤10	0
>10	1

The maximum score is 13; a score of ≥6 should raise suspicion of necrotizing fascitis, and a score of ≥8 is strongly predictive of this disease.

Answer: E

Muizelaar JP, Lutz HA, Becker DP (1984) Effect of mannitol in ICP and CBF and correlation with pressure autoregulation in severely head-injured patients. *Journal of Neurosurgery* **61**, 700.

Vialet R, Albanese J, Thomachot L, *et al.* (2003) Isovolume hypertonic solutes (sodium chloride or mannitol) in the treatment of refractory posttraumatic intracranial hypertension: 2 mL/kg 7.5% saline is more effective than 2 mL/kg 20% mannitol. *Critical Care Medicine* **31**, 1683.

7. *The most common identifiable cause of severe soft-tissue infections is:*

A. *Clostridial infections*

B. *Methicillin-resistant staph aureus infections*

C. *Methicillin-sensitive staph aureus infections*

D. *Acinetobacter*

E. *Streptococcal infections*

In a recent prospective multicenter US study, MRSA was the most common identifiable cause of SSTI. *S. aureus* was isolated from 76% of patients who had SSTIs. The prevalence of MRSA was 59% overall and ranged from 15% to 74% by ED. The spectrum of skin infections caused by community acquired MRSA is wide and can range from simple cutaneous abscesses to large abscesses and more severe forms of soft-tissue infections.

Answer: B

Moran GJ, Krishnadasan A, Gorwitz RJ, *et al.* (2006) Methicillin-resistant S aureus infections among patients in the emergency department. *New England Journal of Medicine* **355** (7), 666–74.

8. *The most common cause of necrotizing fascitis and myonecrosis is:*

A. *Group A Streptococcus*

B. *Clostridium perfringens*

C. *Polymicrobial infection*

D. *Methicillin sensitive staph aureus*

E. *Fungal infections*

Necrotizing fascitis and myonecrosis are *most* commonly caused by aerobic and anaerobic organisms as part of a polymicrobial infections that may include *Staph. aureus*. Other common causes include group A Streptococcus and *Clostridium perfringens*. The most predominant organisms isolated in case series have been community-acquired MRSA, accounting for one-third of isolates from a recent retrospective review.

Necrotizing STIs are commonly categorized into three specific types based upon the microbiologic etiology of the infection: Type 1, or polymicrobial; Type 2, or group A streptoccal; and Type 3, gas gangrene, or clostridial myonecrosis.

Answer: C

Wong CH, Chang HC, Pasupathy S, *et al.* (2003) Necrotizing fascitis: clinical presentation, microbiology, and determinants of mortality. *Journal of Bone and Joint Surgery, American Volume* **85** (8), 1454–60.

Young LM, Price CS (2008) Community-acquired MRSA emerging as an important cause of necrotizing fascitis. *Surgical Infections* **9** (4), 469–74.

9. *Vibrio infections are uncommon but potentially serious causes of necrotizing soft-tissue infections that should be particularly suspected among patients with:*

A. *History of simple soft-tissue CA-MRSA infections*

B. *History of exposure to sea water or shellfish*

C. *History of dog bite*

D. *History of a recent wooden splinter*

E. *None of the above*

Vibrio and Aeromonas species are uncommon causes of NSTIs. Vibrio species thrive in aquatic environments, particularly sea water and in shell fish. Aeromonas species are also rare causes of NSTIs that are associated with contact with fresh or brackish water, soil or wood). The contact history and rapid onset of SSTIs can alert providers to infections from these organisms. At least 64 different species of bacteria can be present in dog saliva, thus infections from canine bites are most likely polymicrobial. Infections associated with splinters are likewise, most commonly polymicrobial.

Answer: B

Tsai YH, Hsu RW, Huang TJ, *et al.* (2007) Necrotizing soft-tissue infections and sepsis caused by Vibrio vulnificus compared to those caused by Aeromonas species. *J Bone Joint Surg Am* **89** (3), 631–6.

10. *Which of the following is true about the use of vacuum-assisted (VAC) wound closure therapy use in the setting of necrotizing soft-tissue infections?*

A. *VAC therapy use negates the need for adequate debridement of dead tissues*

B. *VAC use has been validated by prospective randomized trials*

C. *VAC use decreases mobility post-operatively*

D. *VAC use has been associated with decreased time to wound closure*

E. *VAC therapy is associated with increased patient discomfort*

Several reports have documented the utility of VAC therapy for managing patients who have acute NSTIs. VAC therapy has been associated with reduced time for wound care, improved patient comfort, greater mobility, reduced drainage and decreased time to wound closure compared to traditional wet-to-dry dressings. Although no prospective randomized trials have yet been conducted to compare VAC therapy to traditional techniques, it can be considered, particularly for larger wounds and those patients requiring liberal use of conscious sedation and general anesthesia for wound care. The use of VAC has not been validated in prospective randomized trials to date.

Answer: D

Ozturk E, Ozquc H, Yilmazar T (2009) The use of vacuum-assisted closure therapy in the management of Fournier's gangrene. *American Journal of Surgery* **197**, 660–5.

11. *The potential benefit of intravenous immunoglobulin therapy for treating NSTIs is related to*

A. *Improve glucose control in acute illness*

B. *Bacterocidal activity*

C. *Increased IL-1 production*

D. *Improved tolerance of sepsis-related hypotension*

E. *Binding of gram-positive organism exotoxins*

While the use of intravenous immunoglobulins for treatment of NSTIs remains controversial, the potential benefit of this intervention is related to the binding of gram-positive organism exotoxins. The clinical studies that have been completed are not randomized blinded trials, but some show evidence of improved outcomes with IV IG treatment. The treatment should be restricted, however, to critically ill patients who have either staphylococcal or streptococcal NSTIs.

Answer: E

Alejandria MM, Lansang MA, Dans LF, *et al.* (2002) Intravenous immunoglobulin for treating sepsis and septic shock. Cochrane Database Systematic Reviews 1 DC001090.

Darabi K, Abdel-Wahab O, Dzik WH (2006) Current usage of intravenous immunoglobulin and the rationale behind it: The Massachusetts General Hospital data and review of the literature. *Transfusion* **46,** 741–53.

12. *Which of the following is TRUE regarding hyperbaric oxygen (HBO) therapy for necrotizing soft-tissue infections (NSTIs)?*

A. *The use of HBO has been validated by large prospective randomized control trials*

B. *HBO use has been shown to significantly decrease mortality after NSTIs*

C. *HBO use decreases the number of debridements required for treatment of NSTIs*

D. *HBO use decreases hospital length of stay after NSTIs*

E. *HBO use does not decrease the duration of antibiotic use after for NSTIs*

The benefit of HBO as an adjunctive treatment for NSTIs remains controversial, with no prospective randomized clinical trials having been performed to date. Retrospective reviews have failed to demonstrate a significant decrease in mortality, number of debridements required, length of hospital stay or duration of antibiotic use following HBO use.

Answer: E

George ME, Rueth NM, Skarda DE, *et al.* (2009) Hyperbaric oxygen does not improve outcome in patients with necrotizing soft-tissue infection. *Surgical Infections (Larchmt)* **10** (1), 21–8.

13. *Diabetic foot infections (DFIs) can be a cause of severe SSTIs. These patients:*

A. *Never present with severe sepsis or septic shock*

B. *Rarely require surgical abscess drainage or debridement*

C. *Rarely require vascular examination for improved arterial flow*

D. *May sometimes require amputation for source control of infection*

E. *A and C*

Diabetic foot infections can, and do, cause severe SSTIs. These patients can present with severe sepsis and septic shock, frequently require surgical abscess drainage and debridement, often require vascular evaluation for improved arterial flow, and can require amputation for source control.

Answer: D

Lipsky BA, Berendt AR, Deery HG, *et al.* (2004) Infectious Diseases Society of America. *Clinical Infectious Diseases* **39** (7), 885–910.

14. *The predominant pathogens identified among diabetic foot infections are:*

A. *Aerobic gram-positive cocci*

B. *Gram-negative rods*

C. *Fungal pathogens*

D. *Obligate anerobic pathogens*

E. *None of the above*

Aerobic gram-positive cocci (especially *S. aureus*) are the predominant pathogens in diabetic foot infections. Patients with chronic wounds or who recently have received antimicrobial therapy may also be infected with gram-negative rods, and those with foot ischemia or gangrene may have obligate anaerobic pathogens. Special attention to the potential of concurrent osteomyelitis and the need for potential vascular reconstruction for ischemic arterial disease must be paid in this population.

Answer: A

Lavery LA, Armstrong DG, Murdoch DP, *et al.* (2007) Validation of the Infectious Diseases Society of America's diabetic foot infection classification system. *Clinical Infectious Diseases* **44** (4), 562–5.

15. *An 18-year-old girl presents to the ED with a five-day history of a painful tooth and fevers, followed by 12 hours of progressive neck swelling and mental status changes. WBC is 19000/mm^3. CT demonstrates evidence of deep cervical infection with evidence of necrotic changes in the cervical musculature and significant edema. Which of the following is false regarding this process?*

A. *This represents a type I NSTI*

B. *Airway obstruction is rarely a concern in these patients*

C. *Surgical drainage is a pillar of therapy for this patient*

D. *Common causative organisms include Fusibacterium*

E. *Odontogenic infections are the most common cause of these infections*

Cervical necrotizing fascitis is a type I NSTI that is caused by bacterial penetration into the fascial compartments of the head and neck, resulting in a rapidly progressive infection with life-threatening airway obstruction. It is most often associated with odontogenic infection and is likely to require antibiotics and surgical intervention. Airway obstruction is common, and early intubation and airway protection should always be considered. Both Ludwig's angina (submandibular space infection) and cervical necrotizing fascitis are usually caused by mouth anaerobes, such as *Fusobacterium* species, anerobic Strepococcus, Peptostreptococcus, bacteroides and spirochetes, which are usually susceptible to penicillin and clinidamycin.

Answer: B

Phan HH, Conacour CS (2010) Necrotizing soft-tissue infections in the intensive care unit. *Critical Care Medicine* **38** (9), A460–8.

16. *Invasive zygomycosis has been demonstrated in an ICU patient with onset of profound sepsis and necrotizing soft-tissue infection. Initial treatment should include all of the following except:*

A. *Surgical debridement*

B. *Pressor support and resuscitation per the Surviving Sepsis guidelines*

C. *Amphotericin B or equivalent liposomal formulation*

D. *An Echinocandin class of anti-fungal medications*

E. *Broad-spectrum antibiotics*

When invasive zygomycosis has been demonstrated, amphotericin B or equivalent liposomal formulation should be initiated, along with surgical debridement and appropriate supportive care per the Surviving Sepsis guidelines. The liposomal fomulation allows higher dosing with less nephrotoxicity. Echonocandins have no *in vitro* activity against zygomycetes and should be avoided. Posaconazole, which has broad spectrum activity against zygomycetes may be considered for combination therapy or as a step-down therapy for patients who have responded to amphotericin B. Broad-spectrum antibiotics are not indicated unless associated infection is suspected.

Answer: D

Sun QN, Fothergill AW, McCarthy DI, *et al.* (2002) In vitro activities of posaconazole, itraconazole, voriconazole, amphtericin B, and fluconazole against 37 clinical isolates of zygomycetes. *Antimicrobial Agents and Chemotherapy* **46**, 1581–2.

17. *A 54-year-old diabetic man, who has an anaphylactic allergy to penicillin, present to the ED with bullae along the right lower extremity, hypotension and mental status changes. WBC is 24000/mm^3 and the patient has a temperature of 103.0 F. The decision is made to proceed to the operating room for surgical exploration and potential debridement. What initial antibiotic choices are not appropriate for this penicillin-allergic patient.*

A. *Ampicillin*

B. *Clindamycin*

C. *Aminoglycoside with appropriate renal dosing*

D. *Metronidazole*

E. *Ciprofloxacin*

The initial antibiotic therapy should be broad enough to cover diverse and various causative agents. High-dose penicillin G or ampicillin should be used to cover for potential Clostridium, Streptococcus, and Peptostreptoccos infections. Anaerobes such as Bacteroides, Fusobacterium and Peptostreptococcus should also be covered with clindamycin or metronidazole. Clindamycin is also effective in treating group A beta-hemolytic Streptococcus by suppressing exotoxins. Clindamycin is the drug of choice for patients with allergies to penicillin. Gram-negative coverage can be achieved by adding an aminoglycoside, a third- or fourth-generation cephalosporin, a floroquinolone or a carbapenem. Alternatively, penicillin or ampicillin can be replaced by piperacillin-tazobactam or ticaricillin-clavulanate to include Gram-negative coverage. Given this patient's history of anaphylactic response to penicillin, ampicillin is not a viable option in this scenario.

Answer: A

Phan HH, Conacour CS (2010) Necrotizing soft-tissue infections in the intensive care unit. *Critical Care Medicine* **38** (9), A460–8.

Chapter 40 Obesity and Bariatric Surgery

Stacy A. Brethauer, MD and Carlos V.R. Brown, MD, FACS

1. *Which of the following statements is true regarding the pulmonary pathophysiology of obese individuals as compared to lean individuals?*

A. *Obese individuals have decreased work of breathing*

B. *Obese individuals have higher lung volumes*

C. *Obese individuals have increased minute ventilation*

D. *Obese individuals have a lower respiratory rate*

E. *Obese individuals have decreased work of breathing*

Pulmonary pathophysiology is associated with an increase in the work of breathing. This increase in the work of breathing is due to a variety of factors including increased chest wall resistance, increased abdominal pressure altering diaphragmatic position, and respiratory muscle dysfunction. Pulmonary volumes such as tidal volume, vital capacity, total lung capacity, and functional residual capacity are all decreased in obese individuals during pulmonary function testing. As a response to decreased pulmonary volumes, increased oxygen consumption, and increased carbon dioxide production, obese individuals have an increase in baseline respiratory rate, which in turn leads to higher minute ventilation.

Answer: C

Jubber AS (2004) Respiratory complications of obesity. *International Journal of Clinical Practice* **58**, 573–80.

Kuchta KF (2005) Pathophysiologic changes of obesity. *Anesthesiology Clinics of North America* **23**, 421–429.

Levi D, Goodman ER, Patel M, Savransky Y (2003) Critical care of the obese and bariatric surgical patient. *Critical Care Clinics* **19**, 11–32.

Surgical Critical Care and Emergency Surgery: Clinical Questions and Answers, First Edition. Edited by Forrest O. Moore, Peter M. Rhee, Samuel A. Tisherman and Gerard J. Fulda.

2. *Which of the following room air arterial blood gas results would be most consistent with long-standing obesity hypoventilation syndrome in a patient with a BMI = 60 kg/m^2?*

A. *pH = 7.24, $PaCO_2$ = 60 mm Hg, PaO_2 = 100 mm Hg, HCO_3 = 24 mEq/L*

B. *pH = 7.38, $PaCO_2$ = 58 mm Hg, PaO_2 = 65 mm Hg, HCO_3 = 36 mEq/L*

C. *pH = 7.40, $PaCO_2$ = 40 mm Hg, PaO_2 = 100 mm Hg, HCO_3 = 24 mEq/L*

D. *pH = 7.56, $PaCO_2$ = 32 mm Hg, PaO_2 = 65 mm Hg, HCO_3 = 24 mEq/L*

E. *pH = 7.42, $PaCO_2$ = 32 mm Hg, PaO_2 = 65 mm Hg, HCO_3 = 18 mEq/L*

Two pulmonary complications of obesity that may affect the care of the obese surgical patient include the obesity hypoventilation syndrome and obstructive sleep apnea. The obesity hypoventilation syndrome is usually seen in super-obese individuals and is characterized by hypercapneic respiratory failure and alveolar hypoventilation. Severe, long-standing cases of the obesity hypoventilation syndrome may eventually lead to right heart failure. Obstructive sleep apnea occurs from narrowing of the upper airway due to excess adipose deposition and is relatively common in obese individuals. This narrowing is worsened during sleep or in the recumbent position. Obstructive sleep apnea may increase the risk of respiratory failure (especially in the postoperative period) or extend the need for mechanical ventilation

Answer: B

Kuchta KF (2005) Pathophysiologic changes of obesity. *Anesthesiology Clinics of North America* **23**, 421–9.

Nasraway SA, Hudson-Jinks TM, Kelleher RM (2002) Multidisciplinary care of the obese patient with chronic critical illness after surgery. *Critical Care Clinics* **18**, 643–57.

3. *When writing mechanical ventilation orders for an obese surgical patient, which of the following should be used to determine initial tidal volume settings?*

A. *Total body weight*

B. *Adjusted body weight*

C. *Ideal body weight*

D. *Body mass index*

Weights used in calculations used to care for critically ill obese patients include total body weight (TBW), ideal body weight (IBW), or adjusted body weight (ABW). TBW is the simplest to acquire and is simply the weight recorded when a patient is placed on a scale. IBW is a calculated value and is based on gender and height: Male IBW = 50 kg + 2.3 kg for each inch over 5 feet and Female IBW = 45.5 kg + 2.3 kg for each inch over 5 feet. The definition of ABW varies significantly in the literature, but generally follows the formula ABW = IBS + x (TBW − IBW), where the variable x is equal to a factor ranging from 0.2 − 0.5. When calculating initial tidal volume in obese patients the ideal body weight should be used for calculation.

Answer: C

Levi D, Goodman ER, Patel M, Savransky Y (2002) Critical care of the obese and bariatric surgical patient. *Critical Care Clinics* **19**, 11–32.

4. *A 25-year-old obese woman (BMI = 50 kg/m²) presents to the emergency department with acute appendicitis diagnosed by CT scan. The patient is taken to the operating room for laparoscopic appendectomy. The appropriate dose of succinylcholine for rapid sequence intubation should be:*

A. *1 mg/kg based on ideal body weight*

B. *1 mg/kg based on adjusted body weight*

C. *1 mg/kg based on total body weight*

D. *The "standard" 100 mg dose*

E. *Succinylcholine should not be given to obese individuals*

Dosing of medications for an obese individual varies widely depending on the agent and its pharmacokinetic properties. Medications may be dosed on total body weight, adjusted body weight, or ideal body weight. Succinylcholine is dosed at 1 mg/kg based on total body weight. However, when using nondepolarizing agents such as rocuronium or vecuronium ideal body weight should be used for dosing calculation.

Answer: C

Blouin RA, Warren GW (1999) Pharmacokinetic considerations in obesity. *Journal of Pharmaceutical Sciences* **88**, 1–7.

Lemmens HJM, Brodsky JB (2006) The dose of succinylcholine in morbid obesity. *Anesthesia and Analgesia* **102**, 438–42.

Ogunnaike BO, Whitten CW (2002) Anesthetic management of morbidly obese patients. *Seminars in Anesthesia* **21**, 46–58.

5. *A 41-year-old obese man undergoes laparoscopic Roux-en-Y gastric bypass. The next day, the patient acutely develops a low-grade temperature, tachypnea, and a heart rate of 120 beats per minute. Diagnostic evaluation reveals no obvious leak on a contrast study. The most appropriate next step in management is:*

A. *IV fluids*

B. *IV fluids, IV antibiotics*

C. *IV fluids, IV antibiotics, and urgent abdominal exploration*

D. *Mobilization and incentive spirometry*

E. *Computed tomography of the abdomen*

Anastomotic leak is one of the most dreaded complications following bariatric surgery. Anastomotic leak following Roux-en-Y gastric bypass may occur at the jejunojejunostomy but most commonly occurs at the gastrojejunostomy. Leak rates after Roux-en-Y gastric bypass range from 1.5% to 6.0% and usually occur in the early postoperative period. A high index of suspicion is required due to the lethal nature of anastomotic leak in this setting. Early signs and symptoms include fever, tachypnea, and tachycardia. Radiographic evaluation may include an upper gastrointestinal series or CT scan. However, clinical presentation is nonspecific and contrast studies may be normal in a significant number of patients with a leak. For these reasons, when there is a high clinical suspicion, abdominal exploration (either laparoscopic or open) is an essential part of the algorithm for diagnosis of anastomotic leak after gastric bypass.

Answer: C

Gonzalez R, Sarr MG, Smith CD, *et al.* (2007) Diagnosis and contemporary management of anastomotic leaks after gastric bypass for obesity. *Journal of the American College of Surgeons* **204**, 47–55.

6. *A 38-year-old woman undergoes laparoscopic gastric banding for morbid obesity. She is discharged home after an uneventful hospital course. However, she is brought to the hospital by EMS three days after surgery in extremis and dies in the emergency department soon after arrival. The most likely cause of death in this patient is:*

A. Myocardial infarction

B. Sepsis

C. Pseudotumor cerebri

D. Pulmonary embolism

E. Obesity hypoventilation syndrome

Perioperative mortality following surgery for morbid obesity is uncommon, with a 30-day operative mortality 0.25%–6% depending on the surgical procedure performed. The most common cause of death following bariatric surgery is pulmonary embolism, despite the extreme steps taken to protect against this lethal complication. Other common causes of death include myocardial infarction and technical complications related to the operation such as anastomotic leak, gastric perforation, and bowel obstruction.

Answer: D

Gagner M, Milone L, Young E, Broseus A (2008) Causes of early mortality after laparoscopic adjustable gastric banding. *Journal of the American College of Surgeons* **206**, 664–9.

Mason EE, Renquist KE, Huang YH, *et al.* (2007) Causes of 30-day bariatric surgery mortality: with emphasis on bypass obstruction. *Obesity Surgery* **17**, 9–14.

7. *A 54-year-old severely obese man with hypertension, diabetes, and peripheral vascular disease undergoes a complicated laparoscopic cholecystectomy for acute cholecystitis, which lasts 270 minutes. Six hours postoperatively the patient complains of bilateral buttock pain and has not voided since surgery. A urinary catheter is placed and 30 mL of dark colored urine is collected. Despite crystalloid resuscitation the patient goes on to develop acute renal failure. The most likely cause of this patient's acute renal failure is:*

A. Fat embolism

B. Renal artery stenosis

C. Diabetic nephropathy

D. Rhabdomyolysis

E. Renal vascular injury during surgery

Rhabdomyolysis, or skeletal muscle breakdown, has a variety of causes and most commonly occurs after trauma. An uncommon cause is prolonged immobilization on the operating table during an elective surgical procedure. This leads to continuous muscle compression and necrosis, leading to rhabdomyolysis and subsequent acute renal failure. For lean individuals, operative times of greater than six hours are usually required to cause rhabdomyolysis, but in obese individuals rhabdomyolysis has been reported after procedures lasting less than 90 minutes. Risk factors for postoperative rhabdomyolysis include male gender, older age, higher BMI, and comorbidities such as diabetes, hypertension, and peripheral vascular disease. Intraoperative risk factors include operative time >5 hours, inadequate padding of pressure areas, dehydration, bleeding, and hypotension.

Patients with postoperative rhabdomyolysis may complain of pain in the affected muscle compartment or neurologic symptoms of motor or sensory nerves. They may also manifest amber colored urine, reflecting spillage of myoglobin into the urine. Diagnosis requires a high index of suspicion and is confirmed with serum creatine kinase or urinary myoglobin measurement. Treatment is centered around vigorous hydration with crystalloid solution and the addition of bicarbonate to alkalinize the urine or diuresis with mannitol for severe cases. Postoperative rhabdomyolysis may be prevented by padding pressure areas, limiting operative time, use of pneumatic beds or combined surgical tables, optimal positioning on operating table, repositioning during the procedure, and ensuring adequate hydration.

Answer: D

Ettinger J, Filho P, Azaro E, *et al.* (2005) Prevention of rhabdomyolysis in bariatric surgery. *Obesity Surgery* **15**, 874–9.

Ettinger J, Souza C, Filho P, *et al.* (2007) Rhabdomyolysis: diagnosis and treatment in bariatric surgery. *Obesity Surgery* **17**, 525–32.

8. *A 25-year-old woman three years following a Roux-en-Y gastric bypass presents with an incarcerated inguinal hernia. Preoperative evaluation reveals iron deficiency anemia. Which of the following statements is true regarding iron deficiency following bariatric surgical procedures?*

A. *The majority of iron is absorbed in the terminal ileum*

B. *The majority of iron is absorbed in the mid-ileum*

C. *Iron deficiency does not occur after bariatric surgical procedures*

D. *Fe^{3+} cannot be reduced to the more absorbable Fe^{2+} due to the reduction of gastric acid production*

E. *Iron deficiency never occurs after restrictive procedures, but may occur after malabsorptive procedures*

A variety of nutritional deficiencies may occur after bariatric surgical procedures and may impact care of the surgical patient who has undergone a prior bariatric surgical procedure. In addition to protein deficiency associated with malabsorptive and restrictive bariatric surgical procedures, patients may become deficient in vitamins and minerals including iron, calcium and vitamins A, B_1, B_{12} (and folic acid), D, E, and K. Iron deficiency is one of the most common deficiencies associated with bariatric surgical procedures and can occur after restrictive and malabsorptive procedures. Iron deficiency after bariatric surgery is due to decreased gastric acid production, which limits the ability of the gastrointestinal tract to reduce Fe^{3+} to the more absorbable Fe^{2+} form of iron.

Answer: D

Davies DJ, Baxter JM, Baxter JN (2007) Nutritional deficiencies after bariatric surgery. *Obesity Surgery* **17**, 1150–8.

Schweitzer DH, Posthuma EF (2008) Prevention of vitamin and mineral deficiencies after bariatric surgery: evidence and algorithms. *Obesity Surgery* **18**,1485–8.

9. *A 43-year-old severely obese (BMI = 45 kg/m²) man was involved in a motor vehicle crash and sustained rib fractures, a pulmonary contusion, and a splenic injury requiring laparotomy. He has now been on the ventilator for two weeks and has not made significant progress towards extubation. Which of the following is true regarding tracheostomy in obese individuals?*

A. *Tracheostomy should rarely be performed in obese patients due to the unacceptable risk of complications*

B. *Percutaneous tracheostomy is associated with more complications in obese individuals when compared to lean individuals*

C. *Indications for tracheostomy are different for obese and lean individuals*

D. *Percutaneous dilatational tracheostomy is a safe alternative in obese patients who require a tracheostomy*

E. *Obese individuals who require tracheostomy should receive an open procedure, which is associated with fewer complications than the percutaneous approach*

Obese patients requiring tracheostomy should be evaluated in the same fashion as their lean counterparts, and indications for tracheostomy remain the same for obese individuals. Open tracheostomy in obese individuals is associated with more complications and more life-threatening complications than lean patients. In addition, patients may require longer tracheostomy tubes due to the increased distance between the skin and the airway. Percutaneous dilatational tracheostomy has become standard in the care of critically ill and injured patients. Obesity was initially considered a contraindication but it is now clear that percutaneous dilatational tracheostomy can be safely performed in obese patients as well.

Answer: D

El Solh AA, Jaafar W (2007) A comparative study of the complications of surgical tracheostomy in morbidly obese critically ill patients. *Critical Care* **11**, R3.

Heyrosa MG, Melniczek DM, Rovito P, Nicholas GG (2006) Percutaneous tracheostomy: a safe procedure in the morbidly obese. *Journal of the American College of Surgeons* **202**, 618–22.

10. *A 26-year-old woman who underwent laparoscopic Roux-en-Y gastric bypass three years ago now presents with abdominal pain, nausea, and vomiting intermittently for the past several weeks. At endoscopy for evaluation of her symptoms she is found to have a 1 cm ulceration at her gastrojejunal anastomosis. The best initial management includes:*

A. *Proton pump inhibitors, sucralfate, and repeat endoscopy in several weeks to ensure healing of ulcer*

B. *Urgent surgery and resection of ulcer*

C. *Repeat endoscopy in 4-6 weeks as most of these ulcers heal spontaneously*

D. *Endoscopic ulcer management with sclerotherapy*

E. *Course of oral antibiotics and diet modification*

11. *The same patient presents several weeks later with an acute onset of acute abdominal pain, fever, diffuse abdominal tenderness, and free air on plain films. Surgery is planned for a presumed perforation of her marginal ulcer. All of the following are options for surgical management of a perforated marginal ulcer except:*

A. *Laparoscopic repair of perforation with jejunal or omental patch*

B. *Open repair of perforation with jejunal or omental patch*

C. *Irrigation and wide drainage if primary closure is not possible*

D. *Resection and reconstruction of gastrojejunal anastomosis*

E. *Total gastrectomy and esophagojejunostomy*

Marginal ulceration is an ulcer that develops at a gastrointestinal anastomosis, occurring at the gastrojejunal anastomosis following Roux-en-Y gastric bypass. Although relatively uncommon, occurring after 1–15% of Roux-en-Y gastric bypasses, marginal ulceration can be a challenge to diagnose and treat. Risk factors to develop marginal ulcers after Roux-en-Y gastric bypass include smoking, NSAIDS, large gastric pouches, and failure of staple lines. Symptoms may be vague but patients typically present with abdominal pain, nausea, and vomiting and diagnosis is established by upper endoscopy. Treatment is primarily medical with proton pump inhibitors and sucralfate for 3–6 months, and follow-up endoscopy is essential to confirm ulcer healing. Surgical indications include perforation, obstruction, bleeding, presence of a gastro-gastric fistula, and failure of medical management.

Surgical options for an acutely perforated marginal ulcer include primary repair with jejunal or omental patch, either open or laparoscopic. If primary repair is not possible irrigation and wide drainage is an acceptable option. If ischemia is suspected as the underlying problem then resection and reconstruction of the gastrojejunal anastomosis is advised.

Answers: 10: A 11: E

Racu C, Mehran A (2010) Marginal ulcers after roux-en-y gastric bypass: pain for the patient . . . pain for the surgeon. *Bariatric Times* **7**, 23–5.

12. *Several hours after an uneventful laparoscopic Roux-en-Y gastric bypass a 31-year-old woman begins to have a large amount of hematochezia and tachycardia. A gentle upper endoscopy reveals no blood in the gastric pouch. In addition to resuscitation with fluid and blood products the best initial step in management is:*

A. *Angiography*

B. *Colonoscopy*

C. *Tagged red blood cell scan*

D. *Abdominal exploration*

E. *Computed tomography*

Gastrointestinal bleeding after gastric bypass is an uncommon complication, occurring 1–4% of the time. Postgastric bypass gastrointestinal hemorrhage usually occurs from within hours to a few days after the initial procedure. The most common source of hemorrhage after gastric bypass is from one of the staple lines (gastric pouch, gastrojejunostomy, jejunojejunostomy, and gastric remnant). Bleeding that presents within hours of surgery is almost assuredly bleeding from a staple line and requires prompt intervention without delays caused by additional diagnostic tests. Bleeding from staple lines can be managed via endoscopy or exploration and suture control. Bleeding from the gastric pouch and gastrojejunostomy may be managed with endoscopy and injection of epinephrine solution, clipping of bleeders, or thermal coagulation. The gastric remnant and jejunojejunostomy are not accessible by endoscopy and require abdominal exploration and oversewing of the gastric remnant suture line or revision of jejunojejunal anastomosis.

Answer: D

Nguyen NT, Hinojosa MW, Gray J, Smith BR (2010) Gastrointestinal bleeding after Roux-en-Y gastric bypass. *Bariatric Times* **7**, 20–2.

13. *A 38-year-old man presents to the emergency department two weeks after an uncomplicated laparoscopic Roux-en-Y gastric bypass. Evaluation by CT scan reveals a small bowel obstruction. The most likely etiology of small bowel obstruction in this patient is:*

A. *Intussusception*

B. *Internal hernia*

C. *Ischemic stricture*

D. *Adhesions*

E. *Jejunojejunostomy*

14. *A 38-year-old man presents to the emergency department two years after an uncomplicated laparoscopic Roux-en-Y gastric bypass. Evaluation by CT scan reveals a small bowel obstruction. The most likely etiology of small bowel obstruction in this patient is:*

A. *Intussusception*

B. *Internal hernia*

C. *Ischemic stricture*

D. *Volvulus*

E. *Jejunojejunostomy stenosis*

Mechanical small bowel obstruction can complicate 1–9% of laparoscopic Roux-en-Y gastric bypass operations. Small bowel obstructions may occur early in the postoperative period, usually due to an obstruction at the jejunojejunostomy. While late small bowel obstructions are typically due to adhesions or internal hernia. Clinical presentation of small bowel obstruction may be subtle and nonspecific but patients may present with abdominal pain, distention, nausea, and vomiting. Though CT scan is the diagnostic test of choice for small bowel obstruction in the post-gastric bypass patient, it may be unreliable or misinterpreted in a significant percentage of patients. For these reasons early operative intervention (open or laparoscopic) is often necessary when the clinical index of suspicion for mechanical small bowel obstruction is high.

Answer: 13: E 14: B

Capella RF, Iannace VA, Capella JF (2006) Bowel obstruction after open and laparoscopic gastric bypass surgery for morbid obesity. *Journal of the American College of Surgeons* **203**, 328–35.

Koppman JS, Li C, Gandsas A (2008) Small bowel obstruction after laparoscopic Roux-en-Y gastric bypass: a review of 9527 patients. *Journal of the American College of Surgeons* **206**, 571–84.

15. *Which of the following is true regarding gastric prolapse after lap-band placement?*

A. *Posterior prolapse of the fundus is the most common variety, and is associated with the pars flaccida technique*

B. *Gastric prolapse ("slipped band") can be identified on plain film abdominal X-ray*

C. *Treatment of gastric prolapse includes intravenous fluid resuscitation, electrolyte repletion and nasogastric tube decompression, which usually results in spontaneous "reduction" of the prolapse*

D. *The current incidence of gastric prolapse is approximately 25%*

E. *Gastric prolapse only occurs after Roux-en-Y gastric bypass operations*

There are three types of gastric prolapse: anterior (greater curve/fundus, pars flaccida technique), posterior (lesser curve, peri-gastric technique), and concentric (combination of anterior and posterior slip or band placed too low on stomach). Since the pars flaccida technique has become the standard approach for band placement, the most common type of prolapse is the anterior slip. The diagnosis of gastric prolapse can be detected using plain film abdominal x-ray, esophogram and/or upper endoscopy. The common findings on plain film include a horizontal band (normally should be at a 45-degree angle toward the left shoulder) or a gastric air bubble or air-fluid level above the band. An upper GI contrast study is confirmatory and typically shows downward band rotation, dilated stomach above the band, an air-contrast level, a "wave sign" of the stomach that has prolapsed over the top of the band (see figure), or obstruction of contrast flow. Treatment of an acute, symptomatic prolapse includes intravenous fluids and electrolyte replacement, and removal of all the fluid from the band system at the time of diagnosis. Nasogastric tubes are not routinely used and do not provide definitive reduction of the prolapsed stomach. Most prolapses require operative intervention to reduce the prolapsed stomach and reposition or remove the band. The timing of surgery depends on the patient's clinical condition, the presence of pain (more urgent), and their response to having the band fluid removed. Early studies of laparoscopic adjustable gastric banding reported high prolapse rates, however as surgical techniques and band technology have been refined, current studies report gastric prolapse rates in the range of 2–6%.

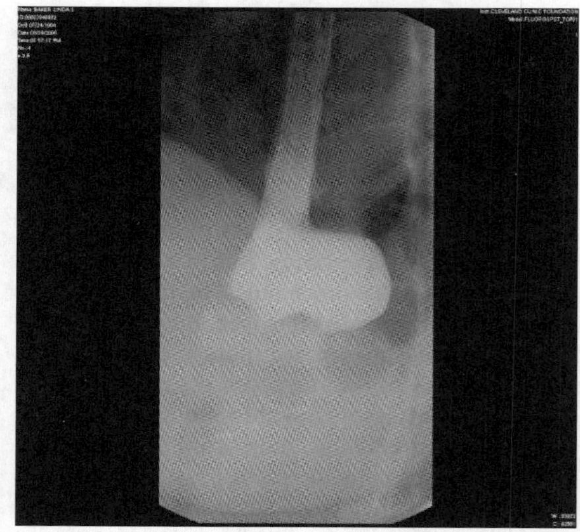

Answer: B

Parikh MS, Fielding GA, Ren CJ (2005) U.S. experience with 749 laparoscopic adjustable gastric bands: intermediate outcomes. *Surgical Endoscopy* **19** (12), 1631–5.

Ponce J, Paynter S, Fromm R (2005) Laparoscopic adjustable gastric banding: 1014 consecutive cases. *Journal of the American College of Surgeons* **201** (4), 529–35.

Ren CJ, Horgan S, Ponce J (2002) US experience with the LAP-BAND system. *American Journal of Surgery* **184** (6B), 46S–50S.

Suter M, Calmes JM, Paroz A, Giusti V (2006) A 10-year experience with laparoscopic gastric banding for morbid obesity: high long-term complication and failure rates. *Obesity Surgery* **16** (7), 829–35.

16. *Which of the following statements regarding laparoscopic adjustable band complications is true?*

A. *The incidence of band erosion is 5–10%*

B. *The recommended treatment for band erosion is emergent removal of the band*

C. *Erosion rates are attributable to technical factors such as suturing the anterior gastro-gastric plication too tightly over the band*

D. *Port-related problems (infection, leak, breakage) occur with a frequency of >10%*

E. *None of the above*

The incidence of band erosion is reported to be approximately 1–4% in recent studies with a median follow-up of three years, although a more current study showed an erosion rate of 9.5% with a 10-year followup period. Band erosion typically occurs late and is related to creation of a tight gastric plication over the band, particularly if it is placed over the buckle of the band. A late infection at the subcutaneous port site may herald a band erosion and should prompt an endoscopic evaluation. The reported erosions rates have declined with improved surgical techniques and the development of high volume, low pressure balloons in the current bands. The recommended management for band erosion includes elective removal. This complication rarely results in sepsis or an acute decompensation as a fibrous capsule encases the band as it slowly erodes into the lumen. Endoscopic removal has been reported but laparoscopic removal of the band through a distal gastrotomy allows removal without the necessity for dissecting out the gastroesophageal junction and repairing the erosion defect. Bands should not be replaced during the same operation; however, it has been shown that band replacement or another procedure can safely be performed 4 to 6 months following removal. Port- and tubing-related complications occur in about 5% of patients and are relatively simple to correct.

Answer: C

Angrisani L, Furbetta F, Doldi SB, *et al.* (2003) Lap Band adjustable gastric banding system: the Italian experience with 1863 patients operated on 6 years. *Surgical Endoscopy* **17** (3), 409–12.

Fielding GA, Rhodes M, Nathanson LK (1999) Laparoscopic gastric banding for morbid obesity. Surgical outcome in 335 cases. *Surgical Endoscopy* **13** (6), 550–4.

Rubenstein RB (2002) Laparoscopic adjustable gastric banding at a U.S. center with up to 3-year follow-up. *Obesity Surgery* **12** (3), 380–4.

Weiner R, Blanco-Engert R, Weiner S, *et al.* (2003) Outcome after laparoscopic adjustable gastric banding—8 years' experience. *Obesity Surgery* **13** (3), 427–34.

17. *Which of the following is/are true regarding gastric perforation during laparoscopic adjustable band placement?*

A. *It is most commonly related to the calibration balloon being overinflated at the gastroesophageal junction*

B. *Intraoperative endoscopy is not useful in detecting a posterior perforation after the band is placed.*

C. *Once the perforation is repaired, band placement should proceed as planned to cover the repaired defect*

D. *If not recognized intraoperatively, it presents as abdominal pain, fever, or sepsis one or two days after band placement.*

E. *If not recognized intraoperatively, it presents as gastric outlet obstruction several months after band placement.*

Most intraoperative gastric perforations during band placement occur during the creation of the retrogastric tunnel. The blunt instrument used to create the tunnel should pass without resistance from the base of the right crus to the angle of His after the appropriate peritoneal surfaces have been dissected. Intraoperative findings that should alert the surgeon to a posterior perforation include unexplained bleeding from the tunnel or bile staining, especially if there have been repeated attempts to pass the instrument through the retrogastric tunnel. When a perforation occurs it should be identified intraoperatively and repaired primarily. Intraoperative endoscopy is a valuable tool to aid in the detection and location of a perforation. In this situation, band placement should be abandoned and not re-attempted for several months. Most patients are discharged within 24 hours of band placement, so a missed perforation will result in abdominal sepsis when the patient returns to the emergency department 24 to 48 hours after discharge. These patients will require aggressive fluid resuscitation, antibiotics, laparoscopic or open removal of the band, primary repair of the perforation if possible, and wide local drainage.

Answer: D

Allen JW (2007) Laparoscopic gastric band complications. *Medical Clinics of North America* **91** (3), 485–97.

O'Brien PE, Dixon JB (2003) Lap-band: outcomes and results. *Journal of Laparoendoscopic and Advanced Surgical Techniques* **13** (4), 265–70.

18. *A 50-year-old woman underwent a laparoscopic Roux-en-Y gastric bypass one year ago and now presents with severe epigastric pain and blood in her stool. Gastroscopy shows a very small proximal gastric pouch (<15 ml) and a gastrojejunal stomal ulcer. Possible contributing factors to marginal ulcer formation include all of the following except:*

A. *Smoking*

B. *Using absorbable suture for anastomosis*

C. *NSAID use*

D. *Helicobacter pylori infection*

E. *Gastro-gastric fistula*

Gastrojejunal ulceration after gastric bypass has been associated with a foreign-body reaction at the anastomosis, particularly when nonabsorbable suture erodes into the lumen. Ulcers at the site of the gastrojejunal anastomosis complicate between 1% to 16% of gastric bypasses with the highest risk in the first three months after surgery. The etiology is often multifactorial and this complication has been associated with use of nonsteroidal anti-inflammatory agents, nonabsorbable suture material, a gastric pouch size larger than 50 ml, *Helicobacter pylori,* and excessive acid exposure in the gastric pouch from a gastro-gastric fistula. In one study, patients who were preoperatively screened and treated for *H. pylori* had a significantly lower incidence of marginal ulcers at three years (2.4%) compared to those who were not screened. Alcohol and smoking have also been causally implicated in patients with marginal ulcers.

Pouch ulceration usually heals with proton pump inhibitors and /or sucralfate along with cessation of NSAID intake and smoking. Foreign material present at the anastomosis can be removed endoscopically to facilitate healing. In patients with a large pouch or gastro-gastric fistula with recurrent ulcers, surgical revision of the gastrojejunostomy and/or pouch may be necessary.

Answer: B

Christou NV, Sampalis JS, Liberman M, *et al.* (2004) Surgery decreases long-term mortality, morbidity, and health care use in morbidly obese patients. *Annals of Surgery* **240** (3), 416–23; discussion 423–4.

Jordan JH, Hocking MP, Rout WR, Woodward ER (1991) Marginal ulcer following gastric bypass for morbid obesity. *American Journal of Surgery* **57** (5), 286–8.

Printen KJ, Scott D, Mason EE (1980) Stomal ulcers after gastric bypass. *Archives of Surgery* **115** (4), 525–7.

Sanyal AJ, Sugerman HJ, Kellum JM, *et al.* (1992) Stomal complications of gastric bypass: incidence and outcome of therapy. *American Journal of Gastroenterology* **87** (9), 1165–9.

Sapala JA, Wood MH, Sapala MA, Flake TM, Jr (1998) Marginal ulcer after gastric bypass: a prospective three-year study of 173 patients. *Obesity Surgery* **8** (5), 505–16.

Schirmer B, Erenoglu C, Miller A (2002) Flexible endoscopy in the management of patients undergoing Roux-en-Y gastric bypass. *Obesity Surgery* **12** (5), 634–8.

19. *Nutritional deficiencies after Roux-en-Y gastric bypass surgery most commonly include all of the following except:*

A. *Vitamin D deficiency leading to metabolic bone disease*

B. *Calcium deficiency manifesting as tertiary hyperparathyroidism*

C. *Iron*

D. *Cobalamin*

E. *Calcium deficiency manifesting as secondary hyperparathyroidism*

The majority of dietary calcium absorption occurs in the duodenum due to the greater density of available transporters in this area. Prolonged poor calcium absorption, in addition to inadequate supplementation, can lead to *secondary* hyperparathyroidism. In addition to all fat soluble vitamins (A, D, E, K), calcium, iron, thiamine, folate, and B_{12} (cobalamin) deficiencies are possible after gastric bypass if appropriate lifelong supplementation and monitoring are not maintained.

Answer: B

Bloomberg RD, Fleishman A, Nalle JE, *et al.* (2005) Nutritional deficiencies following bariatric surgery: what have we learned? *Obesity Surgery* **15**, 145–54.

Youssef Y, Richards WO, Sekhar N, *et al.* (2007) Risk of secondary hyperparathyroidism after laparoscopic gastric bypass surgery in obese women. *Surgical Endoscopy* **21** (8), 1393–6.

20. *Concerning postoperative enteric leaks after gastric bypass, all of the following are true, except:*

A. *Leaks from the jejuno-jejunostomy are typically diagnosed later than leaks at the gastrojejunostomy*

B. *Persistent tachycardia >120 bpm is often the earliest indication of a leak*

C. *A negative upper GI contrast study combined with a negative CT scan are 95% accurate in ruling out a gastrointestinal leak*

D. *Amylase levels from a surgically placed drain can be helpful in early detection of a leak.*

E. *Failure to expeditiously return to the operating room in the setting of an enteric leak is the most common cause of preventable, major long-term disability or death in bariatric surgical patients.*

There are many limitations to radiographic studies and imaging in the postoperative bariatric surgery patient. Studies are often incomplete or suboptimal due to patient body habitus or positioning. Up to one-third of patients found to have a leak at operation will have had a negative upper GI and a negative CT scan. In a patient with a clinical concern for a leak, even with negative imaging studies, the best course of action is to return to the operating room. Diagnostic laparoscopy or laparotomy will allow examination of the gastrojejunostomy, jenuno-jenunostomy, and the remnant stomach. Failure to expeditiously return to the operating room in the setting of an enteric leak is the most common cause of preventable, major long-term disability or death in bariatric surgical patients. If a drain was left in place near the gastrojejunostomy at the time of the initial operation, salivary amylase from a leak will result in an extremely high fluid amylase level and can be an early indicator of a leak. The gastrojejunostomy is the most common site of a postoperative leak with an incidence of 1–4%. Leaks at the gastric remnant staple line or jejuno-jejunostomy are more difficult to diagnose radiographically and have a higher rate of delayed diagnosis and abdominal sepsis.

Answer: C

Gonzalez R, Sarr MG, Smith CD, *et al.* (2007) Diagnosis and contemporary management of anastomotic leaks after gastric bypass for obesity. *Journal of the American College of Surgeons* **204** (1), 47–55.

Livingston, E. Complications of bariatric surgery (2005) *Surgical Clinics of North America* **85**, 853–68.

21. *A 36-year-old woman who underwent a laparoscopic Roux-en Y gastric bypass 18 months ago now presents to the emergency department with sudden onset of severe mid-abdominal pain. Her postoperative course to this point has been uncomplicated and she has lost 160 pounds. She is visibly uncomfortable, her abdomen is diffusely tender without peritonitis, and her heart rate is 122 beats per minute. Her WBC is 15 000/mm^3, serum amylase is 320 units/L, total bilirubin is 2.1 mg/dL and her transaminases are in the 300s. An acute abdominal series is normal. The most likely diagnosis in this patient is*

A. *Acute pancreatitis*

B. *Cholangitis*

C. *Internal hernia with biliopancreatic limb obstruction*

D. *Acute viral hepatitis*

E. *Myocardial infarction*

Bowel obstruction after gastric bypass can result from adhesive disease or internal hernias. Large case series report bowel obstruction rates ranging from 1% to 10.5%. In a collective review of 10 large laparoscopic RYGB series, bowel obstruction occurred in 3% of patients compared to 2% in open RYGB ($P = 0.02$). Fewer intra-abdominal adhesions form after laparoscopic surgery, presumably due to less tissue trauma and bowel manipulation; this may explain the higher incidence of internal hernias relative to adhesive obstructions after laparoscopic RYGB. Hernias can occur at the mesenteric defect of the jejunojejunostomy, between the mesocolon and the Roux limb, or at the mesocolic defect for a retrocolic Roux limb. Retrocolic placement of the Roux limb has a higher internal hernia rate than antecolic Roux limb placement due to the presence of a mesocolic defect and a true Peterson's space between the mesocolon and Roux mesentery. To reduce the incidence of internal hernias, the mesenteric defects are closed during the primary procedure, but massive weight loss and decreases in visceral fat may result in these defects re-opening over time. Patients with intermittent, crampy abdominal pain that occurs months to years after gastric bypass should be evaluated with CT imaging or a small bowel series to evaluate for internal hernia. Gastric bypass patients that present with sudden onset of severe abdominal pain and laboratory findings that suggest pancreatitis should be evaluated promptly with a CT to evaluate for obstruction of their biliopancreatic limb. This problem should be managed with laparoscopic or open reduction of the internal hernia, repair of the mesenteric defect and placement of a gastrostomy tube in the gastric remnant. Radiographic-guided decompression of the gastric remnant may temporize the situation and decompress the biliopancreatic limb in the unstable patient.

Answer: C

Husain S, Ahmed AR, Johnson J, Boss T, O'Malley W (2007) Small-bowel obstruction after laparoscopic Roux-en-Y gastric bypass: Etioology, diagnosis, and management. *Archives of Surgery* **142** (10), 988–93.

Podnos YD, Jimenez JC, Wilson SE, *et al.* (2003) Complications after laparoscopic gastric bypass: a review of 3464 cases. *Archives of Surgery* **138** (9), 957–61.

Rogula T, Yenumula PR, Schauer PR (2007) A complication of Roux-en-Y gastric bypass: intestinal obstruction. *Surgical Endoscopy* **21** (11), 1914–18.

22. *All of the following would be considered severe, comorbid diseases that would create unacceptably high operative risk in bariatric surgery except:*

A. *Cirrhosis with portal hypertension and ascites*

B. *History of unstable angina with coronary stenting five months ago*

C. *Pulmonary embolism two months ago*

D. *Poorly controlled congestive heart failure*

E. *Severe obstructive sleep apnea with mild pulmonary hyptertension*

Although recognition of obstructive sleep apnea (OSA) and subsequent postoperative management are critical, severe OSA should not be considered a contraindication to bariatric surgery, even when the patient has developed early findings of obesity hypoventilation syndrome. There is abundant data demonstrating successful treatment of OSA with surgical weight loss. Conditions such as poorly controlled cardiac disease, recent coronary stenting requiring anti-platelet therapy, recent venous thromboembolism, or end-stage liver failure with portal hypertension and varices are contraindications to bariatric surgery. If these severe comorbidities can be effectively optimized, some of these high risk patients may ultimately be able to safely undergo bariatric surgery.

Answer: E

Fritscher LG, Mottin CC, Canani S, Chatkin JM (2007) Obesity and obstructive sleep apnea-hypopnea syndrome: the impact of bariatric surgery. *Obesity Surgery* **17** (1), 95–9.

Haines KL, Nelson LG, Gonzalez R, *et al.* (2007) Objective evidence that bariatric surgery improves obesity-related obstructive sleep apnea. *Surgery* **141** (3), 354–8.

Hallowell PT, Stellato TA, Schuster M, *et al.* (2007) Potentially life-threatening sleep apnea is unrecognized without aggressive evaluation. *American Journal of Surgery* **193** (3), 364–7; discussion 367.

23. *A 42-year-old man underwent a vertical sleeve gastrectomy one day ago. The intraoperative course was normal and a 34 French calibration tube was used. You are covering for your bariatric colleague who routinely obtains an upper GI contrast study on postoperative day one (see figure, barium tablet also given). Except for some nausea, the patient has no complaints. He looks well and his heart rate is 112 beats per minute at rest. What is the best course of action for this patient?*

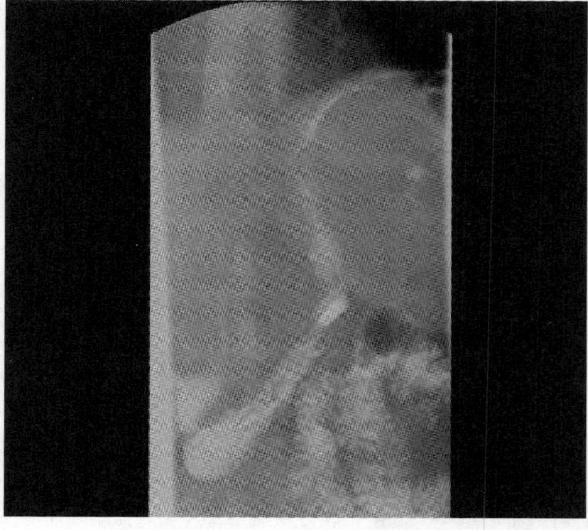

A. *Observe for 24–48 hours and repeat the contrast study*

B. *CT scan of the abdomen*

C. *Start antibiotics and have radiology place drains in the left upper quadrant*

D. *Return to the operating room to manage this problem*

E. *Start a clear liquid diet and monitor closely*

This image shows an early postoperative leak after sleeve gastrectomy. The ingested contrast is freely extravasating into the left subphrenic space. In a systematic review of sleeve gastrectomy literature, the overall leak rate for sleeve gastrectomy was 2.2%. The leak rate differed according to the indication as was 1.2% for first stage operations in high risk patients and 2.7% when the sleeve was used as a primary procedure. Most leaks occur at the proximal staple line near the angle of His. Early postoperative leaks should be managed operatively to control the leak and, if possible, repair the perforation. There can be a role for nonoperative management in the stable patient, but aggressive management and closure of these early postoperative leaks should be undertaken before a chronic abscess cavity or gastrocutaneous fistula develops. Leaks that present several weeks after sleeve gastrectomy as an abscess can be managed with percutaneous drainage, antibiotics, and endoscopic stenting if the patient is stable.

Answer: D

Brethauer SA, Hammel JP, Schauer PR (2009) Systematic review of sleeve gastrectomy as staging and primary bariatric procedure. *Surgery for Obesity and Related Diseases* **5**, 469–75.

Csendes A, Braghetto I, Leon P, Burgos AM (2010) Management of leaks after laparoscopic sleeve gastrectomy in patients with obesity. *Journal of Gastrointestinal Surgery* **14** (9), 1343–8.

Chapter 41 Burns, Inhalation Injury, Electrical and Lightning Injuries

Joseph J. DuBose, MD, FACS

1. *Which of the following is false regarding the initial resuscitation of burn victims?*

A. *Ineffective resuscitation will result in shock among patients with >20% total body surface area burn involvement*

B. *Delays in resuscitation beyond 2 hours have not been associated with increased mortality*

C. *Consequences of over-resuscitation include the need for fasciotomy*

D. *Over-resuscitation may be associated with conversion of superficial into deep burns*

E. *Abdominal compartment syndrome may result from over-resuscitation*

Without effective and rapid initiation of resuscitation, hypovolemia and shock will develop in patients with burns >15% to 20% total body surface area (TBSA) burns. Delay in fluid resuscitation beyond 2 hours of burn injury increases mortality and morbidity after these injuries. Consequences of over-resuscitation following burns include pulmonary edema, conversion of superficial into deep burns, the need for fasciotomy (including unburned limbs), and abdominal compartment syndrome.

Answer: B

Latenser B (2009) Critical care of the burn patient: The first 48 hours. *Critical Care Medicine* **37**, 2819–26.

Surgical Critical Care and Emergency Surgery: Clinical Questions and Answers, First Edition. Edited by Forrest O. Moore, Peter M. Rhee, Samuel A. Tisherman and Gerard J. Fulda.

2. *Burn shock pathophysiology is marked by:*

A. *Neurogenic shock*

B. *High pulmonary artery occlusion pressure*

C. *Decreased cardiac output*

D. *Decreased systemic vascular resistance*

E. *Increased intravascular volume*

Burn shock is the result of distributive and hypovolemic shock, manifested by intravascular volume depletion, low pulmonary artery occlusion pressure, elevated systemic vascular resistance and depressed cardiac output. Reduced cardiac output is a combined result of decreased plasma volume, increased afterload and decreased contractility. Impaired cardiac contractility is likely caused by circulating mediators such as tumor necrosis factor and impaired cellular calcium levels.

Answer: C

Pham TN, Cancio LC, Gibran NS (2008) American Burn Association practice guidelines: burn shock resuscitation. *Journal of Burn Care and Research* **29**, 257–66.

3. *All of the following are sequelae of initial burn injury except:*

A. *Loss of vessel wall integrity with leakage into the interstitum*

B. *Increased intravascular colloid osmotic pressure*

C. *Decreased circulating plasma volume*

D. *Depressed cardiovascular function*

E. *Massive edema formation*

Following burn injury, capillary leak promotes protein and osmotic loss into the interstitial space.

This, in turn, decreases intravascular colloid osmotic pressure. The outcome of the dramatic pouring of fluids, electrolytes and proteins into the interstitum are reflected in the loss of circulating plasma volume, hemoconcentration, massive edema formation, decreased urine output and depressed cardiovascular function.

Answer: B

Barton RC, Saffle JR, Morris SE, *et al.* (1997) Resuscitation of thermally injured patients with oxygen transport criteria as goals of therapy. *Journal of Burn Care and Rehabilitation* **18**, 1–9.

4. *How much fluid should routinely be given to the acutely burned patient?*

A. *2 liters crystalloid over one hour for every patient*

B. *1 mL/kg of lactated ringers for 24 hours*

C. *2 mL/kg per percentage body surface area burned of albumin for the first 24 hours*

D. *2 to 4 mL/kg per percentage body surface area burned of 7.5% hypertonic saline for the first 24 hours*

E. *2 to 4 mL/kg per percentage body surface area burned of lactated ringers for the first 24 hours, half of which is given in the first 8 hours*

Although several resuscitation formulas exist, the Parkland formula is the Consensus formula used by the American Burn Association in the Advanced Burn Life Support Curriculum. This formula calls for 4 mL/kg per percentage TBSA, describing the amount of lactated Ringer's solution required in the first 24 hours after burn injury, where 'kg' represents the patient's weight, and percentage TBSA is the size of the burn injury. Starting from the time of burn injury, half of the fluid is given in the first eight hours and the remaining half is given over the next 16 hours. It is important to note that, while formulas are useful in establishing goals of initial therapy, all therapy should be guided by measured endpoints of resuscitation.

Answer: E

Ahms KS, Harkins DR (1999) Initial resuscitation after burn injury: Therapies, strategies and controversies. *AACN Clinical Issues* **10**, 46–60.

Pham TN, Cancio LC, Gibran NS (2008) American Burn Association practice guidelines: burn shock resuscitation. *Journal of Burn Care and Research* **29**, 257–66.

5. *Which of the following is the most reliable method of monitoring resuscitation of burn injured patients?*

A. *Urine output*

B. *Lactate normalization*

C. *Abdominal compartment pressure monitoring*

D. *Response of measured cardiac index to fluid bolus*

E. *Direct tissue oxygen measurements*

Urine output, although the least technologically advanced of the described measures, remains the best validated method of guiding resuscitation. Abnormal admission arterial lactate and base excess values have been shown to correlate with the magnitude of injury and their failure to correct over time predicts mortality, but there remain no prospective studies to support the use of these parameters to guide fluid resuscitation. Abdominal compartment pressure monitoring can assist in the detection of abdominal compartment syndrome, a possible complication of over-resuscitation, but does not provide a measure of adequate resuscitative efforts. Although several preliminary studies documented successful increases in preload and cardiac index with aggressive fluid resuscitation after burns, a prospective randomized control trial failed to confirm these benefits. Direct tissue oxygen measurements have also been investigated in preliminary studies, but require additional study and are compromised by the edema that is associated with burn injury.

Answer: A

Cancio LC, Galvez E Jr, Turner CE, *et al.* (2006) Base deficit and alveolar-arterial gradient during resuscitation contribute independently but modestly to the prediction of mortality after burn injury. *Journal of Burn Care Research* **27**, 289–96.

Holm C, Mayr M, Tegeler J, *et al.* (2004) A clinical randomized study on the effects of invasive monitoring on burn shock resuscitation. *Burns* **30**, 798–807.

6. *A 70 kg patient with 40% TBSA burn has transferred to your facility after receiving >250 mL/kg of* *crystalloid for the 16 hours prior to transfer. On arrival, his abdomen is tense, his heart rate is 118 beats per minute and his blood pressure is 94/42 mm Hg. He has an elevated CVP and a bladder pressure measurement reveals a pressure of 40 mm Hg. The next appropriate step should be:*

A. *Diuresis*

B. *500 mL of 5% albumin bolus over 5 minutes*

C. *Attempt at percutaneous catheter decompression of the abdomen*

D. *Emergent decompressive laparotomy in the emergency department*

E. *None of the above*

Bladder pressure monitoring should be initiated as part of the burn fluid resuscitation protocol of every patient with >30% TBSA burn. Patients who receive >250 mL/kg of crystalloid in the first 24 hours will likely require abdominal decompression. Percutaneous decompression is a minimally invasive procedure that should be attempted prior to resorting to laparotomy. The International Conference of Experts on Intra-Abdominal Hypertension and Abdominal Compartment Syndrome recommends that if less invasive maneuvers fail, decompressive laparotomy should be performed in patients with ACS that is refractory to other treatment options. The reported mortality rates for decompressive laparotomy for ACS can be as high as 88% to 100%.

Answer: C

Cheatam ML, Malbrain ML, Kirkpatrick A, *et al.* (2007) Results from the International Conference on Experts on Intra-abdominal Hypertension and Abdominal Compartment Syndrome, II: recommendations. *Intensive Care Medicine* **33**, 951–62.

Latenser BA, Kowal-Vern A, Kimball D, *et al.* (2002) A pilot study comparing percutaneous decompression with decompressive laparotomy for acute abdominal compartment syndrome in thermal injury. *Journal of Burn Care Rehabilitation* **23**, 190–5.

7. *Reliable signs of infections among severely burned patients include:*

A. *Fever*

B. *Tachycardia*

C. *Tachypnea*

D. *Leukocytosis*

E. *None of the above*

Current definitions for sepsis and infection have many criteria routinely found in patients with extensive burns without infection/sepsis (e.g. fever, tachycardia, tachypnea, leukocytosis). The inflammatory and hyperdynamic responses associated with burns may result in fever, tachycardia, tachypnea and even leukocytosis—all in the absence of infection. Useful clues of infection may, however, manifest in the form of increased fluid requirements, decreasing platelet counts >3 days after injury, altered mental status, worsening pulmonary status, and impaired renal function.

Answer: E

Latenser B (2009) Critical care of the burn patient: The first 48 hours. *Critical Care Medicine* **37**, 2819–26.

8. *Central line catheters are commonly required for severe burn victims. Given the risk of catheter-related blood stream infections, these lines require special care. Reasonable approaches to minimize the risk and sequelae of infection from these lines include all of the following except:*

A. *Meticulous sterile technique with placement*

B. *Preferential utilization of a subclavian site when possible.*

C. *Avoiding line placement through burn eschar whenever possible*

D. *Prophylactic systemic antibiotics after line placement*

E. *Daily assessment of line need*

Any infection in a burn patient should be considered to be from the central venous catheter until proven otherwise. If no other source is clearly attributable, the line should be removed after new access has been established; always utilizing meticulous sterile technique for every line placement. According to the 2011 NIH consensus statement on central venous catheter utilization, the subclavian site is preferred over jugular or femoral sites to potentially reduce the infection risks associated with these sites. The same guidelines support the daily practice of routine evaluation of line need, and subsequent removal when an indication for central venous catheterization is no longer necessary. It should also be remembered that in the setting of severe burns, many of the traditional markers of infection (fever, tachycardia) may be present without actual infection. Therefore, routine removal of a central line in patients with tachycardia or low grade fever in the setting of a severe burn response, particularly if vascular access options are limited, should be avoided. If infection is documented by gram stain or culture, or if clinical suspicion is strong, then removal and change of a line is indicated. The correct answer is D, as prophylactic systemic antibiotics have not demonstrated a role in the routine care of thermal injury.

Answer: D

Greenhalgh DG, Saffle JR, Holmes JH, *et al.* (2007) American Burn Association consensus conference to define sepsis and infection in burns. *Journal of Burn Care Research* **28**, 71–5.

O'Grady NP, Alexander M, Burns LA, *et al.* 2011 Guidelines for the prevention of intravascular catheter-related infections. *Clin Infect Dis.* **52**(9), e162–93.

9. *Which of the following is false regarding nutrition among burn patients?*

A. *Patients with 20% TBSA burns are unlikely to meet their nutritional needs with native oral intake alone*

B. *Patients fed early after thermal injury have shorter hospital stays*

C. *Parenteral nutrition is the first-line of nutritional delivery in severe burns*

D. *Early feeding is associated with enhanced wound healing*

E. *The hypermetabolism associated with burn injury can lead to a doubling of normal resting energy expenditure and higher caloric requirements*

Hypermetabolism can double energy expenditure and significantly increase caloric requirements of burn patients. Enteral nutrition is the most desirable route, and should be started for these patients as soon as resuscitation is underway. Patients with $> 20\%$ TBSA are not likely to meet their nutritional requirements by mouth alone, and should have a transpyloric feeding tube placed if possible. Patients fed early have significantly enhanced wound healing and shorter hospital stays.

Answer: C

Venter M, Rode H, Sive A, *et al.* (2007) Enteral resuscitation and early enteral feeding is children with major burns: Effect on McFarlane response to stress. *Burns* **33**, 464–71.

10. *Which of the following has not proven potentially beneficial for burn patients?*

A. *Glucose control*

B. *Routine exogenous cortisol*

C. *Oxandralone*

D. *Propanolol*

E. *Topical antimicrobial agents*

Although absolute adrenal insufficiency occurs in up to 36% of patients with major burns, there has not been a correlation between response to corticotropin stimulation or cortisol and survival. Glucose control in burn patients has been shown to be associated with decreased infectious complications and mortality rates. Anabolic steroids, including oxandralone has been shown to promote regain of weight and lean mass two to three times faster than nutrition alone after burn injury. Beta blockers like propanolol have been shown to attenuate hypermetabolism and reverse muscle-protein catabolism. Once a wound is clean, topical antimicrobial agents limit bacterial proliferation and fungal colonization in burn wounds.

Answer: B

Judkins K (2000) Current consensus and controversies in major burns management. *Trauma* **2**, 239–51.

Rose JK, Herndon DN (1997) Advances in the treatment of burn patients. *Burns* **23** (suppl. 1), S19–S26.

11. *Mafenide acetate (sulfamylon acetate) is a topical antimicrobial frequently utilized in burn wound care. This medication is associated with characteristic side effects, including:*

A. *Hyponatremia*

B. *Hypochloremia*

C. *Methemoglobinemia*

D. *Hyperchloremic acidosis*

E. *Leukopenia*

Mafenide acetate (sulfamylon acetate) has broad antimicrobial spectrum of action and excellent eshcar penetration. Some side effects that are worrisome with the use of this topical antimicrobial (either 10% cream or 5% soaks) are burning sensation, allergic reactions and hyperchloremic acidosis. Silver sulfadiazine is essentially a combination of two anti-microbials, silver and a sulfonamide. It has a more moderate eschar penetration ability than mafenide acetate. Complications of silver sulfadiazine include allergic reactions, methemoglobinemia and leukopenia. Silver nitrate also has a broad antimicrobial spectrum of topical action, and can be associated with the side effects of hyponatremia, methemoglobinemia and hypochloremia.

Answer: D

12. *All of the following constitute clear criteria for transfer to a burn center except:*

A. *>10% TBSA partial thickness burns*

B. *Inhalational injury*

C. *Electrical injury*

D. *Serious chemical injury*

E. *6% TBSA partial thickness burn to the back of a previously healthy adult man with a nonoperative scaphoid fracture*

The American Burn Association has established criteria for burn patients who should be acutely transferred to a burn center: >10% TBSA partial thickness burns, any size full thickness burn, burns to special areas of function or cosmesis, inhalational injury including lightning, burns with trauma where burns are the major problem, pediatric burns if the referring hospital has no special pediatric capabilities, and smaller burns in patients with multiple co-morbidities. Patient E meets none of these criteria.

Answer: E

American Burn Association, www.americanburn.org

13. *A 34-year-old man is brought to your emergency department after a house fire. He has a cough productive of carbonaceous sputum and has singed facial hairs and eyebrows. He complains of mild shortness of breath. All of the following have a potential role in the treatment of inhalational injury, except:*

A. *Early intubation for airway protection*

B. *Treatment of bronchospasm with alpha agonists*

C. *N-acteylcysteine nebulized treatments*

D. *Inhaled steroids*

E. *Nebulized heparin*

Inhalational injury can progress very rapidly and the identification of these injuries demands serious consideration of early intubation. Early bronchoscopy provides for diagnosis of inhalational sequelae and documentation of airway ulceration/assessment of severity. Both nebulized heparin and N-acetylcysteine have been used to break down the casts that form following these injuries. Alpha agonists are effective in the treatment of associated bronchospasm. Inhaled steroids have not been shown to be of benefit in inhalational injury and should not be given unless the patient is steroid-dependent before injury or has bronchospasm resistant to standard therapy.

Answer: D

Desai MH, Mlcak R, Richardson J, *et al.* Reduction in mortality in pediatric patients with inhalational injury with aerosolized heparin/N-acetylcysteine. *Journal of Burn Care Rehabilitation* **19**, 210.

14. *A 24-year-old woman is struck by lightning during a golf outing. She has burns on her hands and a separate burn on her right thigh. Initial concerns upon arrival of the patient to the hospital include:*

A. *Initial ECG*

B. *Fluid hydration to maintain urine output at 1.0 to 1.5 mL/kg/hr*

C. *Vigilance for evidence of compartment syndrome*

D. *Early detection of myoglobinuria*

E. *Emperic use of bicarbonate infusions*

High-voltage injuries with electrical transmission from lightening strikes have serious potential sequelae that must be considered. Initial and delayed cardiac and neurogenic abnormalities are frequent manifestations. Compartment syndromes under areas of unaffected skin can complicate the course, particularly if not recognized early. Subsequent muscle injury from the transmission effects as well as compartment pressure elevations can lead to myoglobinuria and renal failure. Urine output should be maintained at 1.0 to 1.5 mL/kg/hr to minimize the renal effects of myoglobinuria. While bicarbonate and mannitol have been used in attempts at renal protection, hydration alone has proven sufficient in the treatment of myoglobinuria that accompanies the deep muscle necrosis and acidosis in these injuries.

Answer: E

Luce EA (2000) Electrical burns. *Clinical Plastic Surgery* **27**, 133.

15. *Central nervous system injury is common in lightning strike victims. These sequelae may be characterized by all of the following except:*

A. *Early symptoms followed by universal resolution within hours*

B. *Loss of consciousness*

C. *Hypoxic ischemic neuropathy*

D. *Epidural hematomas due to associated falls*

E. *Keraunoparalysis*

Neurologic effects of lightning injuries may be both temporary and permanent. These can be classified into four groups. Group 1 effects are immediate and transient, and are very common. These include loss of consciousness (75%), amnesia, paresthesias (80%) and keraunoparalysis. Keraunoparalysis (Charcot's paralysis) is a neurologic disorder specific to lightning victims which features transient paralysis, often predominantly affecting the lower extremities, and accompanied by loss of sensation; it last several hours and the resolves. Group 2 neurologic effects are immediate, prolonged or permanent in nature. These include hypoxic ischemic neuropathies, intracranial hemorrhage, post-arrest cerebral infarctions and cerebellar syndromes. Group 3 neurologic effects are possibly delayed syndromes, including motor neuron diseases and movement disorders. Finally, group 4 injuries such as subdural or epidural hematomas occur as a result of associated falls or blasts.

Answer: A

Cherington M (2003) Neurologic manifestations of lightning strikes. *Neurology* **60** (2), 182–5.

16. *The most common cause of death after lighting strikes are:*

A. *Flash pulmonary edema*

B. *Cardiopulmonary arrest and apnea*

C. *Multi-organ failure*

D. *Grand mal seizures*

E. *Myoglobinuria*

The most common causes of death from lighting injury are cardiopulmonary arrest and apnea. The interruption of normal cardiac conduction by the associated direct current results in asystole, but like a defibrillator, spontaneous cardiac activity typically resumes shortly thereafter. The apnea that results from the same direct current is caused by effects on the brain's respiratory center, however is longer lasting and if left untreated will result in hypoxia, arrythmias and secondary cardiac arrest.

Answer: B

Blumenthal R (2005) Lightning fatalities on the South African Highveld: a retrospective descriptive study for the period 1997 to 2000. *American Journal of Forensic Medicine and Pathology* **26** (1), 66–9.

Ritenour AE, Morton MJ, McManus JG, *et al.* (2008) Lighting injury: A review. *Burns* **34**, 585–94.

17. *Early burn wound excision and grafting, of deep second- and third-degree burns is associated with:*

A. *Increased infection rates*

B. *Increased blood loss*

C. *Improved survival*

D. *Increased length of hospital stay*

E. *All of the above*

Deep second- and third-degree burns do not heal in a timely fashion without autografting. The persistence of these burned tissues serve as a nidus for inflammation and infection that can lead to sepsis and death. Early excision and grafting of these wounds is now practiced in most burn centers, and has been associated with improved survival, decreased blood loss and shorter hospitalizations.

Answer: C

Herndon DN, Parks DH (1986) Comparison of serial debridement and autografting and early massive excision with cadaver skin overlay in the treatment of large burns in children. *Journal of Trauma* **26**, 149–54.

Thompson P, Herndon DN, Abston S, *et al.* (1987) Effect of early excision on patients with major thermal injury. *Journal of Trauma* **27**, 205–9.

18. *For a patient with a localized burn to the ear and exposed cartilage, which topical agent is most likely to be beneficial in minimizing the risk of cartilaginous infection?*

A. *Silver sulfdiazene*

B. *Mafenide acetate*

C. *Bacitracin*

D. *Topical steroids*

E. *All of the above are just as likely to minimize risk*

Mafenide acetate is the best choice for this location, as it has the best eschar or cartilaginous penetration. Silver sulfdiazine, comparatively, has poorer penetration of these tissues. Bacitracin has even less effectiveness in this regard. Steroids are of no benefit in the avoidance of chondritis.

Answer: B

Skedros DG, Goldfarb IW, Slater H, Rocco J (1992) Chondritis of the burned ear: a review. *Ear Nose and Throat Journal* **71** (8), 359–62.

Chapter 42 Urologic and Gynecologic Surgery

Julie L. Wynne, MD, MPH, FACS

1. *When evaluating a patient with suspected Fournier's gangrene, it is important to be aware of all of the following except:*

A. *An etiology can be identified in the majority of cases*

B. *The testis, bladder, and rectum are frequently involved*

C. *The infection is typically polymicrobial*

D. *Involvement of the testicle suggests an intra-abdominal or retroperitoneal source of infection*

E. *Infection does not spread from the anterior to the posterior triangle of the pelvic outlet*

Fournier's gangrene, while initially reported as an infection of men, is now used to describe necrotizing fasciitis of the perineum, genitals, or perianal region of both men and women. However, the disease is ten times as common in men as women. Etiology can be discovered in the majority of cases, and includes urogenital causes (urethral strictures), anorectal processes (abscesses, malignancies), trauma (bites, stings, blunt trauma), cutaneous processes (cellulitis), and retroperitoneal events (psoas and perinephric abscesses, appendicitis, pancreatitis). The infection is typically polymicrobial. Initial antibiotic therapy should cover the commensal flora of the perineum, streptococci, and GI organisms. Diabetes mellitus is the most common underlying systemic disorder but it also may occur in the context of cirrhosis, malnutrition, chemotherapy or steroid use, malignancy, and HIV/AIDS. Knowledge of the anatomy of the pelvic outlet can be helpful in determining the etiology; Colles' fascia, the fascia of the anterior triangle of the pelvic outlet, terminates at the perineal membrane and prevents spread from the anterior to posterior triangle. However, the infection may progress in the reverse direction, from the posterior to the anterior pelvic triangle, as Colles' fascia fenestrates at the level of the bulbocavernosus muscle. Consequently, retroperitoneal infections can spread along the internal and external fascial layers of the spermatic cord. The testis, bladder, and rectum are rarely involved, due to the fact that their blood supply derives from the aorta. Testicular involvement in particular suggests an intra-abdominal or retroperitoneal source on infection.

Surgical Critical Care and Emergency Surgery: Clinical Questions and Answers, First Edition. Edited by Forrest O. Moore, Peter M. Rhee, Samuel A. Tisherman and Gerard J. Fulda.

Answer: B

Eke N (2000) Fournier's gangrene: a review of 1726 cases. *British Journal of Surgery* **87**, 718–28.

Heyns CF, Theron PD (207) Fournier's gangrene. In: Hohenfellner M, Santucci RA (eds) *Emergencies in Urology*, Springer-Verlag, Berlin, pp. 50–60.

2. *Which of the following is false regarding testicular torsion?*

A. *It frequently presents with sudden onset of severe unilateral pain accompanied by nausea and vomiting*

B. *A viable de-torsed testis AND the contralateral testis should undergo orchidopexy*

C. *Irreparable damage occurs within 4-8 hours of ischemia*

D. *History of intermittent pain rather than acute onset of unrelenting pain rules out torsion*

E. *Radionuclide scanning and scrotal ultrasound can confirm the diagnosis*

Testicular torsion is the only cause of the acute scrotum that mandates emergent diagnosis and treatment. Patients typically present with acute onset of unilateral pain, accompanied by nausea and vomiting. Prior operation for torsion does not rule out a subsequent episode. As well, a history of intermittent pain is consistent with the diagnosis, in that serial torsion and spontaneous detorsion may be occurring. The involved testicle may be high riding, or lie transversely rather than vertically. Absence of cremasteric reflex supports the diagnosis. A positive Prehn's sign, relief of pain with elevation of the scrotum towards the abdomen, may suggest epididymitis rather than testicular torsion. The duration of tolerance of the ischemic insult depends on the degree of twisting, but generally torsion must be relieved within four to eight hours. The diagnosis can be made clinically, or with diagnostic imaging. Imaging options include high resolution scrotal ultrasound with color Doppler and radionuclide scanning. Absence of blood flow mandates emergent exploration via a midline raphe incision. The involved testis should be detorsed, and then wrapped in warm sponges. The contralateral testis is then examined and orchidopexy performed with three absorbable sutures. The detorsed testis is then re-examined, and decision made regarding orchidopexy versus orchiectomy.

Answer: D

Gatti JM, Murphy JP (2007) Current management of the acute scrotum. *Seminars in Pediatric Surgery* **16**, 58–63.

Master V (2007) Scrotal emergencies. In: Hohenfellner M, Santucci RA (eds) *Emergencies in Urology*, Springer-Verlag, Berlin, pp. 132–41.

3. *Acute care surgeons may be consulted to manage phimosis and paraphimosis. Which of the following is true regarding these conditions?*

A. Both are urological emergencies

B. Circumcision is ultimately required after all cases of paraphimosis reduction

C. Phimosis is related to presence of concurrent sexually transmitted disease

D. Emergent circumcision is the therapy in both cases

E. Manual reduction is a reasonable first intervention in cases of paraphimosis

Phimosis, or the inability to retract the foreskin beyond the glans penis, presents with symptoms of painful erections, hematuria, recurrent UTI, pain, or weakened urinary stream. Causes include poor hygiene leading to balanoposthitis, repeated episodes of forceful retraction causing microtears and fibrosis, and balanitis xerotica obliterans (BXO), a fibrosing dermatosis. Phimosis is rarely a surgical emergency, and the chief indication for emergency circumcision is obstruction of the urinary stream with inability to pass a Foley catheter. Paraphimosis, or entrapment of a retracted foreskin behind the coronal sulcus, is a surgical emergency, and requires immediate reduction in order to avoid the possible sequellae of ischemia of the foreskin and glans. Common causes of paraphimosis include failure to replace the foreskin after Foley catheterization or voiding/bathing, vigorous sexual activity, or chronic balanoposthitis. The usual first intervention is manual reduction, which may be facilitated by application of ice. The osmotic method involves wrapping the penis in gauze, and applying a hypertonic solution such as 3% saline or 50% dextrose. In austere settings, granulated sugar may be applied. The puncture method involves using a 21–26 gauge needle to make circumferential punctures in the edematous foreskin, releasing the trapped liquid. Injection of hyaluronidase in 1 mL doses into the foreskin is another option; the hyaluronidase is felt to reduce the edema by breaking down the hyaluronic acid in the extracellular fluid. Aspiration of 3–12 mL of blood from the corpora (after initiation of a penile block and placement of a tourniquet) may allow for reduction of the paraphimosis. Finally, a dorsal slit or emergent circumcision may be performed. The dorsal slit is performed after anesthetizing the dorsal aspect of the foreskin with 1% plain lidocaine; placement of a straight hemostat at the 12 o'clock position will render the area hemostatic, facilitating the incision. The majority of patients treated for paraphimosis will not require a formal circumcision.

Answer: E

Cook A, Koury AE (2007) Urologic Emergencies in Children. In: Hohenfellner M, Santucci RA (eds) *Emergencies in Urology*, Springer-Verlag, Berlin, pp. 73–100.

Little B, White M (2005) Treatment options for paraphimosis. *International Journal of Clinical Practice* **59** (5), 591–3.

4. *Which of the following is incorrect regarding the evaluation and management of a man who presents with priapism?*

A. Two etiologies exist, ischemic and non-ischemic

B. A careful history and physical is likely to determine the cause

C. Both ischemic and nonischemic types are considered surgical emergencies

D. Ultrasound is the preferred type of diagnostic imaging

E. Total parenteral nutrition may cause the ischemic type

Priapism is defined as persistence of erection beyond four hours, in the absence of sexual stimulation. Two etiologies exist, termed ischemic and nonischemic. It is important to distinguish between the two due to the difference in management. In ischemic priapism, occlusion of venous outflow leads to cessation of arterial inflow, creating an acidotic and hypoxic milieu within the corpora, which will lead to fibrosis, necrosis, and erectile dysfunction. Intracavernous therapy with papaverine or phentolamine, psychotropic drugs, recreational drugs including cocaine, high lipid content of TPN, and some classes of antihypertensives are known to precipitate this variant of priapism. Physical exam reveals a rigid and painful erection with a soft glans. Ultrasound confirms absence of cavernosal arterial flow. The diagnosis of ischemic priapism mandates emergent therapy. The first maneuver is aspiration of the corpora with a 19 or 21 gauge needle. The corpora may also be irrigated, to encourage release of the clot. Injection of sympathomimetic agents, preferably phenylephrine, is the next step in the algorithm. If these interventions are unsuccessful, a distal fistula is attempted. This procedure can be done at the bedside, using a penile block. Either a biopsy needle or a scalpel is used to create a fistula between the corpus cavernosum and the glans/corpus spongiosum/veins. Non-ischemic, or "high-flow" priapism, on the other hand, is a nonemergent condition. Trauma to the penis, perineum, or pelvis, causes rupture of an artery, typically a branch of the cavernosal artery, resulting in increased arterial inflow to the penis. Appropriate history, physical (perineal bruising and a semi-erect, nonpainful penis), and ultrasound, which demonstrates ruptured cavernosal artery with unregulated blood flow, diagnose this condition. Because the tissue remains well oxygenated, there is limited potential for ischemia or necrosis. Use of ice packs in conjunction with expectant management is a reasonable first approach, and may be successful in up to 62% of cases. If the penis fails to detumesce, angioembolization may be attempted. If this is unsuccessful, open surgical ligation may be indicated.

Answer: C

Brant WO, Bella AJ, Gracia MM, Lue TF (2007) Priapsim. In: Hohenfellner M, Santucci RA (eds) *Emergencies in Urology*, Springer-Verlag, Berlin, pp. 301–12.

Shrewsberry A, Weiss A, Ritenour CWM (2010) Recent advances in the medical and surgical management of priapism. *Current Urology Reports* **11**, 405–13.

5. *A C5 quadriplegic patient is brought to the emergency department three weeks after discharge from the trauma service. The patient reports a sense of anxiety, as well as onset of headaches accompanied by nausea. On exam, his vital signs include: BP 160/90 mm Hg, HR 50 beats/minute, RR 20 breaths/minute, temperature 98.5 °F. Physical exam reveals a slightly anxious patient lying in supine position, with possible mild distention of the lower abdomen. Which initial intervention is most likely to eliminate the trigger for this disorder?*

A. Digital rectal exam with lubricant

B. Removal of any tight clothing

C. Transitioning the patient to the upright position

D. Catheterization of the urinary bladder

E. Resection of ingrown toenail

Patients with spinal cord injury (SCI) may acutely develop autonomic dysreflexia in response to a wide variety of stimuli. The syndrome is typically seen in patients with injury at or above T6, and is more common with cervical rather than thoracic spine injuries. Stimuli including bladder distention, urinary tract infection, bowel distention, fecal impaction, perianal processes, ingrown toenails, pressure sores, and fractures send a stimulus to the spinal cord via peripheral nerves. Sympathetic discharge is evoked, and because the descending inhibitory pathways have been disrupted by the injury, vasoconstriction and hypertension result. The signs and syndromes of this disorder include hypertension, bradycardia, headaches, flushing, upper truncal paresthesias, blurred vision, nausea, anxiety, penile erection, and piloerection below the level of the injury. Of note, the baseline blood pressure for SCI patients is in the range of 90s/60s, and an increase in systolic blood pressure of 20–30 mm Hg is considered to be consistent with the diagnosis, i.e., systolic blood pressures in the 110–120 mm Hg range represent hypertension. If untreated, this condition may lead to sequellae such as seizures, subarachnoid hemorrhage, encephalopathy, neurogenic pulmonary edema, and death. Fully 90% of such episodes have a genitourinary etiology (bladder distention, urinary tract infection, stones), and the highest yield maneuver is to ensure that the bladder is adequately drained. The second most common etiology is bowel distention, and fecal impaction should be ruled out, taking care to use ample amount of lubrication. Sitting the patient upright while attempting to identify the trigger will typically normalize the blood pressure. If the trigger is not identified, and the blood pressure remains elevated, antihypertensive therapy with nifedipine or nitrates should be initiated. It is noted that patients should be queried as to possible concomitant use of phosphodiesterase-5 inhibitors before utilizing nitrates.

Answer: D

Krassioukov A, Warburton DE, Teasell R, Eng JJ (2009) A systematic review of the management of autonomic dysreflexia after spinal cord injury. *Archives of Physical Medicine and Rehabilitation* **90**, 682–95.

Wefer B, Junemann KP (2007) autnomic dysreflexia and emergencies in neurogenic bladder. In: Hohenfellner M, Santucci RA (eds) *Emergencies in Urology*, Springer-Verlag, Berlin, pp. 101–3.

6. *A 75-year-old man underwent an uncomplicated transurethral resection of the prostate. The patient was initially alert, appropriate, and mildly hypertensive on admission to the ICU. Six hours later, he is somewhat lethargic, and nauseated. He is hypotensive and bradycardic, with an oxygen saturation of 87%. A chest radiograph demonstrates interstitial pulmonary edema. What additional information is most likely to explain the change in this patient's condition?*

A. *Computed tomography of the chest*

B. *Electrocardiogram*

C. *Arterial blood gas*

D. *Hemoglobin*

E. *Serum electrolytes*

Endourologic procedures such as cystoscopy and transurethral resection (TUR) of the prostate and bladder require continuous irrigation to optimize visibility. This may result in the absorption of up to several liters of fluid, resulting in dilutional hyponatremia. The resultant clinical findings have been called the TUR syndrome. Almost all endourologic procedures result in absorption of irrigating fluid but patients develop TUR syndrome less than 7% of the time, usually as a result of longer or more complicated procedures. The water is typically absorbed via transected veins in the operative field. A second mechanism for absorption of large volumes of irrigant is undetected perforation of the bladder or prostatic capsule, or misplacement of the catheter, resulting in instillation of irrigant within the retroperitoneum. The TUR syndrome may manifest intraoperatively, but usually within 24 hours of the procedure. Expansion of the intravascular volume caused by absorption of the irrigating solution leads to hypoosmolarity. The fluid then transitions to the extravascular interstitial space, resulting in hyponatremia, hypovolemia, and, potentially, cerebral and pulmonary edema. Clinical manifestations may include confusion/agitation, nausea/vomiting, seizures, hypotension with bradycardia, and hypoxia. Hypertension may also be seen. The diagnosis of this syndrome is made within the appropriate clinical context, and is supported by serum electrolytes demonstrating hyponatremia. Treatment is supportive, and requires expeditious correction of the hyponatremia and fluid status.

Answer: E

Hahn RG (2006) Fluid absorption in endoscopic surgery. *British Journal of Anaesthesia* **96** (1), 8–20.

Zantl N, Hartung R (2007) TUR-related complications. In: Hohenfellner M, Santucci RA (eds) *Emergencies in Urology*, Springer-Verlag, Berlin, pp. 335–48.

7. *A 40-year-old man on antiretroviral therapy for HIV infection presents to the emergency department with complaint of colicky left flank pain radiating to the groin, accompanied by nausea/vomiting and fevers. He appears acutely ill, and his temperature is 102.5°F. Labs reveal a significant leukocytosis. Urinalysis reveals turbid urine with microscopic hematuria. Noncontrasted computed tomography of the abdomen/pelvis is obtained; no stones are seen, though proximal ureteral dilation is noted. Which of the following is correct?*

A. *Because of the high sensitivity and specificity of non-contrasted CT scan for urinary tract calculi, this diagnosis is ruled out*

B. *A contrasted CT scan should be obtained immediately to evaluate for non-urologic causes of flank pain*

C. *An upper urinary tract obstruction with infection is a urologic emergency warranting prompt drainage*

D. *Due to the high clinical suspicion for urinary stones, an MRI should be obtained to rule in the diagnosis*

E. *Retrograde stenting, rather than percutaneous nephrostomy tube, is the preferred intervention for temporary drainage for ureteral obstruction*

While the etiologies of upper urinary tract obstruction are numerous, patients typically present with a similar set of symptoms: severe flank pain radiating to the groin, external genitalia, or thigh, accompanied by fevers/chills and nausea/vomiting. A CT scan of the abdomen/pelvis without IV contrast is extremely accurate for the diagnosis of urinary stones (sensitivity >95%, specificity >98%) but will miss noncalcified stones, or obstruction due to crystallized protease inhibitors, as is the diagnosis in this patient. However, additional CT findings, within the appropriate clinical context, can secure the diagnosis. These include proximal ureteral dilation, hydronephrosis, perinephric fat stranding, and asymmetric appearance of renal parenchymal density. If the scan does not demonstrate stones, and the patient's history and physical are not specific for urinary stones, repeating the scan with IV contrast can help with the diagnosis of nonurologic sources of flank pain, including adnexal masses, appendicitis, and diverticulitis. Ultrasound is a reasonable study for use in pediatric or pregnant patients, as it can diagnose stones, pyelonephritis, hydronephrosis, and sedimentation. Magnetic resonance imaging is unlikely to help with this diagnosis, as it does not reliably detect calcified stones. Indications for emergent temporary drainage procedures include unilateral or bilateral urinary obstruction, obstruction with acute renal failure, obstruction in a renal allograft or solitary native kidney, or obstruction in a pregnant woman. Obstruction with infection, as in this scenario, is regarded as a urologic emergency. There is no definitive evidence to support use of percutaneous nephrostomy drains over retrograde stents; this decision is patient and physician specific.

Answer: C

Gettman MT, Segura JW (2007) Failure of urinary drainage: upper urinary. In: Hohenfellner M, Santucci RA (eds) *Emergencies in Urology*, Springer-Verlag, Berlin, pp. 104–17.

8. *Following an uncomplicated open inguinal herniorrhaphy, a 62-year-old man is unable to void in the recovery room. The most appropriate approach is:*

A. *Perform a digital rectal exam to rule out benign prostatic enlargement and prostatitis*

B. *Obtain a urinalysis to rule out infection*

C. *Administer an alpha antagonist*

D. *Bladder scan the patient and perform in-out catheterization if the residual is >300 ml*

E. *Obtain metabolic panel and prostate-specific antigen (PSA)*

The experience of undergoing surgery is a known precipitant of acute urinary retention. The incidence ranges from 4% to 29%, depending on the type and context of the surgery. Of ambulatory patients, those who undergo inguinal herniorrhaphy and anal surgery have the highest rates. Inpatients undergoing complex pelvic or rectal surgeries also have a high incidence of postoperative urinary retention. The type of anesthesia is a factor, as general and neuraxial anesthetics are associated with postoperative urinary retention, while local anesthesia is not. Multiple additional factors, such as medications, volume of fluids, operative time, control of postoperative pain, use of opioids, and patient age, are all felt to play a role. Normal bladder capacity is 400–600 mL, and optimal bladder emptying is felt to occur at 300 mL; the point at which patients feel the urge to micturate varies. Patients with failure to void postoperatively should undergo portable ultrasound scan of the bladder, and consideration for in-out catheterization when the residual is >200–300 mL. A recent Cochrane review identified no evidence to support use of pharmacologic management of postoperative urinary retention. Patients who present with "spontaneous" acute urinary retention (AUR) should undergo digital rectal exam to assess for the most common etiology, benign prostatic enlargement, and to rule out rarer causes such as malignant prostatic disease and prostatitis. Physical examination should also rule out phimosis as the etiology for the lower urinary tract obstruction. Urinalysis is useful to rule out urinary tract infection as the cause. Metabolic panel results are important to identify patients with renal insufficiency, in whom additional studies such as renal ultrasound may be useful. PSA measurement is not recommended during episodes of acute urinary retention, as it may be falsely elevated. Pharmacologic management, particularly with alpha antagonists, is most likely to be useful in the subset of patients with AUR due to benign prostatic enlargement.

Answer: D

Buckley BS, Lapitan MCM (2010) Drugs for treatment of urinary retention after surgery in adults (review). The Cochrane Collaboration 10.

Darrah DM, Griebling TL, Silverstein JH (2009) Postoperative urinary retention. *Anesthesiology Clinics* **27**, 465–84.

Patterson JM, Chapple CR (2007) Failure of urinary drainage: lower tract. In: Hohenfellner M, Santucci RA (eds) *Emergencies in Urology*, Springer-Verlag, Berlin, pp. 118–31.

9. *A 63-year-old obese woman with a medical history significant for diabetes mellitus and hypertension, presents to the emergency room with a complaint of a 24-hour history of left-flank pain, fevers, and dysuria. She has not had these symptoms before. She appears ill and she is tender to palpation on the left flank. Vital signs are temperature 103°F, BP 90/60 mm Hg, HR 120 beats/minute, RR 25 breaths/minute, and room air oxygenation saturation is 92%. Patient states she has had an abdominal ultrasound in the past, and has two kidneys; she does not have a history of renal insufficiency. The ED staff has obtained a kidneys, ureters and bladder radiograph (KUB), which demonstrates pockets of gas within the left renal parenchyma and collecting system. Your recommendation for management includes resuscitation, antibiotics, and*

A. Observation

B. Obtain noncontrasted computed tomography of the abdomen/pelvis

C. Emergent nephrectomy

D. Placement of a ureteral stent

E. Percutaneous drainage of localized pockets of gas or abscesses

Emphysematous pyelonephritis is a urologic emergency that occurs almost exclusively in diabetic patients, with a 4:1 woman-to-man ratio, and is frequently associated with urinary tract obstruction. Gram negative bacteria such as *E. coli*, Klebsiella, and Proteus cause a necrotizing infection of the renal parenchyma, collecting system, and/or perinephric space. This condition is to be distinguished from emphysematous pyelitis, in which gas formation is limited to the collecting system; this condition is successfully treated medically. In contrast, patients with emphysematous pyelonephritis typically progress to multi-system organ failure, and the mortality rate is 50% for medical management. The diagnosis may be made with plain films, as in this patient, or by ultrasound. However, the accuracy with CT scan is 100%, and allows for percutaneous drainage maneuvers. IV-contrasted scans should be obtained unless contraindicated. In the past, emergent nephrectomy was the standard of care, but current recommendations are for aggressive resuscitation with support of blood pressure, initiation of antibiotics, and glycemic control. Percutaneous drainage of gas pockets in conjunction with aggressive physiologic support has a mortality rate of 13.5%. Patients who do not respond to these efforts will require nephrectomy. The subset of patients who require initial nephrectomy are those with a nonfunctioning kidney. This condition may occur in renal allografts, and limited data suggests that medical management with percutaneous drainage is a viable option.

Answer: E

Al-Geizawi SM, Farney AC, Rogers J, *et al.* (2010) Renal allograft failure due to emphysematous pyelonephritis: successful non-operative management and proposed new classification scheme based on literature review. *Transplant Infectious Diseases* **12**, 543–50.

Pontin AR, Barnes RD (2009) Current management of emphysematous pyelonephritis. *Nature Reviews Urology* **6**, 272–9.

Somani BK, Nabi G, Thorpe P, *et al.* (2008) Is percutaneous drainage the new gold standard in the management of emphysematous pyelonephritis? Evidence from a systematic review. *Journal of Urology* **179**, 1844–9.

10. *A 32-year-old woman with history of right ovarian cysts presents to the emergency department with complaint of sudden onset of intense right-sided pelvic pain; she has never had this type of pain before. She denies fevers, but reports nausea and vomiting. She states that the pain radiates to the right lumbar area. Vital signs are normal. Her abdominal and pelvic exams reveal only focal tenderness in the right lower quadrant. β-human chorionic gonadotropin (HCG) is negative, the urinalysis is normal, and WBC is 8500/mm^3. Regarding further evaluation, which of the following is true regarding adnexal torsion?*

A. *The patient should undergo immediate laparoscopy*

B. *Ultrasound can rule out adnexal torsion*

C. *The absence of fever is consistent with the diagnosis*

D. *Adnexal torsion rarely occurs on the right, and this diagnosis should not be pursued*

E. *CT Scan and MRI provide no useful information with regards to the diagnosis*

Adnexal torsion may involve twisting of the ovary alone, the ovary and fallopian tube together, or the fallopian tube alone. This entity is rare in postmenopausal women. In children and adolescents, the cause is usually increased mobility of the pedicle, while in adult women a cyst is typically the precipitant. Torsion is more likely to occur on the right than the left, as the right-sided utero-ovarian ligament is longer. Some authors speculate that the presence of the sigmoid colon reduces space of the left pelvis, and decreases the likelihood of left sided torsion. Any condition that results in increased adnexal weight is a risk factor for torsion. These include ovarian cysts and tumors, corpus luteum cysts, tubal pregnancies, and hemo and hydrosalpinx. Patients undergoing ovarian stimulation for *in vitro* fertilization are at increased risk. The patients present with sudden onset of intense unilateral pelvic pain, which may radiate to the lumbar area. The pain episodes may be intermittent, if the adnexal structures spontaneously torse and detorse. Nausea and vomiting, but not fevers, are common. Physical examination may reveal the presence of a tender adnexal mass. In a patient with a negative β-HCG, adnexal torsion, pelvic inflammatory disease and even appendicitis remain in the differential. Ultrasound is the next best step, as it may identify pathologic adnexa, abscess, or appendicitis. However, it is specific but not sensitive for adnexal torsion, as pathologic adnexa may be undetected in up to 25% of cases. Doppler investigation of the presence or absence of venous or arterial flow is useful only when the flow is absent; the presence of flow does not rule out partial or intermittent torsion. A CT scan can be helpful in identifying abnormal ovaries and associated findings of loss of fat planes and ascites, but is less useful in determining ischemia. Contrast-enhanced MRI may identify nonenhancement of the ovary consistent with infarction, but this would not be helpful in early torsion. The diagnosis is definitively made with diagnostic laparoscopy. Detorsion is performed, and ischemic or necrotic appearing structures are resected. Oophoropexy is an option if the ovary appears viable.

Answer: C

Huchon C, Fauconnier A (2010) Adnexal yorsion: a literature review. *European Journal of Obstetrics and Gynecology and Reproductive Biology* **150**, 8–12.

McWilliams GDE, Hill MJ, Dietrich CS (2008) Gynecologic Emergencies. *Surgical Clinics of North America* **88**, 265–83.

Vandermeer FQ, Wong-You-Cheong JJ (2009) Imaging of Acute Pelvic Pain. *Clinical Obstetrics and Gynecology* **52** (1), 2–20.

11. *A 22-year-old woman, with past medical history remarkable only for previously treated sexually transmitted disease, presents with a complaint of acute onset of severe pelvic pain. She denies a history of trauma, and states that there is no possibility of pregnancy. She cannot recall the date of her last menses. On exam, she is mildly hypotensive; her abdomen is soft but moderately distended, and she has nonfocal pain to palpation, without peritoneal signs. Pelvic exam reveals exquisite tenderness to palpation at the left adnexa, but no cervical motion tenderness. Stat labs reveal a positive β-HCG, hemoglobin of 6 gm/dL, and normal urinalysis. Which of the following does not support the diagnosis of ruptured ectopic pregnancy as the cause of this patient's abdominal pain and anemia?*

A. *Sonographic finding of complex adnexal mass*

B. *Sonographic finding of echogenic free fluid*

C. *History of irregular vaginal bleeding*

D. *History of neck and shoulder pain*

E. *Absence of intrauterine pregnancy by ultrasound, with quantitative β-HCG of 500 mIU/mL*

Patients with ectopic pregnancy typically present with history of abdominal pain and amenorrhea. Irregular vaginal bleeding may also occur. The presence of rupture is suggested by a history of severe, stabbing pelvic pain. Irritation of the diaphragm by hemoperitoneum may also result in complaint of neck or shoulder pain. Abdominal exam is typically remarkable for ipsilateral pelvic tenderness, and bimanual exam is painful. In a hemodynamically normal patient, the diagnosis is secured with a pregnancy test and transvaginal ultrasound. The first goal of sonography is to identify the presence or absence of an intrauterine pregnancy, and this should be possible if the quantitative β-HCG is >2,000 mIU/mL. With levels of β-HCG greater than 1500 mIU/mL (and definitely 800 mIU/mL), an intrauterine gestational sac is typically detected with a normal pregnancy. Absence of an intrauterine pregnancy, along with findings of a complex adnexal mass and echogenic free fluid (blood) supports the diagnosis of ruptured ectopic pregnancy. In austere settings, culdocentesis can be used to make the diagnosis. In this procedure, the posterior lip of the cervix is retracted anteriorly, and a needle is passed parallel to the cervix through the posterior vaginal fornix in order to aspirate the posterior cul-de-sac; the presence of non-clotting blood is consistent with bleeding secondary to ruptured ectopic pregnancy. However, hypotensive patients with (+) β-HCG should be taken directly to the operating room. The decision for laparoscopy versus laparotomy rests on the comfort level of the surgeon. Either salpingostomy (opening of the salpinx), salpingotomy (opening of the salpinx followed by suture closure), or salpingectomy may be performed. Salpingectomy is indicated if needed for hemostasis, if the salpinx has had prior damage, or if the patient does not desire the option of future fertility. Risk factors for ectopic pregnancy include prior episodes of salpingitis, prior tubal surgeries, or history of assisted reproduction.

Answer: E

Cunningham FG, Leveno KJ, Bloom SL, *et al.* (2005) Ectopic pregnancy. In: Cunningham FG (ed.) *Williams Obstetrics*, 22nd edn, McGraw-Hill, New York, pp. 253–72.

McWilliams GDE, Hill MJ, Dietrich CS (2008) Gynecologic emergencies. *Surgical Clinics of North America* **88**, 265–83.

Vandermeer FQ, Wong-You-Cheong JJ (2009) Imaging of acute pelvic pain. *Clinical Obstetrics and Gynecology* **52** (1), 2–20.

12. *Regarding pelvic inflammatory disease (PID), which of the following is incorrect?*

A. *Mild-to-moderate PID may be treated on an outpatient basis*

B. *Transvaginal ultrasound has excellent specificity but poor sensitivity*

C. *Laparoscopy is the gold standard for diagnosis*

D. *Tubo-ovarian abscess is an indication for hospital admission*

E. *Surgery is indicated for tubo-ovarian abscess that fails to respond to medical therapy*

Pelvic inflammatory disease is a polymicrobial infection of the upper genital tract that typically occurs in young women of reproductive age, secondary to sexually transmitted organisms or lower genital tract flora. The symptoms may be gradual in onset, with pelvic pain and fevers being the most prominent complaints. Exam typically reveals an ill-appearing young woman, with abdominal tenderness to palpation, as well as cervical motion tenderness and bilateral adnexal tenderness on pelvic exam. Laboratories reveal leukocytosis. The diagnosis can be difficult, and requires the abdominal and pelvic exam findings, as well as one of the following secondary findings: $T > 38.3\,°C$, purulent cervical drainage, elevated erythrocyte sedimentation rate or C-reactive protein, *C. trachomatis* or *N. gonorrhoeae* cervical infection, or presence of adnexal mass on sonography. Transvaginal ultrasound has excellent specificity, and can distinguish uncomplicated PID from tubo-ovarian abscess. However, it has poor sensitivity. Oral and IV-contrasted CT scan is useful in the face of an unremarkable ultrasound. It may identify early inflammatory changes as well as delineate the architecture of the complex adnexal masses and fluid collections that comprise tubo-ovarian abscess. An MRI may be a useful alternative in the context of a pregnant patient. (β-HCG should be obtained, as early pregnancy and pelvic inflammatory disease co-exist in 3–4% of patients.) Laparoscopy is regarded as the gold standard for diagnosis. Patients with mild to moderate disease may be treated as outpatients; coverage should include agents active against *C. trachomatis* and *N. gonorrhoeae*. Tubo-ovarian abscess is an indication for hospitalization. Patients who fail to respond to medical management may be considered for percutaneous drainage. Surgical intervention is reserved for patients with life-threatening infection, ruptured tubo-ovarian abscess, or symptomatic/recurrent adnexal masses.

Answer: E

Eckert LO, Lentz GM (2007) Infections of the upper genital tract. In: Katz V (ed.) *Comprehensive Gynecology*, 5th edn, Mosby, Philadelphia PA, Chapter 23.

Lareau SM, Beigi RH (2008) Pelvic inflammatory disease and tubo-ovarian abscess. *Infectious Disease Clinics of North America* **22**, 693–708.

McWilliams GDE, Hill MJ, Dietrich CS (2008) Gynecologic emergencies. *Surgical Clinics of North America* **88**, 265–83.

Vandermeer FQ, Wong-You-Cheong JJ (2009) Imaging of acute pelvic pain. *Clinical Obstetrics and Gynecology* **52** (1), 2–20.

Chapter 43 Cardiovascular and Thoracic Surgery

Jared L. Antevil, MD and Carlos V.R. Brown, MD, FACS

1. *A 63-year-old woman is admitted to the surgical intensive care unit with acute respiratory failure two days after total hip arthroplasty. On admission, the patient is intubated and sedated with a paO_2 of 180 mm Hg on 100% FiO_2. She requires infusions of dopamine (10 μg/kg/min) and norepinephrine (20 μg/min) to maintain adequate hemodynamics. A bedside echocardiogram reveals moderate to severe right ventricular dysfunction, moderately depressed left ventricular function and no obvious intracardiac thrombus. In addition to anticoagulation, which of the following interventions would be appropriate in this patient?*

A. *Surgical or transvenous pulmonary embolectomy*

B. *Anticoagulation alone*

C. *Systemic intravenous thrombolytic therapy*

D. *Venovenous extracorporeal membrane oxygenation (ECMO)*

E. *Anticoagulation and IVC filter placement*

Immediate and aggressive anticoagulation with either intravenous unfractionated heparin or subcutaneous low-molecular-weight heparin is the mainstay of treatment for acute pulmonary embolism. By accelerating the action of circulating antithrombin III, heparin permits more rapid endogenous thrombolysis and retards the propagation of pulmonary arterial thrombus.

When associated with significant hemodynamic compromise acute pulmonary embolism (PE) carries a mortality rate in excess of 50%. Accordingly, more aggressive treatment with thrombolytic therapy or surgical embolectomy should be considered for any patient with massive PE presenting in shock. There are no large-scale prospective

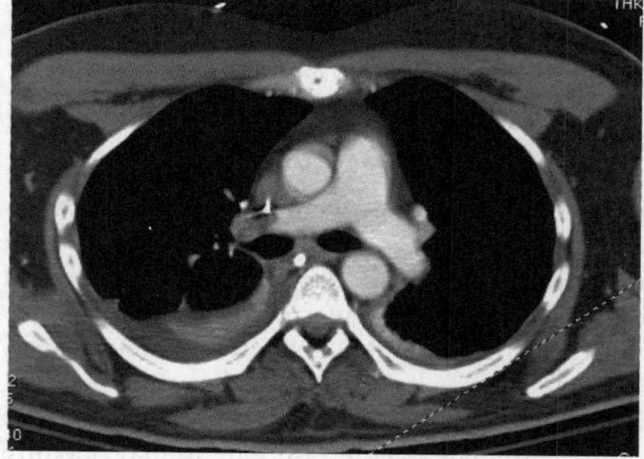

Large right pulmonary embolus on CT scan

studies demonstrating a mortality benefit for either of these modalities compared to anticoagulation alone. However, evidence from numerous case series and the high historical mortality in patients with acute PE and hypotension have led to consensus that anticoagulation alone is not optimal treatment for this small subset of patients. The use of surgical embolectomy or thrombolytics for PE patients with right ventricular dysfunction in the absence of hemodynamic instability is not well established, although these modalities may improve outcome.

The choice between thrombolysis and surgical embolectomy is controversial and often driven by institutional resources and experience. However, systemic thrombolytics are contraindicated in the setting of recent major surgery or trauma and thrombolytics introduce a significant risk of intracranial hemorrhage or other bleeding complications even in the absence of a known contraindication. More recently, catheter-based embolectomy has been reported for PE with encouraging results.

The current patient presents with a massive pulmonary embolism and hemodynamic instability after adequate resuscitation. Her recent major

Surgical Critical Care and Emergency Surgery: Clinical Questions and Answers, First Edition. Edited by Forrest O. Moore, Peter M. Rhee, Samuel A. Tisherman and Gerard J. Fulda.

orthopedic operation represents a contraindication to systemic thrombolytic treatment. If available, surgical embolectomy is indicated on an emergent basis. Percutaneous catheter-direct embolectomy would be a reasonable alternative treatment, although less well established. Importantly, surgical embolectomy is only appropriate for patients such as this with a large central thromboembolic burden. When not contraindicated, thrombolysis may have a relative advantage over embolectomy in patients with more distal or diffuse embolization.

Extracorporeal membrane oxygenation may be appropriate in select patients with massive PE and shock, with reports of its successful use as a temporary stabilizing measure to allow more definitive treatment or as a bridge to recovery by maintaining oxygenation and perfusion and unloading the right ventricle during the period of native thrombolysis. However, ECMO support for the present patient would require venoarterial rather than venovenous circuitry. Venovenous ECMO would allow for better oxygenation but would not address this patient's hemodynamic compromise.

Answer: A

Aklog L, Williams CS, Byrne JG, Goldhaber SZ (2002) Acute pulmonary embolectomy: a contemporary approach. *Circulation* **105**, 1416–19.

Buller HR, Agnelli G, Hull RD, *et al.* (2004) Antithrombotic therapy for venous thromboembolic disease: the seventh ACCP conference on antithrombotic and thrombolytic therapy. *Chest* **126**, 401S-428S.

Goldhaber SZ, Visani L, De Rosa M (1999) Acute pulmonary embolism: clinical outcomes in the International Pulmonary Embolism Registry (ICOPER). *Lancet* **353**, 1386–9.

Goldhaber SZ (1998) Pulmonary embolism. *New England Journal of Medicine* **339**, 93–104.

Hsieh C-H, Wang S-S, Ko W-J, *et al.* (2001) Successful resuscitation of acute massive pulmonary embolism with extracorporeal membrane oxygenation and open embolectomy. *Annals of Thoracic Surgery* **72**, 266–7.

Kolvekar SK, Peek GJ, Sosnowski AW, Firmin RK (1997) Extracorporeal membrane oxygenator for pulmonary embolism. *Annals of Thoracic Surgery* **64**, 883–4.

Konstantinides S, Geibel A, Olschewski M, *et al.* (1997) Association between thrombolytic treatment and the prognosis of hemodynamically stable patients with major pulmonary embolism: results of a multicenter registry. *Circulation* **96**, 882–8.

Kucher N (2007) Catheter embolectomy for acute pulmonary embolism. *Chest* **132**, 657–63.

2. *A 64-year-old diabetic, hypertensive man was admitted to the hospital with an acute ST-elevation myocardial infarction (STEMI) after emergent angioplasty and stent placement. He is being treated with aspirin, clopidogrel and subcutaneous low-molecular-weight heparin. On the third hospital day, the patient develops sudden hypotension associated with acute pulmonary edema and respiratory failure. Physical examination reveals distended neck veins, pulmonary rales, and a previously undetected prominent systolic murmur. Which of the following is/are a likely explanation for this patient's sudden hemodynamic compromise?*

A. *Ventricular free wall rupture with cardiac tamponade*

B. *Atrial septal rupture*

C. *Papillary muscle rupture with acute mitral regurgitation*

D. *Acute stent thrombosis*

E. *Stent migration*

Mechanical complications after acute myocardial infarction include papillary muscle rupture, ventricular septal rupture, and ventricular free wall rupture. The majority of patients with post-infarct mechanical complications present within two weeks of an ST-elevation myocardial infarction in the setting of anatomically limited coronary artery disease with inadequate collateral blood flow. All of these complications must be considered in any post-infarct patient presenting with new hypotension or shock, as all three mandate urgent surgical correction.

Ventricular free-wall rupture is the most common mechanical complication of acute myocardial infarction, and typically results in immediate death. In some cases, a controlled state of tamponade may ensue allowing time for emergent surgical repair. Although a patient with contained ventricular rupture and cardiac tamponade could certainly present with new hypotension and distended neck veins, pulmonary rales and a prominent systolic murmur are not typical features of patients with tamponade.

Papillary muscle rupture typically occurs in association with an inferior myocardial infarction.

Because of its acute nature, the severe mitral regurgitation seen after papillary muscle rupture is generally associated with fulminant heart failure and pulmonary edema. As opposed to atrial septal rupture, which does not occur in this setting, ventricular septal rupture after myocardial infarction results in an acute left-to-right intracardiac shunt with associated pulmonary vascular congestion and a variable degree of systemic hypoperfusion. It is associated with a new pansystolic murmur in the majority of cases.

Although acute thrombosis is a known complication of coronary stent placement and could manifest as sudden, severe left ventricular dysfunction, this would be a highly unlikely event within the first several days of stenting, particularly in a fully anticoagulated patient.

Answer: C

Reeder S (1995) Identification and treatment of complications of myocardial infarction. *Mayo Clinic Proceedings* **70**, 880–4.

3. *A 74-year-old man was admitted to the intensive care unit for unstable angina and left main coronary artery stenosis. He is presently pain free and hemodynamically stable with an intra-aortic balloon pump (IABP) in place via a right femoral arterial sheath. The patient is awaiting planned coronary artery bypass. After the patient complains of new pain in his right foot, your physical examination reveals absent right pedal pulses with an otherwise stable neurovascular examination. Appropriate intervention(s) at this point would include which of the following?*

A. *Reduction from 1:1 to 1:2 IABP pulsation*

B. *IABP removal and replacement in the left leg*

C. *Downsizing of IABP*

D. *Leave IABP in place and schedule emergent coronary artery bypass*

E. *IABP removal and immediate four-compartment fasciotomy*

Limb ischemia is the most common complication of IABP counterpulsation and is associated with significant morbidity and mortality. Other less common complications of IABP use include bleeding, paraplegia, and arterial dissection.

All patients undergoing IABP treatment must be assessed with frequent neurovascular examinations. Any significant distal pulse deficit necessitates immediate balloon pump removal. If IABP removal does not restore adequate distal perfusion, emergent bidirectional thromboembolectomy is indicated. Concomitant arterial bypass and/or limb fasciotomy may be indicated in selected cases.

Reducing the rate of IABP counterpulsation would have no effect on distal limb ischemia and is not indicated in this case. In the above clinical scenario, immediate IABP removal is indicated. If continued IABP therapy is absolutely required, the balloon pump may be placed via the contralateral femoral artery. Fasciotomy is not indicated in the absence of clinical evidence of lower extremity compartment syndrome. Emergent coronary bypass in this stable patient would be inappropriate without first addressing his acute limb ischemia.

Answer: B

Arafa OE, Pedersen TH, Svennevig JL, *et al.* (1999) Vascular complications of the intraaortic balloon pump in patients undergoing open heart operations: 15-year experience. *Annals of Thoracic Surgery* **67** (3), 645–51.

Baskett RJF, Ghali WA, Maitland A, Hirsch GM (2002) The intraaortic balloon pump in cardiac surgery. *Annals of Thoracic Surgery* **74**, 1276–87.

4. *A 64-year-old man underwent right pneumonectomy for non-small cell lung carcinoma five days earlier suddenly develops respiratory distress associated with severe tachypnea and copious frothy pink respiratory secretions. Which of the following interventions represent(s) appropriate initial treatment?*

A. *Placement of a large-bore right tube thoracostomy to 20 cm H_2O suction*

B. *Tracheostomy*

C. *Immediate reoperation*

D. *Immediate CT scan of the chest*

E. *Placement of a large-bore right tube thoracostomy to water seal*

The above description is the classic presentation for acute bronchopleural fistula (BPF) after lung resection, which occurs most frequently after right pneumonectomy. BPF after pneumonectomy indicates a loss of bronchial stump integrity. Although this is an uncommon complication, it carries a mortality in excess of 30% and demands immediate recognition and treatment.

The greatest immediate risk in a patient with early BPF after pneumonectomy is soilage of the remaining lung and subsequent aspiration pneumonia or acute lung injury. Initial treatment is therefore predicated upon immediate drainage of the affected pleural space and protection of the contralateral lung by way of either postural maneuvers or endotracheal intubation (ideally with the cuff distal to the affected bronchial stump). A tube thoracostomy after pneumonectomy should not be placed to suction until the mediastinum has stabilized (typically at about two weeks). The use of suction prior to mediastinal stabilization may result in mediastinal herniation and acute hemodynamic compromise. Immediate tube thoracostomy is indicated in the patient above, but the tube should be placed to water seal rather than suction.

After these initial measures and the initiation of broad-spectrum antibiotic therapy, bronchoscopy is performed to evaluate the degree of bronchial stump disruption and to plan appropriate treatment. Although CT scan may be a useful diagnostic adjunct in these patients after initial evaluation and treatment it has no role in the acute setting. Reoperation with reinforced closure of the fistula is likely the treatment of choice for early BPF after pneumonectomy, but should not be performed until the immediate risk of aspiration has been addressed and the patient adequately stabilized.

Answer: E

Darling GE, Abdurahman A, Yi Q-L, *et al.* (2005) Risk of a right pneumonectomy: role of bronchopleural fistula. *Annals of Thoracic Surgery* **79**, 433–7.

Hollaus PH, Huber M, Lax F, *et al.* (1999) Closure of bronchopleural fistula after pneumonectomy with a pedicled intercostal muscle flap. *European Journal of Cardiothoracic Surgery* **16**, 181–6.

Hollaus PH, Lax F, El-Nashef BB, *et al.* (1997) Natural history of bronchopleural fistula after pneumonectomy: a review of 96 cases. *Annals of Thoracic Surgery* **63**, 1391–6.

Miller JI (2005) Postsurgical empyema. In: Shields TW (ed.) *General Thoracic Surgery*, 7th edn, Wolters Kluwer, Philadelphia, PA, pp. 781–7.

Puskas JD, Mathisen DJ, Grillo HC, *et al.* (1995) Treatment strategies for bronchopleural fistula. *Journal of Thoracic Cardiovascular Surgery* **109**, 989–95.

5. *A 44-year-old man with longstanding hypertension presents to the ED with acute chest pain. CXR reveals a markedly widened mediastinum and CT scan of the chest reveals an acute aortic dissection. The cardiac surgical team is en route for planned emergent operative repair. The patient presently has a heart rate of 96 beats per minute with a systolic blood pressure of 86 mm Hg. Plausible explanations for this patient's hypotension include all of the following except:*

A. *Cardiac tamponade*

B. *Acute coronary occlusion*

C. *Free thoracic aortic rupture*

D. *Acute aortic valve insufficiency*

E. *Proximal propagation of aortic dissection*

As patients with acute aortic dissection typically present with hypertension and tachycardia, the finding of hypotension in a patient with known aortic dissection is highly suggestive of a secondary complication. Proximal propagation of an aortic dissection may lead to hemopericardium with cardiac tamponade, coronary ostial disruption with myocardial ischemia, or aortic annular dilatation with valvular insufficiency and associated malperfusion. All three of these scenarios are plausible explanations for hypotension in the above patient. Free thoracic aortic rupture would normally lead to immediate exsanguination and death.

Answer: C

Nienaber CA, Eagle KA (2003) Aortic dissection: new frontiers in diagnosis and management; part II: therapeutic management and follow-up. *Circulation* **108**, 772–8.

Reece TB, Green GR, Kron IL (2008) Aortic dissection. In: Cohn L (ed.) *Cardiac Surgery in the Adult*, 3rd edn, McGraw-Hill, New York, pp. 1195–222.

6. *A 60-year-old woman is admitted to the intensive care unit with an acute dissection limited to the descending thoracic aorta. Her admission blood pressure is 185/110 mm Hg with a heart rate of 110 beats per minute. There is no evidence of end-organ malperfusion. Which of the following would constitute appropriate management?*

A. *Immediate operative repair*

B. *Initial blood pressure control with intravenous sodium nitroprusside infusion alone*

C. *Initial blood pressure control with intravenous esmolol infusion alone*

D. *Heart rate control with intravenous infusions of amiodarone*

E. *Initial blood pressure control with nitroglycerine*

Patients with acute aortic dissection limited to the descending thoracic aorta ("Stanford" Type B, "Debakey" Type III) are treated non-surgically in the absence of rupture, malperfusion, or refractory pain. The mainstay of medical treatment for these patients is strict control of blood pressure and heart rate to reduce aortic sheer forces and minimize the risk of propagation or rupture. Beta-blockers or calcium channel blockers are the appropriate initial therapy (in addition to intravenous narcotics), with the addition of vasodilatory agents such as sodium nitroprusside for patients with persistent hypertension. The use of a pure vasodilator alone in patients with acute aortic dissection may lead to an increase in the rate of rise of aortic pressure with a concomitant increase in aortic shear stress. An infusion of nitroprusside alone would therefore not be appropriate therapy in this patient.

Answer: C

Nienaber CA, Eagle KA (2003) Aortic dissection: new frontiers in diagnosis and management; part II: therapeutic management and follow-up. *Circulation* **108**, 772–8.

Reece TB, Green GR, Kron IL (2008) Aortic dissection. In: Cohn L (ed.) *Cardiac Surgery in the Adult*, 3rd edn, McGraw-Hill, New York, pp. 1195–222.

7. *A 48-year-old woman develops new relative hypotension, oliguria and dyspnea two days after aortic valve replacement with a mechanical valve. Bedside echocardiography reveals a large pericardial effusion. Which of the following measures would constitute appropriate treatment?*

A. *Urgent bedside sub-xiphoid pericardial window*

B. *Image-guided catheter drainage of the pericardium*

C. *Urgent reoperation*

D. *Aggressive diuresis*

E. *NSAIDs*

Cardiac tamponade must be an immediate consideration in any patient with malperfusion after cardiac surgery. The risk of tamponade is increased in patients on anticoagulant medications. The echocardiogram above depicts a large pericardial effusion, confirming this diagnosis. When diagnosed and treated promptly, postoperative cardiac tamponade should not significantly affect mortality.

Early tamponade (within the first several days of surgery) is generally indicative of a surgical source of bleeding and is best addressed with an urgent reoperation. Bedside drainage would be ill-advised in a patient with early postoperative tamponade as drainage of the effusion in such patients often leads to profound hemodynamic derangement and one must be prepared to immediately address the source of bleeding. In patients with profound hemodynamic collapse or if an operating theatre is not immediately available, bedside reoperation is a treatment option. However, this operation would be approached by reopening the patient's sternotomy rather than via a subxiphoid incision.

Image-guided catheter drainage is likely the treatment of choice for patients with delayed pericardial effusion after cardiac surgery, but is not indicated for early postoperative tamponade. Diuretics have no role in the treatment of patients with postoperative tamponade.

Answer: C

Kuvin JT, Harati NA, Pandian NG, *et al.* (2002) Postoperative cardiac tamponade in the modern surgical era. *Annals of Thoracic Surgery* **74**, 1148–53.

Mangi AA, Palacios IF, Torchiana DF (2002) Catheter pericardiocentesis for delayed tamponade after cardiac valve operation. *Annals of Thoracic Surgery* 1479–83.

8. *A 22-year-old otherwise healthy man is admitted to the intensive care unit with chest pain, dyspnea and a CT scan that reveals a large anterior mediastinal mass with >50% tracheal compression. After a non-diagnostic CT-guided core biopsy, a surgical biopsy is planned. Which of the following would be appropriate anesthetic strategies for this operation?*

A. *Conventional general anesthesia with the use of inhaled agent and intravenous neuromuscular blockade*

B. *Local anesthesia with intravenous sedation*

C. *Anesthesia with neuromuscular blockers and intravenous sedation*

D. *Definitive resection using adjunctive cardiopulmonary bypass*

E. *Definitive resection using left-heart bypass*

In patients with anterior mediastinal masses, a tissue diagnosis is essential prior to resection, as lymphoma and most germ-cell tumors are not optimally treated with primary resection. Pretreatment of patients with massive anterior mediastinal masses with steroids, empiric radiotherapy or chemotherapy may alleviate airway obstruction but may also adversely affect the accuracy of subsequent tissue diagnosis. The risks of anesthesia in patients with anterior mediastinal masses can be estimated based on the presence of symptoms such as stridor, dyspnea at rest, or dyspnea in the recumbent position. Airway compression of greater than 50% on CT imaging also indicated an increased risk of airway obstruction during general anesthesia.

Muscular relaxation causes loss of chest wall tone and reduces the external support of narrowed airways. Therefore, most advocate the maintenance of spontaneous respiration and the avoidance of muscular relaxation during general anesthesia in patients with large anterior mediastinal masses. Conventional general anesthesia in the upright position followed by rigid bronchoscopy to maintain airway patency has also been advocated for these patients, although this is probably a more appropriate approach in patients for whom definitive resection rather than biopsy is planned.

Wherever possible, biopsy for large anterior mediastinal masses should be attempted under local anesthetic with intravenous sedation. Anterior mediastinotomy and biopsy for the patient above could likely be performed in this manner. If general anesthesia was felt to be required, it would optimally be performed under spontaneous ventilation without the use of paralytics. Cardiopulmonary bypass may be indicated for extreme cases in patients with massive anterior mediastinal masses, but resection of this mass without prior tissue diagnosis would not be an appropriate therapeutic strategy.

Answer: B

Goh MH, Goh YS (1999) Anterior mediastinal masses: an anaesthetic challenge. *Anaesthesia* **54**, 670–2.

Gothard JWW (2008) Anesthetic considerations for patients with anterior mediastinal masses. *Anesthesiology Clinics* **26**, 305–14.

9. *A 44-year-old man with known metastatic small-cell lung cancer is admitted to the intensive care unit with worsening hemoptysis. He has expectorated approximately 400 mL of blood over the past six hours. He was mildly hypotensive on presentation but stabilized with intravenous resuscitation. Which of the following would constitute appropriate therapeutic considerations at this time?*

A. *Emergent rigid and flexible bronchoscopy in the operating room*

B. *Emergent bronchial artery embolization (BAE)*

C. *Immediate tracheostomy*

D. *Immediate bedside flexible bronchoscopy*

E. *Thoracotomy for lung resection*

The definition of "massive" hemoptysis varies in the literature, but hemoptysis of greater than 600 mL in 24 hours is a widely accepted criterion. Certainly any patient presenting with hemoptysis and associated hypotension meets the criteria of massive hemoptysis, which is associated with a mortality rate of 25–50%. Patients with massive hemoptysis typically die of asphyxiation rather than exsanguination. Airway control is therefore of paramount importance and endotracheal intubation would be appropriate in the case above. If the source of hemoptysis is known a double-lumen endotracheal tube or bronchial blocker may be useful for temporary isolation of the bleeding source.

Bronchoscopy is indicated in all patients with hemoptysis to localize the source of bleeding and for local control. In all but the most unstable patients, bronchoscopy should be preceded by chest imaging to aid in the identification of a bleeding source. For patients with massive hemoptysis, rigid bronchoscopy is the initial procedure of choice as it allows greater suctioning ability and maintenance of airway patency compared to flexible bronchoscopy. After placement of a rigid bronchoscope (through which ventilation may be maintained), the flexible scope can be introduced to assess the more distal airways as needed. Bedside flexible bronchoscopy is not an appropriate initial procedure for a patient with massive hemoptysis. After a bleeding source is localized by rigid bronchoscopy, bleeding can often be controlled with a combination of mechanical tamponade or dilute epinephrine injection.

Bronchial artery embolization (BAE) is highly effective in the initial management of hemoptysis with control rates consistently greater than 80%. It is not indicated or effective when the source of bleeding is not from the bronchial circulation. For patients with massive hemoptysis with a known resectable source and suitable reserve, surgical resection is likely the treatment of choice, although surgery may optimally be delayed until the patient has been stabilized and airway patency ensured. Surgery would not be appropriate in a patient with a known terminal malignancy unless all available nonsurgical means for control had been exhausted.

Answer: A

Ayed A (2003) Pulmonary resection for massive hemoptysis of benign etiology. *European Journal of Thoracic Surgery* **24**, 689–93.

Endo S, Otani S, Saito N, *et al.* (2003) Management of massive hemoptysis in a thoracic surgical unit. *European Journal of Thoracic Surgery* **23**, 467–72.

Jean-Baptiste E (2000) Clinical assessment and management of massive hemoptysis. *Critical Care Medicine* **28**, 1642–7.

Shigemura N, Wan IY, Yu SCH, *et al.* (2008) Multidisciplinary management of life-threatening massive hemoptysis: a 10-year experience. *Annals of Thoracic Surgery* **87**, 849–53.

10. *A 35-year-old woman with metastatic renal cell cancer presents with worsening dyspnea and CXR with complete opacification of the left chest. A left tube thoracostomy is placed with the immediate drainage of two liters of straw-colored pleural fluid. During preparations to replace the patient's full pleural drainage chamber for continued chest tube output, the patient develops a refractory cough, worsening tachypnea and the expectoration of copious frothy white sputum. Which of the following constitute appropriate maneuvers at this time?*

A. *Immediately clamping the patient's chest tube*

B. *Placement of a second left chest tube*

C. *Replacement of the patient's pleural drainage chamber and continued suction evacuation*

D. *Intravenous fluid challenge*

E. *None of the above*

Re-expansion pulmonary edema (RPE) is a rare complication from drainage of a large pleural effusion, but is associated with mortality as high as 20%. It may occur with lung re-expansion after pneumothorax in addition to after the drainage of a large pleural effusion, and patients with a longstanding effusion are likely at higher risk. Although expert consensus suggests limiting drainage in one setting to 1L to avoid this complication or the monitoring of pleural pressures during drainage, there is little scientific evidence to support the efficacy of these practices in reducing the risks of RPE.

Patients with RPE may experience dyspnea, pain, cough with or without pink/foamy sputum or cyanosis. Symptoms typically occur within the first two hours of lung expansion, but may be delayed by as many as 24 to 48 hours.

The mainstay of therapy for RPE is supplemental oxygen, a low threshold for mechanical ventilation with positive end-expiratory pressure, diuresis, and hemodynamic support as needed. For this patient with RPE, drainage of her pleural effusion should be immediately halted with the institution of supplemental oxygen, intravenous diuretic therapy and airway/hemodynamic support as needed. Placing an additional chest tube would have no effect on this complication.

Answer: A

Feller-Kopman D, Berkowitz D, Boiselle P, Ernst A (2007) Large-volume thoracentesis and the risk of reexpansion pulmonary edema. *Annals of Thoracic Surgery* **84**, 1656–62.

Mahfood S, Hix WR, Aaroon BL *et al.* (1997) Reexpansion pulmonary edema. *Annals of Thoracic Surgery* **63**, 1206–7.

Stawicki SP, Sarani B, Braslow BM (2008) Reexpansion pulmonary edema. *OPUS 12 Scientist* **2**, 29–31.

11. *A 22-year-old man with multi-organ injury and paraplegia due to a high-speed motor vehicle accident underwent tracheostomy ten days ago. You are called to the bedside because of a report of bright red blood from the tracheostomy site and tube, but are unable to detect any bleeding on your assessment. Appropriate diagnostic maneuvers would include which of the following?*

A. *Rigid bronchoscopy after tracheostomy removal in the operating room*

B. *Urgent angiography*

C. *Bedside examination during bag-mask ventilation after tracheostomy removal*

D. *CT Scan of the neck and chest*

E. *Flexible bronchoscopy at the bedside*

Any patient with bleeding from a tracheostomy tube after the first 48 hours of placement must be suspected of having a tracheoinnominate fistula (TIF), an uncommon but highly lethal complication of open or percutaneous tracheostomy.

An episode of transient, low-volume minor bleeding ("herald" or "sentinel" bleed), as described above, is a common feature in patients with TIF and must be addressed immediately. The diagnostic procedure of choice is flexible and/or rigid bronchoscopy in the operating room, allowing immediate subsequent repair if needed.

Angiography and CT imaging have no role in the diagnosis of TIF. Bedside tracheostomy removal without definitive airway control and preparations for an immediate operation would be contraindicated.

Answer: A

Ailawadi G (2009) Technique for managing tracheo-innominate arterial fistula. *Operative Techniques in Thoracic and Cardiovascular Surgery* **2**, 66–72.

Thorp A, Hurt TL, Kim TY, Brown L (2005) Tracheoinnominate artery fistula. A rare and often fatal complication of indwelling tracheostomy tubes. *Pediatric Emergency Care* **21**, 763–6.

12. *A 64-year-old woman presents with ongoing bright red hemorrhage from her tracheostomy tube site 14 days after percutaneous tracheostomy. Which of the following would constitute appropriate initial management?*

A. *Urgent angiography and embolization*

B. *Deflation of the tracheostomy cuff*

C. *Endotracheal intubation, tracheostomy removal and digital compression*

D. *Immediate flexible bronchoscopy*

E. *Urgent cervical exploration*

Massive bleeding from a tracheostomy site must be assumed to be associated with a tracheoinnominate fistula (TIF). The immediate goals in treating such patients involve airway protection and temporary control of active bleeding. After these initial measures, the patient should be resuscitated, blood products made available, and the patient taken to the operating room to investigate for TIF and perform definitive repair if identified.

Overinflation of the tracheostomy cuff is successful in temporarily arresting bleeding in 85% of cases. If this is unsuccessful, the inominate artery may be digitally compressed against the sternum after tracheostomy removal and endotracheal intubation. Flexible bronchoscopy prior to the use of these initial measures and transport to the operating room is not advised as it often fails to visualize the area of concern and may exacerbate bleeding by destabilizing clot.

Definitive repair after initial stabilization is approached via upper hemisternotomy or more often complete sternotomy. Cervical exploration is never indicated as it does not allow vascular control of the inominate artery prior to encountering the fistula site. Angiographic embolization is not an appropriate treatment for TIF.

Answer: C

Ailawadi G (2009) Technique for managing tracheo-innominate arterial fistula. *Operative Techniques in Thoracic and Cardiovascular Surgery* **2**, 66–72.

Thorp A, Hurt TL, Kim TY, Brown L (2005) Tracheoinnominate artery fistula. A rare and often fatal complication of indwelling tracheostomy tubes. *Pediatric Emergency Care* **21**, 763–6.

13. *A 36-year-old woman with recently diagnosed non-Hodgkin's lymphoma is awaiting planned initiation of systemic chemotherapy. In the interim, she is transferred to the intensive care unit for worsening facial and upper extremity edema, mild dyspnea and CT scan revealing a large anterior mediastinal mass. Which of the following modalities are appropriate for immediate management?*

A. *Immediate institution of chemotherapy*

B. *Immediate angiographic stent placement*

C. *Urgent surgical bypass between the inominate vein and the right atrium*

D. *Vigorous intravenous hydration*

E. *No management necessary due to collateral circulation*

Superior vena cava (SVC) syndrome is characterized by SVC obstruction due to either external compression or internal thrombus. Patients may present with edema of the head, neck and arms, with cyanosis or plethora, respiratory symptoms, or in extreme cases with signs of cerebral edema. Although this condition may present in a clinically dramatic fashion, mortality from SVC obstruction alone is extremely rare and most patients have developed significant collateral venous flow by the time of presentation.

Malignancy is the most common contemporary etiology of SVC syndrome, most often bronchogenic carcinoma or lymphoma. Benign etiologies include SVC thrombosis, mediastinal fibrosis, and complications of intravascular devices and catheters.

In the absence of hemodynamic compromise or evidence of cerebral edema, most cases of SVC syndrome associated with intrathoracic malignancy as best managed by the immediate institution of specific cancer treatment. In the case presented above, this patient's planned chemotherapy should be instituted immediately and will likely ameliorate her SVC syndrome in short order. Although of unproven benefit, steroids and diuretics are generally instituted for the initial treatment of patients with SVC syndrome.

For the rare patient with SVC syndrome presenting in extremis, endovascular therapy is very effective for treatment. Endovascular treatment is also indicated for patients with malignant SVC syndrome due to malignancy without available effective medical therapies. For the stable patient presented above, immediate invasive treatment is not indicated. Surgical bypass of the SVC is a treatment option for cases not amenable to medical or percutaneous therapies or in particular for SVC syndrome of benign etiology, for whom a durable modality is needed.

Answer: A

Cheng S (2009) Superior vena cava syndrome. A contemporary review of a historic disease. *Cardiology in Review* **17**, 16–22.

Yu JB, Wilson LD, Detterbeck FC (2008) Superior vena cava syndrome—a proposed classification system and algorithm for management. *Journal of Thoracic Oncology* **3**, 811–14.

14. *A 50-year-old man is transferred to the intensive care unit for new dyspnea and pleuritic right chest pain after an attempted right internal jugular venous catheter placement. On physical examination his respirations are rapid and labored. Right-sided breath sounds are absent. His heart rate is 126 beats per minute and his blood pressure is 88/60 mm Hg. Which of the following measures constitute appropriate immediate therapy?*

A. *Two liters warm lactated ringers*

B. *Endotracheal intubation*

C. *Portable chest radiography (CXR)*

D. *Placement of a right tube thoracostomy*

E. *Initiation of vasoactive support*

This patient's presentation is consistent with a pneumothorax related to attempted central venous line placement. The presence of tachycardia and hypotension in this setting is indicative of tension pneumothorax, a life-threatening condition requiring immediate treatment. Tension pneumothorax is a clinical diagnosis. There is no indication for a CXR prior to treatment as this would introduce an unnecessary delay in therapy.

Tension pneumothorax may be treated by needle thoracostomy with a needle or cannulae of at least 4.5 cm length (followed by tube thoracostomy) or by immediate tube thoracostomy. The patient's hypotension and respiratory distress will likely be immediately resolved by treatment of his pneumothorax. Intubation or vasoactive support would not be indicated unless the patient manifested persistent cardiopulmonary compromise after appropriate treatment of his mechanical complication.

Answer: D

Henry M, Arnold T, Harvey J (2003) BTS guidelines for the management of spontaneous pneumothorax. *Thorax* **58**, ii39–ii52.

Hoyt DB, Coimbra R, Acosta J (2007) Management of acute trauma. In: Townsend CM (ed.) *Sabiston Textbook of Surgery*, 18th edn, WB Saunders, Philadelphia, PA.

Zenergink I, Brink PR, Laupland KB, *et al.* (2008) Needle thoracostomy in the treatment of a tension pneumothorax in trauma patients: what size needle? *Journal of Trauma* **64**, 111–14.

15. *A 54-year-old diabetic man without prior cardiac disease presented to the hospital four days ago with fevers and new left arm weakness. A noncontrast CT scan of the head reveals an acute right thalamic hemorrhage. Echocardiography revealed multiple 3–5 mm vegetations on the mitral valve and severe mitral valve regurgitation. His admission blood cultures grew out Streptococcus viridans. The patient has manifested a steady hemodynamic and respiratory decline since admission. As of this morning, he required intubation and is requiring infusions of vasopressin (0.04 units/min), milronone (0.5 μg/kg/min), and escalating doses of epinephrine (currently 12 μg/min) to maintain acceptable hemodynamics. Which of the following is an appropriate course of action at this point?*

A. *Urgent mitral valve repair*

B. *Urgent mitral valve replacement with prosthetic valve*

C. *Urgent mitral valve repair with biologic valve*

D. *Continuation of intravenous antibiotics and respiratory/hemodynamic support*

E. *Mitral valve debridement only*

Approximately 50% of patients with bacterial endocarditis will require surgical treatment. Indications for surgery in endocarditis include refractory bacteremia or sepsis, recurrent embolic phenomena, congestive heart failure, and myocardial extension. Congestive heart failure from endocarditis that is severe and refractory to medical treatment is the most common indication for surgery for endocarditis, and early surgical intervention has the potential to substantially reduce mortality in this group of patients.

The patient above has evidence of cardiogenic shock due to acute severe mitral valve regurgitation from his endocarditis. This is a clear surgical indication. Mitral valve repair or replacement may be performed, although repair is preferred whenever this can be achieved in concert with the complete eradication of all infected tissues. Unfortunately this patient's acute hemorrhagic cerebrovascular accident (CVA) presents an absolute contraindication to mitral valve surgery at this time. The requirement for high-dose anticoagulation during cardiopulmonary bypass would present prohibitive risk and would likely be associated with a dismal neurological outcome.

This patient's prognosis is extremely poor but there is no role for surgery at this time. He should be treated with continued antibiotic therapy and respiratory/hemodynamic support. Given his requirement for escalating doses of inotropic and vasopressor support, IABP placement would be a reasonable adjunct (although not optimal in a patient with recent bacteremia). If he survives, surgical intervention could be contemplated after an interval of four weeks from his hemorrhagic event.

Answer: D

Feringa HHH, Shaw LJ, Poldermans D, *et al.* (2007) Mitral valve repair and replacement in endocarditis: a systematic review of literature. *Annals of Thoracic Surgery* **83**, 564–71.

Lester SJ, Wilansky S (2007) Endocarditis and associated complications. *Critical Care Medicine* **35**, S384–S391.

Prendergast BD, Tornos P (2010) Surgery for infective endocarditis. Who and when? *Circulation* **121**, 1141–52.

16. *A 68-year-old man developed a leak with sepsis and multi-organ dysfunction after sigmoid colectomy for diverticulitis. He has been ventilator-dependent for 14 days and is receiving enteral nutrition via a nasogastric (NG) tube. Over the past two days he has developed increasing pulmonary secretions, progressive abdominal distension, and loss of ventilatory volumes. Panendoscopy confirms a moderate-size tracheoesophageal fistula (TEF). Which of the following would represent appropriate management at this time?*

A. *Immediate repair by fistula division and repair of trachea and esophagus*

B. *Decompressing gastrostomy, feeding jejunostomy, placement of endotracheal tube cuff distal to fistula*

C. *Immediate esophageal exclusion/diversion*

D. *Esophagectomy and spit fistula*

E. *Observation*

Cuff-related tracheal injury due to prolonged intubation is the most common cause of acquired nonmalignant TEF. In general, this complication may be prevented by close scrutiny of endotracheal tube (ETT) and tracheostomy cuff pressures and avoiding the use of stiff, indwelling NG tubes in ventilated patients. Spontaneous fistula closure is rare.

The optimal management for most patients with acquired nonmalignant TEF is fistula division with primary repair of the trachea and esophagus and the interposition of viable tissue. In the case of more extensive TEF, tracheal resection and end-to-end anastomosis may be indicated.

However, TEF repair should only be applied in patients who can be immediately extubated after repair, as there is otherwise a prohibitive risk of recurrence or failure of repair.

Until patients with TEF can be weaned from mechanical ventilation, this complication should be treated conservatively, with placement of the ETT or tracheostomy cuff distal to the fistula site, NG tube removal, a decompressive gastrostomy, and feeding jejunostomy tube placement. Antibiotics are also appropriate. Single-stage repair is performed after the patient is weaned from mechanical ventilation.

For patients with a fistula in close proximity to the carina in whom effective distal ventilation cannot be achieved, cervical esophageal exclusion may be applied. Esophageal stenting may be an option for the management of patients with TEF, but is probably not the treatment of choice for most patients.

Answer: B

Landreneau RJ, Hazelrigg SR, Boley TM, *et al.* (1991) Management of an extensive tracheoesophageal fistula by cervical esophageal exclusion. *Chest* **99**, 777–80.

Marzelle J, Dartevelle P, Khalife J, *et al.* (1989) Surgical management of acquired post-intubation tracheoesophageal fistulas: 27 patient. *European Journal of Cardiothoracic Surgery* **3**, 499–502.

Mathisen DJ, Grillo HC, Wain JC, Hilgenberg AD (1991) Management of acquired nonmalignant tracheoesophageal fistula. *Annals of Thoracic Surgery* **52**, 759–65.

Yeh C-M, Chou C-M (2008) Early repair of acquired tracheoesophageal fistula. *Asian Cardiovascular and Thoracic Annals* **16**, 318–20.

17. *A 35-year-old man with a traumatic brain injury and dysphagia undergoes a difficult esophagogastroduodenoscopy (EGD) for placement of a percutaneous endoscopic gastrostomy (PEG) tube. Several hours after the procedure the patient develops fever, tachycardia, and crepitance in the neck. The best next steps in management include:*

A. *IV antibiotics, fluid resuscitation, contrast swallow, attempted nonoperative management*

B. *IV antibiotics, fluid resuscitation, and immediate cervical exploration*

C. *IV antibiotics, fluid resuscitation, and left thoracotomy*

D. IV antibiotics, fluid resuscitation, and right thoracotomy

E. IV antibiotics, fluid resuscitation, and laparotomy

This patient sustained a perforation of the cervical esophagus as a complication of his upper endoscopy. Esophageal perforation can result from iatrogenesis, trauma, malignancy, inflammatory process, or infection. Iatrogenic injury is the most common cause of esophageal perforation, usually as a result of an upper endoscopy. The diagnosis of esophageal perforation is suspected with history of prior esophageal instrumentation or trauma, but the diagnosis is usually confirmed with a contrast swallow.

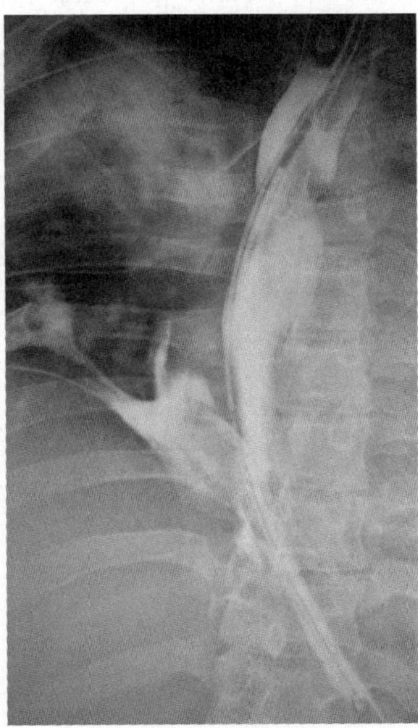

Free esophageal perforation into the right pleural cavity.

General management of esophageal perforation includes broad-spectrum intravenous antibiotics and fluid resuscitation. Decision for operative versus nonoperative management depends on several factors including location of perforation, cause of perforation, time since perforation occurred, whether or not the leak is contained, and overall status of the patient. In general, patients with a localized perforation (particularly of the cervical esophagus after instrumentation), who have the leak identified in a timely fashion and are clinically stable, are potential candidates for nonoperative management. If operative management is required the surgical approach depends on the location of perforation, and may require a cervical incision, left or right thoracotomy, or laparotomy.

Answer: A

Altorjay A, Kiss J, Bohak A (1997) Nonoperative management of esophageal perforations. Is it justified? *Annals of Surgery* **225**, 415–21.

DeMeester SR (2008) Esophageal perforation. In: Cameron JL (ed.) *Current Surgical Therapy*, 9th edn, Mosby, Philadelphia, PA, pp.16–20.

18. *A 17-year-old girl who ingests laundry bleach in a suicide attempt presents to the emergency department with oropharyngeal pain, difficulty swallowing, and excessive drooling. Management priorities include which of the following:*

A. *Placement of a nasogastric tube for activated charcoal administration.*

B. *Airway evaluation.*

C. *Ingestion of agents to neutralize or dilute the acid.*

D. *Upper endoscopy within 1–2 weeks to evaluate the extent of injury.*

E. *Neck x-rays to rule out perforation*

Caustic injuries of the esophagus usually result from an accidental ingestion in children or a suicide attempt in adults. The severity of injury to the esophagus depends on the type of agent ingested and the amount and concentration of the agent. Most common ingestions involve acid or alkaline substances, with an alkali ingestion leading to more extensive injury and associated mortality. Acids have a low viscosity leading to rapid transit time through the esophagus and cause a coagulation necrosis that causes a more superficial injury to the esophagus. In contrast, ingested alkalis cause a liquefactive necrosis and deep esophageal injury. Furthermore, alkali substances have higher viscosity, slowing transit time and prolonging exposure to the esophagus.

Clinical presentation after caustic ingestion typically includes oropharyngeal pain, dysphagia, salivation, and may include chest or abdominal pain. However, presenting symptoms are poor predictors for extent of injury. Essential in evaluation and treatment of a patient with a caustic ingestion includes early identification of the ingested agent and the amount ingested. Initial evaluation should focus on the airway by physical exam for direct visualization with laryngoscopy or fiber optic nasopharyngoscopy, and with any suspicion of airway compromise the patient should be endotracheally intubated. Further evaluation with chest or abdominal x-rays may indicate evidence of full thickness perforation. The mainstay of diagnosis and evaluation of extent of injury is early endoscopic evaluation within 12–24 hours.

Treatment for mild injury seen by endoscopy includes antibiotics, acid suppression therapy, and nutritional support if needed. Patients with moderate to severe injury seen on endoscopy require the same therapy as those with mild injury but the physician must maintain a high index of suspicion for progression of injury during the next 24–48 hours. Patients initially managed nonoperatively need a gastrograffin swallow or upper endoscopy several weeks after injury to evaluate for stricture formation. Patients with evidence of perforation require emergent surgery via thoracotomy, laparotomy, or both. Blind passage of nasogastric tubes or any attempt to neutralize or dilute the offending agent should be avoided.

Answer: B

Fischer AC (2008) Chemical esophageal injuries. In: Cameron JL (ed.) *Current Surgical Therapy*, 9th edn, Mosby, Philadelphia, PA, pp. 49–52.

Hugh TB, Kelly MD (1999) Corrosive ingestion and the surgeon. *Journal of the American College of Surgeons* **189**, 508–22.

Chapter 44 Extremes of Age: Pediatric Surgery and Geriatrics

Michael C. Madigan, MD and Gary T. Marshall, MD, FACS

1. *Which of the following is an important consideration when managing the airway of pediatric trauma patients?*

A. *The length of the trachea in children results in more left main stem intubations than in adults*

B. *The vocal cords are the narrowest portion of the pediatric airway and are commonly the site of obstruction*

C. *Cricothyroidotomy in children has a similar risk of complications as in adults*

D. *The larynx in children sits higher and more anterior than that in adults*

E. *Children have an increased functional residual capacity as compared to adults, giving them increased reserve during respiratory compromise*

Management of the pediatric airway can represent a unique set of challenges. The airway diameter in younger children is typically smaller, the larynx is higher and more anterior, the tongue is proportionally larger, and the trachea is shorter than in adults. Children's airways are relatively narrower than those of adults, leading to an increased resistance that makes them more prone to respiratory failure. The narrowest portion of the airway is at the cricoid ring as opposed to the vocal cords in adults, making this a common location for obstruction. The shortened trachea predisposes to a right mainstem intubation that is poorly tolerated in these patients. Typically, children >8 years have an airway similar to adults. Many of the same principles in airway management are similar in children, including supplemental oxygenation, suctioning, and use of oral and nasal airway adjuncts. These are, however, tailored to the pediatric airway. Infants preferentially are nasal breathers and nasal suctioning can be of great benefit. Care must be exercised in using nasal airways due to the acute angle between the nasopharynx and oropharynx. Surgical airways are avoided in children less than 12 years of age due to collapsibility of the airway and high complication rate.

Answer: D

Gaines BA, Scheidler MG, Lynch JM, Ford HR (2008) Pediatric trauma. In: Peitzman AB, Rhodes M, Schwab CW, *et al.* (eds) The Trauma Manual: Trauma and Acute Care Surgery, 3rd edn, Lippencott Williams & Wilkins, Philadelphia, PA, pp. 499–514.

Santillanes G and Gausche-Hill M (2008) Pediatric airway management. *Emergency Medical Clinics of North America* **26**, 961–75.

2. *Spinal cord injury without radiographic abnormality (SCIWORA) is characterized by which of the following?*

A. *SCIWORA injuries typically show no abnormalities on magnetic resonance imaging (MRI), which is of no benefit in predicting the prognosis of the injury*

B. *SCIWORA lesions in younger children (<9 years) often occur at higher cervical level and are more severe than SCIWORA injuries in older children (9–16 years)*

C. *A SCIWORA injury does not require further immobilization because the child is at minimal risk for a further injury since there is lack of fracture or ligamentous damage*

D. *SCIWORA is a more common injury in older children, ages 9–16 years, due to decreased elasticity of the spinal cord*

E. *The lumbar spine is the most common location for a SCIWORA injury*

Surgical Critical Care and Emergency Surgery: Clinical Questions and Answers, First Edition. Edited by Forrest O. Moore, Peter M. Rhee, Samuel A. Tisherman and Gerard J. Fulda.

SCIWORA is an injury that occurs primarily in people 17 years of age or younger, and is most common in those younger than 9 years. It was first described in 1982 as a spinal cord injury in the absence of abnormality on plain x-ray and tomography. This was prior to MR imaging as a common modality to evaluate spinal cord injury and the definition is somewhat antiquated. Patients with SCIWORA who have a normal MRI, minor hemorrhage, or edema only, have an improved prognosis compared to that predicted by the initial neurological examination. It is thought to occur through hyperextension, flexion, distraction, and spinal-cord ischemia. The hypermobility of the juvenile spinal column allows for the spinal cord to stretch beyond its ability to withstand injury. Pooled data from multiple studies estimates that 63.1% of children with spinal cord injury (SCI) age 0–9 have SCIWORA whereas 19.7% of children with SCI age 10–17 have SCIWORA. In children age 0–9, 77.5% of these injuries were classified as severe, whereas only 12.5% of injuries were severe in those 10–17 years old. Younger children also have a higher incidence of level C1–C4 injury. Although no radiographic spinal column injury instability is noted, recurrent injury has been documented up to ten weeks after initial injury prompting some to recommend three months of immobilization.

Answer: B

Pang D (2004) Spinal cord injury without radiographic abnormality in children, 2 decades later. *Neurosurgery* **55**, 1325–43.

Liao CC, Lui TN, Chen LR, *et al.* (2005) Spinal cord injury without radiological abnormality in preschool-aged children: correlation of magnetic resonance imaging findings with neurological outcomes. *Journal of Neurosurg (Pediatrics 1)* **103**, 17–23.

3. *A 6-year-old 22 kg boy who was a restrained passenger in the back seat of a car involved in a two-vehicle collision has a grade III splenic laceration. He was transiently hypotensive, requiring two fluid boluses and a single transfusion of pRBCs. Which of the volume is most appropriate?*

A. *660 mL normal saline × 2, 220 mL pRBCs*

B. *440 mL lactated Ringers × 2, 440 mL pRBCs*

C. *660 mL lactated Ringers × 2, 440 mL pRBCs*

D. *440 mL lactated Ringers × 2, 220 mL pRBCs*

E. *1000 mL normal saline × 2, 1 unit pRBCs*

The Advanced Trauma Life Support guidelines for initial adult resuscitation begins with 2L of crystalloid (either normal saline or lactated Ringers) followed by pRBC based on response to fluids and anticipation of ongoing blood loss. In contrast, fluid and pRBC resuscitation in a child is based on weight. Often, this is unknown and can be best estimated using the Breslow Pediatric Emergency Tape. Initial boluses of warm, isotonic crystalloid are given in 20 mL/kg volumes. After two boluses, packed red blood cells should be considered based on the child's response to the initial fluid volume and anticipation of ongoing bleeding. Packed red cells are given in 10 mL/kg boluses. For a 22 kg male, 22 kg × 20 mL/kg or 440 mL boluses of crystalloid plus 22 kg × 10mL/kg or 220 mL pRBCs are recommended by the 2008 ATLS guidelines as the initial transfusion. Guidelines for massive transfusion in pediatric patients are less well defined. In adults, massive transfusion can be defined by the loss of one or more circulating volume in 24 hrs, loss of half of the circulating volume in 3 h, or ongoing loss of greater than 150 mL/hr. Often, a transfusion ration of 1:1:1 (pRBCs to FFP to platelets) is used, however the optimal ratio is still under investigation.

Answer: D

Pediatric trauma (2008) In: Advanced Trauma Life Support, 8th edition. American College of Surgeons, Chicago, IL pp 225–246.

Dehmer JJ, Adamson WT (2010) Massive transfusion and blood product use in the pediatric trauma patient. *Seminars in Pediatric Surgery* **19**, 286–91.

4. *The leading cause of pediatric trauma death is . . .*

A. *Motor vehicle crash*

B. *All-terrain vehicle accident*

C. *Non-accidental trauma*

D. *Burn-related injury*

E. *Falls*

Blunt injury is much more common than penetrating injury in pediatric patients, making up approximately 86% of all injuries. The most common presenting mechanism for trauma is falls. Motor-vehicle accidents are the leading cause of pediatric deaths, followed by drownings, house fires, homicides, and falls. Similar to adults, males comprise approximately 60% of all pediatric trauma admissions.

Answer: A

Pediatric trauma (2008) In: Advanced Trauma Life Support, 8th edition. American College of Surgeons,Chicago, IL, pp 225–246.

Cooper A, Barlow B, DiScala C, String D (1994) Mortality and truncal injury: the pediatric perspective. *Journal of Pediatric Surgery* 33–8.

Guice KS, Cassidy LD, Oldham, KT (2007) Traumatic injury and children: a national assessment. *Journal of Trauma* **63**, S68–S80.

5. *Which child below would be considered hypotensive and tachycardic?*

A. 4-year-old boy with HR 148 beats/minute, SBP 69 mm Hg

B. 8-month-old girl with HR 156 beats/minute, SBP 63 mm Hg

C. 2-year-old girl with HR 149 beats/minute, SBP 73 mm Hg

D. 10-year-old boy with HR 115 beats/minute, SBP 85 mm Hg

E. 7-year-old girl with HR 116 beats/minute, SBP 84 mm Hg

When caring for pediatric trauma patients, it is important to know the ranges for normal vital signs at a given age. Of note, tachycardia is the most important early indicator of hypovolemic shock in the pediatric patient. Systolic blood pressure can give a false sense of security and may not be significantly low until almost 50% of the blood volume is lost. A 4-year-old boy should have a HR less than 140 beats/minute and a SBP >75 mm Hg.

Answer: A

Pediatric trauma (2008) In: Advanced Trauma Life Support, 8th edition. American College of Surgeons, Chicago, IL, pp 225–246.

Gaines BA, Scheidler MG, Lynch JM, Ford HR (2008) Pediatric trauma. In Peitzman AB, Rhodes M, Schwab CW, *et al.* (eds) The Trauma Manual: Trauma and Acute Care Surgery, 3rd edn, Lippencott, Williams & Wilkins, Philadelphia, PA, pp. 499–514.

6. *A 5-year-old 22 kg boy presents after falling 10 feet off a deck. He was immobilized on a spine board before transport by medics. His workup reveals a fractured left radius. The AP cervical spine film is normal and his lateral cervical spine film reveals mild anterior displacement (1 mm) of C2 on C3. His cranial nerves are intact and he has no peripheral weakness or sensory deficits. He denies pain in his neck with palpation. What is the next appropriate step in management?*

A. Flexion and extension c-spine x-rays

B. CT scan to evaluate for a missed c-spine fracture

C. MRI to evaluate for cervical spinal cord injury

D. Cervical collar immobilization and repeat x-rays in 4–6 weeks

E. Observation

An appreciation of the normal variation of c-spine anatomy is important in caring for children. Pseudosubluxation of C2 on C3 is a common variant. Reviews of normal, uninjured children reveal that this variation occurs in 22–46% of children <8 years old. A true dislocation of C2 on C3 can be differentiated from pseudosubluxation by drawing Swischuk's line. Swischuk's line is drawn along the anterior aspect of the spinous processes of C1 and C3. If the line is more than 2 mm anterior to the anterior process of C2, then it suggests a true dislocation. Because the patient has no neurological symptoms or neck pain, further x-rays or immobilization are not necessary. Routine CT in pediatric patients following trauma is not recommended unless x-ray studies are inadequate, show suspicious findings, or are abnormal. Magnetic resonance imaging would be recommended if neurological symptoms were present, x-rays were abnormal, or the c-collar could not be cleared due to neck pain or instability.

Answer: E

Easter JS, Barkin R, Rosen CL, Ban K (2010) Cervical spine injuries in children, part II: management and special considerations. *Journal of Emergency Medicine* **41** (2), 142–50.

Shaw M, Burnett H, Wilson A, Chan O (1999) Pseudosubluxation of C2 on C3 in polytraumatized children—prevalence and significance. *Clinical Radiology* **54** (6), 377–80.

7. *A 6-year-old, 25 kg girl who was a back seat passenger involved in a motor vehicle crash is diagnosed with a severe splenic laceration. Which of the following would mandate surgical exploration and splenectomy?*

A. *Tachycardia and hypotension prior to resuscitation*

B. *Transfusion requirement of 1 unit of pRBCs within the first 8 hours*

C. *Transfusion requirement of 1L of pRBCs within the first 24 hours*

D. *Grade IV or V splenic laceration on CT scan*

E. *Grade IV or V splenic laceration with blush on CT scan*

Splenic preservation has become the standard of care for management of blunt splenic injuries. Nonoperative management avoids complications associated with laparotomy as well as overwhelming postsplenectomy infection. This is most important in children less than five years of age who have a serious infection rate of greater than 10%. The risk for postsplenectomy sepsis in adults is around 1% or less. Nonoperative management of blunt splenic injury is successful in greater than 90% of all children, and is influenced by the grade if injury. Grade III injury and above has been shown to be an independent risk factor for splenectomy. Despite this, a study by Potoka *et al.* found splenic preservation to be as high as 82% for grade IV and 52% for grade V splenic injury at pediatric trauma centers. Hemodynamic instability is an absolute indication for splenectomy, but splenectomy is also indicated when blood transfusion of greater than half the blood volume (40 mL/kg) is anticipated or when other significant intra-abdominal injuries are present. A 25 kg child has an approximate blood volume of 80 mL/kg × 25 or 2 L. A transfusion requirement of 1 L of pRBCs would be a significant enough transfusion requirement to mandate splenectomy.

Answer: C

Jim J, Leonardi MJ, Cryer HG, *et al.* (2008) Management of high-grade splenic injury in children. *American Journal of Surgery* **74** (10), 988–92.

Mooney DP, Downard C, Johson S, *et al.* (2005) Physiology after pediatric splenic injury. *Journal of Trauma* **58**, 108–11.

Potoka DA, Schall LC, Ford HR (2002) Risk factors for splenectomy in children with blunt splenic trauma. *Journal of Pediatric Surgery* **37**, 294–9.

8. *A 2-year-old boy apparently fell down the stairs a few days ago. Areas of bruising of varying age are suspicious of non-accidental trauma. Which of the following actions should be taken?*

A. *Notify child protection services*

B. *Obtain a skeletal survey, CT head, and ophthalmological exam, and notify child protection services only if additional injuries are found*

C. *Consult the hospital ethics committee for advise*

D. *Notify child protection services only if the child has a history of prior visits for trauma*

E. *Defer to the child's own pediatrician who knows his full history*

Health professionals caring for pediatric trauma patients should remain on alert for potential signs of child abuse. Laws in all 50 states require the examining physician to report all suspicious cases of child abuse to the child protective services for review. Red flags include an inconsistent history, inconsistent mechanism, repeated ED visits, significant delay between injury and presentation, bruises or fractures in different stages of healing, long bone fractures in children <3 years, and multiple subdural hematomas. The workup includes an admission to the hospital, CT scan of the head, skeletal survey for patients under 2 years, optical exam for those under 3 years, and any additional studies tailored to specific clinical concern. Child protective services should be notified for all cases of suspected nonaccidental trauma. An ethics consult or a consultation with the child's pediatrician are not necessary.

Answer: A

Adamsbaum C, Mejean N, Merzoug V, Rey-Salmon C (2010) How to explore and report children with suspected non-accidental trauma. *Pediatric Radiololgy* **40**, 932–8.

Tuggle DW, Garza J (2008) Pediatric trauma. In Feliciano DV, Mattox KL, Moore EE (eds) *Trauma*, 6th edn, McGraw-Hill, New York, pp. 987–1002.

9. *An 8-year-old, 28 kg boy was shot with a stray bullet in the right chest while riding his bike. En route to the hospital he was transiently hypotensive, but responded to infusion of 1 L normal and 250 mL pRBCs. His workup in the ED has revealed a right sided hemopneumothorax for which a right-sided chest tube was placed. Approximately 600 mL of blood was evacuated from the right chest. Which of the following is the most appropriate treatment course?*

A. *Obtain a CT of the chest to further evaluate the intrathoracic injury*

B. *Transfer directly to the OR for thoracic exploration*

C. *Transfer to the ICU for close evaluation and take to the OR if bloody output exceeds 3 mL/kg over the next 4 h*

D. *Transfer to the ICU for close evaluation and take to the OR if requires more than 40 mL/kg of pRBCs within 24 h*

E. *Transfer to the ICU. Operative management would only be necessary if the child becomes hemodynamically unstable*

Penetrating thoracic trauma in the pediatric patient is a relatively infrequent occurrence. A single institutional study found the incidence to be around 1–2%. Of these, 54% ($n = 7$) required operative intervention. As with any penetrating trauma, low threshold for operative intervention should be maintained. Hemodynamic instability unresponsive to resuscitation or a significant bloody chest tube output (>15 mL/kg initially) or 2–3 mL/kg over the next 4 hours would mandate operative intervention. The above patient, greater than 28 × 15 mL/kg or 420 mL of blood would be significant enough to justify operative intervention. A CT scan of the chest in this situation would delay intervention and put the patient at risk for decompensating during the scan. If the patient had minimal chest tube output initially and was hemodynamically stable, then a CT of the chest and close observation of chest tube output, oxygenation, and hemodynamic stability in the ICU would be reasonable.

Answer: B

Peterson RJ, Tiwary AD, Kissoon N, *et al.* (1994) Pediatric penetrating thoracic trauma: a five-year experience. *Pediatric Emergency Care* **10** (3), 129–31.

Tuggle DW, Garza J (2008) Pediatric trauma. In Feliciano DV, Mattox KL, Moore EE (eds) *Trauma*, 6th edn, McGraw-Hill, New York, pp. 987–1002.

10. *Which of the following statements regarding comparing adult and pediatric nutrition is true?*

A. *Pediatric patients have a similar overall energy expenditure compared to adults*

B. *Pediatric patients have a greater energy reserve due to proportionally larger fat stores*

C. *Unlike adults, pediatric patients do not increase total energy expenditure after traumatic injury*

D. *Children are at minimal risk for gut mucosal atrophy and bacterial translocation and therefore TPN is a good alternative to enteral feeding*

E. *Pediatric patients have a lower daily protein requirement per kilogram than adults*

As with adults, optimal nutrition is an important component of treatment for pediatric trauma patients. While many of the aspects of nutritional support are similar with adults and children, some important distinctions exist. One of the main distinguishing characteristics in pediatric nutrition is that children do not increase their overall energy consumption after trauma as seen in adults. Instead, they shift their energy from growth support to the hypermetabolic response. Children also have higher baseline energy expenditure per kilogram and a higher protein requirement per kilogram compared to adults. Protein support becomes vital in children because they have a higher requirement, decreased stores, and decrease ability to tolerate protein deficiency without complications of infection, respiratory failure, and wound healing. Most recommend supplemental enteral or parenteral feedings to commence if more than three days without a diet is anticipated. As with adults, enteral feeding is recommended if it can be tolerated due to risk of central venous catheter complications, infection, and bacterial translocation from gut mucosal atrophy. It is recommended that children fed enterally have a 10% increase in calorie content due to obligate intestinal malabsorption.

Answer: C

Cook RC, Blinman TA (2010) Nutritional support of the pediatric trauma patient. *Seminars in Pediatric Surgery* **19**, 242–51.

Jaksic T (2002) Effective and efficient nutritional support for the injured child. *Surgical Clinics of North America* **82**, 379–91.

The following vignette applies to questions 11–14. A 76-year-old woman is admitted to the intensive care unit following a fall down stairs. Her injuries include a 6 mm subdural hematoma, a type II odontoid fracture, and fractures of left ribs 3–9 with moderate hemopneumothorax. On presentation, she has a blood pressure of 160/96 mm Hg, heart rate of 70 beats/minute, and oxygen saturation of 91% on 6 L of oxygen by nasal cannula. Her GCS is 14. Her medical history is significant for the use of warfarin for paroxysmal atrial fibrillation, with a presenting international normalized ratio (INR) of 3.1.

11. *All of the following statements regarding this patient's cardiovascular system are true except:*

A. *There is a significant loss of elasticity in the arterial tree during the course of normal aging with a corresponding increase in afterload*

B. *The volume of crystalloid, blood, and blood products should be minimized to avoid congestive heart failure in the elderly patient*

C. *Diastolic compliance is reduced and diastolic filling delayed*

D. *There is more than 40% chance that this patient has had unrecognized or silent myocardial infarction*

E. *Ventricular filling is more dependent on the atrial kick at the end of diastole than in the younger patient*

There are numerous age-related changes in the heart. The replacement of normal elastin fibers and the deposition of calcium contribute to progressive loss of distensibility in the arterial tree. The results in increased afterload and early transmission of pulse pressure to the coronary tree during late systole rather than diastole. Similarly, the heart itself becomes increasingly stiff. There can be as much as a 30% increase in ventricular wall thickness. The Framingham heart study found that more than 40% of subjects over the age of 75 years had silent or unrecognized ischemia. All of these factors contribute to the elderly heart being much more reliant on preload, rather than heart rate, to maintain adequate cardiac output. For this reason careful attention must be paid to adequately restore circulating volume and maintain sinus rhythm to maximize diastolic filling and cardiac output.

Answer: B

Kannel, WB, Bannenberg, AL, Abbott, RD (1985) Unrecognized myocardial infarction and hypertension: The Framingham Study. *American Heart Journal* **109**, 581–5.

London GM, Marchais SJ, Guerin AP, *et al.* (2004) Arterial stiffness: pathophysiology and clinical impact. *Clinical and Experimental Hypertension* **26**, 689–99.

Oxenham H, Sharpe N (2003) Cardiovascular aging and heart failure. *European Journal of Heart Failure* **5**, 427–34.

12. *Because of the patient's rib fractures and intracranial hemorrhage she is admitted to the ICU for close observation and treatment. A chest tube has been placed on the left and drained 200 ml of blood. She is requiring 6 L's oxygen by nasal cannula to maintain her oxygen* *saturation above 90%. Multiple rib fractures in an elderly patient:*

A. *Result in the same risk for mortality as seen in younger patients*

B. *Lead to pneumonia twice as often as in younger patients with similar injury*

C. *Usually result in mortality in the first 72 hours after injury*

D. *Result in complications with the same frequency whether epidural analgesia or opioids are used for pain control*

E. *Require significant mechanism of injury to occur*

In the geriatric population, rib fractures and other chest trauma are frequent, and can occur in two thirds of blunt injured trauma patients, and up to 35% of these may have pulmonary complications. Mechanism of injury is frequently misleading. Elderly patients with same level falls had much higher injury severity than younger patients with the same mechanism of injury, and the injury from falls is much more likely to result in death. Death from isolated chest trauma occurs late; in one study, an average of 23 days after trauma. Pneumonia is frequent in the elderly after fib fractures, occurring in nearly one-third of patients, a rate much higher than younger patients. Epidural and other regional anesthesia offers significant benefit for patients and has been shown to both reduce the number of ventilator days and the rate of pneumonia.

Answer: B

Bergeron E, Lavoie A, Clas D, *et al.* (2003) Elderly trauma patients with rib fractures are at greater risk of death and pneumonia. *Journal of Trauma* **54**, 478–85.

Bulger EM, Arneson MA, Mock CN, Jurkovich GJ (2000) Rib fractures in the elderly. *Journal of Trauma* **48** (6), 1040–6.

Bulger EM, Edwards T, Klotz P, Jurkovich GJ (2004) Epidural analgesia improves outcome after multiple rib fractures. *Surgery* **136** (2), 426–30.

13. *Despite aggressive pulmonary hygiene measures and adequate pain control she eventually progresses to respiratory failure, is intubated, and placed on mechanical ventilation. When managing mechanical ventilation in the elderly:*

A. *Position will have little effect, as the work of breathing will be the same in the supine and upright positions*

B. *Chest wall compliance will be increased due to weakening of connective tissue and loss of muscle strength*

C. *The use of positive end-expiratory pressure (PEEP) is important to overcome the greater tendency of the lungs to collapse at higher volumes*

D. *Higher tidal volumes should be used in order to overcome the loss of elasticity in the alveoli*

E. *Standard weaning parameters for extubation show the same predictive power as in younger patients*

The elderly patient has numerous changes in pulmonary physiology. Declines in vital capacity, forced expiratory volume in one second, arterial oxygen tension and maximal oxygen consumption are all clinically relevant. Chest wall compliance is also decreased in the elderly due to calcification of the ribs and spine. Upright positioning has been shown to decrease oxygen consumption compared to the sitting position. PEEP is helpful in elderly patients, as the loss of elasticity in the airways results in closure of the lung at much higher volumes. The tendency of the airways to close, and the use of high tidal volumes, results in over aeration of the healthy lung and begins a cycle of progressive lung injury and decline. Standard weaning parameters have been shown to be less accurate in predicting successful weaning from mechanical ventilation in geriatric patients.

Answer: C

Brandi LS, Bertoline R, Janni A, *et al.* (1996) Energy metabolism of thoracic surgical patients in the early postoperative period. Effect of posture. *Chest* **109**, 630–7.

Gee MH, Gottlieb JE, Albertine KH, *et al.* (1990) Physiology of aging related to outcome in the adult respiratory distress syndrome. *Journal of Applied Physiology* **69**, 822–9.

Krieger BP, Ershowsky PF, Becker DA, Gazeroglu HB (1989) Evaluation of conventional criteria for predicting successful weaning from mechanical ventilatory support in elderly patients. *Critical Care Medicine* **17**, 858–61.

14. *The patient has a subdural hematoma in the setting of warfarin use with an INR of 3.1. Which statement is most accurate for trauma patients on pre-injury warfarin?*

A. *All trauma patients on warfarin have a greater incidence of death and disability than patients with no history of warfarin use*

B. *Presenting INR and Glasgow Coma Score can be used to accurately identify patients with intracranial hemorrhage in trauma*

C. *Warfarin use is present in less than 5% of geriatric trauma patients*

D. *Rapid reversal of anticoagulation with vitamin K and fresh frozen plasma can decrease the intracranial hemorrhage progression and reduce mortality*

E. *Elderly trauma patients on warfarin with no CT evidence of intracranial hemorrhage can safely be discharged from the emergency department*

Warfarin use in elderly patients is quite common, and may be present in as many as 9% of patients presenting after trauma. Despite this, multiple studies have seen no change in mortality in the absence of traumatic intracranial hemorrhage. Intracranial hemorrhage is only reliably detected in these patients by liberal use of CT scans. The rate of significant bleeding may approach 7–14% with absent or minimal symptoms. In addition, decompensation after minor injury is common, and patients require monitoring as an inpatient for at least 24 hours, although the INR does not need to be corrected unless intracranial hemorrhage is present. In conjunction with rapid detection of injury, rapid reversal of anticoagulation with FFP has been shown to reduce expansion of the intracranial hemorrhage and reduce mortality.

Answer: D

Ivascu FA, Howells GA, Junn FS, *et al.* (2005) Rapid warfarin reversal in anticoagulated patients with traumatic intracranial hemorrhage reduces hemorrhage progression and mortality. *Journal of Trauma* **59**, 1131–9.

Li J, Brown J, Levine M (2001) Mild head injury, anticoagulants, and risk of intracranial injury. *Lancet* **357**, 771–2.

Mina AA, Bair HA, Howells GA, Bendick PJ (2003) Complications of preinjury warfarin use in the trauma patient. *Journal of Trauma* **54**, 842–7.

The following vignette applies to questions 15 and 16. An 84-year-old patient with a history of mild Alzheimer's disease was admitted to the ICU after undergoing emergent colectomy for complications of diverticular disease. He was successfully weaned from mechanical ventilation on post operative day # 2. Since extubation he has been intermittently confused and at times agitated, usually at night.

15. *Delirium in the ICU:*

A. *Is easily identified and diagnosed in the critically ill patients*

B. *Is unavoidable due to required sedation and analgesia*

C. *Is minimized by use of constant infusions of sedatives to prevent the detrimental cognitive effects of sleep loss*

D. *Is best managed by restraints and immobilization to prevent injury during exacerbations*

E. *Can be reduced by the use of gamma-aminobutyric acid (GABA) receptor sparing agents such as opioids and dexmedetomidine instead of benzodiazepines*

Answer: E

16. *Which of the following medications should be avoided in the elderly, delirious patient?*

A. *Haldol*

B. *Risperidone*

C. *Benadryl*

D. *Fentanyl*

E. *Quetiapine*

Delirium in the ICU is frequent and is often under recognized by the treatment team. The classic presentation of agitation and confusion at night makes up less than half of the patients with delirium. Daily screening measures should be employed such as the Confusion Assessment Method for the

ICU (CAM-ICU) assessment. Sedation and analgesia are, of course, required in the mechanically ventilated patient, but techniques are available to avoid delirium. Intermittent, rather than continuous infusions can result in less delirium, and the duration of the first episode may be shorter. Daily sedation interruptions are an essential part of critical care. Sleep disturbance is almost uniform in the ICU, with the average patient getting only 2 hours of sleep over 24 hours. In addition the time spent in rapid eye movement (REM) sleep is reduced. Restraints are a last resort, and should only be employed when medically needed to protect the patient and medically necessary devices. The immobilization actually contributes to delirium. Newer GABA-sparing agents such as dexmedetomidine have less incidence of delirium than benzodiazepines.

After ruling out metabolic sources of delirium, pharmacologic treatment of delirium is employed. Haldol is the recommended drug of choice for the treatment of ICU delirium by Society of Critical Care Medicine. Use of other newer antipsychotics, such as risperidone, ziprasidone and quetiapine, can be useful in the treatment of delirium, but are not as useful for treatment of acute exacerbations. Anticholinergic drugs should be avoided in elderly patients. Atypical reactions are common and can exacerbate alterations in mental status.

Answer: C

Girard TD, Pandharipande PP, Ely EW (2008) Delirium in the intensive care unit. *Critical Care* **12** (suppl. 3), S3.

Jacobi J, Fraser GL, Coursin DB, *et al.* (2002) Clinical practice guidelines for the sustained use of sedatives and analgesics in the critically ill adult. *Critical Care Medicine* **30** (1), 119–41.

Ouimet S, Kavanagh BP, Gottfried SB, Skrobik Y (2007) Incidence, risk factors and consequences of ICU delirium. *Intensive Care Medicine* **33**, 66–73.

The following vignette applies to questions 17 and 18. A 65-year-old woman has been transferred to the ICU from the surgical floor for respiratory insufficiency. She underwent repair of pelvic fractures two days ago and had been recovering well until this morning, when she became hypoxic, tachycardic and tachypnic. A presumptive diagnosis of pulmonary embolism is made, and a CT pulmonary angiogram has been ordered. She has a baseline creatinine of 1.1 mg/dL.

17. *To prevent contrast-induced nephropathy in this patient:*

A. *Normal creatinine levels indicate that renal function is preserved and no measures are needed*

B. *Dopamine should be administered to vasodilate the renal bed and promote renal function*

C. *Fluid use should be minimized prior to CT scan to prevent volume overload*

D. *Hydration with sodium chloride prior to contrast administration should be utilized*

E. *The use of antioxidants such as N-acetylcysteine is indicated*

Answer: D

18. *Following the CT scan the patient is noted to have, which eventually progresses to anuria. In an elderly patient with acute renal failure (ARF) in the ICU:*

A. *There is little chance of return to normal renal function if renal replacement therapy is required*

B. *Is most commonly due to prerenal factors*

C. *Furosemide should be administered to convert anuric renal failure to oliguric renal failure*

D. *Protein administration should be limited to prevent further damage to the kidney*

E. *Renal replacement therapy will be required in up to 85% of patients with oliguric renal failure, and should follow the same medical indications as younger patients*

The risk of contrast-induced nephropathy (CIN) is relatively low overall but the risk factors for renal dysfunction are much more prevalent in the geriatric patient, and efforts should be made to avoid this adverse effect. Creatinine should be assessed in all patients prior to administration of contrast. Normal creatinine is not always indicative of normal glomerular filtration rate and age is a determinant. Optimization of fluids and the avoidance of dehydration remain important. Additional strategies including the use of non-ionic contrast media and avoiding repeated exposures at close intervals. Numerous studies have been conducted on various other strategies. Prophylaxis with sodium bicarbonate has been shown to reduce the incidence of CIN, though the studies have been considered of poor quality. Therefore bicarbonate is currently not recommended. Vasodilators such as dopamine and fenoldopam, and antioxidants such as N-acetylcysteine have not proven to be beneficial in preventing renal dysfunction.

In the elderly, pre-renal ARF is the predominant type seen in hospitalized patients, usually secondary to dehydration. Acute tubular necrosis, however, is the most frequent cause of intrinsic ARF, and accounts for up to 76% of ARF in the in intensive care unit. Furosemide is frequently administered in an effort to increase urine output. Although urine output may be increased this does not translate into any improvement in clinical outcome or mortality, and is not recommended. The initiation of renal replacement is a complex decision, but the medical indications are the same as in younger patients, and the decision should be made according to the patient's directives. Many elderly patients, up to 57%, have complete return of renal function to baseline. The elderly are frequently malnourished and hypermetabolic in the setting of critical illness. Adequate nutrition is important to overall care and protein should not be withheld.

Answer: E

Cheung CM, Ponnusamy A, Anderton JG (2008) Management of acute renal failure in the elderly patient. *Drugs and Aging* **25** (6), 455–76.

Merten GJ, Burgess P, Gray LV (2004) Prevention of contrast-induced nephropathy with sodium bicarbonate. *JAMA* **291** (19), 2328–34.

Pannu N, Weibe N, Tonelli M, *et al.* (2006) Prophylaxis strategies for contrast-induced nephropathy. *JAMA* **295** (23), 2765–79.

Chapter 45 Telemedicine and Surgical Technology

Rifat Latifi, MD, FACS

1. *Telemedicine and telepresence can be performed though:*

A. *Local area networks (LAN) and wide area networks (WAN)*

B. *Private networks, closed or restricted networks such as a corporate network*

C. *Virtual private networks (VPN)*

D. *Wired network, network transmissions via fiber or copper cabling*

E. *All of the above*

Telemedicine requires electronic data communications networks to facilitate the exchange of patient information between two or more parties. Each network technology has its own unique features that distinguish it from other technologies. These should be carefully considered in accordance with the needs and future plans of any telemedicine program. The type of network that is needed will depend on the specific needs for the telemedicine service, but bandwidth, security, and mobility requirements, the initial and recurring costs of the network, and in some cases, the distances between networked locations, are important factors. There are numerous networks that make possible completion of telemedicine programs

Answer: E

Hadeed HG, Holcomb M, Latifi R (2010) Communication Technologies—An Overview of Telemedicine Connectivity. In Latifi R (ed.) *Telemedicine for Trauma, Emergency and Disaster Management*, Artech, Norwich, MA. pp 37–52.

SNMPTools.net *Network Basics: LAN, WAN, VPN*, http://www.snmptools.net/netbasics/lanwan/ (accessed February, 2010).

2. *Telesurgery has evolved to an important field of telemedicine as we know it today, and involves surgical telementoring, teleproctoring and other education activities as well as actual performance of the operation at the distance. Which of the following statement is not true?*

A. *Several studies have demonstrated the practicality, effectiveness and safety of surgical telementoring*

B. *Two- and three-dimensional video-based laparoscopic procedures, are an ideal platform for real-time transmission, and development of telesurgery*

C. *An experienced surgeon at a remote site can be safely guided and supervised by an expert*

D. *When comparing the traditional presence of the mentor with "telepresence" of the mentor from the distance, there are no significant differences in the performances of the operating surgeons or in outcomes of the operations*

E. *Laparoscopic training cannot be done via distance*

Real-time interactive long-distance teaching of surgical techniques was performed many decades ago but it was not until the late 1990s that telesurgical mentoring was reported as feasible, useful and acceptable teaching technique and practice. As advances in technologies and communications progressed, telesurgery was popularized by "live demonstrations" at many of the various annual surgical societies meetings, supported by industry and commercially available surgical systems. Now we are at the point where telesurgery has expanded and one can see this in the literature reports from educational and clinical telesurgical programs around the world. This is a remarkable progress in surgery and medicine overall, but we have still

Surgical Critical Care and Emergency Surgery: Clinical Questions and Answers, First Edition. Edited by Forrest O. Moore, Peter M. Rhee, Samuel A. Tisherman and Gerard J. Fulda.

a long road ahead of us before we can declare telesurgery as a common practice in our professional lives. This is despite that fact that numerous studies have demonstrated that an inexperienced surgeon at a remote site can be safely guided and supervised by an expert, and when comparing the traditional presence of the mentor with "telepresence" of the mentor from the distance there are no significant differences in the performances of the operating surgeons or in outcomes of the operations. Furthermore, the safety and potential cost-effectiveness of advanced training in laparoscopic procedures from the distance was demonstrated. An experienced surgeon can guide a less experienced surgeon to perform advanced laparoscopic procedures using simple technologies such as the telephone with a baud of 12 kbps even from extreme conditions. While the real long-term value of application of telementoring is not established, this represents a new means of educating surgeons throughout the world in the latest surgical practices and technology. Accordingly, these and other studies have led to establishment of clinical telesurgical programs for real rural world.

Answer: E

Anvari M, McKinley C, Stein H (2005) establishment of world's first telerobotic surgical service: for provision of advanced laparoscopic surgery in a rural community. *Annals of Surgery* **241**, 460–4.

Bauer JJ, Lee BR, Bishoff JT, *et al.* (2000) International surgical telementoring using a robotic arm: our experience. *Telemedicine Journal* **6**, 25–31.

Cubano M, Poulose B, Talamini M, *et al.* (1999) Long distance telementoring: A novel tool for laparoscopy aboard the *USS Abraham Lincoln. Surgical Endosccopy* **13**, 673–8.

Janetschek G, Bartsch G, Kavoussi LR (1998) Transcontinental interactive laparoscopic telesurgery between the United States and Europe. *Journal of Urology* **160**, 1413.

Lee BR, Bishoff JT, Janetschek G, *et al.* (1998) A novel method of surgical instruction: international telementoring. *World Journal of Urology* **16**, 367–70.

Lee BR, Png DJ, Liew L, *et al.* (2000) Laparoscopic telesurgery between the United States and Singapore. *Annals, Academy of Medicine, Singapore* **29**, 665–8.

Marescaux J, Leroy J, Rubino F, *et al.* (2002) Transcontinental robot-assisted remote telesurgery; feasibility and potential applications. *American Journal of Surgery* **235**, 487–92.

Rosser J, Bell R, Harnett B, *et al.* (1999) Use of mobile low-bandwidth telemedical techniques for extreme telemedicine applications. *Journal of American College of Surgeons* **189**, 397–404.

Rosser J, Gabriel N, Herman B, *et al.* (2001) Telementoring and teleproctoring. *World Journal of Surgery* **25**, 1438–48.

3. *Which of the following is true regarding virtual intensive care?*

A. *The critical care specialist is confined in the intensive care unit of the hospital*

B. *There is no need for nursing staff*

C. *There is better compliance with evidence based medicine and guideline compliance using telemedicine and e-health tools*

D. *It is not expensive and has become very common practice already*

E. *Most common technology is "open source."*

Telemedicine application in the intensive care units has become a reality in many institutions in the USA. There are multiple reports that suggest better compliance with evidence-based medical guidelines and protocols when a centralized telemedicine process is in place. In one study, a remote care program used intensivists and physician extenders to provided supplemental monitoring and management of ICU patients for 19 h/day (noon to 7 a.m.) from a centralized, off-site facility (eICU). Supporting software, including electronic data display, physician note-writing and order-writing applications, and a computer-based decision-support tool, were available both in the ICU and at the remote site. They reported lower hospital mortality for ICU patients and ICU length of stay. In another study by the same group, lower variable costs per case and higher hospital revenues (from increased case volumes) generated financial benefits in excess of program costs were reported. The cost savings were associated with a lower incidence of complications. More recently, other studies by Thomas *et al.* and Morrison *et al.* did not demonstrate mortality benefit.

Virtual intensive care unit management is most commonly done through a proprietary technology and not an open source. The installation and running cost remain expensive.

Answer: C

Breslow, MJ, Rosenfeld, BA, Doerfler, M, *et al.* (2004) Effect of a multiple-site intensive care unit telemedicine program on clinical and economic outcomes: An alternative paradigm for intensivists staffing. *Critical Care Medicine* **32**, 31–8.

Morrison JL, Cai Q, Davis N, Yan Y, (2010) Clinical and economic outcomes of the electronic intensive care unit: Results from two community hospitals. *Critical Care Medicine* **38**, 2–8.

Rosenfeld BA, Dorman T, Breslow MJ *et al.* (2000) Intensive care unit telemedicine: alternate paradigm for providing continuous intensivists care. *Critical Care Medicine* **28** (12), 3925–31.

Thomas, EJ, Lucke JF, Wueste L, *et al.* (2009) Association of Telemedicine for Remote Monitoring of Intensive Care Patients With Mortality, Complications, and Length of Stay. *Journal of the American Medical Association* **302** (24), 2671–8.

4. *Which of the following about the telemedicine for trauma and emergency management is true?*

A. *It is performed on a secured virtual private network under Health Insurance Portability and Accountability Act (HIPAA) regulations*

B. *Should be used only amongst small hospitals in order that they can help each other*

C. *When it comes to teletrauma, HIPAA regulations do not apply*

D. *You need to complete a fellowship in telemedicine in order to be able to get privileges for telemedicine*

E. *The best technology is an open source*

Technologies used for teletrauma and telepresence vary; in a way, each of them is in a constant experimental phase. Some systems may be more feature packed than others. One element, however, is important for all such technologies: the network connectivity is the backbone. Dedicated telemedicine networks, such as the Arizona Telemedicine Program, use dedicated T1 lines for its connectivity, while others rely on a combination of technologies. Some programs use integrated services digital network (ISDN), digital subscriber lines (DSL), or cable in the home. Yet others prefer satellite, since it provides a mobile and reliable source for connectivity during times of uncertainty. It is important for reliable technology to be in place, for policies and procedures to be well rehearsed, and for all personnel to be well-versed in the use of the technology. It should be "on line" 24/7 and can be used for any other conditions. The HIPPA regulations apply as in any other patient relationship and care situation. There is no extra fellowship but training should be taken before the teletrauma is practiced. Most programs do not use an open source currently. A secured network is a must.

Answer: A

Hadeed HG, Holcomb M, Latifi R (2010) Communication Technologies—An Overview of Telemedicine Connectivity. In Latifi, R (ed.) *Telemedicine for Trauma, Emergency and Disaster Management*, Artech, Norwich MA. pp. 37–52.

5. *Which of the following describes best teletrauma?*

A. *The telepresence of trauma surgeons through the teletrauma system is unable to provide care in rural hospitals*

B. *During teletrauma sessions, experts cannot identify knowledge gaps of providers in remote areas*

C. *The acceptance of teletrauma by trauma surgeons, referring physicians, nurses, and other providers, as well as by patients, has been reported*

D. *As technology becomes friendlier and cheaper, the concepts of teletrauma, telepresence, and teleresuscitation will not be needed any more*

Recent advances in technology, coupled with the decreasing cost of equipment, have opened the door for wider adoption of teletrauma. Robust systems can now be implemented that bring the telepresence of trauma surgeons and other emergency specialists into any rural hospital emergency room, allowing definitive trauma care to begin almost immediately after a patient's arrival at a rural hospital. Trauma surgeons can now assist in the evaluation, resuscitation, and care of the patient—a process that is often difficult to accomplish over the telephone alone. The ability to completely visualize the patient in real time is invaluable, enabling first-hand assessment by the surgeon as well as constant monitoring of the patient while the emergency team is at work. Telepresence can help prevent departures from the standard of care and avoid errors experienced in low-volume rural emergency centers. The field of trauma and emergency care management is ripe with opportunities for using telemedicine as patient care is complex and time-sensitive, whereas the ability of the health care providers of a small hospital to remain equipped with the capacity, knowledge, and ability to deliver the timely care is limited.

Teletrauma may be able to prevent numerous deaths. Often, intervention, even if minor, will have a significant impact on the outcome of the patient. Teletrauma may not only be able to decrease mortality, but it may decrease the morbidity and cost associated with suboptimal (or no) care. The biggest promise of teletrauma is the transformation of the concept of intervention from the *golden hour* to the *golden minutes,* during which the patient is stabilized through appropriate teleresuscitation and then safely transported, if need be, to a trauma center. Initial experiences with teletrauma in saving lives of trauma patients, and in reducing the overall cost of trauma care have been reported. The acceptance of teletrauma by trauma surgeons, referring physicians, nurses, and other providers, as well as by patients, has been excellent. The telepresence of trauma surgeons through the teletrauma system is providing the missing segment of care in rural hospitals. Furthermore, during teletrauma sessions, experts can often identify significant knowledge gaps and the need for instituting new outreach educational programs in such hospitals. As technology becomes more user friendly and cheaper, the concepts of teletrauma, telepresence, and teleresuscitation continue to evolve and to become more integrated into the modern care of trauma and surgical patients.

Answer: C

Baker SP, Whitfield RA, O'Neil B (1987) Geographic variation from mortality from vehicle crashes. *New England Journal of Medicine* **316**, 1384–7.

Flow KM, Cunningham PRG, Foil MB (1995) Rural trauma. *Annals of Surgery* **27**, 29–39.

Latifi R, Hadeed GJ, Rhee P, *et al.* (2009) Initial experiences and outcomes of telepresence in the management of trauma and emergency surgical patients. *American Journal of Surgery* **198** (6), 905–10.

Ricci MA, Caputo M, Amour J, *et al.* (2003) Telemedicine reduces discrepancies in rural trauma care. *Telemedicine Journal and e-Health* **9**, 3–11.

Rogers F, Ricci M, Shackford S, *et al.* (2001) The use of telemedicine for real-time video consultation between trauma center and community hospital in a rural setting improves early trauma care. Preliminary results. *Journal of Trauma* **51** (6), 1037–41.

6. *Which of the following is true about real-time trauma resuscitation?*

A. *Reduces the unnecessary transport of trauma patients and may prevent preventable deaths*

B. *Does not helps with resuscitation when there is no trauma surgeon present in the remote site*

C. *Has never proved to be useful in the rural setting*

D. *Staff privileges in a remote hospital to practice telemedicine are not needed since the physician is not physically present*

E. *There is high rate of malpractice law suits in teletrauma*

The first attempt to simulate the use of telemedicine in real-time trauma resuscitation was in 1978 by Dr R. Adams Cowley, who staged a disaster exercise at Friendship Airport in Baltimore, in an aged DC-6 aircraft, using old cumbersome satellite technology. Rogers *et al.* reported their use of a teletrauma service in rural Vermont; 68% of that state's population lives in rural areas. Their initial experience with 41 teletrauma consultations was very encouraging. Of 41 patients seen via the teletrauma system, 31 were transferred to a tertiary care center. For 59% of the patients, transfer was recommended immediately, because of their critical condition; 41% of transfers were accomplished by helicopter. In three patients, teletrauma consultation was considered lifesaving. The most common recommendations from the teletrauma consultant concerned patient disposition; for example, for 15% of the patients, the consultant recommended keeping them at the referring facility. Other recommendations included suggestions for diagnostics (such as obtaining or foregoing a computed tomography scan) and for additional therapeutics (such as placement of a nasogastric tube, placement of a chest tube, or transfusion of blood). Other investigators have described various applications of teletrauma in rural settings, such as the management of orthopedic injuries, including the evaluation and treatment of extremity and pelvic injuries. In one study, 68 of 100 patients referred for teletrauma were able to remain in the rural community hospital with pelvic fractures. That outcome certainly has major cost implications, minimizing the number of costly transfers to major medical centers, increasing the use of local health-care facilities, and avoiding the array of social and financial issues involved with treating patients away from their families. The clinical accuracy of teletrauma has also been affirmed. Of our own first 59 patients evaluated, 35 (59%) were treated for trauma and 24 (41%) for general surgery. Of the 35 trauma patients, 32 (91%) suffered blunt injuries; 3 (9%), penetrating injuries. Policies and procedures need to be in place in order to practice telemedicine for trauma. Privileges, usually limited ones, must be obtained in each of the hospitals that one practices telemedicine. Today there is no report of malpractice involving telemedicine for trauma. Most commonly telemedicine for trauma is practiced between the rural hospital and urban trauma center.

Answer: A

Aucar J, Granchi T, Liscum K, *et al.* (2000) Is regionalization of trauma care using telemedicine feasible and desirable? *American Journal of Surgery* **180**, 535–9.

Duchesne, JC, Kyle, A, Simmons, J, *et al.* (2008) injury, infection, and critical care: impact of telemedicine upon rural trauma care. *Journal of Trauma* **64** (1), 92–8.

Latifi R, Peck K, Porter JM, *et al.* (2004) Telepresence and telementoring in trauma and emergency care management. In: Latifi R (ed.) *Establishing Telemedicine in Developing Countries: From Inception to Implementation,* IOS Press, Amsterdam, pp. 193–9.

Latifi R, Weinstein RS, Porter JM, *et al.* (2007) Telemedicine and telepresence for trauma and emergency care management. *Scandinavian Journal of Surgery* **96** (4), 281–9.

Latifi R, Weinstein RS, Porter JM, Ziemba M, *et al.* (2007) Telemedicine and telepresence for trauma and emergency care management. *Scandinavian Journal of Surgery* **96** (4), 281–9.

Latifi R (2008) The dos and don'ts when you establish telemedicine and e-health (not only) in developing countries. *Studies in Health Technology and Informatics* **131**, 39–44.

Maull K (2002) The Friendship Airport disaster exercise: pioneering effort in trauma telemedicine. *European Journal of Medical Research* **7** (suppl.), 48.

Rogers FB, Shackford SR, Osler TM *et al.* (1999) Rural trauma: the challenge for the next decade. *Journal of Trauma* **47**, 801–21.

Chapter 46 Statistics

Randall S. Friese, MD, MSc, FACS, FCCM

1. *All of the following are best classified as descriptive statistics except:*

A. *Z-score*

B. *Mean*

C. *Median*

D. *Mode*

E. *Standard deviation*

Statistics involves the analysis and interpretation of data with the goal of quantifying uncertainty. It can be grouped into two broad categories, descriptive and inferential (also called comparative). Descriptive statistics are used to describe a single variable, such as a baseball player's batting average or the consumer price index, while inferential statistics are used to explore the relationship between two or more variables.

Descriptive statistics include a point estimate of the measured variable as well as a measure of the variation or dispersion around that point estimate. Examples of point estimates include the mean (average), median (middle measurement in an order set of data), and mode (most frequently occurring measurement in a data set). The two most commonly employed measures of variation around point estimates are the standard deviation (SD) and the interquartile range (IQR). The standard deviation is used in conjunction with the sample mean while the IQR is used in conjunction with the sample median. Other commonly seen measures of variation are the standard error of the mean (SEM) and the confidence interval. The SEM represents the measure of variation around the point estimate of the mean of a group of sample means. This should only be used when describing the characteristics of *more than one sample*. Otherwise, the SEM should not be utilized. By convention the confidence interval is usually described at the 95% level. Fundamentally, a 95% confidence interval means that the true value of the measured variable has a 95% probability of lying within the stated interval.

A *z*-score is determined using the normal distribution and is not a descriptive statistic.

Answer: A

2. *Data generated from measurements made on an ordinal scale are best described using:*

A. *Mean and standard deviation*

B. *Median and inter-quartile range*

C. *Both*

D. *Neither*

Quantitative data are generally classified into three major types: continuous, ordinal, or categorical (also called nominal).

Continuous data are positions on a scale, such as a person's weight. These positions can be as close to one another as the user is able to discern. There is always a possible value between any other two values. Additional characteristics of continuous data include: (i) there is a constant size interval between any adjacent units on the measurement scale. (ii) continuous data have a nonarbitrary zero point enabling the conclusions that 160 pounds is twice as heavy as 80 pounds. Discrete data are a special subset of continuous data. Discrete data are recorded only as distinct values, usually integers. Due to these characteristics, the descriptive statistics of choice for point estimates and measures of variation around the point estimate for continuous (and discrete) data are mean and standard deviation, respectively.

Ordinal data express relative differences between subjects when actual numerical differences are not known, such as in rank order. An important

Surgical Critical Care and Emergency Surgery: Clinical Questions and Answers, First Edition. Edited by Forrest O. Moore, Peter M. Rhee, Samuel A. Tisherman and Gerard J. Fulda.

distinction between ordinal data and continuous data is that quantitative comparisons are not possible for ordinal data. A patient with a GCS of 12 does not have twice as severe a brain injury as a patient with a GCS of six. Due to the characteristics of ordinal data the descriptive statistics of choice for point estimates and measures of variation around the point estimate are median and inter-quartile range (IQR), respectively. The IQR is simply the 25th percentile through the 75th percentile ranking while the median is simply the 50th percentile rank.

Categorical or nominal data represent some quality or attribute that a subject possesses rather than a measured numerical value. These data may occur in any sequence and are nonorderable. Statistical methods applicable to continuous and ordinal data are not useful for categorical/nominal data. Therefore, it is important to recognize when this data type is utilized.

Answer: B

3. *A researcher wishes to study patients with papillary thyroid cancer. Since the research staff is unavailable on other days, the researcher only enrolls patients seen in the surgical endocrine clinic on the second and fourth Thursday of each month. This type of sampling from the population of all patients with papillary thyroid cancer is called a*

A. *Random sample*

B. *Probability sample*

C. *Convenience sample*

D. *Limited sample*

E. *None of the above*

The basic tenet of statistics involves inferring conclusions from multiple measurements of variables of interest. The entire collection of measurements from the variables of interest about which conclusions are drawn constitutes the population of interest. Populations of interest are infrequently small enough to allow for the inclusion of all measurements into the analysis. When populations are so large that obtaining all of the measurements of interest is unfeasible, a subset of the measurements in the population is obtained and analyzed. This subset is called a sample, and conclusions about population characteristics can be drawn from the analysis of sample characteristics.

In order to reach valid conclusions and generalizations about a population from a given sample of that population, the sample must accurately represent the population. A random sample is more likely to be representative of any given population. A random sample is one in which each member of the population has an equal and independent chance of being included in the sample. In our example above the researcher did not design a random sample because every patient with thyroid cancer seen in the surgical endocrine clinic does not have an equal chance of getting enrolled. Only those seen on certain clinic days will have an opportunity to enter the trial. This type of sample, called a convenience sample, leads to the introduction of bias into the results.

Answer: C

4. *When utilizing inferential parametric statistical methods to draw conclusions on continuous data which of the following is not a type of distribution that could apply:*

A. *Normal distribution*

B. *T-distribution*

C. *F-distribution*

D. *Binomial distribution*

E. *Chi-square distribution*

The most basic yet fundamental description of a group of observed measurements is a description of the distribution of the data. A frequency distribution, describing the proportion of sample measurements falling within intervals of interest, allows one to summarize large amounts of data by tabulating the number of times each measurement of an observation occurs.

The six distributions commonly used in statistics are the normal or Gaussian distribution, the *t*-distribution, chi-square distribution, the *F*-distribution, the binomial distribution and the Poisson distribution. Continuous data depend mostly on the normal distribution, the *t*-distribution, the *F*-distribution, and sometimes the chi-square distribution. Categorical or nominal data depend mostly on the chi-square distribution, the binomial distribution, and the Poisson distribution. Statistical tests which are dependent upon the assumption that the sample data approximates one of these probability distributions are referred to as parametric tests.

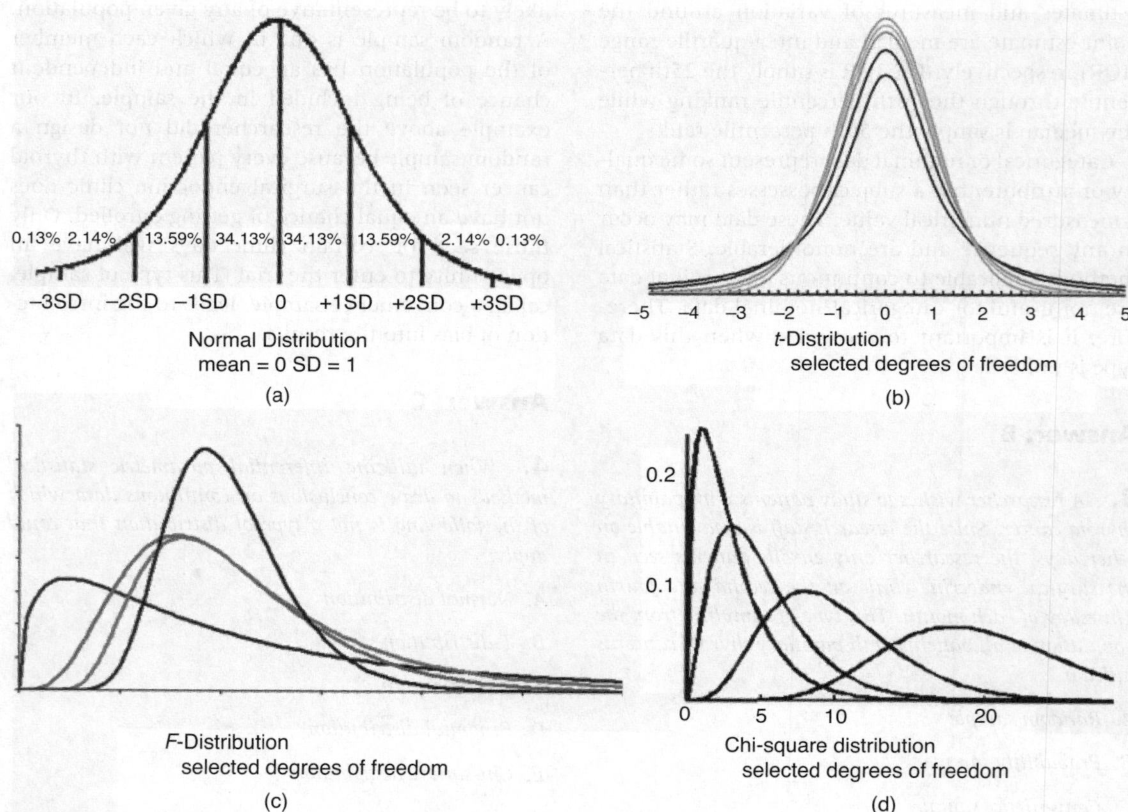

Figure 46.1 Examples of Normal or Gaussian distribution, *t*-distribution, chi-square distribution, and *F*-distribution. Figure (b) modified from www.weibull.com/DOEWeb/students_t_distribution.htm with permission from ReliaSoft Corporation. Figure (c) modified from www.vosesoftware.com/ModelRiskHelp/index.htm#Distributions/Continuous_distributions/F_distribution.htm with permission from Vose Software BVBA. Figure (d) modified from www.jrigol.com/Statistics/AboutChiSquare.htm with permission from Dr Jorge Rigol.

Answer: D

5. *Which of the following inferential statistical tests is not an example of a distribution free or nonparametric test?*

A. Mann-Whitney U

B. Kruskal-Wallis

C. ANOVA

D. Sign test

E. Wilcoxon matched pairs

When using parametric testing one makes the assumption that the sample distribution closely approximates the probability distribution of the statistical test in use. However, this assumption is frequently violated with small sample sizes, skewed data, and non-normally distributed biological data. In these cases, distribution-free tests are warranted.

In distribution free statistical testing the actual measurements themselves are not utilized in the analysis. Instead, the rank order of the measurements is used to test the null hypothesis of no difference.

Statistical tests based on the rank order of measured values are distribution free and are referred to as nonparametric analyses. ANOVA uses the *F*-distribution and is not distribution free.

Answer: C

6. *Which of the following are probabilities?*

A. Alpha

B. Beta

C. Power

D. None of the above

E. A, B, and C

Alpha (α) represents the probability that a null hypothesis, which is in fact true, will be rejected. In other words, a difference is concluded to exist when, in fact, there is none. By convention alpha is set at a maximum of 5% (0.05), meaning that there is a 5% probability that chance alone will result in an erroneous rejection of the null hypothesis. This fact is an important one to consider when performing multiple comparisons using a group of data.

Beta (β) represents the probability of not rejecting the null hypothesis when it is in fact false. In other words the investigator has failed to find a difference when one truly exists. By convention beta is set at 10% to 20% (0.10–0.20) based on the amount of resources available to the investigator. A beta of 10% will require more subjects and therefore more resources (time and money). A beta of greater than 0.20 is not acceptable.

Power (1– β) represents the probability of rejecting the null hypothesis when it is in fact false, and should be rejected. In other words, a study with a power of 0.90 has 90% probability of detecting a difference if one truly exists.

Answer: E

7. *Sometimes an error in drawing conclusions about the sampled population may occur. When the null hypothesis (no difference between groups) is incorrectly rejected, meaning a difference was determined to exist when in reality there is none, which type of error has occurred?*

A. Type I error

B. Type II error

C. Beta error

D. No error has occurred

E. Gamma error

When the null hypothesis is incorrectly rejected, a type I error has occurred. Type I error is also referred to as alpha error because it occurs at the frequency of alpha. When the null hypothesis is incorrectly retained, a type II error has occurred. Type II error is also referred to as beta error because it occurs at the frequency of beta. Type II errors are frequently due to very small effect size for the intervention or predictor variable under study as well as small sample sizes.

Answer: A

8. *Regarding sensitivity and specificity which of the following statements is incorrect?*

A. Both are conditional probabilities

B. High sensitivity means a negative result rules out disease

C. High specificity means negative result rules in disease

D. Sensitivity = true positives/(true positives + false negative)

E. Specificity = true negatives/(false positives + true negatives)

Sensitivity and specificity are conditional probabilities. The basic principle of a conditional probability is determining the probability of X given that Y is true. For sensitivity we are determining the probability of *test positive* given that *disease is present*. And for specificity we are determining the probability of *test negative* given that *disease is absent*. These conditional probabilities are determined by constructing a 2 × 2 contingency table.

		Reality (or GOLD STANDARD TEST)	
		Disease Present	*Disease Absent*
	Test (+)	True Positive (TP)	False Positive (FP)
Test Outcome	*Test (–)*	False Negative (FN)	True Negative (TN)
		Sensitivity = TP/(TP + FN)	Specificity = TN/(FP + TN)

Answer: C

9. *The positive predictive value of a screening test is the*

A. *Probability of disease present given test positive*

B. *probability of disease absent given test negative*

C. *probability of disease negative given test positive*

D. *probability of disease present given test negative*

Positive predictive value (PPV) and negative predictive value (NPV) are also conditional probabilities. For PPV we are determining the probability of *disease present* given that the *test is positive*. And for NPV we are determining the probability of *disease absent* given that the *test is negative*.

		Reality (or GOLD STANDARD TEST)		
		Disease Present	*Disease Absent*	
	Test (+)	True Positive (TP)	False Positive (FP)	PPV = TP/(TP + FP)
Test Outcome	*Test (–)*	False Negative (FN)	True Negative (TN)	NPV = TN/(FN + TN)

Answer: A

10. *Hypothesis-driven study designs include all of the following except:*

A. *Case-control studies*

B. *Cohort trials*

C. *Case series*

D. *Experimental trials*

There are three basic clinical research designs; descriptive, observational, and experimental.

The descriptive study design allows for the description of characteristics or outcomes in a single patient (case study) or a group of patients (case series). This design is not hypothesis based. There is no intervention or predictor variable (risk factor). There is no analytical plan or inferential statistical testing. However, there is a detailed use of descriptive statistics in describing patient characteristics and outcomes. This study design is very useful in that it can fully characterize diseases and their treatments, generate hypotheses to be tested in further studies, and generate estimates of effect sizes which are critical for sample size calculations for experimental trials.

Answer: C

11. *When utilizing a case-control study design the investigator is able to calculate which of the following:*

A. *Disease prevalence*

B. *Disease incidence*

C. *Effect size of an intervention*

D. *Odds ratio of a risk factor*

The case-control study design is a type of hypothesis-driven observational trial. More simply put, the case-control design is a case series with a control group. One fundamental distinction of this study design is that the cases (those with the disease under study) and controls (those without the disease under study) are drawn from two distinctly separate populations.

Samples are taken from each separate population and the presence or absence of risk factor (predictor variable) is assessed at a single point in time. The odds of the predictor variable in each group is calculated from a 2 × 2 contingency table. The odds ratio, defined as the odds of exposure given disease/odds of exposure given no disease, can then be determined.

When the odds ratio is greater than 1.0 the predictor variable (risk factor) is associated with the presence of the disease. When the odds ratio is less than 1.0, the predictor variable is associated with the nondisease state (protective). When the odds ratio is equal to 1.0 (or when the 95% confidence interval contains unity) no association exists between predictor variable and disease state. Since the data is collected from two distinct and separate populations, disease prevalence (number with disease at a single point in time) cannot be determined. Since the data is collected at one point in time disease incidence (number that develop disease over time) cannot be determined.

Answer: D

12. *All of the following statements are true regarding cross sectional study design except:*

A. *It could become a longitudinal study if data is collected over time*

B. *It allows the investigator to determine prevalence*

C. *It allows the investigator to determine incidence*

D. *Data is collected from each patient at a single point in time*

E. *Data is collected from patients belonging to a single population*

The cross sectional study design is a type of hypothesis-driven observational trial with two groups (cases and controls) coming from a single population. A major distinction of this design from the case-control design is that all subjects are recruited from a *single* population. However, the data is collected from each subject at a single point in time. In other words, the study subject is contacted only once and no follow up data collection occurs after the initial contact.

Since the two groups (cases and controls) come from the same population, disease prevalence can be determined. However, as the data collection occurs at a single point in time, disease incidence cannot be determined.

Unlike odds ratios, which give information only on the presence and directionality of an association of the predictor variable with the disease state, relative prevalence describes the magnitude of the association. In other words, if the relative prevalence is ten then exposure to the predictor variable results in a tenfold increase in disease prevalence. Additionally, if the relative prevalence is 0.50 then exposure to the predictor variable results in a 50% reduction in disease prevalence (protective effect). Similar to odds ratio the relative prevalence is reported with a 95% confidence interval. When the 95% confidence interval includes unity no change in disease prevalence occurs with exposure to the predicator variable.

Answer: C

13. *An important distinction of the cohort study design is that*

A. *It allows the investigator to determine whether an intervention causes a particular outcome*

B. *It allows the investigator to calculate the relative risk of a disease process related to exposure to a predictor variable of interest*

C. It is easier to perform (requires less resources) than a case-control study

D. It does not require Institutional Review Board approval (IRB)

E. None of the above is true of the cohort study design

The cohort study design is a type of hypothesis driven observational trial. A sample of patients is taken from a single population and baseline data is collected on the exposure to predictor variables of interest. Follow up data is later collected on the development of the outcome of interest (disease process). A major distinction of the cohort study design is that time is passing between periods of data collection allowing the investigator to determine disease incidence and relative risk. Observational study designs can only identify associations between predictor variables and outcomes. No observational study design allows the investigator to conclude causation.

Answer: B

14. *Which of the following determines group assignment in a randomized controlled (experimental) trial?*

A. The subjects themselves

B. Time

C. The investigator

D. Presence of the disease being studied

E. Presence of a risk factor being studied

The major distinction between an observational trial and an experimental trial is that in experimental trials the investigator determines group assignment for all subjects. This significant distinction allows the investigator to establish causation between the intervention and the outcome of interest. The protocol for group assignment may be randomized or nonrandomized, blinded or unblinded. However, a protocol that allows the investigator to determine group assignment directly will introduce bias into the results. The aim of randomization in group assignments is to produce equality of baseline characteristics between groups. Specifically, the only difference that should exist between the groups is the presence of the intervention in the experimental group.

Answer: C

15. *When performing a sample size calculation for an experimental trial one must take into account the limits of alpha and beta as well as which of the following:*

A. The outcome measure of interest

B. The magnitude and variability of the expected effect size of the intervention on the primary outcome

C. The magnitude and variability of the expected effect size of the intervention on the secondary outcome

D. All of the above

E. None of the above

The important considerations for sample size calculation include the limits of alpha and beta, an estimate of the magnitude and variability of the expected effect size of the intervention on the primary outcome, as well as the statistical plan (which test will be used to analyze data for the primary outcome). The limits of alpha and beta are set by convention at 0.05 and 0.10–0.20, respectively. The magnitude and variability of the effect size are estimated by the investigator based on a literature review, prior studies performed, or a pilot trial.

Answer: B

References for all questions were the following texts:

Haynes R, Sackett DL, Guyatt GH, Tugwell P (2006) *Clinical Epidemiology*, 3rd edn, Lippincott Williams & Wilkins, Philadelphia, PA.

Riffenburgh RH (1999) *Statistics in Medicine*. Academic Press, San Diego, CA.

Zar J (1999) *Biostatistical Analysis*, 4th edn, Prentice Hall, Upper Saddle River, NJ.

Chapter 47 Ethics, End-of-Life, and Organ Retrieval

Lewis J. Kaplan, MD, FACS, FCCM, FCCP and Felix Lui, MD, FACS

1. *An elderly woman is brought to the emergency department from her nursing home with obvious septic shock. She is intubated, fluid resuscitated and placed on a norepinephrine infusion. Her husband is dead and her sole surviving relative is her daughter. When the daughter arrives, she indicates that her mother would not want all of the care she is currently receiving and would wish to pursue comfort care. Which of the following principles is the care team using in pursuing the daughter's statement of her mother's wishes for comfort care?*

A. *Substituted judgment*

B. *Distributive justice*

C. *Ethical parity*

D. *Nonmalfeasance*

E. *Respect*

Since the patient is intubated, and cannot state her desires if she knew all of the information that the care team knows, one must obtain outside input. Using a family member who is more likely to understand the patient's desires is appropriate. Accepting that family member's input is termed substituted judgment. Distributive justice is the principle that applies the concept of justice across several individuals or groups of individuals instead of a single person. Ethical parity implies the equally appropriate application of ethical principles across different cultures and circumstances. Nonmalfeasance indicates a lack of wrongdoing by a public official, often in a financial undertaking. Respect is linked with the concept of autonomy, but does not address accepting another's representation of what individuals' wishes would be if they were only able to share them.

Answer: A

Thompson IE (1987) Fundamental ethical principles in healthcare. *British Medical Journal* **295**, 1461–5.

2. *A 67-year-old man has a potentially resectable colon cancer and has a tumor type that is thought to be favorably responsive to chemotherapy administration. After a lengthy discussion with you, his surgeon, he declines operative therapy as well as chemotherapy. What principle is being utilized in his decision to decline indicated and potentially life-saving therapy?*

A. *Nonrational thinking*

B. *Deontology*

C. *Autonomy*

D. *Munificence*

E. *Principlism*

This question addresses the role of patient autonomy in medical decision making. Autonomy is a key principle in Western medical ethics, which preserves a patient's ability to engage in self-determination with regard to goals of therapy, as well as diagnostic or therapeutic undertakings. If the physician believes that the patient has appropriate decisional capacity and understands the implications of the decisions being made, then respecting their informed and autonomous decision to decline medically indicated therapy is appropriate. Nonrational thinking is decision making based on obedience, imitation, feeling, desire, intuition, or habit. Deontology is rules-based decision-making. Munificence is generosity in giving and does not apply here. Principlism, generally a Western approach,

Surgical Critical Care and Emergency Surgery: Clinical Questions and Answers, First Edition. Edited by Forrest O. Moore, Peter M. Rhee, Samuel A. Tisherman and Gerard J. Fulda.

embraces beneficence, nonmaleficence, and autonomy as well as justice, and as such is too broad an answer.

Answer: C

Limentani AE (1999) The role of ethical principles in health care and the implications for ethical codes. *Journal of Medical Ethics* **25**, 394–8.

Thompson IE (1987) Fundamental ethical principles in healthcare. *British Medical Journal* **295**, 1461–65.

3. *A 24-year-old man motorcyclist arrives with a severe traumatic brain injury (TBI) and within 48 hours has an examination and supportive investigations consistent with brain death. Which of the following strategies is associated with the greatest likelihood that his family's legally authorized representative will consent to organ donation on his behalf?*

A. *A structured interview with an organ donation recipient and family*

B. *Approach and consent obtained by the physician and nurse care team*

C. *Approach and consent by the organ procurement surgeon*

D. *Combined approach by the care team and organ procurement network team*

E. *Combined approach by nursing, social service, and chaplaincy representatives*

One of the challenges in organ procurement has been obtaining consent from the legally authorized representative of a potential donor patient. Components cited as contributing to failure in obtaining consent are: lack of consistent message between clinicians, lack of an appropriately constructed message based that would render donation process easily understood, lack of understanding of organ donation in general, concerns regarding costs of organ donation, concerns regarding mutilation as well as religious concerns. Perhaps the most readily addressable set of concerns are those that address communication. A prefamily meeting "huddle" consisting of physicians, nurses, and representatives of the organ procurement organization at a minimum to discuss the best approach for a given family has been demonstrated to significantly improve consent rates. Other members of the care team may also participate in the "huddle" as needed or appropriate. Engaging a donor recipient and family is appropriate for recipients and families but not the donor family. The organ procurement surgeon is ethically constrained from participating in the consent process due to a conflict of interest.

Answer: D

Rady MY, Verheijde JL, McGregor JL (2010) Scientific, legal and ethical challenges of end-of-life organ procurement in emergency medicine. *Resuscitation* **81** (9), 1061–2.

4. *The ethical and humane treatment of prisoners of war (POW) by physicians is specifically addressed by which of the following:*

A. *Hastings Center report*

B. *Nuremberg proceedings*

C. *North Atlantic Treaty Organization*

D. *World Health Organization*

E. *Geneva Convention*

The ethical treatment of POWs is laid out in detail within the Geneva Convention. The tenets are embraced and further articulated within a variety of military field manuals as well. Physicians are specifically constrained from being active combatants but are expected to be able to defend themselves and the patients for whom they are providing care. The Geneva Convention also prohibits the deliberate attack of medical care providers, and torture of prisoners. Provision of nourishment, medical and surgical care, and humane holding conditions are also explicitly required within the document. The Hastings Center mission is to address fundamental ethical issues in the areas of health, medicine, and the environment as they affect individuals, communities, and societies. This center focuses ethical issues centered about end-of-life, public health issues and new and emerging technology. Periodic reports are generated on these topics, but not treatment of POWs. The Nuremberg

Proceedings addressed war crimes. NATO is a collection of allied countries with similar aims and who have signed mutual aid and intent treaties. The WHO is an organization that addresses world health issues. NATO and the WHO both endorse the Geneva Convention.

Answer: E

Carter BS (1994) Ethical concerns for physicians deployed to Operation Desert Storm. *Military Medicine* **159** (1), 55–9.

www.wma.net/en/30publications/10policies/c8/; accessed January 21, 2012.

5. *If one argues that principles and moral rules are not absolutely binding, but are instead prima facie, this means that the principles and moral rules are:*

A. *Self-evident and are context independent when rendering moral judgment*

B. *Duties that are binding unless in conflict with an equal or stronger duty*

C. *Unable to be equally applied across the same circumstance in different cultures*

D. *Only able to be understood within the context of virtue ethics and behavior*

E. *Rooted in Western culture and interwoven within the rules for social behavior*

Prima facie means that principles and moral rules are duties that are binding unless in conflict with an equal or stronger duty. In this way, *prima facie* recognizes that principles may come into conflict with one another and there is a context-sensitive nature to principles that may not translate from one culture to another. Therefore, *prima facie* allows one to allow contextual influences to help shape a moral judgment, instead of strictly adhering to a single set of rules. Thus, a need for overall balance is embedded in the concept of *prima facie.* Virtue ethics asserts that decision-maker characteristics are reflected in their behavior and ethics may be interpolated from a behavior set. This type of ethics implies that virtuous behavior is a type of moral excellence.

Answer: B

Limentani AE (1999) The role of ethical principles in health care and the implications for ethical codes. *Journal of Medical Ethics* **25**, 394–8.

6. *Which of the following ethical principles may be used as a justification for performing scientific and medical research?*

A. *Nonmaleficence*

B. *Distributed justice*

C. *Beneficence*

D. *Autonomy*

E. *Pluralism*

Beneficence is acting for the greater good, and implies a sense of moral and ethical correctness in the assignation of good to a particular behavior or activity. Research may be justified using this concept in that the discovery of new knowledge may be applied to others with similar conditions to enable recovery, survival, or mitigate consequences of that particular, and other related, illnesses. Nonmaleficence is different in that it constrains one from willfully doing harm. Distributed justice implies equality in a particular element in either equal share, or in proportion to need, effort, contribution or merit. Autonomy relates to an individual's right to self-determination. Pluralism is the philosophy that it is desirable and beneficial to have several distinct ethnic, religious, or cultural groups thrive within a single society. Pluralism also holds that no single explanatory or belief system may reliably and definitively account for all the phenomena of life. In this way pluralism supports many different ethical viewpoints and contextually specific moral judgments.

Answer: C

Limentani AE (1999) The role of ethical principles in health care and the implications for ethical codes. *Journal of Medical Ethics* **25**, 394–8.

Beauchamp TL, Childress JF (eds) (2009) *Principles of Biomedical Ethics,* 6th edn, Oxford University Press, New York.

7. *A patient with metastatic colorectal cancer, with symptomatic bony and brain metastases, is critically ill in the ICU with severe sepsis and impending acute respiratory failure. As the intensivist, you have a discussion with the patient regarding his goals of therapy. He states that although he is aware that he has only a limited time to live based on his malignancy, he wishes to receive intubation, mechanical ventilation and CPR if he has a pulmonary or cardiac arrest. His wife is on her way to the ICU but has not yet arrived. As the intensivist, you do not believe that those therapies are reasonable to pursue for this patient. The next most appropriate course of action is to:*

A. *Accept the patient's decisions to respect his autonomy*

B. *Enter a DNR/DNI order to respect your autonomy*

C. *Contact the hospital legal/risk management department*

D. *Discuss with the wife and accept her substituted judgment*

E. *Convene an ethics committee consultative visit*

This patient is critically ill and has brain metastasis. Therefore, his judgment may be compromised and he may not be able to appropriately interpret the consequences of his decisions. Moreover, as it is an emergency situation, asking a patient to articulate goals of therapy may be viewed as coercive. Furthermore, since you do not believe that intubation will help the patient achieve a reasonable goal, it is appropriate to discuss goals of therapy with an individual who is not in severe sepsis and with impending respiratory failure. The next most appropriate individual is his wife. Were she not alive, then the oldest son or daughter would be the next most appropriate individual. Others may have a legally authorized representative empowered by a durable healthcare power of attorney designation. Still others have a court appointed conservator when there is no kin to help make healthcare decisions—or when those who are present are unwilling or incapable of making such decisions. Accepting the goals as articulated by the most appropriate individual as those of the patient is known as substituted judgment. Substituted judgment relies on the perspective that the goals being related are those that the patient would most likely share with the care team if they were able to do so. The clinician must be careful to ensure that the goals do not instead reflect what the individual stating the goals wants for the patient, but rather what the patient would want for his or herself. Respecting autonomy also implies that the patient is competent to render a decision. Entering a DNR/SNI order to respect your autonomy is inappropriate and violates the patient's right to self-determination—either autonomously or via substituted judgment. Hospital agencies generally act to slowly to render a rapid decision regarding care, but are very helpful when there is the luxury of time to have an outside agency (not the primary healthcare team) review the case and share input regarding difficult ethical decisions.

Answer: D

Mazur DJ (2006) How successful are we at protecting preferences? Consent, informed consent, advance directives and substituted judgment. *Medical Decision Making* **26** (2), 106–9.

Seckler AB, Meier DE, Mulvihill M, Paris BE (1991) Substituted judgment: how accurate are proxy predictors? *Annals of Internal Medicine* **115** (2), 92–8.

8. *While on call at night in the ICU, one of the surgeon's brings up a patient from the OR after performing an adhesiolysis and small bowel resection for a small-bowel obstruction. The operation went smoothly and appears to have been performed in the usual fashion without complication. As the surgeon is discussing the patient with you in the ICU, it is clear to you that the surgeon's breath smells of alcohol and the surgeon appears to be intoxicated. You most appropriate course of action is to:*

A. *Have a private conversation with the surgeon once sober*

B. *Do nothing as you do not have laboratory evidence of intoxication*

C. *Immediately contact your Chairman with your concerns*

D. *Disenfranchise the surgeon from the patient's care due to incompetence*

E. *discuss your observations with the patients family to provide full disclosure*

Using the principle of nonmaleficence (do no harm), one is compelled to act in order to preserve patient safety. Operating while under the influence of alcohol is clearly unsafe, unethical and morally unsupportable. The most appropriate action is to engage the hierarchical power structure that can directly intervene to protect patient's from harm. From the standpoint of beneficence (doing good), one must also act in the surgeon's best interest as if the surgeon is operating while intoxicated, it is a powerful marker of a personal health issue. While "blowing the whistle" may be superficially construed as damaging, it is the most appropriate action to undertake from any perspective. A private conversation will not support patient safety, and nor will taking no action. One cannot unilaterally disenfranchise a surgeon from their patient's care. Providing disclosure without evidence that supports your suspicion of intoxication is also not appropriate at this time, especially if there is no direct evidence of harm.

Answer: C

Beauchamp TL, Childress JF (eds) (2009) *Principles of Biomedical Ethics*, 6th edn, Oxford University Press, New York.

9. *A 36-year-old woman was involved in a motorcycle crash two days ago. She has severe TBI and the neurosurgeon believe it to be a nonsurvivable injury. She has a physical examination that describes the absence of brain stem reflexes by two physicians, and has a transcranial Doppler assessment through an ocular insonation window that demonstrates no optic flow. Her temperature is 32.8C, HR 102 beats/minute, BP 96/42 mm Hg (MAP = 60 mm Hg), SaO_2 98% on AC/VCV and FIO_2 0.40 on fentanyl at 0.5 µg/kg/hour and midazolam at 2 mg/hour. She breathes only with the ventilator. The next most appropriate action is to:*

A. *Start a norepinephrine infusion to raise her MAP*

B. *Perform an apnea test to assess CO_2 responsivity*

C. *Disconnect her from the ventilator as she is brain dead*

D. *Obtain a radionuclide cerebral blood flow scan*

E. *Change to fentanyl and propofol to minimize sedation*

This patient may have a nonsurvivable brain injury in the neurosurgeon's opinion, but she does not meet criteria for the declaration of brain death. The absence of brainstem reflexes is supportive, but she is still on sedating agents that need to be discontinued to render the examination valid. Transcranial Doppler examination is similarly insufficient to determine cerebral blood flow as a universally agreed upon standard. Universal standards include four-vessel cerebral angiography and cerebral radionuclide scanning. There remains controversy regarding cerebral computed tomogram angiography for the declaration of brain death. One does need to be warm as well to be declared brain dead. Given the low temperature and the analgesic and sedative agents, a radionuclide scan is the most appropriate method of supporting the determination of brain death of the choices offered as it is temperature and sedative independent, unlike an apnea test—which may be significantly influenced by sedative agents. Raising the MAP will also not help address whether or not she is brain dead, and MAP manipulation is best done in conjunction with determining cerebral perfusion pressure (MAP – ICP) and there is no ICP monitor in this patient.

Answer: D

Greer DM, Straczyk D, Schwamm LH (2009) False positive CT angiography in brain death. *Neurocritical Care* **11** (2), 272–5.

Tibbalis J (2010) A critique of the apneic oxygenation test for the diagnosis of "brain death". *Pediatric Critical Care Medicine* **11** (4), 475–8.

Zuckier LS, Kolano J (2008) Radionuclide studies in the determination of brain death: criteria, concepts and controversies. *Seminars in Nuclear Medicine* **38** (4), 262–73.

10. *A patient is declared brain dead and you have shared the news with the family. It is Wednesday evening and they request that you do not remove their father from the ventilator until Saturday as they want family to arrive from across the country. However, Friday is their father's wedding anniversary and their mother died only eight months ago. Which of the following paradigms best described the basis for the family members' thought process in requesting the three-day delay?*

A. *Consequentialism*

B. *Principlism*

C. Nonrationalism

D. Virtue ethics

E. Deontologism

This patient's family is making an unsupportable request. It is superficially logically to the family but is inconsistent with appropriate medical care and legal rulings. Once one is declared brain dead then one is legally dead and may be disconnected from life support devices. The family has articulated a desire to delay disconnection, which is a nonrational request as they apparently understand that he is medically and legally dead. Nonrationalism identifies that decision and requests stem from feelings, desires, intuition, habit, obedience, or imitation. Consequentialism renders decisions based on the downstream effects of each individual decision. Principlism frames decisions within autonomy, beneficence, nonmaleficence, justice, and respect. Virtue ethics derives ethical values from the behavior of an individual who is believed to be virtuous as a kind of moral excellence. Deontologism renders ethical decisions based adherence to predefined and accepted rules.

Answer: C

Limentani AE (1999) The role of ethical principles in health care and the implications for ethical codes. *Journal of Medical Ethics* **25**, 394–8.

Thompson IE (1987) Fundamental ethical principles in healthcare. *British Medical Journal* **295**, 1461–5.

11. *A 72-year-old man is admitted to the surgical service after undergoing a left inguinal hernia as he had hypoxemia in the PACU and is now oxygen requiring. He has underlying COPD, CAD, DM and CRI (baseline creatinine 2.4); he is DNR but not DNI. You are called at 02:00 as part of your hospital's rapid response team for severe hypoxemia. When you arrive, the patient has a HR of 126 beats/minute, RR of 36 breaths/minute, A BP of 98/52 mm Hg (baseline 142/82 mm Hg) and a SaO_2 of 90% on 100% O_2 by nonrebreather while sitting bolt upright. Before proceeding with intubation, the anesthesiologist wants to obtain consent from the patient. Which of the following is the most appropriate course of action?*

A. Engage in a discussion of intubation to obtain an informed consent

B. Obtain a CXR to look for treatable causes of hypoxemia

C. Administer furosemide 80 mg IVP as well as nebulized albuterol

D. Establish phone contact with a family member to obtain consent

E. Proceed with intubation as consent in this situation is coercive

The concept of informed consent embraces a plethora of issues including the clarity and scope of the discussion, the patient's ability to comprehend the discussion, the ability of the clinician to explain the procedure, and the ability of the patient to understand the consequences of agreeing or disagreeing to the intended procedure. Truly informed consent must allow for adequate time for questions, answers, discussion, and perhaps reflection as well. Emergency situations such as the one described preclude that process in large part with the patient as well as with family members. It also underscores the importance of having discussions that impact goals of therapy prior to elective hospitalization and early within the course of unplanned admission. Diagnostic or therapeutic undertakings that do not immediately address impending respiratory arrest are inappropriate compared with rapid airway and work of breathing control.

Answer: E

Brendel RW, Wei MH, Schouten R, Edersheim JG (2010) An approach to selected legal issues: confidentiality, mandatory reporting, abuse and neglect, informed consent, capacity decisions, boundary issues, and malpractice claims. *Medical Clinics of North America* **94** (6), 1229–40.

12. *You are caring for an injured patient who is being nonoperatively managed for a grade II liver injury and a grade III splenic injury but who also has a right femur fracture. The orthopedic surgeon on call, and who is ready to operate on the patient, is one whom you believe is less technically and cognitively competent than any of the other surgeons who take orthopedic trauma panel call. The patient's family asks you for your opinion of* *the orthopedic surgeon who is intending to operate on their mother. Your most appropriate course of action is to:*

A. *Reassure the family that they should feel comfortable with the surgeon*

B. *State the since you are not an orthopedist, you cannot comment*

C. *Suggest that the family might want to obtain a second opinion*

D. *Find a reason to delay the OR until a better surgeon is responsible*

E. *Offer that it is their comfort with the surgeon that is important*

This question addresses both patient autonomy (the right to choose therapy and who will deliver it) and surgeon autonomy (the right to practice in an unrestricted fashion) in the setting of medical professionalism (professional conduct in patient care). Reassuring the family that "all is well" if one does not believe it to be so is patently lying and not to be condoned as appropriate behavior. Declining to comment about the surgeon since you have expertise in different aspects of the field is similarly untruthful and deceitful. Suggesting a second opinion may also infringe upon the orthopedist's practice autonomy. Delaying an indicated operation on the basis of personal bias is medically inappropriate, and morally incorrect. Therefore, the only appropriate answer is to identify that it is not your opinion that matters, but rather the family's comfort and confidence in the surgeon that is paramount. If you truly believe that the orthopedist is practicing below an acceptable standard of care, then there are performance improvement data-driven mechanisms that one may engage to evaluate performance. Engaging your hospital's peer-review process is the professional and appropriate means to address your concerns regarding the orthopedist's skill set and professional judgment.

Answer: E

Lantos J, Matlock AM, Wendler D (2011) Clinical integrity and limits to patient autonomy. *Journal of the American Medical Association* **305** (5), 495–9.

13. *A 14-year-old boy is struck by a vehicle at high speed and brought into the emergency department. On evaluation, the child has a GCS of 4, no pupillary responses and a palpable open, depressed skull fracture. While the trauma team does not feel that there is a reasonable hope of survival, the patient is intubated and resuscitated in the hopes that he could be an organ donor. Which of the following is true?*

A. *Providing futile care to the child is unethical, and all efforts should be halted*

B. *Resuscitative efforts should be provided to give the family a chance to come to terms with the prognosis and decide on organ donation*

C. *The local organ procurement organization (OPO) should be immediately called for consultation*

D. *Resuscitation should proceed with set limits to give the appearance to the family that every effort was made*

E. *The parents should be informed that their son will die and the decision left to them as to how to proceed*

The appropriateness of continuation of care is predicated on the determination of futility in further care of this patient and the intent of the actions behind those actions. Given the lack of certainty in the patient's prognosis in the acute setting, discontinuation of care would be premature at this stage. Similarly, contacting the OPO at this stage is premature as one is still engaged in actively providing care for a patient in whom the outcome is uncertain. Such contact may be construed as a conflict of interest in certain circumstances. When prognosis is definitively established, nonbeneficial procedures such as CPR may be considered in limited circumstances as a compassionate act for the benefit of the family, providing comfort and reassurance that everything possible was done for their child. For patients in whom organ transplantation is considered, the United States Uniform Anatomic Gift Act was revised in 2006 to permit the use of life support systems at or near death in order to maximize the potential for organ procurement. The revised act presumes donation intent and the use of life support systems, overriding expressed intent, but has not yet been universally adopted among all states.

Answer: B

Sachdeva R, Jefferson L, Coss-Bu J, *et al.* (1996) Resource consumption and extent of futile care among patients in a pediatric intensive care unit setting. *Journal of Pediatrics* **128** (6), 742–7.

Truog RD (2010) Is it always wrong to perform futile CPR? *New England Journal of Medicine* **362**, 477–9.

Verheijde JL, Rady MY, McGregor JL (2007) The United States Revised Uniform Anatomical Gift Act (2006): new challenges to balancing patient rights and physician responsibilities. *Philosophy, Ethics, and Humanities in Medicine* **2**, 19.

14. *During a routine preoperative chest x-ray in a 68-year-old woman, a suspicious nodule is found. The reviewing physician feels that a CT scan is warranted, and she refers her to a radiology center that her husband owns and manages. Which of the following is true?*

A. *The patient can be referred so long as the physician's financial ties are disclosed to the patient*

B. *There is no violation of conflict of interest since the physician herself has no direct financial ties to the center*

C. *The patient can referred since the center is an external facility, and regulations against self-referral only apply to internal facilities*

D. *Referring to this center is a violation of Stark laws unless no other nearby facilities exist*

E. *The physician cannot make the referral herself, but can have her physician's assistant fill out the referral*

Physician self-referral occurs when physicians refer patients to medical facilities in which they have a financial interest. Such arrangements are ethically questionable due to the potential for overutilization of medical resources and subsequently, increased healthcare costs for society. The Stark laws, enacted in 1992, state that a physician cannot refer a Medicare or Medicaid patient to a facility in which he or she (or an immediate family member) has a financial relationship. An exception to this rule exists for rural settings in which no other facility is conveniently available. A midlevel practitioner operates under the supervision of the physician within the practice and therefore is not exempt.

Answer: D

Department of Health and Human Services, Centers for Medicare & Medicaid Services (2007) 42 CFR Parts 409, 410, *et al.* Medicare Program; Proposed Revisions to Payment Policies Under the Physician Fee Schedule, and Other Part B Payment Policies for CY 2008; July 12.

Manchikanti L, McMahon EB (2007) Physician refer thyself: is Stark II, phase III the final voyage? *Pain Physician* **10** (6), 725–41.

15. *A 45-year-old man suffers a massive intracranial hemorrhage from a previously undiagnosed aneurysm and despite aggressive medical and surgical management, is deemed unsalvageable. The surgical critical care fellow has been taking care of this patient and is very involved in the discussions with the family. The family eventually decides to withdraw care and consents to organ donation. At the time of organ harvest, the transplant surgeon invites the fellow to join them in the operating room since this is a good "teaching opportunity." The fellow should do which of the following?*

A. *Accepting this could be seen as a conflict of interest, and he should therefore decline*

B. *Accept this because as a trainee, there is no conflict of interest, and this would be an educational opportunity*

C. *Accept this but as an observer only since he is a critical care fellow and not a transplant fellow*

D. *Accept but go to the operating room only with the written consent of the family*

E. *Accept and participate in the procedure since it is educational, but without informing the family*

Perceived conflict of interest can occur when there is overlap or confusion between the treating team and the transplantation team. Indeed, consent rates have been shown to be up to three times greater when an optimal request pattern was pursued, including clear separation between the treatment team and the donation requester. The surgical critical care fellow is a member of the treatment care team, and although he may not be involved in the discussion of organ donation and obtaining consent for transplantation, is at risk of appearing to have conflicting motivations.

Answer: A

Siminoff LA, Arnold RM, Hewlett J (2001) The process of organ donation and its effect on consent. *Clinical Transplantation* **15**, 39–47.

16. *A surgery resident places an enteral access catheter to provide nutritional support in an elderly, debilitated patient in the ICU. On followup chest X-ray, the catheter is found to have gone down the right mainstem bronchus and to be in the right pleural space with a large pneumothorax. The family is informed, the catheter is removed, and a chest tube is placed. The patient remains stable throughout, and the chest tube is removed five days later without complications. The family is irate and threatens to sue. Which is the best course of action?*

A. *Conduct further discussions only in the presence of the Legal department*

B. *Request the input of the hospital Ethics committee to determine the best course of action and to counsel the family*

C. *Say as little as possible since the resident was unsupervised at the time*

D. *Ignore the family's threat, since there is no medical liability due to the fact that no harm was done*

E. *Schedule a family meeting to ensure that the family is fully informed and to discuss their concerns*

Mistakes are common in medicine. Full disclosure of medical errors can be difficult due to embarrassment and concerns over legal liability and erosion of the patient-physician relationship. However, studies have shown that when a policy of full disclosure is followed, no clear increases in lawsuits or healthcare costs occur. Moreover, the provider-patient relationship is strengthened with a policy of openness and honesty. Models for medical error compensation have been proposed and may lead to decreases in overall healthcare costs.

Answer: E

Hebert PC (2001) Disclosure of adverse events and errors in healthcare: An ethical perspective. *Drug Safety* **24** (15), 1095–104.

Kachalia A, Kaufman SR, Boothman R *et al.* (2010) Liability claims and costs before and after implementation of a medical error disclosure program. *Annals of Internal Medicine* **153** (4), 213–21.

O'Connor E, Coates HM, Yardley IE *et al.* (2010) Disclosure of patient safety incidents: a comprehensive review. *International Journal for Quality in Health Care* **22** (5), 371–9.

17. *During the hernia repair of a patient with a history of IV drug use, the surgeon accidentally sticks himself with a 2-0 suture needle and breaks the skin. Which of the following is true?*

A. *Consent for HIV testing is not required, and the patient can be tested confidentially based on medical necessity*

B. *The patient may refuse to consent to testing and consent is required for HIV testing*

C. *If the patient refuses to be tested for HIV, the patient can be legally mandated to submit to testing*

D. *Nothing needs to be done since the risk of HIV transmission from non-hollow bore needlesticks is negligible*

E. *Testing of the patient without consent is allowable so long as test results are confidential and anonymous*

Testing for HIV without the patient's consent or knowledge is a violation of the patient's rights to privacy, self-determination and autonomy. Patients must have the freedom and capacity to make an informed decision regarding testing and dealing with the emotional, personal and structural consequences of an HIV-positive diagnosis. While there are no reported cases of HIV transmission from suture-related needlestick injuries, clinicians need to assess the severity of exposure and characterize the risk of HIV transmission to determine the appropriateness of anti-retroviral prophylaxis. If testing of the source patient cannot be performed, then prophylactic treatment should be initiated and serial testing of the exposed surgeon performed.

Answer: B

Centers for Disease Control and Prevention (1995) Case-control study of HIV sero-conversion in health care workers after exposure to HIV infected blood—France, United Kingdom, and United States, January 1988–August 1994. *Morbidity and Mortality Weekly Report* **44**, 929–33.

Hanssens C (2007) Legal and ethical implications of opt-out HIV testing. *Clinical Infectious Diseases* **45** (suppl 4), S232–9.

18. *At the end of a routine orthopedic procedure, a patient is accidently given a large dose of a benzodiazepine instead of the narcotic she was supposed to receive for pain. As a consequence, she was unable to be extubated at the end of the case, and was left intubated overnight. She was subsequently extubated the next morning and went home without incident. What is the best course of action?*

A. *Nothing, since prolonged recovery from anesthesia is a known complication and covered in the initial consent*

B. *The anesthesia team should fully disclose to the patient what occurred and admit that a mistake was made*

C. *Tell the family that this is a known risk of anesthesia, and that it is not uncommon after operation*

D. *It is unnecessary to inform the family, but the hospital legal department needs to be informed of the incident*

E. *The family should be told about the details of the case without admission of fault*

While the patient suffered no long-term effects from her prolonged intubation, increased length of stay and risks of sedation cannot be dismissed as expected consequences of her procedure, and can be considered harmful. Often patients and families perceive adverse effects in a more broad sense than clinicians. Full disclosure of unexpected events and medical errors fosters communication and trust in the physician-patient relationship.

Answer: B

Gallagher TH, Waterman AD, Ebers AG, *et al.* (2003) Patients' and physicians' attitudes regarding the disclosure of medical errors. *Journal of the American Medical Association* **289**, 1001–7.

Institute of Medicine (2000) *To Err Is Human: Building A Safer Health System*, National Academy Press, Washington, DC.

O'Connor E, Coates H, Yardley I, *et al.* (2010) Disclosure of patient safety incidents: a comprehensive review. *International Journal of Quality in Health Care* **22** (5), 371–9.

19. *A 12-year-old girl falls onto a glass table with a deep laceration to her thigh and loses a significant volume of blood before being found. She is brought into the emergency department tachycardic, hypotensive, and profoundly anemic. Her parents, who are Jehovah's Witnesses, refuse to consent to blood transfusion based on their religious beliefs. What is the most appropriate course of action?*

A. *Try to obtain the patient's consent to transfusion*

B. *Respect the wishes of the parents since the patient is a minor*

C. *Transfuse the patient, since her condition is life-threatening*

D. *Obtain a court order to override the wishes of the parents*

E. *Contact the congregation elder to negotiate with the family*

The Jehovah's Witness Society is notable for their religious stance against transfusion of blood, even in the face of life-threatening anemia. In the competent adult patient, adherence to the patient's wishes is in accordance with *respect for persons* and the patient's right to self-determination. However, in the case of the child, the patient is incapable of formulating a rational, informed choice and expressing those views, therefore transfusion is justified by our societal obligation to the child's best interests, based on the principle of *beneficence.*

Answer: C

Gillon R (1994) Medical ethics: four principles plus attention to scope. *British Medical Journal* **309**, 184–8.

Gillon R (2003) Four scenarios. *Journal of Medical Ethics* **29** (5), 267–8.

Woolley S (2005) Children of Jehovah's Witnesses and adolescent Jehovah's Witnesses: what are their rights? *Archives of Disease in Childhood* **90** (7), 715–19.

Woolley S (2005) Jehovah's Witnesses in the emergency department: what are their rights? *Emergency Medicine Journal* **22** (12), 869–71.

20. *On review of his monthly billings, a physician notices that he billed for the incorrect procedure on a patient. The claim had already been accepted and paid* *out by the insurance company. What is the appropriate course of action?*

A. *Nothing, since the RVUs between the two procedures is similar*

B. *If the claim amount is less than $10 000, no correction is necessary*

C. *Report the error, refund the monies, and resubmit with justification*

D. *Report the error to the insurance company and refund the claim*

E. *Nothing can be done since the claim is already paid to the physician*

Policies differ between insurance carriers and Medicare/Medicaid in terms of correction of incorrect claims. Review and understanding of these agreements is important in minimizing your exposure to liability and prosecution. In general, failure to report errors in billing is subject to repayment of claims and imposed fines. Reporting, refunding and resubmitting an honest error with justification will cover all of the requirements for full disclosure and accuracy in correcting incorrect billing claims. This strategy may not ensure that there is not an associated fine, but is consistent with the concept of distributed justice across the healthcare system, and is internally consistent with the concept of virtuous behavior. The worst course of action is to do nothing and hope that the incorrect billing is not noticed.

Answer: C

Vogel RL (2010) The False Claims Act and its impact on medical practices. *Journal of Medical Practice Management* **26** (1), 21–4.

Index

Surgical Critical Care and Emergency Surgery: Clinical Questions and Answers, First Edition. Edited by Forrest O. Moore, Peter M. Rhee, Samuel A. Tisherman and Gerard J. Fulda.